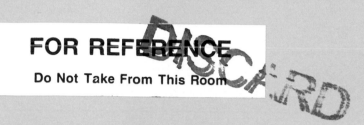

Atlas of Sexually Transmitted Diseases and AIDS

Third Edition

Edited by

Stephen A Morse MSPH PhD

Associate Director of Science
Division of AIDS, STDs and TB Laboratory Research
Centers For Disease Control and Prevention
Atlanta, GA, USA

Ronald C Ballard PhD

Branch Chief
Division of AIDS, STDs and TB Laboratory Research
Centers for Disease Control and Prevention
Atlanta, GA, USA

King K Holmes MD PhD

Professor of Medicine
Director, Center for AIDS and STD
University of Washington
Seattle, WA, USA

Adele A Moreland MD

Countryside Dermatology and Laser Center
Clearwater, FL, USA

Mosby

Edinburgh London New York Oxford Philadelphia St Louis Sydney Toronto 2003

MOSBY
An affiliate of Elsevier Science Limited

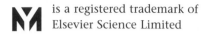 is a registered trademark of
Elsevier Science Limited

First edition 1990
Second edition 1996
Third edition 2003

ISBN 0 7234 3227 9

British Library Cataloguing in Publication Data
A catalogue record for this book is available from the British Library

Library of Congress Cataloging in Publication Data
A catalog record for this book is available from the Library of Congress

Notice
Medical knowledge is constantly changing. Standard safety precautions must be followed, but as new research and clinical experience broaden our knowledge, changes in treatment and drug therapy may become necessary or appropriate. Readers are advised to check the most current product information provided by the manufacturer of each drug to be administered to verify the recommended dose, the method and duration of administration, and contraindications. It is the responsibility of the practitioner, relying on experience and knowledge of the patient, to determine dosages and the best treatment for each individual patient. Neither the Publisher nor the editor/contributor assumes any liability for any injury and/or damage to persons or property arising from this publication.

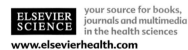 your source for books,
journals and multimedia
in the health sciences
www.elsevierhealth.com

Printed in Spain by Grafos SA

Commissioning Editor: *Kim Murphy/Jill Day*
Project Development Manager: *Martin Mellor*
Project Manager: *Rory MacDonald*
Designer: *Andy Chapman*
Illustrations: *MTG*

The
publisher's
policy is to use
**paper manufactured
from sustainable forests**

Contents

Contributors

RHODA L ASHLEY PHD
Professor of Laboratory Medicine
Children's Hospital and Regional Medical Center
Seattle, WA, USA

RONALD C BALLARD PHD
Division of AIDS, STDs and TB Laboratory Research
Centers for Disease Control and Prevention
Atlanta, GA, USA

CONSUELO BECK-SAGUE MD
Division of Reproductive Health
Centers for Disease Control and Prevention
Atlanta, GA, USA

FRANCIS BOWDEN MBBS, MD, FRACP, FACSHP
Professor of Medicine, Australian National University
Canberra Sexual Health Centre
The Canberra Hospital
Canberra, Australia

WILLIAM A BOWER, MD
Division of Hepatitis
Centers for Disease Control and Prevention
Atlanta, GA, USA

GAIL H CASSELL MS, PHD
Vice President
Scientific Affairs and Distinguished Lilly Research Scholar
for Infectious Diseases
Eli Lilly & Company
Indianapolis, IN, USA

ROBERT COOMBS MD, PHD, FRCP(C)
Professor of Laboratory Medicine and Medicine
Department of Laboratory Medicine
Harborview Medical Center
Seattle, WA, USA

DAVID L COX PHD
Division of AIDS, STDs and TB Laboratory Research
Centers for Disease Control and Prevention
Atlanta, GA, USA

KENNETH L DOMINGUEZ
Division of HIV/AIDS Prevention
Centers for Disease Control and Prevention
Atlanta, GA, USA

JOHN M DOUGLAS MD
Director of STD Control and Professor of Medicine
and Preventative Medicine
Denver Public Health
Denver, CO, USA

PATRICIA L FLEMING MS, PHD
Division of HIV/AIDS Prevention
Centers for Disease Control and Prevention
Atlanta, GA, USA

ROBERT D HARRINGTON MD
Associate Professor of Medicine
Division of Infectious Diseases
University of Washington Medical Center
Seattle, WA, USA

SHARON HILLIER PHD
Professor of Obstetrics, Gynecology and
Reproductive Sciences
Department of Obstetrics and Gynecology
Magee-Womens Hospital
Pittsburgh, PA, USA

KING K HOLMES MD, PHD
Professor of Medicine
Director, Center for AIDS and STD
University of Washington
Seattle, WA, USA

CATHERINE A ISON PHD, FRCPATH
Reader in Medical Microbiology
Department of Infectious Diseases and Microbiology
London, UK

PETER KOHL MD, PHD
Professor of Dermatology, Venereology and Allergology
Department of Dermatology and Venereology
Neukölln Academic Hospital
Berlin, Germany

HELEN H LEE PHD
Associate Professor of Medical Biotechnology
Department of Haematology
University of Cambridge
Cambridge, UK

WILLIAM C LEVINE MD, MSC
Global AIDS Program/Thailand
National Center for HIV, STD and TB Prevention
Centers for Disease Control and Prevention
Atlanta, GA, USA

JOEL S LEWIS
Division of AIDS, STDs and TB Laboratory Research
Centers for Disease Control and Prevention
Atlanta, GA, USA

HSI LIU DVM, PHD
Microbiologist
Division of AIDS, STDs and TB Laboratory Research
Centers for Disease Control and Prevention
Atlanta, GA, USA

JOHN LONG MD, MPH
Consulting Physician
Division of Pediatric Infectious Diseases
Scottish Rite Children's Medical Center
Atlanta, GA, USA

LOURDES MAHILUM-TAPAY PHD
Research Associate
Department of Haematology
University of Cambridge
Cambridge, UK

DAVID H MARTIN MD
Harry E Dascomb, MD Professor of Medicine and
Microbiology
Department of Medicine
Louisiana State University Health Sciences Center
New Orleans, LO, USA

MARILYNNE MCKAY
Professor Emerita of Dermatology, Emory University, Atlanta;
Chairman of Dermatology, Lovelace Health System,
Albequerque, NM, USA

ADELE MORELAND MD
Countryside Dermatology and Laser Center
Clearwater, FL, USA

STEPHEN A MORSE MSPH, PHD
Division of AIDS, STDs and TB Laboratory Research
Centers For Disease Control and Prevention
Atlanta, GA, USA

ELPIDIO CESAR B NADALA PHD
Senior Research Associate
Department of Haematology
University of Cambridge
Cambridge, UK

FRANCIS J NDOWA MBCHB, DIP GU MED, DIP DERM
Specialist
Department of Reproductive Health and Research
World Health Organisation
Geneva, Switzerland

JORMA PAAVONEN MD
Professor of Obstetrics and Gynecology
Department of Obstetrics and Gynecology
University of Helsinki
Helsinki, Finland

PHILIP PELLETT PHD
Division of Viral and Rickettsial Diseases
Centers for Disease Control and Prevention
Atlanta, GA, USA

ANGELA J ROBINSON MBBS
Consultant in Sexual Health
Department of Genitourinary Medicine
Mortimer Market Centre
London, UK

JULIUS SCHACHTER PHD
Professor of Laboratory Medicine
Chlamydia Laboratory
UCSF
San Francisco, CA, USA

DAVID A SCHWARTZ MD
Visiting Professor of Pathology
Vanderbilt University School of Medicine
Nashville, TN, USA
Guest Scientist, Centers for Disease Control and Prevention
Atlanta, GA, USA

CRAIG SHAPIRO MD
Division of Hepatitis
Centers for Disease Control and Prevention
Atlanta, GA, USA

JACK D SOBEL MD
Professor of Medicine
Chief Division of Infectious Diseases
Department of Internal Medicine
Harper Professional Building Suite 2140
Detroit, MI, USA

DAVID H SPACH MD
Associate Professor of Medicine
Division of Infectious Diseases
Harbourview Medical Center
Seattle, WA, USA

RICHARD S STEPHENS PHD
Professor
School of Public Health
University of California
Berkeley, CA, USA

DAVID TAYLOR-ROBINSON MD, MRCP, FRCPATH
Emeritus Professor of Genitourinary Microbiology
and Medicine
Division of Medicine
Imperial College of Science, Technology and Medicine
St Mary's Hospital
London, UK

KEN B WAITES MD, FAAM
Professor of Pathology and Microbiology
Director of Clinical Microbiology
Department of Pathology
University of Alabama at Birmingham
Birmingham, AL, USA

ANNA WALD MD, MPH
Assistant Professor of Medicine
University of Washington
Seattle, WA, USA

Preface

Even a lifetime of clinical experience does not produce an expert clinician. The expert must be able to sort out the wheat from the chaff in the accelerating number of changes in many clinical and laboratory disciplines. The bewildered beginner needs a practical synthesis of the essential facts, the classical and typical clinical manifestations and the most useful techniques, tests and therapy. This third edition of the Atlas of Sexually Transmitted Diseases and AIDS again presents an enormous amount of well-illustrated, up-to-date and practical material on the most common (and several uncommon) sexually transmitted infections. The first chapter reviews genital anatomy and examination, and includes dermatological conditions which may be confused with STDs. The chapters following cover the etiologic agents, epidemiology, clinical manifestations, laboratory diagnosis and current treatment recommendations for sexually transmitted infections, including opportunistic infections associated with AIDS.

We thank each of the authors of this edition of the Atlas, who were selected on the basis of their outstanding reputations as clinicians and teachers. It is gratifying how they have been able to combine succinct text with a wealth of photographs and helpful illustrations to distill essential, practical information into a uniquely accessible format. Specialists and generalists alike can literally complete the book in a day and, like the editors, will learn dozens of important new findings and approaches (while relearning many old ones!). They will find this a very useful resource to return to, again and again. The student or trainee will be surprised at how easy it is to understand and assimilate new information, because it is so richly illustrated and so clearly presented. When finished with the Atlas, they will have acquired a broad and solid foundation from which to pass board examinations and to go on to become expert clinicians themselves.

Stephen A Morse, Ronald C Ballard,
King K Holmes and Adele A Moreland

Acknowledgements

We would like to recognize and express deep gratitude to the late Sumner E (Sam) Thompson, MD and Sidney Olansky, MD, for their inspiration, teaching, clinical expertise and hard work. Dr Thompson inspired us to tackle the project and was a co-editor of the first edition of this Atlas of Sexually Transmitted Diseases. His clinical vision inspired physicians, medical students and clinicians at Emory University and it's affiliates. Dr Sidney Olansky transmitted his vast knowledge and love of dermatology and syphilology to all those he taught. His long associations at the Fulton County Health Department in conjunction with his teaching in the dermatology department at Emory University provided a great deal of the inspiration and interest in STDs at Emory that ultimately resulted in this book. We would also like to express our thanks to the authors of the previous editions for their contributions, which were responsible for the success of the Atlas. We would also like to acknowledge Samuel K Sarafian, PhD (d.1996) for his contributions to the first two editions.

Stephen A Morse, Ronald C Ballard,
King K Holmes and Adele A Moreland

Genital and Dermatologic Examination

A Moreland, M McKay and P Kohl

INTRODUCTION

Skin changes (cutaneous disorders) of the genital skin may be assumed either by patient or physician to be of a sexually transmitted nature because of their location. This chapter will review genital anatomy and examination, and general principles of dermatologic examination. The latter will include common cutaneous disorders of the genitalia that are not sexually transmitted, but that may be seen in a sexually transmitted disease (STD) clinic or be mistaken for a STD.

GENITAL ANATOMY AND EXAMINATION

The examination of both the male and female genital region should begin below the umbilicus at the mons pubis. It is generally unsatisfactory to try to evaluate a partially clothed patient, because important ancillary findings (e.g. lymph nodes) may be missed. The patient should be undressed below the waist and gowned or draped; the gloved physician then exposes the lower abdomen and genitalia in a systematic manner. Inspect the inguinal folds, noting erythema or scaling and palpating for nodes. Exam table stirrups afford better visualization of the genitalia and perianal area in either sex, and should be used if available. Examine pubic hair for nits and look for papules of molluscum contagiosum, folliculitis, human papillomavirus (HPV), or scabies burrows. Other skin lesions such as blisters (herpesvirus, HSV) or scaly plaques (tinea, syphilis) should be noted, as well as ulcerations anywhere on the genitalia. At the inferior midline near the male penis or female clitoris, the hair becomes more sparse.

MALE GENITAL EXAMINATION

PENIS AND SCROTUM

Male genital anatomy is shown in *Fig. 1.1*. Deep pigmentation is usual on the shaft of the penis and the hair is almost absent. A few minute yellowish papules may be seen (*Fig. 1.2*). These are pilosebaceous units (sometimes a vestigial hair and its associated oil gland). Sweat glands are also present on the base, shaft and glans of the penis.

Fig. 1.1 Male genitals.

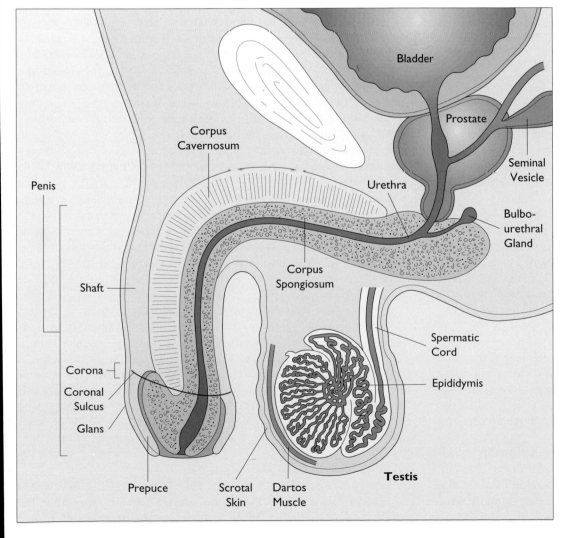

Bladder

Corpus Cavernosum

Prostate

Urethra

Seminal Vesicle

Penis

Bulbo-urethral Gland

Corpus Spongiosum

Shaft

Spermatic Cord

Epididymis

Corona

Coronal Sulcus

Glans

Prepuce

Scrotal Skin

Dartos Muscle

Testis

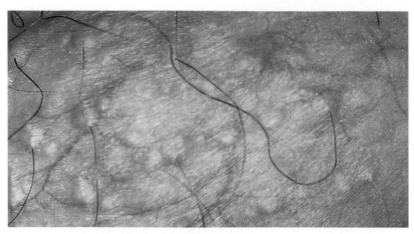

Fig. 1.2 Sebaceous glands. Penile sebaceous glands appear as yellowish papules on shaft of penis and may also be present on the scrotum. These may be quite prominent on some individuals.

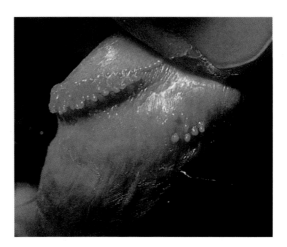

Fig. 1.3 'Pearly penile papules.' A normal variant, these tiny papules are sometimes mistaken for condylomata.

The redundant prepuce (foreskin) projects over the glans where sebaceous glands (of Tyson) secrete a keratinous material called smegma which may accumulate between the prepuce and gland in an uncircumcised male.[1] The inner surface of the prepuce has a moist appearance, much like a mucous membrane. Scattered sebaceous glands empty directly to the surface of the glans and are not associated with hair follicles.

The ridge encircling and bordering the glans is called the corona and the sulcus below it the coronal sulcus. A varying number of smooth or slightly pebbly flesh-colored papules in one or two orderly rows may rim some or all of the corona; these are a normal variant called 'pearly penile papules'. They may be mistaken for condylomata (HPV) but histologically are angiofibromas (*Fig. 1.3*).[2] The urethral meatus is usually located on the posterior or undersurface of the glans and should be carefully examined for discharge, ulcers, or growths such as condylomata.

The skin of the scrotum is thin and more deeply pigmented than the surrounding skin. Scrotal skin is closely adherent to the underlying dartos muscle, which gives it a rugose wrinkled appearance with contraction of the muscle (e.g. at rest in younger individuals, and in the cold at all ages). The scrotum has numerous pilosebaceous, eccrine and apocrine glands. Hair is sparse and coarse.[3]

Gentle palpation of the testes, spermatic cord and epididymis within the scrotal sac will reveal any tenderness or masses which may indicate infection. Raise the scrotum to examine the perineal skin between the scrotum and the anus. Sparse, coarse hair covers the skin up to the anal mucosa and sweat and sebaceous glands are present.

ANUS AND RECTUM

The folds of the anus are hairless and pale and should be examined for hemorrhoids, fissures, ulcers, erosions, and growths. By gentle pressure with a gloved finger the rectal mucosa can be palpated for tenderness, ulcers, discharge, or masses beyond the anal sphincter.

FEMALE GENITAL EXAMINATION

THE VULVA

The female genitalia are shown in *Fig. 1.4*. The commonest diagnostic error in evaluation of the vulva is failure to systematically examine the area. Proceed from the labia majora inward, and routinely perform the examination in the same way for all genital complaints to assure recognition of the range of normal anatomic variations. During the examination, the physician can reassure the patient by verbalizing normal findings, and an office hand-mirror may help communication between patient and physician regarding specific areas of concern.

THE LABIA MAJORA

The plump paired labia majora fuse anteriorly at the mons pubis and posteriorly merge with the perineal area. They are bounded laterally by the intertriginous folds and are covered by coarse hair. Sweat and sebaceous glands are present. Abnormal findings or signs of infection may be difficult to see because of the pubic hair.

THE LABIA MINORA

In addition to the pigmentation of the outer labia minora, there are two other normal findings which can confuse the untrained examiner. First are the normal smooth yellowish 'pebbly' papules that are most numerous at the outer edges of the labia minora. These are sebaceous glands and normally occur along the outer minora and inner majora (*Fig. 1.5*). Under the clitoral hood, sebaceous secretions called smegma may accumulate. The sebaceous glands usually stop about halfway along the surface of the inner minora, and this line (Hart's line) demarcates mucosal from squamous epithelium (*see Fig. 1.4*).[4] Patients sometimes mistake these papules for vesicles or pustules and become concerned. In some cases, the sebaceous glands give rise to inclusion cysts; small ones are called milia and larger ones develop into epidermoid cysts. If they are not symptomatic, they can be ignored.

The second normal variant is the presence of small, often asymptomatic, cutaneous papillae on the inner labia minora, especially at the posterior vaginal introitus (*Fig. 1.6*). Longer papillae in the posterior introitus have been described as a normal variant and a rough, papillomatous labial mucosal surface often becomes more prominent in inflammatory conditions or lichenification. The clinician should be careful not to overdiagnose benign papillomatosis as 'subclinical HPV.' Condylomatous HPV lesions in the posterior introitus are typically plaque-like and are relatively easy to differentiate from the delicate stalk-like papillae.[5,6]

Some investigations of vulval mucosal papillae initially implicated HPV infection, especially when magnified inspection of papillomatous epithelium revealed an associated mosaic or punctate vascular pattern with capillaries extending into individual papillae. Since there might not have been either a history of previous infection nor obvious condylomata acuminata, it was suggested that papillomatosis represented 'subclinical' HPV infection. Research studies using polymerase chain reaction (PCR) technology, Southern blot or other molecular biologic techniques have made this assumption valid.[7]

THE VULVAR VESTIBULE

The vestibule is the inner portion of the vulva extending from Hart's line on the labia minora inward to the hymenal ring. Within the vestibule are located the urethral meatus and the openings of Skene's

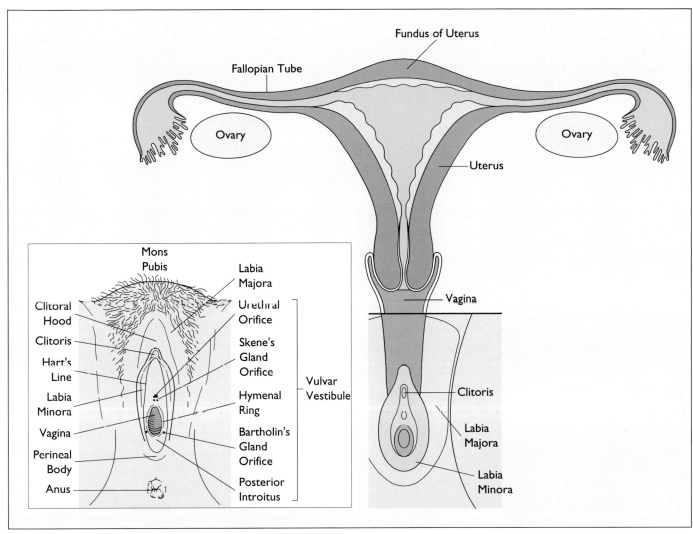

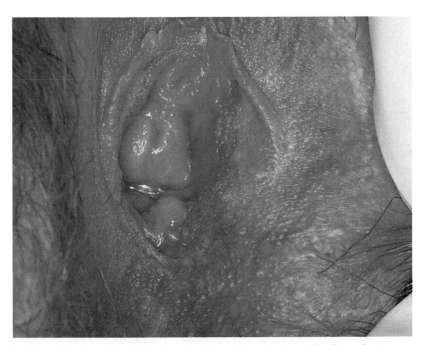

Fig. 1.4 Female genitalia. Courtesy of Stevens A, Lowe J, Histology. London, Mosby, 1992.

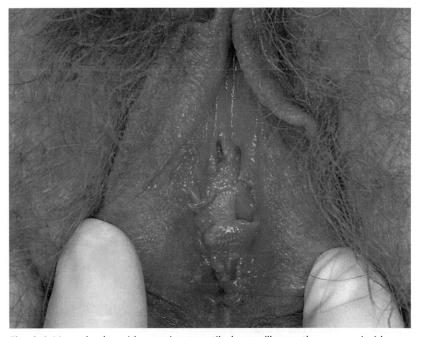

Fig. 1.5 Normal vulva with finely textured papular sebaceous glands on the inner labia majora and labia minora. In this case, glands are confluent over the outer minora, producing an almost white appearance. By contrast, the vestibular mucosa inside Hart's line appears red, although this is normal coloration. There is much individual variation in the size and distribution of genital sebaceous glands, but in general, they decrease in number with age.

Fig. 1.6 Normal vulva with prominent vestibular papillae on the mucosa inside Hart's line and at the posterior fourchette. Although they are frequently mistaken for condylomata, biopsied papillae are typically negative for human papillomavirus (HPV). HPV lesions are usually more keratotic and less translucent than papillae; the latter are often symmetrical and/or linear on both sides of the vulva, unlike condylomata. No treatment is necessary.

and Bartholin's glands (*Fig. 1.4*). Smaller minor mucous glands are found throughout the vestibule, mostly in the posterior fourchette and in the groove at the base of the hymenal ring, where they may be seen as tiny pit-like openings. Vulvar vestibulitis should be suspected by the patient's complaint of significant and persistent entry dyspareunia and discomfort at the opening of the vagina. The diagnosis is made by finding erythema and point tenderness upon palpation of the gland orifice with a cotton-tipped applicator.[8]

Visible changes (plaques, scarring, thickening) should be biopsied, preferably in the thickest portion of a lesion. Acetowhitening (application of vinegar or 3–5% acetic acid for 1–2 minutes) can be used to highlight thickened areas if there is a history of HPV. If HPV infection is found on the vulva, colposcopy of the vagina and cervix is recommended; if on the anus, proctoscopy. Biopsies should be performed on any diagnostically questionable areas, especially if intraepithelial neoplasia is suspected, but biopsies are rarely helpful for nonspecific inflammation or vestibulitis. Findings such as koilocytosis without obvious condylomata should be considered nonspecific; many women with this histology are asymptomatic and others with vulvar burning have no evidence of HPV.

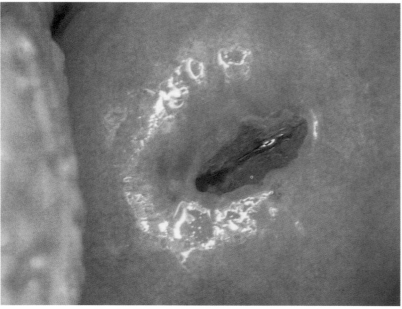

Fig. 1.7 Normal cervix. The squamocolumnar junction is seen and also the lower part of the endocervical canal. (See also **4.26**.) Courtesy of Mr Peter Greenhouse.

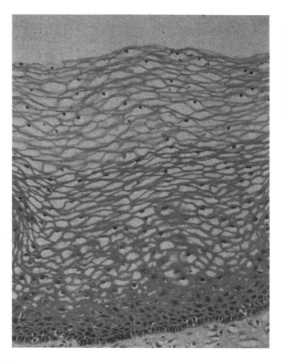

Fig. 1.8 Stratified squamous epithelium covers the ectocervix. Like those of the vagina, the cells are rich in glycogen during the period of sexual maturity. Courtesy of Stevens A, Lowe J, Histology. London, Mosby, 1992.

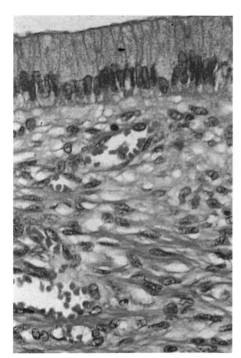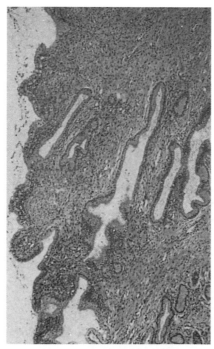

Fig. 1.9 (Left) the endocervical canal is lined by a single layer of tall columnar mucus-secreting epithelium. (Right) Numerous deep invaginations of the mucus-secreting epithelium extend into the cervical stroma and greatly increase the surface for mucus production. Courtesy of Stevens A, Lowe J, Histology. London, Mosby, 1992.

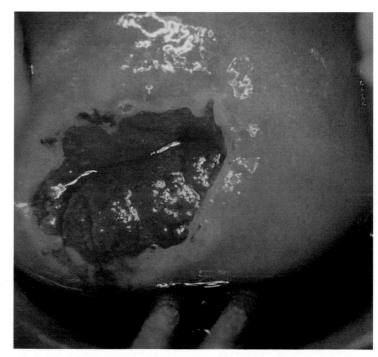

Fig. 1.10 Colposcopy. Ectopy showing early squamous metaplasia. (See also Fig. 4.24.) Courtesy of Mr Peter Greenhouse.

THE VAGINA AND CERVIX

Before inserting a speculum into the vagina, gentle pressure with two fingers on the posterior fourchette relaxes the muscles at the vaginal opening. To view the vagina, a warm speculum of proper size, moistened with water, should be inserted with the blades closed and positioned obliquely. The blades are then slipped horizontally and opened slowly.

The moist vaginal mucosal lining is erythematous and has a slightly irregular surface. Numerous transverse and longitudinal folds give the vaginal canal a rugose appearance. The cervix appears at the end of the vaginal vault as a firm, smooth, somewhat circular or dome-shaped mass with a central concavity, the os (Figs 1.7–1.10), which is the entrance to the endocervical canal. Notations of vaginal discharges, lesions, or ulcers, and cervical mucosal abnormalities, ectropion, or lacerations should be made. Before the speculum is removed, samples can be obtained for cytology, cultures, and other diagnostic tests, and direct microscopy of vaginal and cervical secretions.

Bimanual Examination

The middle and index fingers of one hand should be inserted along the posterior vaginal wall after the speculum is withdrawn. The cervix is then lifted toward the abdominal wall and the opposite hand presses down to palpate the uterus, which can be gently moved to determine presence of tenderness or tumors. The ovaries and Fallopian tubes (adnexa) are found laterally or posterolaterally to the uterus. Bimanual palpation will usually ascertain tenderness and presence of masses. A clean glove should be used for the rectovaginal examination. The examining finger is gently placed into the anal opening and when the sphincter is relaxed the examination can comfortably proceed. The index finger is placed into the vagina and the middle finger into the rectum to palpate the posterior uterine and vaginal structures. Rectal hemorrhoids, polyps, and tumors can be observed and noted.

PRINCIPLES OF DERMATOLOGIC EXAMINATION OF THE GENITALIA

Although it is traditional to classify and discuss infectious diseases and conditions with respect to etiology, this approach has significant shortcomings when applied to cutaneous disorders. A 3 mm papule, for example, can be a congenital nevus, a benign or malignant neoplasm, or the result of infection with a bacteria, a virus, or a fungus. Since the skin lesion itself is the usual starting point for the development of a differential diagnosis, the traditional dermatologic approach is to seek out a so-called 'primary lesion,' one that recreates the pathophysiology of the disease process. This usually implies a search for a fresh, fully developed lesion, rather than one that has dried, crusted, been scratched, or become secondarily infected. In addition to describing the morphology of the primary process, observation of the distribution and configuration of the lesions on the skin helps to identify the disorder, as it may be one of many dermatoses that are more easily identified by finding similar lesions on other areas of the body.

With these principles in mind and for the purpose of this discussion, the nonvenereal genital dermatoses will be grouped into seven different morphologic categories. Six of these are defined by the primary lesion, such as pustules, pigmentary disorders, and dermatitis. The seventh category, erosions and ulcers, deals with the so-called 'minus' lesions, wherein the original morphology has been altered by the loss of superficial epidermis (erosion) or of the entire skin surface itself (ulcer). This latter category may be difficult to assess, for normal morphologic clues to differential diagnosis frequently are absent.

The final category is itching, defined by the symptom. This section will discuss evaluation of pruritus ani, scrota, and vulvae.

DERMATITIS/ECZEMA

The term dermatitis simply means inflammation of the skin. The Greek root eczema, which means 'boiling over or out,' is remarkably descriptive of the oozing, wet appearance of dermatitic skin. Eczemas characteristically are pruritic. The patient complains of itching, and scratch marks (excoriations) may be seen on the skin surface. Dermatitis typically changes its appearance over time. The first sign simply may be erythema, which is followed by a pebbly appearance to the skin surface that rapidly evolves into small blisters which may ooze and crust (Fig. 1.11). As dermatitis evolves, the skin becomes thickened, leathery, and often scaly, with increased skin markings. These findings are the hallmark of lichenification (Fig. 1.12) and are even more important than scaling in making this diagnosis. The patient's rubbing or scratching of the initial condition will increase the likelihood of lichenification, which persists long after the original insult has been removed. Acute dermatitis, then, is seen as a plaque that is erythematous, edematous, and oozing; chronic dermatitis is a plaque that may be purplish, hyperpigmented, and lichenified. In the latter case, the patient is said to have lichen simplex chronicus, a descriptive term that indicates only that the patient has a plaque of thickened skin that has been rubbed or scratched. Any area of the body may be involved (Fig. 1.13), but genital

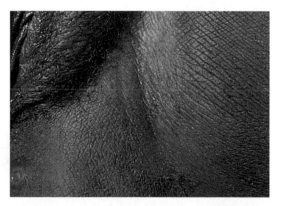

Fig. 1.11 Allergic contact dermatitis of the penis due to spermicidal jelly. Note the typical appearance of microvesicles on the glans penis. This patient complained of pruritus and rash developing approximately 2 days after use of the product.

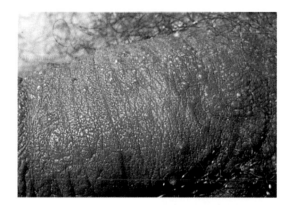

Fig. 1.12 Lichenification of intertriginous skin as a result of chronic rubbing and scratching with an ulcer due to scratching (excoriation).

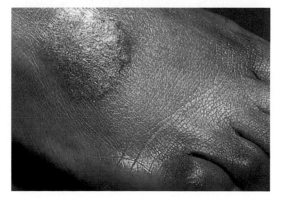

Fig. 1.13 Lichen simplex chronicus on the foot. The hallmark of this diagnosis is the leathery appearance of the skin.

skin is a common area of involvement (*Figs 1.14* and *1.15*). Some underlying skin conditions, such as atopic dermatitis, may make it more likely that the patient will develop areas of lichen simplex chronicus. In other cases, the skin reaction is due to something that has come in contact with the epidermis. The offending substance may be an irritant such as urine or a true allergen. Neomycin and benzocaine are relatively common allergens found in nonprescription topical medications. These medications may be self-prescribed by patients or prescribed by physicians to treat both pruritus and any type of irritation, abrasion, or ulcer.[9]

PAPULOSQUAMOUS DISORDERS

The papulosquamous dermatoses, as the name implies, are characterized by papules and plaques that typically have a scaly surface. While a plaque of lichen simplex chronicus might fit this description, it should be noted that lichenification is secondary to rubbing and scratching of the affected skin. The papulosquamous dermatoses, on the other hand, begin with a scaly papule as the primary lesion. Of all dermatologic disorders, probably the most commonly encountered are those in the papulosquamous category, and it is important for the clinician to develop a logical approach to the differential diagnosis of these problems (*Table 1.1*).

The acute onset of a pruritic annular lesion anywhere on the body, especially in intertriginous areas, should raise the suspicion of a dermatophyte (*Fig. 1.16*) infection. Scraping a bit of scale from the border of a lesion and examining it under 10–20% potassium hydroxide (KOH) solution will allow the visualization of fungal hyphae (*Figs 1.17–1.20*). Dermatophyte infections are more common in men than in women, but the latter are more likely to develop candidal infections, usually as a result of spread from the vagina (see section on pustular

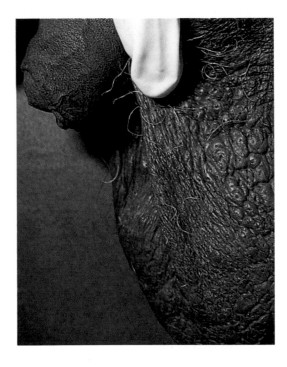

Fig. 1.14 Lichen simplex chronicus of the scrotum. The accentuation of normal skin markings is shown clearly. The inguinal area is hyperpigmented — a milder sign of continuous rubbing.

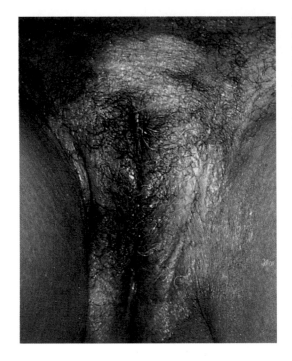

Fig. 1.15 Vulvar lichen simplex chronicus. The extensiveness of the area involved suggests that pruritus has been present for several months or more. The skin is lichenified, scaly, and in some areas hyperpigmented.

Condition	Erythema	Thickening	Pruritus	Associated lesions
Psoriasis	++	+++	+/−	Red plaques with silvery scale on knees, elbows, scalp. Nail pitting. Little or no scaling on genital psoriasis.
Seborrheic dermatitis	++	+	+	Scaling/erythema on eyebrows, nasolabial folds, hairline, occasionally on axillae, inguinal folds, or genitals.
Dermatophyte (tinea cruris)	++	Raised border	++	Annular plaque with central clearing and peripheral scale. KOH shows hyphae.
Candidiasis	++	Edema	+++	Acute erythema, edema, peeling, satellite pustules. Gram stain shows budding yeast.
Lichen simplex chronicus	++	+++	+++	May be limited to vulva; other common sites are ankle, nape of neck, arm.
Chronic dermatitis (contact or irritant)	+++	++	++	Often eczematous and oozing. May involve congruent areas, eyelids. May generalize.
Lichen planus	Violaceous	++	++	Purple polygonal papules and plaques, especially on wrists and legs. Lacy white pattern on buccal mucosa.
Lichen sclerosus and mixed dystrophy	+	−	+/−	Usually limited to vuvla, anus ('keyhole' pattern). White, and nonscaly. Dermis thick, epidermis atrophic.

Table 1.1 Differential diagnosis of common papulosquamous dermatoses.

disorders, p. 12–14). Griseofulvin is effective only for dermatophytes and nystatin only for *Candida*, but the imidazole antifungals are effective treatment for both dermatophyte and candidal infections.[10] Annular lesions also may occur in secondary syphilis, but syphilis only rarely itches, and no hyphae can be seen on KOH and, of course, the serology is positive. Psoriasis is another commonly encountered papulo-squamous disorder with a distinct familial association, even though many patients are unaware of family members with psoriasis. Typically seen as thick, red plaques with adherent white scales, psoriasis occurs most commonly on the arms (*Fig. 1.21*), knees, elbows, trunk, and sacrum, as well as the scalp. Genital lesions, however, are apt to have little if any scale, and may be seen simply as persistent intertriginous erythema (*Figs 1.22* and *1.23*). Scaly plaques may be seen on the penis and scrotum as well as on the pubic area, and in some cases may closely resemble the papulosquamous form of secondary syphilis, with minimal involvement of the rest of the body. Fingernail pitting may lead one to suspect the diagnosis of psoriasis in a persistent genital papulosquamous disorder. A mild topical corticosteroid (hydrocortisone 1%) generally is effective in treating genital psoriasis. The use of strong fluorinated steroids on genital skin may lead to the development of striae, which are permanent and unsightly.

Seborrheic dermatitis usually is seen as scaling in the hairy areas of the body, with a more or less prominent erythematous and papular component. Most commonly diagnosed in the scalp as 'dandruff', seborrheic dermatitis also affects the eyebrows, nasolabial folds (*Fig. 1.24*), axillae, central chest, and genital region. Women usually experience only mild erythema and scaling on the mons pubis (*Figs 1.25* and *1.26*), but men may have erythematous plaques on the penis (*Fig. 1.27*) that are difficult to differentiate from psoriasis or secondary syphilis. Treatment with mild corticosteroids is effective in this condition, as well.

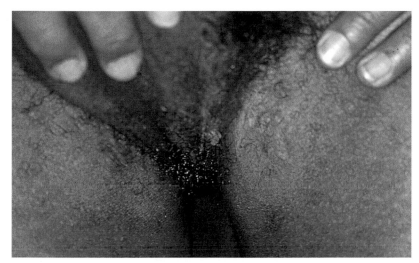

Fig. 1.16 Tinea cruris. Erythema and scaling associated with pruritus are typical features of a dermatophyte infection. Scrapings for potassium hydroxide (KOH) and fungal cultures should be taken from the leading edge of the involved skin, even though scaling there may be minimal.

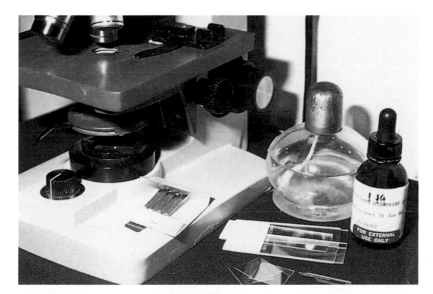

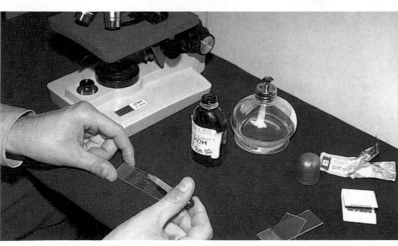

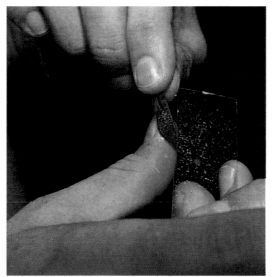

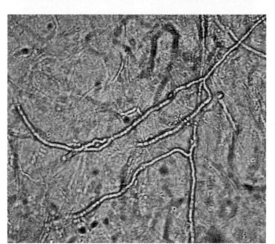

Fig. 1.17 (top left) Equipment needed for KOH examination. Curved scalpel blades, glass microscope slides, 10 to 20% KOH, glass coverslips, heat source, and microscope are shown.
Fig. 1.18 (top right) A curved scalpel blade allows gentle scraping of the skin with minimal trauma. The scale should be collected directly onto a glass slide and the coverslip applied.
Fig. 1.19 (lower left) KOH applied by dropper to the edge of the covered specimen allows it to penetrate under the coverslip by capillary action. The slide is gently warmed, without boiling, to allow clearing of the specimen. The alcohol lamp produces a cleaner flame than do matches.
Fig. 1.20 (lower right) Microscopic view of branched hyphae among cleared keratinocytes as they appear in a positive KOH preparation.

Figs 1.17–1.20 Examination of skin scraping for fungal infection with potassium hydroxide (KOH) solution.

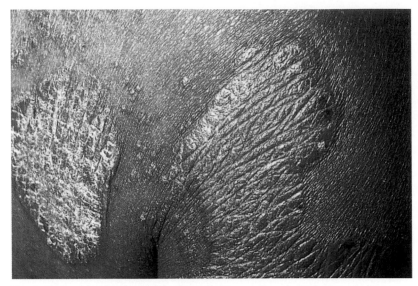

Fig. 1.21 Psoriasis. Thick reddish plaques with an adherent thick white scale are typical on nongenital skin such as the arms, elbows, knees, and scalp.

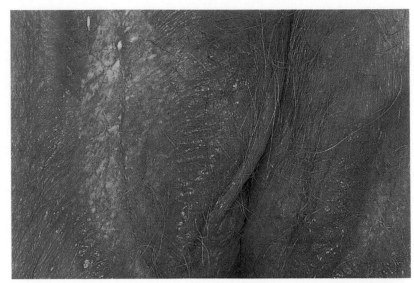

Fig. 1.22 Psoriasis of the vulva. The typical thick scale seen here is sometimes absent when psoriasis occurs on the genital skin, leaving erythematous patches and plaques with a more macerated and moist scale, or with no scale at all.

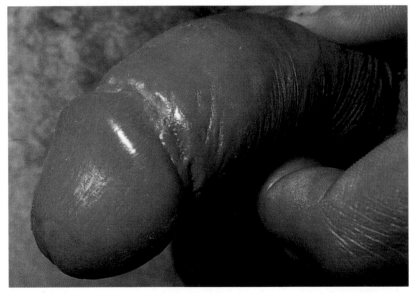

Fig. 1.23 Psoriasis of the penis. The typical intense erythema of psoriatic plaques, but with complete lack of scale, is seen in this largely intertriginous plaque of psoriasis under the foreskin.

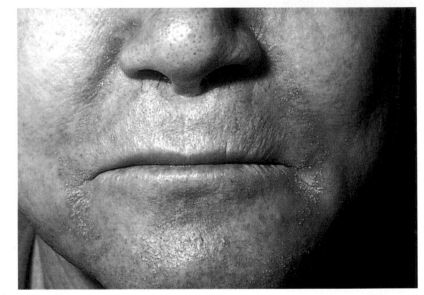

Fig. 1.24 Typical seborrheic dermatitis in the nasolabial crease. Erythema with mild scaling is seen.

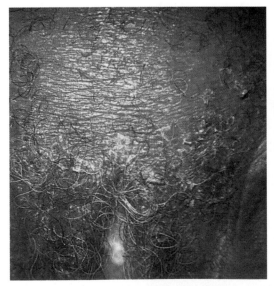
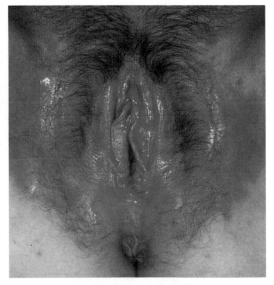

Figs. 1.25 (left) and 1.26 (right) Seborrheic dermatitis of the vulva may present as pruritus of the vulva or mons. The skin appears red or slightly pigmented and thick 'dandruff' scales may be seen. Courtesy du Vivier A.: Atlas of Clinical Dermatology. New York, Gower Medical Publishing, 1986.

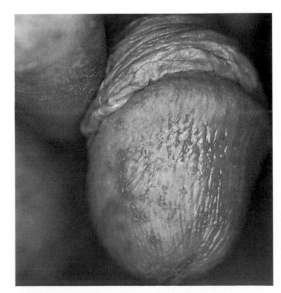

Fig. 1.27 Seborrheic dermatitis on the penis. Erythematous changes are sometimes difficult to differentiate from psoriasis, and may resolve with a mottled hypopigmentation.

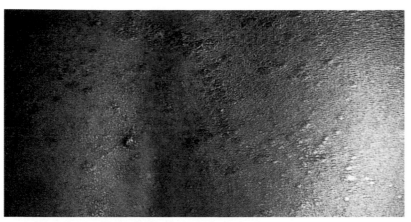

Fig. 1.28 Lichen planus on the trunk. Typical violaceous flat-topped papules are seen, some with angular borders and adherent scale in the form of Wickham's striae.

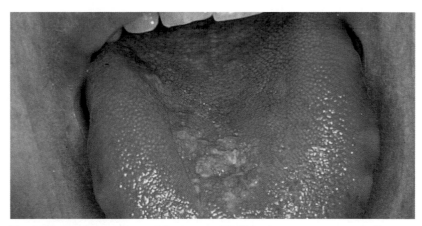

Fig. 1.29 Oral lichen planus of the tongue. Whitish plaques are seen centrally. Courtesy of Emory University School of Dentistry.

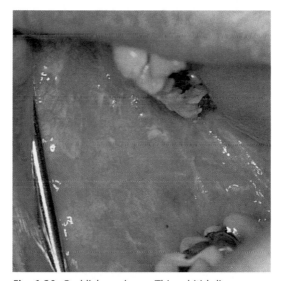

Fig. 1.30 Oral lichen planus. Thin whitish linear streaks or Wickham's striae are seen on the buccal mucosa. This is not symptomatic unless it is erosive. Courtesy of Emory University School of Dentistry;

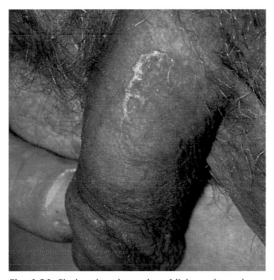

Fig. 1.31 Flesh-colored papules of lichen planus have a lacy white surface and assume an annular configuration. Courtesy du Vivier A.: Atlas of Clinical Dermatology. New York, Gower Medical Publishing, 1986.

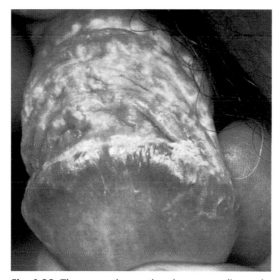

Fig. 1.32 These papules on the glans are scalier and more extensive than those in **1.31**. Courtesy du Vivier A.: Atlas of Clinical Dermatology. New York, Gower Medical Publishing, 1986.

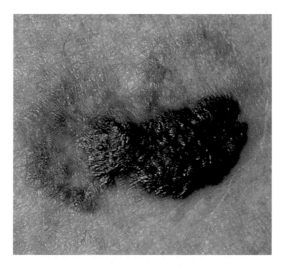

Fig. 1.33 Malignant melanoma. Note the asymmetry, irregular contours, and variable pigmentation that are the hallmarks of this malignancy.

and sometimes erosions difficult to distinguish from *Candida* or thrush. This lacy white pattern also may be seen on genital mucosal surfaces, but violaceous papules with or without scale (*Figs 1.31* and *1.32*) also may be seen. Treatment of lichen planus is symptomatic, with corticosteroids and, if necessary, antipruritic agents. Lichen sclerosus and the so-called mixed dystrophies (see below) may be responsible for thickened, scaly plaques appearing on the genitalia. Although these disorders are not always pruritic, itching may occur primarily or may be secondary to medications that have been applied to the affected area. A biopsy may be necessary to differentiate lichenified dermatitis from a primarily papulosquamous disorder.

PIGMENTARY DISORDERS

Hyperpigmentation

A black macule on the genitalia is an obvious lesion of concern, for it is important to rule out malignant melanoma as a diagnostic possibility.[11,12] Typically, however, a melanoma (*Fig. 1.33*) is a single lesion with an irregular 'notched' border with variable hyperpigmentation, which also may show areas of depigmentation within the larger macule. This malignant change should be distinguished from that of freckle or lentigo (*Fig. 1.34*) — benign macules having regular borders and smooth pigmentation. Diffuse hyperpigmentation as a

Lichen planus (classically described as purple, pruritic, polygonal papules and plaques) is not as scaly as are the above disorders. The typical areas of involvement are the flexor surfaces of the wrists, the trunk (*Fig. 1.28*), and the anterior shins. An examination of the tongue (*Fig. 1.29*) or buccal mucosa (*Fig. 1.30*) may show a lacy white pattern

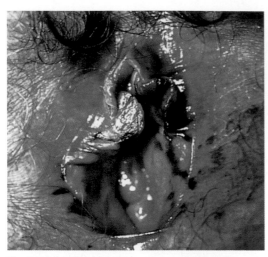

Fig. 1.34 Lentigines of the vulva. Multiple dark macules or freckles on the labia minora and vaginal introitus may appear as a result of previous inflammation, but single lesions should be evaluated carefully to rule out the possibility of malignant melanoma.

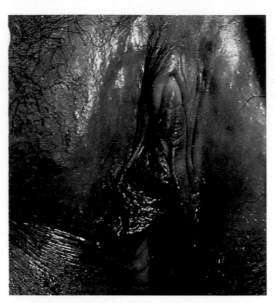

Fig. 1.35 Postinflammatory hyperpigmentation of the vulva. The spotty hyperpigmentation on the right labium majus and left labium minus seen in association with a more diffuse hypopigmentation around the clitoris and the lower introitus.

Fig. 1.36 Pseudoacanthosis nigricans of the neck. The finely papillated surface of the skin gives it a velvety appearance. This feature, in combination with hyperpigmentation, is the cardinal sign of acanthosis nigricans of any etiology.

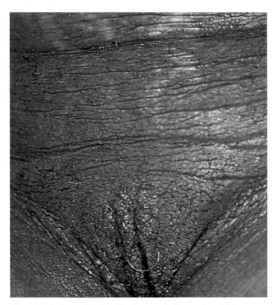

Fig. 1.37 Acanthosis nigricans of the vulva. This patient, who has extensive involvement of all intertriginous skin and of the hands and mouth, was found to have gastric adenocarcinoma — the most common cancer associated with this disorder. The acute onset of thick, velvety intertriginous plaques, hyperpigmented or not, should prompt a thorough evaluation for internal malignancy.

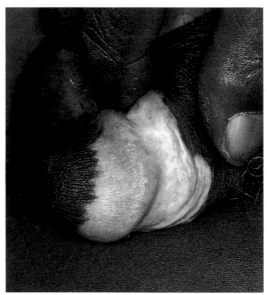

Fig. 1.38 Vitiligo of the glans penis. This is a relatively common condition, which, although asymptomatic, may be a source of great anxiety for the patient.

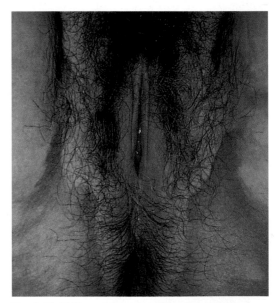

Fig. 1.39 Vitiligo of the vulva. This photograph shows the typical symmetric loss of pigmentation from the periorificial skin. Notice that the epidermis is quite normal in appearance. There is no sign of the atrophy usually associated with lichen sclerosus, which also may be hypopigmented.

result of chronic inflammation, postinflammatory hyperpigmentation, also can occur as multiple macules, giving a 'spotty' appearance to genital skin, especially around the vaginal introitus (*Fig. 1.35*).

Another form of diffuse hyperpigmentation, but with a thickened velvety appearance to the skin, is that of acanthosis nigricans. This pigmentary change may be seen around the neck (*Fig. 1.36*), genitalia (*Fig. 1.37*), and the axillae of genetically predisposed obese individuals or in some patients with endocrine abnormalities. This 'benign' or pseudoacanthosis nigricans cannot be distinguished clinically or histologically from the form that is associated with internal malignancy, usually a gastric adenocarcinoma. Thus a thorough evaluation for

malignancy should be made in patients who present with new-onset acanthosis nigricans. Unfortunately, the malignancy may be well established by the time the cutaneous changes are seen.[13]

Hypopigmentation

By far the most common color change on the genitalia is the loss of pigment in the form of vitiligo. This pigment loss is quite remarkable in persons with dark complexions and may be overlooked entirely in fair-skinned people. Characteristically symmetric in distribution, it may be seen as white patches on the glans penis (*Fig. 1.38*) or as a 'keyhole' pattern around the vagina (*Fig. 1.39*) and anus. When it occurs on other

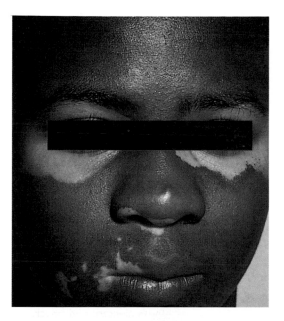

Fig. 1.40 Periorificial facial vitiligo. The patchy symmetric loss of pigmentation in vitiligo may be localized to one area of the body or it may involve many sites. In this patient, the vitiligo was confined to the face and extremities.

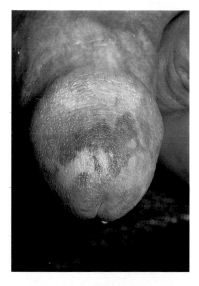

Fig. 1.41 Postinflammatory hypopigmentation and hyperpigmentation of the penis. This finding may be caused by a balanitis or a syphilitic chancre may have been the cause of the spotty pigmentation of the glans that appeared months prior to the development of a generalized papular eruption. This generalized eruption proved to be a manifestation of secondary syphilis.

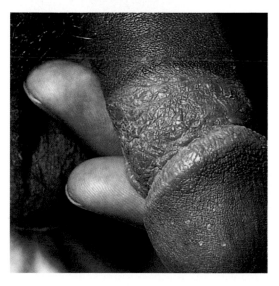

Fig. 1.42 Postinflammatory hypopigmentation of the foreskin and corona of the penis. Seborrheic dermatitis caused the pigment changes in this patient, who visited the STD clinic for this problem.

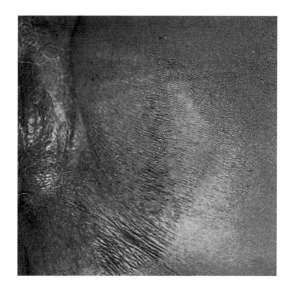

Fig. 1.43 Postinflammatory hypopigmentation and hyperpigmentation of chronic intertrigo. Pigment variations may be seen as inflammatory cutaneous conditions flare and resolve.

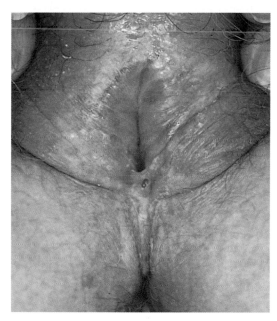

Fig. 1.44 Lichen sclerosus of the vulva. Thinning and atrophy of epidermal skin are seen with loss of architecture of the labia minora, including adhesion formation at the posterior introitus. Note the presence of erosions and petechiae secondary to mild trauma of the fragile skin.

areas of the body, it also is often periorificial, around the mouth, eyes (*Fig. 1.40*), and nares. Vitiligo also may develop distally over the fingers and toes, again, in a typically symmetric pattern. Asymmetric vitiligo is unusual but does occur, often in a dermatomal distribution. Some vitiligo patients have autoimmune thyroid disorders or diabetes, but many have no systemic abnormalities.[14,15] Treatment should be directed to a dermatologist, but spontaneous repigmentation has been known to occur. Post-inflammatory hypopigmentation may be seen after an episode of primary or secondary syphilis (*Fig. 1.41*), any form of genital ulcer, a dermatophyte infection, or chronic dermatitis or intertrigo (*Figs 1.42* and *1.43*).

ATROPHY

Itching or burning may be the presenting symptom in lichen sclerosus (lichen sclerosus et atrophicus). Occurring more commonly on female genitalia, this condition is seen clinically as depigmentation of the skin (*Fig. 1.44*). The atrophic epidermis shows fine 'cigarette paper' wrinkling, while the sclerotic or thickened dermis obscures normal capillary filling, giving a white appearance to the skin. Severe cases may result in complete resorption of the labia minora, and vulvar adhesions are not uncommon. The etiology of this condition is unknown, and occasionally it may be seen in young girls, in some cases resolving at puberty. Symptoms vary in such cases of lichen sclerosus, ranging from the patient's complete unawareness of the problem to severe itching and burning. The thinned epidermis is extremely friable, and petechiae or purpura may be seen as a result of scratching. When seen in the male, lichen sclerosus may cause the glans penis to have an extremely white, scarred-down appearance known as balanitis xerotica obliterans (*Fig. 1.45*). As with lichen sclerosus in the female, balanitis xerotica may respond to topical treatment with glucocorticoids.

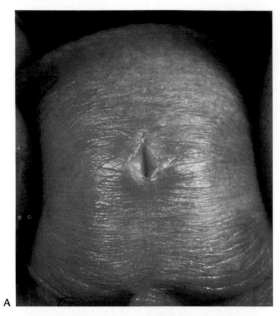

Fig. 1.45A Balantis xerotica obliterans. Lichen sclerosus on the glans penis exhibits white atrophic patches similar to those seen on the vulva. Meatal stenosis may occur.

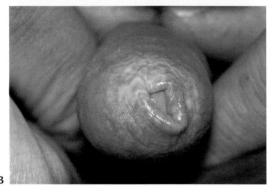

Fig. 1.45B Absolute phimosis caused by lichen sclerosus of the foreskin. This finding needs surgical intervention.

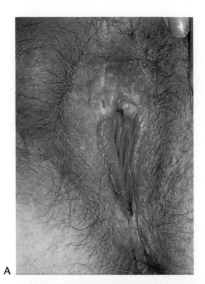

Fig. 1.46 (A) Early changes in lichen sclerosus. White thickened areas of vulva caused by lichen sclerosus. (B) More advanced vulvar lichen sclerosis showing hypertrophic plaques, edema, loss of normal architecture, introital narrowing and perineal involvement. This patient has biopsy-proven lichen sclerosus with areas of cutaneous hyperplasia. There was no evidence of malignancy.

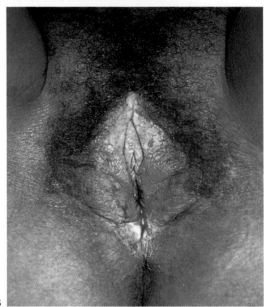

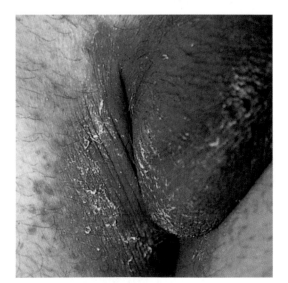

Fig. 1.47 *Candida* infection showing the intense inflammation with satellite pustules. Note that the pustules are superficial and not located at the base of hairs.

PUSTULES

Most physicians regard the presence of pustules on the skin as prima facie evidence of infection. In most cases this is true, and infection certainly should be ruled out when pus-containing papules are seen. The presence of pus generally implies infection; however, there are certain cutaneous conditions that are characterized by the presence of aggregates of white cells that are sterile to culture for bacteria, fungi, or viruses. In the following section, we will discuss the pustular conditions of the genitalia (*Tables 1.2* and *1.3*).

Infectious pustules

One of the most common causes of genital pustules, especially with inflammation, is cutaneous candidiasis or monilia (*Fig. 1.47*). Skin lesions generally are seen in conjunction with a candidal vaginitis in the female (*Fig. 1.48*). Males may also harbor the organism (*Candida albicans*) in the inguinal or gluteal folds, on the scrotum, and, especially if uncircumcised, on the penis (*Fig. 1.49*). Factors predisposing to cutaneous candidiasis include immunosuppression, diabetes mellitus, and the administration of systemic antibiotics.[17] While candidal pseudohyphae sometimes may be seen on KOH examination of material from superficial intertriginous erosions, the better diagnostic tests for this organism are a Gram or PAS stain of material from a pustule. The typical budding yeast forms are Gram-positive and somewhat larger than lymphocytes (*Fig. 1.50*).

In some cases, lichen sclerosus may develop discrete areas of thickened hyperkeratotic stratum corneum (*Fig. 1.46*). Several biopsies should be taken from different areas of thickened dystrophic skin to rule out the possibility of vulvar intraepithelial neoplasia (VIN).[16] Atrophic vaginitis may be seen in the postmenopausal woman, though cutaneous changes may consist only of mild thinning and loss of subcutaneous substance.[17]

Condition	Findings	Treatment
Candida	Most common, itches and burns. Intense erythema; often edema, satellite lesions.	Imidazole or azole creams and suppositories. Nystatin vaginal suppositories. Oral ketoconazole or fluconazole in resistant cases — short courses.
Tinea	Serpiginous 'active' border, itchy, relatively unusual in women.	Oral griseofulvin. Topical imidazoles.
Impetigo	Usually secondary to pruritic dermatitis, excoriations, secondary bacterial colonization.	Topical antibacterial scrubs. Erythromycin or dicloxacillin.
Folliculitis	Pustules at base of hairs (rule out Gram-negative infection if patient is on antibiotics).	Erythromycin or dicloxacillin unless Gram-negative; then according to sensitivities.
Furunculosis ('boils')	Painful, deep-seated nodules may be topped by pustules; may suppurate; recurrent lesions may indicate transmission by close contact	Early treatment with erythromycin or dicloxacillin may abort early lesions and prevent suppuration.
Herpes simplex	WBCs in old intact vesicles may cause lesions to look pustular.	Antivirals or topical antibiotics in mild cases. (See Chapter 13.)
Syphilis	Scattered scaly pustules may be seen in secondary syphilis.	Penicillin: see treatment schedule in Chapter 2.

Table 1.2 Infectious pustular conditions occurring on the genitalia.

Condition	Findings	Treatment
Pseudofolliculitis	Ingrown hairs indicate mechanical trauma.	Stop shaving.
Acneiform rashes	Withdrawal of potent topical steroids; contact with oils, hydrocarbons.	Wean off with hydrocortisones. Eliminate work-related industrial exposure.
Hidradenitis suppurativa	Chronic acneiform condition with sinus tracts and scarring.	Minocin, 100 mg po daily. Surgical excision of affected area.
Pustular psoriasis and/or Reiter's	Often associated with arthritis; usually a previous history of disease.	Methotrexate or retinoid therapy. Refer to dermatologist.
Pemphigus	Chronic familial form (Hailey–Hailey) or acquired (pemphigus vulgaris).	Antibiotics and oral corticosteroids. Refer to dermatologist.

While the presence of pus generally implies infection, this finding is not specific. Just as there are nonpyogenic infections, there are certain pustular skin conditions not at all associated with infectious organisms. Gram stains of pustule contents should be examined for bacteria and Gram-positive budding yeast forms; KOH of the pustule roof may reveal fungal hyphae; and bacterial cultures should be done on material from cleaned, intact lesions. If lesion morphology suggests herpes, Tzanck smears and viral cultures should also be performed; dark-field examination should be done if syphilis is suspected.

Table 1.3 NonInfectious pustular conditions occurring on the genitalia.

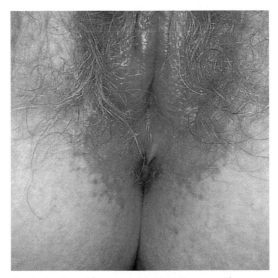

Fig. 1.48 *Candida* vulvovaginitis. Intense erythema and edema appear around the introitus, perineum, and perianal areas. The discrete erythematous macules at the active borders are resolving pustules.

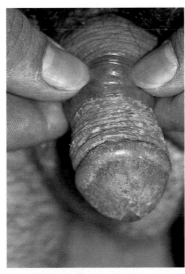

Fig. 1.49 *Candida* balanitis showing edema and erythema in a diabetic. This is seen most commonly in uncircumcised males. Candidiasis should be considered a sexually transmissible disease, treatment with topical antifungal creams may be adequate but systemic antifungals may at times be necessary.

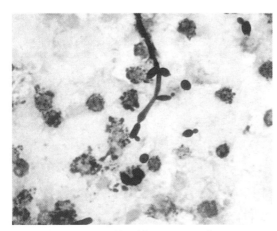

Fig. 1.50 PAS stain of budding yeast and pseudohyphae seen in *Candida albicans*.

Acute inflammatory tinea infections may have a vesiculopustular scaly border (*Fig. 1.51*). KOH of blister or pustule roof will demonstrate fungal hyphae. In the presence of a chronic intertrigo, foci of dermatophyte infections may remain deep in follicles, which can occasionally become nodular (Majocchi's granuloma). The diagnosis of fungal folliculitis should be considered when the patient fails to respond to systemic antibiotics.

Discrete, scattered pustules in hairy areas of the body generally are caused by staphylococci and streptococci (Bockhart's impetigo). Since many cutaneous staphylococci are penicillinase producers, treatment should be with erythromycin or with penicillinase-resistant penicillins such as dicloxacillin.

In susceptible individuals, folliculitis may develop into a larger cutaneous abscess called a carbuncle or a furuncle (*Fig. 1.52*). Typically caused by *Staphylococcus aureus*, early lesions will respond to systemic antibiotics. Most later lesions benefit from application of warm compresses until spontaneous rupture of the abscess occurs, but fully developed walled-off abscesses may require incision and drainage. Recurrent furunculosis does not necessarily imply that a patient has an immune deficiency. Phage-typing of staphylococci has been used to identify cluster groups of patients who pass the infection back and forth, usually in a close-living or sexually active situation. Pustules also

may be seen in mixed bacterial impetigo (*Fig. 1.53*), an extremely common skin infection that may be the result of secondary bacterial colonization of a pre-existing dermatitis.[18,19]

While the umbilicated papules of molluscum contagiosum (*Figs 1.54* and *1.55*) are not actually pustules, the initial appearance of these lesions may mislead the patient and physician. Since usually they are pale or flesh-colored, they can give the appearance of pustules; however, they are actually rather sturdy papules, which may persist for many weeks. The central dell or umbilication is characteristic of the viral etiology of these lesions, which are caused by a pox virus. Therapy is directed toward destruction of the lesion, with curettage or blistering agents applied to the lesions.

Noninfectious Pustules

In most clinical situations, the presence of pus implies infection, and it is entirely appropriate to obtain bacterial, fungal, and/or viral cultures in this setting. There are certain dermatologic conditions, however, in which pustules or the accumulation of white cells in the epidermis is initiated by stimuli other than bacterial infection.

While bacterial superinfection can play an important part in hidradenitis suppurativa also termed acne inversa (*Figs 1.56* and *1.57*), the mechanism of this severe acneiform eruption in the groin and/or

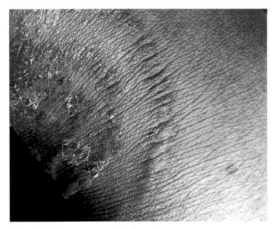

Fig. 1.51 Tinea corporis showing vesicles and pustules at the active advancing edge of a typical scaly plaque.

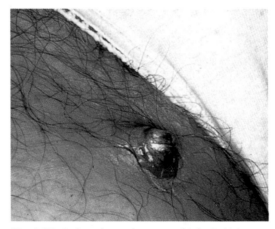

Fig. 1.52 Carbuncle on the upper thigh. A thick crust with surrounding erythema and tenderness is characteristic.

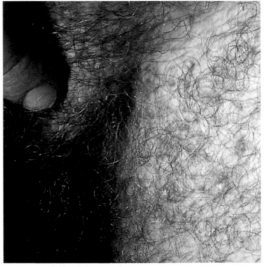

Fig. 1.53 Impetigo. Pustules, pus-filled bullae, crusts, and erosions are all present in this superficial bacterial skin infection, which may be localized to the groin in sexually active patients.

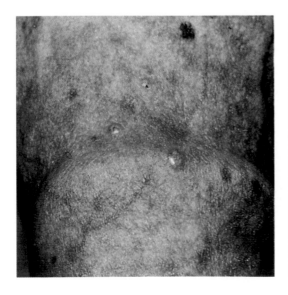

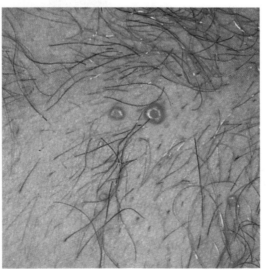

Figs 1.54 (left) and 1.55 (right) Molluscum contagiosum. Flesh-colored papules of molluscum may be distinguished by their umbilicated centers. The papules contain a white cheesy substance, which may be stained for the presence of viral inclusion bodies. Courtesy du Vivier A.: Atlas of Clinical Dermatology. New York, Gower Medical Publishing, 1986.

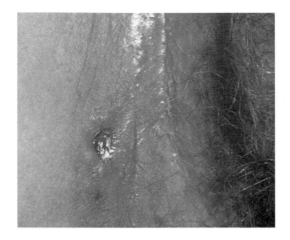

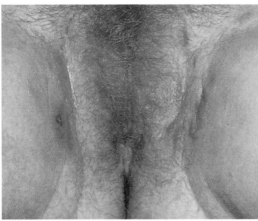

Figs 1.56 (left) and **1.57 (right)** Hidradenitis suppurativa of the vulva. Indolent painful pustules and nodules are associated with this chronic disorder. Sinuses and scars result. Courtesy du Vivier A.: Atlas of Clinical Dermatology. New York, Gower Medical Publishing, 1986.

axillae is related to occlusion of hair follicles and retention of follicular contents, resulting in an inflammatory process that includes hair follicles and sweat glands. Secondary bacterial infection is common. The presence of multiple papules, pustules, cysts, and sinus tracts is the cutaneous constellation common to cystic acne, hidradenitis, and dissecting folliculitis of the scalp, which may occur together. In some chronic cases, keloid formation may be the most prominent feature of a 'burned-out' case of hidradenitis. Antibiotic therapy can be helpful in acute flares of this disease, and resistance to tetracycline or erythromycin should raise the suspicion of superinfection with Gram-negative organisms. Surgical excision and grafting remains the treatment of choice for recalcitrant cases, although the retinoids have shown some promise in the treatment of this distressing condition.[20]

Pustular psoriasis (Fig. 1.58) may begin as groups of sterile pustules in intertriginous areas. These rapidly enlarge and spread across the trunk and extremities in waves that coalesce, forming 'lakes' of pus in the superficial epidermis. This severe form of psoriasis is associated with high fevers and malaise. It occurs primarily in patients already diagnosed with psoriasis and is seen sometimes as a result of systemic steroid therapy. Acute episodes may be difficult to manage, and generally respond best to systemic therapy with antimetabolites such as methotrexate or cyclosporin or with systemic retinoids.[21]

Reiter's syndrome is an uncommon condition in which urethritis and arthritis may be associated with psoriasis-like lesions on the skin, including an inflammatory condition of the penis or vulva known as circinate balanitis or vulvitis.[22,23] The urethritis and involvement of genital mucosa make the STD clinic a likely setting in which to diagnose this disease. The circinate balanitis *(Fig. 1.59)* may appear as nonscaly erythematous plaques, or the eruption may be more pustular, crusted, and scaly. On nongenital skin, it is very similar in appearance to pustular psoriasis *(Fig. 1.60)*. Arthritis is also a typical feature, and conjunctivitis also may be seen. Patients with Reiter's disease usually have histocompatibility antigen HLA-B27,[24] with a high risk of developing ankylosing spondylitis. A link to infections caused by *Chlamydia trachomatis* has been postulated. Fortunately, skin lesions often respond to low-potency topical corticosteroids. The arthritis may be more difficult to treat and can be disabling.[25]

Benign familial pemphigus (Hailey–Hailey disease) frequently presents as pustules and erosions in intertriginous areas *(Fig. 1.61)*, but this inherited disorder can easily become widespread or superinfected with *Candida* or bacteria, which may obscure the initial diagnosis. The familial occurrence and chronicity, as well as a typical histologic picture, make diagnosis relatively easy, although the varied spectrum of lesions from hyperkeratotic papules to erosions may mislead the clinician who looks for fluid-filled vesicles in this so-called 'bullous disease.' Treatment must include appropriate antibiotics or antifungals and if necessary, corticosteroids, retinoids, antimetabolites or surgery.[26]

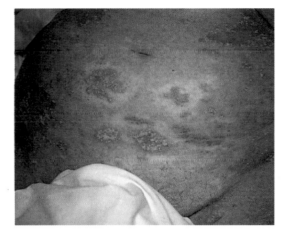

Fig. 1.58 Pustular psoriasis. Typical clusters of pustules arise in intertriginous areas and spread outward, forming 'lakes' of pus at the periphery of the eruption. Patients are febrile and ill, though the pustules are sterile. This form of psoriasis is relatively rare but may be precipitated by systemic corticosteroid therapy.

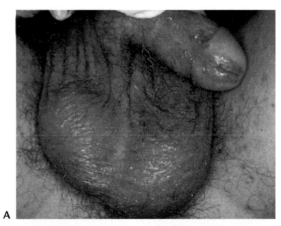

A

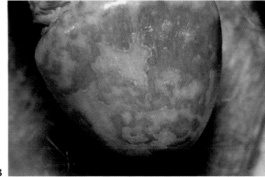

B

Fig. 1.59A and B Balanitis circinata. Reiter's disease presented in this patient with an erythematous circinate eruption on the glans penis resembling psoriasis. This disorder is associated with HLA-B27, and symptoms of arthritis are extremely common.

NODULES AND TUMORS

Epidermoid cysts are firm, yellow, subcutaneous nodules that may occur singly or, in some cases, prolifically over the vulva or scrotum (*Fig. 1.62*). Treatment usually is sought when the cysts rupture or become secondarily infected. Although cutaneous crusting and erosion may be present over the cyst, the nodular nature of the lesion is unlike other sexually transmitted genital ulcers, which are more superficial. Antistaphylococcal antibiotics and sitz baths usually resolve the secondary infection, and, if necessary, the cyst may later be removed. In most cases, the patient is aware of the diagnosis, although with multiple lesions one also should consider the possibility of steatocystoma multiplex. The latter cysts extrude a clear to yellowish gel-like material when punctured, and often appear on the face, neck, upper trunk, and axillae as well. This condition is a hereditary disorder, primarily of cosmetic concern.

Fox–Fordyce disease is characterized by aggregations of tiny 1–2 mm papules in the groin or axilla. This hereditary condition affects the apocrine sweat ducts and is much more common in women than in men. The most common complaint is severe pruritus, which may respond to systemic estrogen therapy.[27]

Keloids (*Fig. 1.63*) are irregular, often linear, firm nodules, seen most often in patients with recurrent episodes of folliculitis or hidradenitis. They should be differentiated from epidermoid cysts, for they will often respond to intralesional steroid therapy, and excision may worsen the condition.

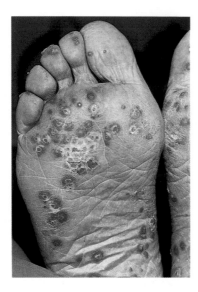

Fig. 1.60 Reiter's disease. Scaly papules cover the instep and heel. Palmar and plantar involvement is termed keratoderma blenorrhagica.

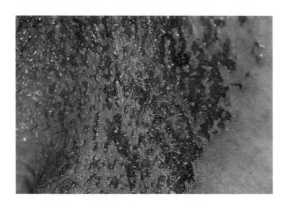

Fig. 1.61 Erosive lesions of benign familial pemphigus (Hailey–Hailey disease) on the scrotum and groin. Traumatic loss of the blister roof in an intertriginous area may cause an otherwise typical bullous disease to appear as multiple erosions.

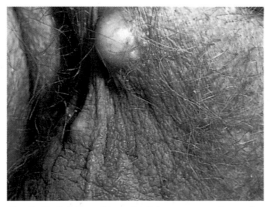

Fig. 1.62 Epidermoid cysts of the scrotum. Generally asymptomatic, these lesions occasionally may rupture and cause discomfort to the patient. They should be differentiated from steatocystoma multiplex, which contain a gel-like material rather than the thick, yellow, sebaceous substance typical of the epidermoid cyst.

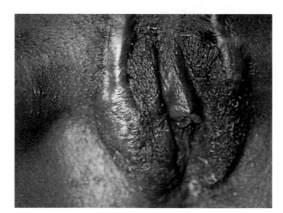

Fig. 1.63 Vulvar keloids. Thickened, linear nodular scars are present on both labia majora. Inciting factors in susceptible individuals include any inflammation or infectious or traumatic insult to skin.

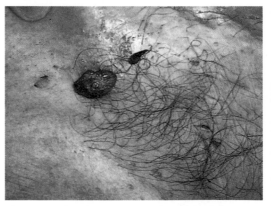

Fig. 1.64 Seborrheic keratosis. This thickened, warty lesion has a typical 'stuck-on' appearance. Similar lesions may be found elsewhere on the trunk.

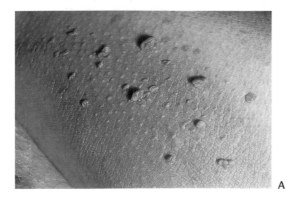

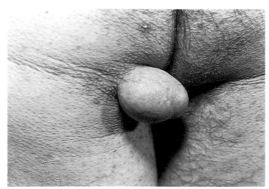

A   B

Fig. 1.65 (A) Acrochordons. 'Skin tags' are often found in intertriginous areas. They usually are asymptomatic unless traumatized. (B) Huge gluteal fibroma.

Seborrheic keratoses are elevated 'stuck-on' growths that may be pigmented or flesh-colored, which most often appear on the trunk (*Fig. 1.64*) but may occur on the genitalia. These warty growths are quite benign, and similar lesions are usually found elsewhere on the body.

They require removal only if they occur in areas where friction from clothing causes irritation. In intertriginous areas, seborrheic keratoses or even simple acrochordons (skin tags) may, with time, become pedunculated and prominent (*Fig. 1.65*). When one of these lesions becomes twisted on its stalk the entire lesion may infarct, becoming black and alarming the patient.

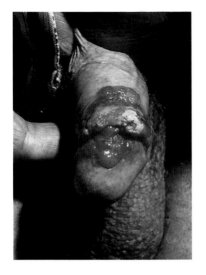

Fig. 1.66 Squamous cell carcinoma of the penis. This large chronic ulcer had been present for over a year. Patients may delay consultation with a physician because they are afraid that a malignancy will be diagnosed. Biopsy proved sqamous cell carcinoma.

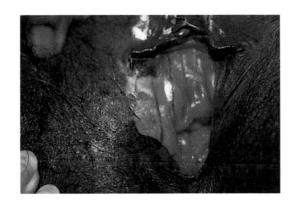

Fig. 1.67 Carcinoma in situ of the vulva. Note the asymmetric, rough, whitish, eroded, thickened appearance of this malignancy on the labium.

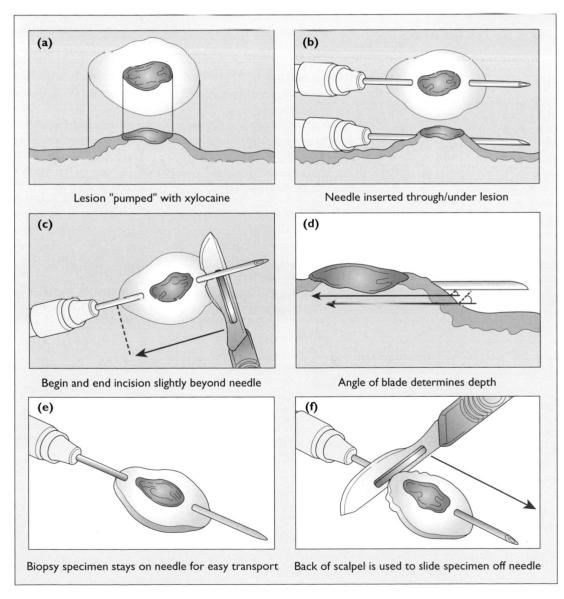

(a) Lesion "pumped" with xylocaine

(b) Needle inserted through/under lesion

(c) Begin and end incision slightly beyond needle

(d) Angle of blade determines depth

(e) Biopsy specimen stays on needle for easy transport

(f) Back of scalpel is used to slide specimen off needle

Fig. 1.68 Needle shave technique for skin biopsy.
(a) Using a small (27–30 gauge) needle, a wheal is formed under and around the lesion with local anesthetic (generally less than 1 ml of 1% xylocaine with epinephrine). For the biopsy, a half-inch 25-gauge needle is preferable, as a 30-gauge needle tends to bend when lifting up on the skin. Place the needle on a syringe for better control.
(b) The orientation of needle insertion is not critical, but a good guide might be the direction of what is to be the long axis of the biopsy. The needle is inserted just proximal to the lesion, advanced just under it, and exited just distal to it.
(c) The scalpel blade (#15 is small and manageable) should also be mounted on a handle for good control. The long axes of the scalpel and the needle are maintained at approximate right angles to one another, and the blade is inserted under the point of the needle, with the back of the blade actually touching the distal needle shaft. The biopsy incision is begun slightly distal to the exit point of the needle, and is directed toward the hub for maximum control.
(d) The angle of the blade should be determined before beginning the incision — a shallow angle for a superficial incision and a wider angle for a deeper specimen. The blade angle (depth of cut) should be maintained as consistently as possible, as the scalpel is drawn toward the hub of the syringe. Running the blade along the undersurface of the needle should be avoided as the incision will be too shallow and tissue immobilization will be lost as the specimen shifts off the needle. 'Scooping' with the blade also should be avoided since the incision will then be wider and deeper than necessary, and wound edges will be ragged.
(e) The incision is begun and ended slightly beyond the needle entrance and exit. The skin is lifted gently with the needle, as the blade slices underneath; the specimen on the needle should not 'pop' free as the biopsy is completed. The biopsy specimen should come smoothly free of the surrounding skin, impaled neatly on the needle for ease of handling. The biopsy specimen may be left on the needle and set aside briefly until bleeding is stopped, or it may be placed directly into fixative.
(f) To remove the biopsy specimen from the needle, use the back of the scalpel blade to slide the specimen off into the bottle of fixative.

Hyperkeratotic or ulcerated lesions that are asymmetrically located on the genitalia should be evaluated carefully for the possibility of squamous cell carcinoma (*Figs 1.66* and *1.67*). The lesions may be asymptomatic, and patients may be unaware of them or deny the chronicity of the problem. Biopsy is recommended for suspicious lesions, and multiple biopsies should be taken of all suspicious areas. In some forms of squamous cell carcinoma, such as Bowen's disease of the vulva and Bowenoid papulosis, the presence of certain human papillomaviruses (HPV 16 and 18) has been reported. Evaluation of the patient with a suspicious lesion should include palpation of regional lymph nodes. It may be appropriate to refer the patient directly to a specialist for evaluation and biopsy, although physicians should be aware that apprehension may make the patient reluctant to seek appropriate and timely health care. For this reason it may be expeditious to perform a biopsy on the first visit so that the correct diagnosis may be made (*Fig. 1.68*).

EROSIONS AND ULCERS

An erosion is defined as the loss of epidermis, while an ulcer extends through the epidermis into the dermis. The lack of a primary lesion makes evaluation of erosions and ulcers extremely difficult for most physicians, and biopsies rarely are helpful unless taken from the edge of a fresh lesion. Infectious ulcers will be covered in other chapters, so this discussion will be limited to noninfectious genital erosions and ulcers.

Bullous Diseases

The fragility of a blister roof in an intertriginous area makes erosions the most common presentation of the bullous diseases, which classically appear as blisters elsewhere on the skin. Erythema multiforme (EM) typically appears as 'target' or 'bull's-eye' lesions on the extremities (*Fig. 1.69*). Involvement of the oral mucosa (*Fig. 1.70*), palms, soles, and glans penis (*Fig. 1.71*) is seen most often in the bullous form called the Stevens–Johnson syndrome. EM often is associated with ingestion of drugs or a preceding HSV infection; however, other infections such as mycoplasmal pneumonia, or other viral or bacterial infections may be associated with the occurrence of this disorder.[28,29] Recurrent episodes are not uncommon and may be limited to mucous membranes such as the mouth and genitalia. It is important to ask the patient whether or not there has been an episode of HSV preceding the outbreak of EM, for control of HSV recurrences with acyclovir may lead to control of EM as well.[30,31]

As mentioned previously in the section on pustular dermatoses, benign familial pemphigus is most commonly seen as localized erosions in the groin. Pemphigus vulgaris, however, also may present with similar ulcers or erosions. Chronic pemphigus may even result in somewhat heaped-up, friable papules (pemphigus vegetans).

Ulcerative Dermatoses

Ulcerative forms of dermatoses may occur when a dermatologic condition makes the skin exceptionally fragile and easily traumatized. When these conditions occur in the genitalia, their presentation may be obscured by their erosive appearance.

Seen most commonly on the glans penis or hands, the fixed drug eruption (*Fig. 1.72*) has been linked with tetracycline therapy,

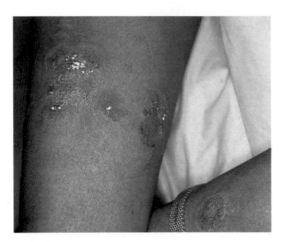

Fig. 1.69 Erythema multiforme (EM) on the arms. The concentric shape ('target' lesions) and presence of bullae are helpful clues to the recognition of this skin disorder, in which many different morphologic types of lesions may be present.

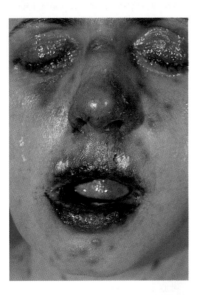

Fig. 1.70 Stevens–Johnson syndrome. This patient's lips and conjunctivae exhibit painful erosions and crusting. There were multiple tender erythematous plaques on the palms and soles.

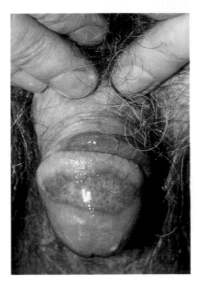

Fig. 1.71 Penile erosion in erythema multiforme. These painful shallow erosions developed after a herpesvirus infection of the mouth — a relatively common association.

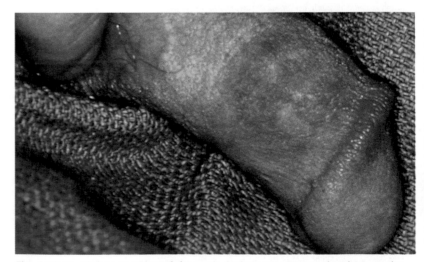

Fig. 1.72 Fixed drug eruption of the penis. Lesions may appear elsewhere on the body as hyperpigmented round macules or bullae that flare with readministration of the offending drug.

phenolphthalein that is found in certain laxatives, and several other drugs (*Table 1.4*).[32] Typically appearing as hyperpigmented round macules on the skin, acute lesions may be eczematous, bullous, or erosive in appearance. The appearance of genital lesions in a patient who is being treated with tetracycline for an STD may cause that patient to believe that he or she is experiencing a relapse of the disease or has another STD (see Chapter 2, Differential Diagnosis).

Lichen planus was discussed under its most typical presentation as a papulosquamous disorder, but ulcerative forms of this disorder do occur on mucous membranes (*Figs 1.73* and *1.74*) and can be extremely difficult to manage. Vulvovaginal erosions may be extensive, and their chronicity may cause the physician to consider the possibility of malignancy. Superinfection with *Candida* may also occur in this disorder, and should be considered and treated, if present. Treatment for ulcerative lichen planus generally is symptomatic, and topical steroids may be necessary.

Lichen sclerosus was discussed under the category of atrophy (p.11), but the extreme friability of the epidermis in this condition makes the presence of erosions, petechiae, and purpura a common occurrence. The patient should be examined carefully for the typical white atrophic epidermis occurring symmetrically around the rectum and perineum.

Cutaneous trauma is an often overlooked source of genital ulceration. A relatively innocuous dermatitis on the genitalia may be extremely pruritic and bothersome, and may result in the patient traumatizing the skin during bouts of itching and scratching. Erosions can be deep and severe (*Fig. 1.75*), and secondary infection may make evaluation difficult. Questioning the patient about his underlying symptoms will frequently evoke an admission of intractable pruritus, and therapy should be directed toward alleviation of symptoms. Trauma induced by the patient's sexual partner also should be considered, especially following oral sex. Human bites (*Fig. 1.76*) are notoriously infectious, and cultures may be necessary to determine appropriate broad-spectrum antibiotic therapy. The presence of symmetric bruises or cuts encircling the penis should lead the physician to suspect cutaneous trauma as a likely etiology; this becomes especially important in the evaluation of children for possible sexual abuse.

Systemic Diseases

Systemic diseases also may lead to secondary genital ulcers. Behçet's disease is a multisystem disorder that may present with skin involvement in a majority of cases. In the full-blown syndrome, oral and genital ulcerations are present (*Figs 1.77–1.79*), as well as a pustular eruption, which may involve the genitals. A spectrum of ocular involvement includes conjunctivitis, photophobia, uveitis, and optic neuritis. Central nervous system changes are variable and can be severe,

Barbiturates
Chlordiazepoxide
Dapsone
Oxyphenbutazone
Phenolphthalein
Quinine and derivatives
Sulfonamides
Tetracycline

Table 1.4 Drugs commonly causing fixed drug eruptions.

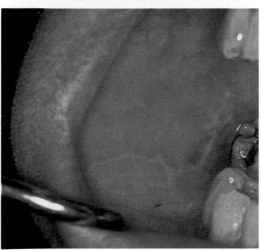

Fig. 1.7 Buccal mucosa with thin whitish linear streaks.

Fig. 1.74 White striae are seen on buccal mucosa. Courtesy of Emory University School of Dentistry.

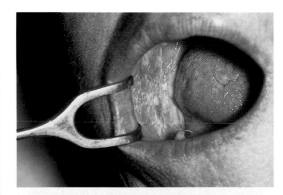

Figs 1.73 and 1.74 Erosive lichen planus on the oral mucous membrane.

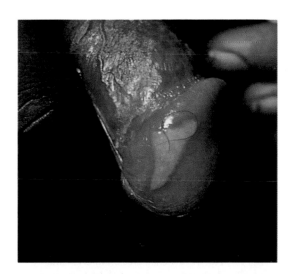

Fig. 1.75 Traumatic ulcer of the penis. The sharply angled borders of this lesion are a clue to its traumatic rather than infectious etiology.

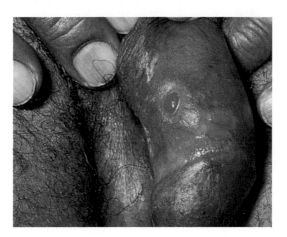

Fig. 1.76 Ulcer secondary to human bite of the penile shaft. Secondary infection is a common sequela of human bite wounds and cultures may be necessary for appropriate antibiotic therapy.

thus frequently dominating the clinical picture. Fever, arthralgias, and cardiac or pulmonary involvement also may be present. The mucosal ulcerations are nonspecific, and more common causes should be excluded before a diagnosis of Behçet's is made on the basis of oral and genital ulcers alone.[33,34]

Pyoderma gangrenosum (*Fig. 1.80*) is a shaggy, painful, 'dirty' looking ulcer with a bluish overhanging border. The name reflects the exceptionally infectious appearance of this actually noninfectious ulcer. It is seen most commonly in patients with inflammatory bowel disease, but also may be seen with multiple myeloma or other hematologic or immunologic disorders.[35]

Although pyoderma gangrenosum may be seen with gastrointestinal disease, cutaneous Crohn's disease classically presents long 'knife-cut' ulcers along the intertriginous groin folds. Flares of these cutaneous lesions often parallel the course of the gastrointestinal disease, and control of one often will lead to control of the other.[36,37]

Asymmetric ulcers of the genitalia that do not heal with appropriate therapy should be biopsied to rule out carcinoma. Biopsies should be multiple and taken from the thickest part of a lesion and the edge of an ulcer. Squamous cell carcinoma was discussed under nodules and tumors (p. 18). Extramammary Paget's disease, an uncommon disorder frequently associated with an underlying adenocarcinoma, presents as a chronic eczematous plaque. Pruritus or pain may be present. Hallmarks of this diagnosis are its chronicity, asymmetry, and lack of response to topical therapy. The vulva is one of the most common sites for extramammary Paget's disease, but it also occurs on the penis, scrotum and perianal region. Biopsy is essential for diagnosis.[38,39]

ITCHING (PRURITUS ANI, SCROTI, VULVAE)

Acute-onset perineal itching or burning should take the physician through a standard differential diagnosis, including *Candida* infection, irritant and contact dermatitis, urinary tract infection, hemorrhoids, pinworms, and condylomata. It is a different challenge to evaluate chronic cutaneous symptomatology, and this problem is not within the scope of this text. However, a few points should be made: lichen simplex chronicus (LSC) (see earlier section on dermatitis/eczema, pp. 5 and 6) is thickening of the skin in response to chronic scratching, and several underlying causes of pruritus must be considered. On the genitalia, maceration and intertriginous rubbing contribute to flares and continuation of symptoms, and infections are particularly likely to initiate itching. Cultures should be done for yeast and fungus as tinea and *Candida* are the most common offenders, and may be primary or secondary to the process. Vigorous scratching or eczematous change disturbs the skin barrier, allowing the development of secondary bacterial infection. In many cases of LSC, the initiating cause cannot be identified; the patient should be reassured that this is probably of no consequence, because the problem is now only the secondary change which has developed as a result of scratching.

In childhood, genital pruritus is often the result of irritant dermatitis, although STDs are an obvious consideration. Young girls may have fecal contamination of the vulva from careless hygiene, or conversely may irritate the skin from vigorous scrubbing or washing with soap. Pinworms are more common in childhood and typically involve the anus, but may also be seen at the vaginal opening. Vaginal or rectal discharge in childhood should be evaluated for evidence of possible sexual abuse, and genital lesions should be examined carefully. Lichen sclerosus (see below) can occur in childhood, and traumatic-appearing purpuric lesions are typical with the fragile epithelium of this cutaneous condition.

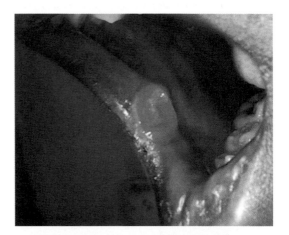

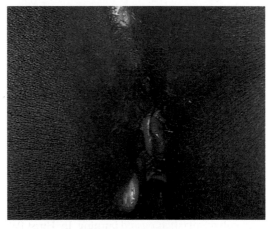

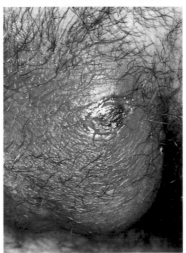

Figs 1.77–1.79 Behçet's disease. Nonspecific painful recurrent ulcers of the oral and genital mucosa were the presenting complaints in these young patients in whom Behçet's disease was diagnosed. Fig. 1.79 shows scrotal ulcer caused by Behçet's disease.

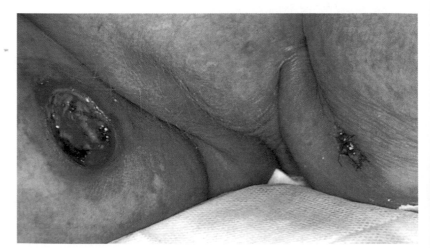

Fig. 1.80 Pyoderma gangrenosum. Multiple deep necrotic ulcers with dusky overhanging margins are characteristic of pyoderma gangrenosum. These lesions may be seen in patients with various systemic diseases.

The symptomatic patient should be asked about pre-existing dermatoses (including oral mucosal lesions), *Candida*, condylomata, methods of cleansing, and the use of topical and systemic medications. Previous treatments should be explored, especially if they resulted in a clearly allergic response (vesicles or erosions lasting for two weeks) rather than local irritation (stinging and burning on application). The patient should be asked specifically about risk factors: for example, the *Candida*-prone patient may receive frequent rounds of antibiotics for sinusitis, urinary tract infections, or acne; steroids or other immunosuppressants may be prescribed for a variety of disorders. Estrogen deficiency may be important if the patient is perimenopausal. On the genitalia, erythematous papules and pustules may develop as a complication of topical steroid use, as well as with cutaneous infections.

While some patients will describe elements of itching and burning, the two conditions can usually be differentiated on physical examination. Cutaneous changes of lichenification (leathery thickening) or excoriation (scratch marks) are more typical of pruritus, because the patient with burning skin rarely rubs or scratches the affected area. Without evidence of scratching, the patient with cutaneous burning or dysesthesia may appear to have a normal examination.[40]

References

1. Hewan-Lowe K, Moreland A, Finnerty DP. Penis and Scrotum. In: Someren, AE Ed. *Urologic Pathology with Clinical and Radiologic Correlations*. MacMillan Publishing Co., 1989; p. 616.
2. Ackerman AB, Kornberg R. Pearly penile papules – acral angiofibromas. *Arch Derm* 1973; **108**:673.
3. Hewan-Lowe K, Moreland A, Finnerty DP. Penis and Scrotum. In: Someren AE, Ed. *Urologic Pathology with Clinical and Radiologic Correlations*. MacMillan Publishing Co., 1989; p. 613.
4. Wilkinson EJ. Normal histology and nomenclature of the vulva, and malignant neoplasms, including VIN. *Dermatol Clin* 1992; **10**:283–296.
5. Bergeron C, Ferenczy A, Richart RM *et al*. Micropapillomatosis labialis appears unrelated to human papillomavirus. *Obstet Gynecol* 1990; **76**:281–286.
6. Moyal-Barracco M, Leibowitch M, Orth G. Vetsibular papillae of the vulva. Lack of evidence for human papillomavirus etiology. *Arch Dermatol* 1990; **126**:1594–1598.
7. Turner MC. Genital Disorders. In: *Cutaneous Medicine and Surgery* Vol. 2. Arndt KA, Le Boit PE, Robinson JK, Wintroub BU Eds: W.B. Saunders, Philadelphia, 1996; pp 1340–1359.
8. Bergeron S, Binik YM, Khalife S *et al*. Vulvar vestibulitis syndrome: Reliability of diagnosis and evaluation of current diagnostic criteria. *Obstet Gynecol* 2001; **98**:45–51.
9. Reitschel RL, Fowler JF, Fischer A, Eds. *Contact Dermatitis*, 4th ed. Baltimore, Williams & Wilkins, 1995; pp 78–82, 118.
10. Rand S. Overview: The treatment of dermatophytosis. *J Am Acad Dermatol* 2000; **43** (Supplement): s104–112.
11. Landthaler M, Braun-Falco O, Richter K *et al*. Malignant melanomas of the vulva. *Dtsch Med Wochenschr* 1985; **110**:789–794.
12. Rock B. Pigmented lesions of the vulva. *Dermatol Clin* 1992; **10**:361–370.
13. Hall J, Moreland A, Cox J *et al*. Oral acanthosis nigracans: Report of a case and comparison of oral and cutaneous pathology. *Am J Dermatopathol* 1988; **10**:68–73.
14. Kemp EH, Waterman EA, Weetman AP. Autoimmune aspects of vitiligo. *Autoimmunity* 2001; **34**:65–77.
15. Betterle C, Caretto A, DeZio A *et al*. Incidence and significance of organ-specific autoimmune disorders (clinical, latent, or only autoantibodies) in patients with vitiligo. *Dermatologica* 1985; **171**:419–423.
16. Meffert JJ, Davis BM, Grimwood RE. Lichen sclerosus. *J Am Acad Dermatol* 1995; **32**(3):393–416.
17 Sobel JD. Vulvovaginitis. *Dermatol Clin* 1992; **10**(2):339–359.
18 Odom RB, James WD, Berger TG. Bacterial Infections. In: *Andrews' Diseases of the Skin*, 9th Ed. W.B. Saunders Co., Philiadelphia, 2000; pp 307–317.
19. Dahl MV. Strategies for the management of recurrent furunculosis. *South Med J* 1987; **80**:352–356.
20. Boer J, van Giemert MJP. Long term results of isotretinoin in the treatment of 68 patients with hidradenitis suppurativa. *J Am Acad Dermatol* 1999; **40**:73–76.
21. Lebwohl M, Ali S. Treatment of psoriasis. Part 2. Systemic therapies. *J Am Acad Dermatol* 2001; **45**:649–661.
22. Lynch PJ, Edwards L. *Genital Dermatology*. Churchill Livingstone, New York, 1994; pp 61–63.
23. Thambar IV, Dunlop R, Thin RN *et al*. Circinate vulvitis in Reiter's Syndrome. *Br J Vener Dis* 1977; **53**:1260–1262.
24. Brewerton DA, Nicholls A, Oates JK *et al*. Reiter's disease and HL-A 27. *Lancet* 1973; **2**:996–998.
25. Kiyohara A *et al*. Successful treatment of severe recurrent Reiter's syndrome with cyclosporin. *J Am Acad Dermatol* 1997; **36**:482–483.
26. Burge SM. Hailey–Hailey disease: The clinical features, response to treatment and prognosis. *Br J Dermatol* 1992; **126**:275–282.
27. Miller ML, Harford RR, Yeager JK. Fox–Fordyce disease treated with topical clindamycin solution. *Arch Derm* 1995; **131**:1112–1113.
28. Lyell A, Gordon A, Dick HM *et al*. Mycoplasma and erythema multiforme. *Lancet* 1967; **ii**:1116–1118.
29. Huff JC, Weston WL, Tonnesen MG. Erythema Multiforme: A critical review of characteristics, diagnostic criteria, and causes. *J Am Acad Dermatol* 1983; **8**:763–775.
30. Lemak MA, Duvic M, Bean SF. Oral acyclovir for the prevention of herpes-associated erythema multiforme. *J Am Acad Derm* 1986; **15**:50–54.
31. Cheriyan S, Patterson R. Recurrent Stevens-Johnson syndrome secondary to herpes simplex: a follow up on a successful management program. *Allergy Asthma Pro* 1996; **17**:71–73.
32. Sehgal VH, Gangwani OP. Genital fixed drug eruptions. *Genitourin Med* 1986; **62**:56–58.
33. Tokoro Y, Seto T, Abe Y *et al*. Skin lesions in Behçet's disease. *Int J Derm* 1977; **16**:227–244.
34. Jorizzo JL, Abernathy JL, White WL et al. Mucocutaneous criteria for the diagnosis of Behçet's disease: an analysis of clinicopathologic data from multiple international centers. *J Amer Acad Dermatol* 1995; **32**:968–976.
35. Powell FC, Schroeter AL, Su WPD, Perry HO. Pyoderma gangrenosum: A review of 86 patients. *Q J Med* 1985; **55**:173–186.
36. Slaney G, Muller S, Clay J *et al*. Crohn's disease involving the penis. *Gut* 1986; **27**:329–333.
37. Reyman L, Milano A, Demopoulos R *et al*. Metastatic vulvar ulceration in Crohn's disease. *Am J Gastro* 1986; **81**:16 49.
38. Odom RB, James WD, Berger TG Extramammary Paget's Disease. In: *Andrews' Diseases of the Skin*, 9th Ed. W.B. Saunders Co., Philiadelphia, 2000; pp 843–844.
39. Wilkinson EJ. Normal histology and nomenclature of the vulva, and malignant neoplasms, including VIN. *Dermatol Clin* 1992; **10**:283–296.
40. McKay M. Pruritus vulvae and vulvodynia: itching and burning. In: Hurst JW (ed): *Medicine for the Practicing Physician*, 3rd ed. Boston, Butterworth-Heinemann, Ch 10–15, 1992; pp 678–680.

Syphilis

D Cox, H Liu, A Moreland and W Levine

2

INTRODUCTION

Syphilis is a chronic systemic infectious disease that is transmitted during sexual intercourse or other intimate contact; it also can be transmitted from a pregnant woman to her fetus *in utero* or by the infant having contact with maternal lesions during birth. The causative agent of syphilis is *Treponema pallidum* subspecies *pallidum*, a spirochete (*Fig. 2.1*). This agent has never been cultured successfully on artificial media, and does not take up the Gram stain. Three other treponemes (subspecies *T. pertenue*, subspecies *T. endemicum*, and *T. carateum*) are also pathogenic for humans (*Table 2.1*). Infection with these organisms will cause serologic tests for syphilis to be reactive, although the infections are not sexually transmitted.

THE BIOLOGY OF *TREPONEMA PALLIDUM*

T. pallidum is a spirochete or spiral-shaped bacterium with cellular dimensions of 0.20 μm in diameter by 5–15 μm in length. The spiral of the organism has a wavelength and amplitude of approximately 1.1 μm and 0.4 μm, respectively. The cell envelope architecture of the organism is quite unique (*Fig. 2.2*). It has an outer membrane (OM) but it is unlike that of typical Gram-negative organisms.[1–4] First, lipopolysaccharide (LPS) is absent. Second, although investigated by several laboratories, the presence of porins has not been demonstrated and therefore the treponemal OM is presumed to be devoid of these structures. Third, freeze-fracture electron microscopy has revealed that there are very few intramembranous proteins in its OM.[5,6] The number has been estimated to be around 100 per cell compared to several thousand for *E. coli* and other typical Gram-negative bacteria. To date, none of these rare OM proteins have been identified or characterized.[7] Last, the organism possesses flagella for locomotion (referred to as endoflagella), but these are located in the periplasmic space instead of externally as in typical motile bacteria. These characteristics demonstrate that the surface of the treponemal OM has very few exposed antigens and therefore this lack of antigenicity gives it 'stealth' properties. This inability to be readily recognized by the human immune system helps to explain how, despite a mounted immune response, some organisms escape to cause the secondary and tertiary stages of syphilis.

T. pallidum is fully capable of DNA, RNA, and protein synthesis. Its replication is restricted to a very narrow temperature range (30–35°C) and the generation time in rabbits has been reported to be about 35 hours. In vitro cultivation of *T. pallidum* is available but limited in scope. Five to six generations of treponemes can be propagated in tissue cultures of cotton-tail rabbit epithelial cells (Sf1Ep), but continuous serial passage has yet to be attained.[8] The inability to achieve a practical cultivation system is a reflection of the unusual and fastidious metabolism of this human pathogen.

In 1998, the complete sequence for the genome of *T. pallidum* was published.[9] The genome, which was determined to be 1.14 Mb and encode for 1040 genes or open reading frames (ORFs), is about 25% the size of the *E. coli* genome. Of those, 577 (55%) have predicted biological roles; 287 (28%) are novel genes; and the remaining have unknown functions.

Documented by many physiological studies in the late 1970s and early 1980s, the genome of *T. pallidum* lacks the genes for the biosynthesis of fatty acids, amino acids, nucleotides, and enzyme

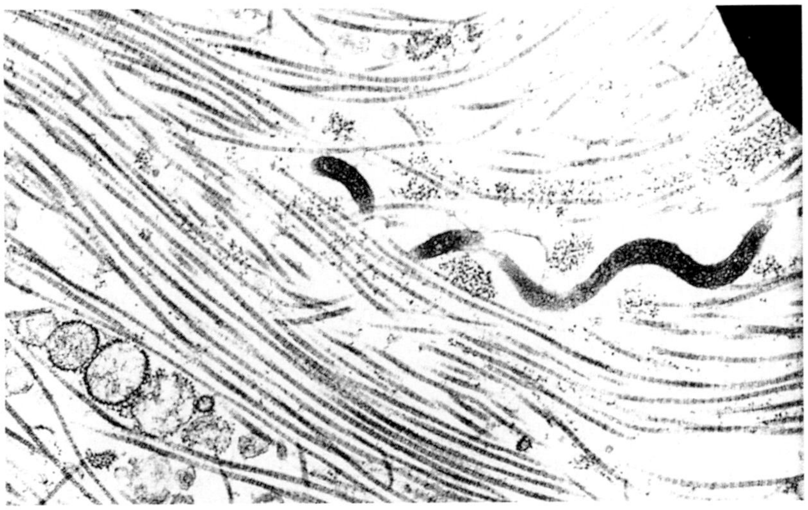

Fig. 2.1 Transmission electron micrograph of *Treponema pallidum* subspecies *pallidum* in tissue.

	Syphilis	Yaws	Bejel	Pinta
ORGANISM	T. pallidum subspecies pallidum	T. pallidum subspecies pertenue	T. pallidum subspecies endemicum	T. carateum
TRANSMISSION	Sexual contact	Skin contact	Skin contact Oral	Skin contact
LESION TYPE				
PRIMARY	Chancre	Crusted papules	Oral mucosal lesions	Crusted papules and plaques
SECONDARY	Macular or papulosquamous	Papillomatous, and scarring	Mucous patches and condylomata lata	Scaly plaques
LATE	Gummata and endarteritis	Gummata of bone and skin	Gummata of cartilage, bone, and skin	Dyschromia

Table 2.1 Diseases caused by pathogenic treponemes of humans.

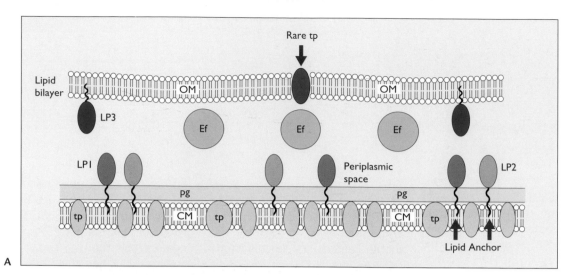

Fig. 2.2 Cell envelope architecture of *T. pallidum*. A. Model of *T. pallidum* cell envelope. tp, transmembrane proteins; OM, outer membrane; Ef, endoflagella in cross-section; LP 1, 2, 3, lipoproteins; pg, peptidoglycan layer; CM, cytoplasmic membrane. B. Freeze fracture electronmicrograph of *T. pallidum* outer membrane. Red circles enclose rare transmembrane proteins. Courtesy of Dr J D Rudolf.

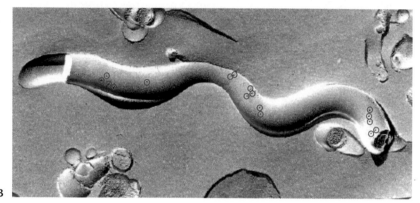

Present
  Glycolysis
  Hexose monophosphate pathway
  Cell wall synthesis
  Lipid modification of proteins
  Transport systems for amino acids, carbohydrates and cations
  DNA, RNA, and protein synthesis
  Minimal DNA repair

Absent
  Fatty acid biosynthesis
  Amino acid biosynthesis
  Nucleotide biosynthesis
  Vitamin biosynthesis
  TCA cycle
  Electron transport
  Phosphate uptake system
  Protein secretion systems
  DNA restriction-modification
  PEP-dependent phosphotransferase systems

Table 2.2 Metabolic capabilities of *T. pallidum*.

co-factors. However, the genome contains 57 ORFs that encode for 18 distinct ABC transporters with specificities for carbohydrates, amino acids, cations and thiamine. Surprisingly, there are no genes for a phosphate uptake system. For energy production, the genome contains all the genes for glycolysis, but none for the TCA cycle or an electron transport system. A summary of the metabolic capabilities of *T. pallidum* is provided in *Table 2.2*.

With respect to cell envelope structure and function, the organism has the complete machinery for peptidoglycan synthesis and protein secretion. Genome analysis indicates the presence of 22 putative lipoproteins; however no pathway for the synthesis of lipopolysaccharide is present. One remarkable find was a family of 12 genes (*T. pallidum* repeat, Tpr), which are paralogs to the major surface protein (msp) of *T. denticola*.[9]

The sequence of the *T. pallidum* genome revealed that the organism possesses a *recF* recombination pathway but lacks *recB*, *recC*, and *recD*.[10] It has a minor pathway for *uvr* excision repair but has no recognizable system for DNA restriction-modification. These findings may explain why there is so little variability in the *T. pallidum* genome, especially with respect to the development of resistance to antibiotics.

In summary, the genome sequence reveals that *T. pallidum* is highly adapted to a parasitic life style. As an obligate parasite, there is little need to synthesize all of the common biological building blocks like amino acids, fatty acids, and nucleotides when they are readily available from the host. The metabolic capabilities of *T. pallidum* are more tailored to acquisition and uptake than to actual synthesis.

EPIDEMIOLOGY

Syphilis is a disease of worldwide importance (*Fig. 2.3*).[11] In contrast with the decline in rates observed in Western Europe during the last decade, there has been a marked increase in syphilis rates in the newly independent states of the former Soviet Union (*Fig. 2.4A* and *B*). In the USA, primary and secondary (infectious) syphilis rates were at a peak in 1947, declined sharply over the following 10 years, and then gradually increased over each succeeding decade to reach a post-World War II peak of 50,578 in 1990 (*Fig. 2.5*). The annual number of cases has subsequently declined sharply, to 6657 cases in 1999, and a renewed

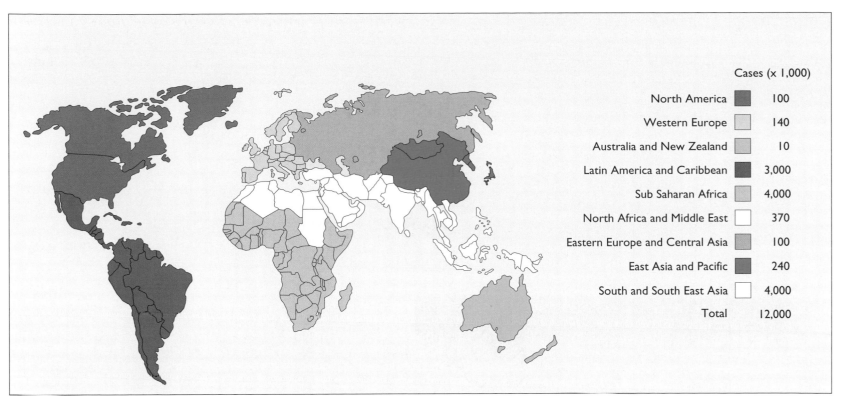

Fig. 2.3 Estimated new cases of syphilis amongst adults by region, 1999. Courtesy of JPA, WHO.

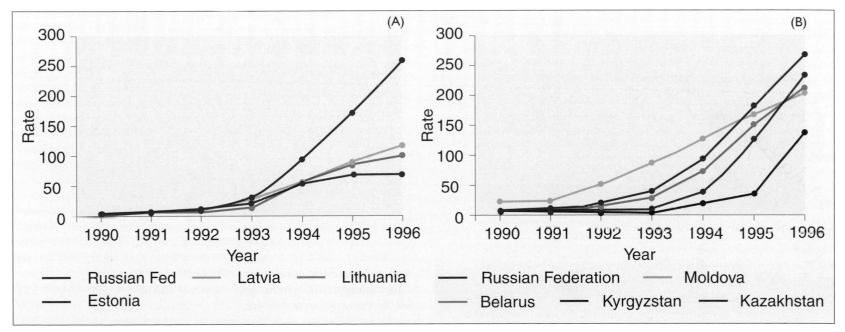

Fig. 2.4 (A) Syphilis prevalence rates (%) in Baltic countries, 1990–1996; (B) Syphilis prevalence rates (%) in former Soviet Union countries, 1990–1996. Courtesy of JPA, WHO.

effort to eliminate syphilis in the United States has been initiated by the Public Health Service.[12]

In the 1970s, syphilis was predominantly a disease of gay men, but the advent of AIDS and the subsequent practice of safer sex has led to a decrease in the incidence of syphilis in this population. A shift of syphilis to the heterosexual population began in 1984 and can most probably be attributed to the practice of exchanging sex with multiple partners for drugs, particularly for crack cocaine. The spread of acquired syphilis to heterosexual populations, with poorer access to medical treatment, has been paralleled by an increase in the number of cases of congenital syphilis; this increase was magnified by a new reporting system for congenital syphilis that was more sensitive, and which led to reports of more presumptive (versus confirmed) cases. Recently, new outbreaks of syphilis have appeared among gay and bisexual men, which are thought to reflect an increase in risk behavior related to the availability of more effective therapies for treatment of HIV infection.[13]

Individuals are infectious for their sex partners during the primary and secondary stages, when skin or mucosal lesions are present. Women are most likely to transmit the infection to their unborn infants during the early stages of the disease when they are spirochetemic, but infection of the fetus during early latency is also possible.

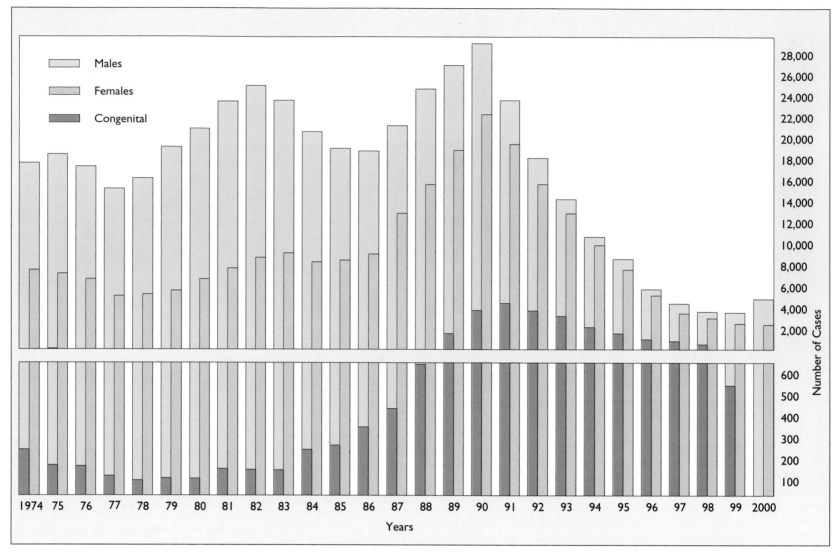

Fig. 2.5 US rates of primary and secondary syphilis in men and women compared with the rates of congenital syphilis (CDC Surveillance Report 2000). Numbers of cases of congenital syphilis are a highly sensitive indicator of the amount of infectious syphilis in a population and the need for control activities. In 1989, in addition to the reporting of symptomatic cases of congenital syphilis, asymptomatic babies born to mothers with reactive serologic tests for syphilis and without a history of adequate treatment for syphilis, and syphilitic stillborns were included in the surveillance case definition.

CLINICAL MANIFESTATIONS

Untreated, syphilis is a chronic disease that is spread throughout the body hematogenously and which can produce manifestations in virtually every organ system (*Fig. 2.6*).[14] The infectious, clinical manifestations, namely primary and secondary syphilis, are transient events. During latency, by definition, there are no clinical signs or symptoms of infection, despite the fact that *T. pallidum* can be demonstrated in some tissues. Clinical history and serology is currently the only available method for accurate diagnosis during this stage of the disease. The clinical course and serologic changes of untreated syphilis are summarized in *Figs 2.7* and *2.8*.

PRIMARY SYPHILIS

The first clinical manifestation of syphilis, the chancre, develops on average about 3 weeks after infection (10–90 days). The chancre appears at the site where treponemal invasion of the dermis first occurred, usually on or near the genitals. However, it may occur on any skin or mucous membrane. Usually, chancres are single lesions and are painless (*Fig. 2.9*) unless superinfected; hence, they may be missed by the patient if they occur in an inaccessible region, such as the cervix, pharynx, or rectum. Nontender regional adenopathy is also common. If untreated,

the chancre will persist for 2–6 weeks and heal without scarring. Occasionally, a relapsing chancre will occur at the same site. Motile spirochetes should be demonstrable in untreated chancres during most stages of their evolution. They may be difficult to demonstrate in late, healing lesions, and are usually absent if the patient has applied local medications or taken antibiotics.

The typical chancre is indurated, has a clean base, and rolled edges (*Fig. 2.10*). Secondary infection with bacteria or even herpesviruses can occur, and may cause the ulcer to appear somewhat atypical (*Fig. 2.11*). The differential diagnosis includes chancroid, donovanosis, and occasionally herpes. The labia and fourchette are the most typical areas for chancres to occur in women (*Fig. 2.12*). Perianal, anal or rectal chancres occur primarily in gay men, and in women who have a history of rectal intercourse (*Fig. 2.13*). While single lesions are seen most commonly, multiple primary chancres are not uncommon (*Fig. 2.14*). Healing lesions may present problems in diagnosis, particularly in their later stages when they are dark-field negative, and adenopathy may not be prominent (*Fig. 2.15*). Acquired syphilis can occur in infants and children (*Fig. 2.16*). Syphilitic chancres occasionally may occur in extragenital sites, such as the fingers (*Fig. 2.17*) or the oral cavity (*Fig. 2.18*). Clinical findings in cases of primary syphilis are summarized in *Table 2.3*.

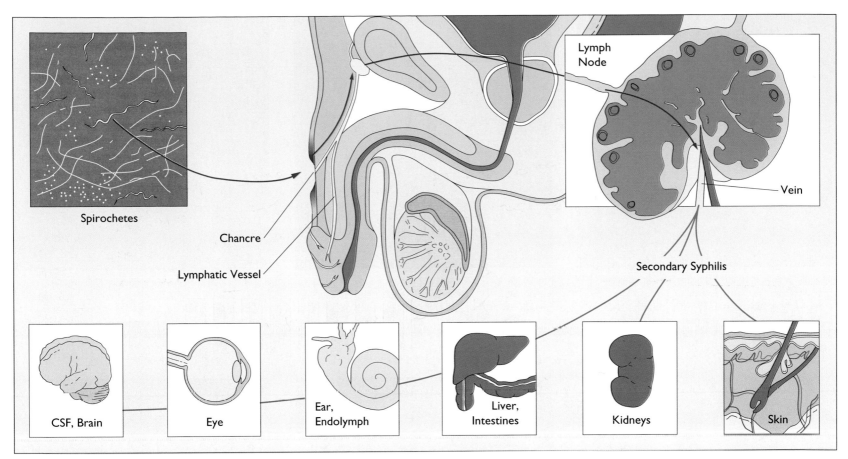

Spirochetes

Chancre

Lymphatic Vessel

Lymph Node

Vein

Secondary Syphilis

CSF, Brain

Eye

Ear, Endolymph

Liver, Intestines

Kidneys

Skin

Fig. 2.6 Schematic diagram to show how spirochetes enter regional lymph nodes from a skin chancre, and then enter the bloodstream. Organ systems that are involved are shown: CSF, brain, eye, ear endolymph, liver, intestines, kidneys, skin.

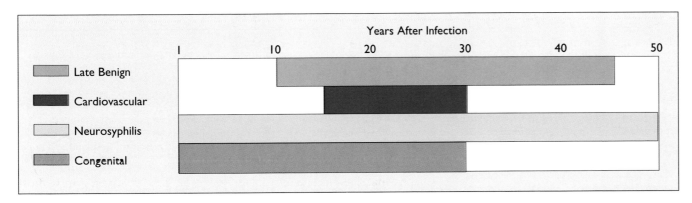

Fig. 2.7 The clinical course of untreated syphilis. Courtesy of Hans Ristow, MD (adapted from unpublished work).

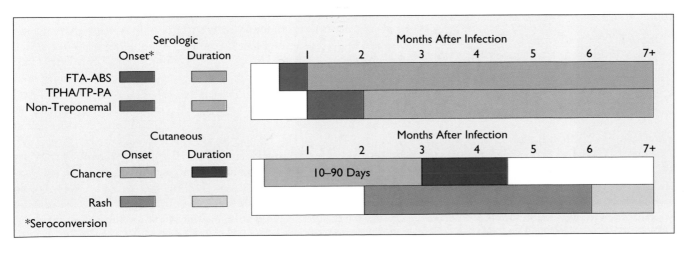

Fig. 2.8 Correlation of serologic and cutaneous changes in untreated syphilis. Courtesy of Hans Ristow, MD (adapted from unpublished work).

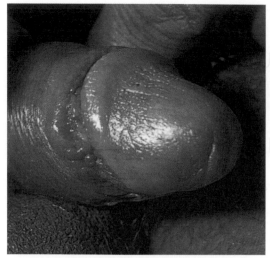

Fig. 2.9 Typical syphilitic chancre of the coronal sulcus. This early asymptomatic chancre in the coronal sulcus shows characteristic induration and a 'clean' base. Dark-field examination will almost always be positive if no medication has been given or applied topically.

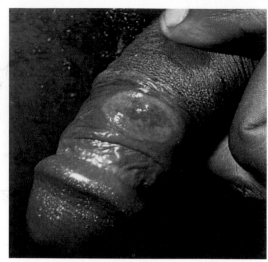

Fig. 2.10 Large, indurated primary chancre of the penile shaft. This penile chancre has been present for several weeks, but it is still painless and large. The induration produces a cartilaginous quality.

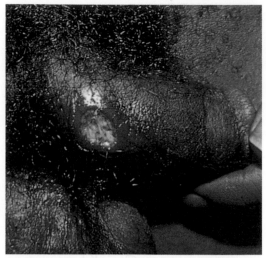

Fig. 2.11 Atypical penile chancre. This chancre appears atypical because it has become secondarily infected with bacteria. Dark-field examination may be difficult because of the presence of nonpathogenic treponemes.

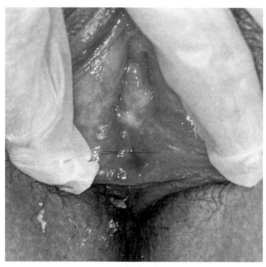

Fig. 2.12 Painless button-like syphilitic chancre of the posterior forchette, a common site for chancres in women. Courtesy of Barbara Romanowski, M.D.

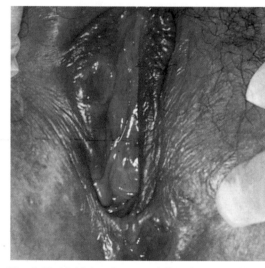

Fig. 2.13 Multiple primary syphilitic chancres of labia and perineum. Typical induration and edema of the chancres are easily seen. Courtesy of Barbara Romanowski, M.D.

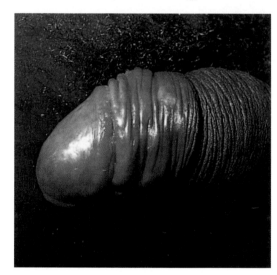

Fig. 2.14 Multiple chancres of primary syphilis. Multiple primary chancres are not uncommon in primary syphilis. They occur most frequently on the penis and vulva.

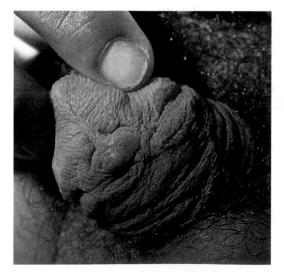

Fig. 2.15 Healing chancre. Primary chancres heal spontaneously, as seen here in this almost resolved penile chancre.

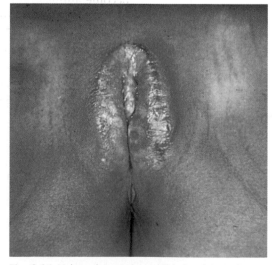

Fig. 2.16 Vulvar chancre in a child. A painless ulcer found on the genitals of a child should always raise the possibility of syphilis, but also may be acquired through nonsexual means. Courtesy of Centers for Disease Control in Atlanta, Georgia.

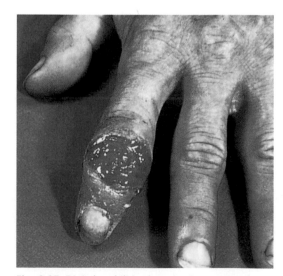

Fig. 2.17 Digital syphilitic chancre. Occupational exposure of health care workers may be the cause of chancres on the hands. Courtesy of Centers for Disease Control in Atlanta, Georgia.

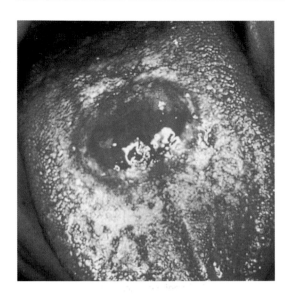

Fig. 2.18 Chancre of the tongue. Dark-field examination of mouth lesions may not be reliable due to the presence of saprophytic spirochetes. However, the direct FA test is useful in this situation. Courtesy of Centers for Disease Control in Atlanta, Georgia.

I. ULCER
    Single genital ulcer most common
    Diameter of lesion usually > 0.5 cm
    Nonpainful
    Indurated, rolled edges
    Clean lesion base
    Dark-field (+) for motile spirochetes

II. ADENOPATHY
    Inguinal, ipsilateral to ulcer
    Nontender
    Nonfluctuant

III. CONSTITUTIONAL SYMPTOMS
    None

Table 2.3 Synopsis of clinical findings of primary syphilis.

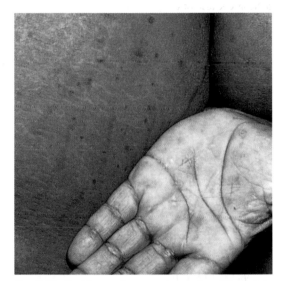

Fig. 2.19 Oval hyperpigmented macules of the trunk and extremities in early secondary syphilis. The eruption was generalized, but not readily visible, and therefore unnoticed by the patient.

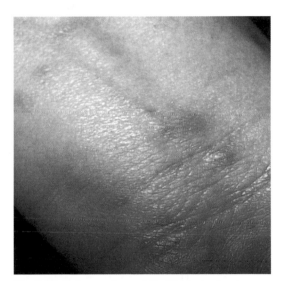

Fig. 2.20 Early papular syphilis. The lack of scale suggests that this is an early form of papular syphilis. Erythema and firmness of the papules on palpation are characteristic.

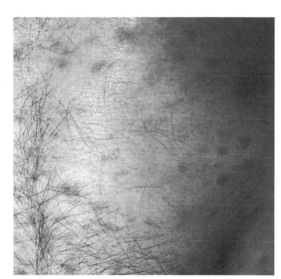

Fig. 2.21 Macular and papulosquamous forms of syphilis coexisting in syphilis of 1 month's duration. This eruption was completely asymptomatic.

SECONDARY SYPHILIS

Onset of the secondary stage of disease ranges from 6 weeks to 6 months after infection in the untreated patient.[14] The primary chancre may still be present when clinically apparent secondary lesions occur. In this phase of the disease, spirochetes enter the bloodstream from their dermal and lymph node foci and are distributed to most tissues and organs (see Fig. 2.6). After a suitable period of multiplication, generalized but nonspecific symptoms occur, such as fever, malaise, headache, sore throat, arthralgias, and anorexia. Generalized adenopathy occurs in more than 50% of patients. Hepatomegaly and occasionally splenomegaly may also occur. There may be leukocytosis, anemia, and an elevated erythrocyte sedimentation rate. Syphilitic hepatitis is characterized by mild derangement of liver enzymes and a markedly elevated alkaline phosphatase. An acute, 'viral type' of meningitis may complicate the picture.

A rash, which is sometimes called a syphilid, occurs in about 75% of patients and is extremely variable in appearance. It may be localized or generalized. Symmetric discrete erythematous, brown or hyperpigmented macules are the earliest generalized syphilid (Fig. 2.19). This eruption commonly begins on the trunk. The macules may enlarge or become annular; and scaling and pruritus are absent. As the eruption progresses, some of the macules may become thickened and papular (Fig. 2.20), and thus a macular syphilid may coexist with the papular forms (Fig. 2.21). Papular syphilids (Fig. 2.22) appear to be more common than macular eruptions, perhaps because they are easier to see. If the disease remains untreated for several weeks, the papules may develop a dry, thin collarette of scale, which peels off easily (Figs 2.23 and 2.24).

Frequent involvement of the palms and soles with macular and papular syphilids may help to distinguish them from other dermatoses (see Fig. 2.25 and the following section on Differential Diagnosis). Many varieties of papular syphilid have been described, and include, among others, the papulosquamous (Fig. 2.26), annular (Fig. 2.27), lenticular (Fig. 2.28), syphilis cornee, in which the lesions resemble clavi (see Figs 2.23 and 2.24), psoriasiform (Fig. 2.29), and framboesiform (Fig. 2.30) types.

Moist hypertrophic papular lesions, known as condylomata lata, occur in intertriginous areas, such as the genitals (Figs 2.31 and 2.32) and gluteal folds (Fig. 2.33). Occasionally, they may become hyperplastic or verrucous, and as such may very closely resemble condylomata acuminata (Fig. 2.34). These lesions may also be seen in extragenital

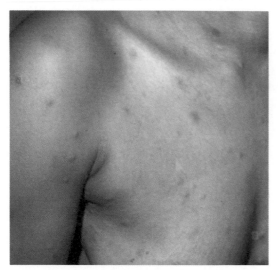

Fig. 2.22 Papular secondary syphilis. The generalized erythematous papules are quite obvious to both patient and physician.

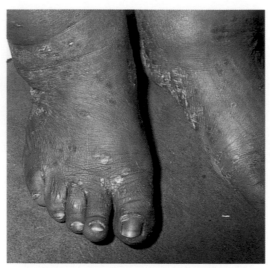

Fig. 2.23 Papulosquamous secondary syphilis. The annular scaling seen here had been present for several weeks. It is quite common.

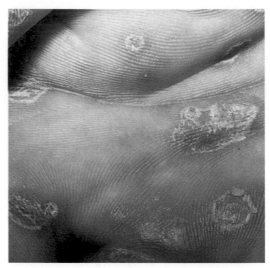

Fig. 2.24 A close-up view of the characteristic colarette of scale and hyperpigmentation seen in untreated secondary syphilis.

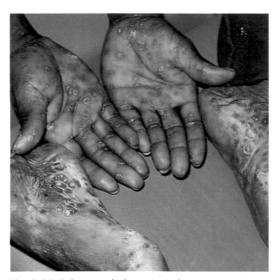

Fig. 2.25 Palmar and plantar papulosquamous secondary syphilis.

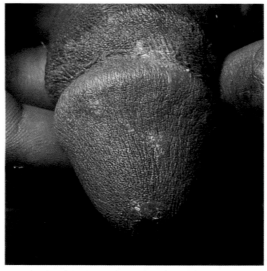

Fig. 2.26 Papulosquamous syphilids are typically flat papules, which are red, indurated, and slightly scaly. Lesions may be limited to the genital region.

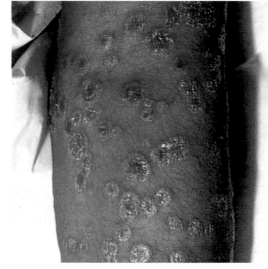

Fig. 2.27 Annular syphilids are florid annular scaly plaques, some with a targetoid hyperpigmented center.

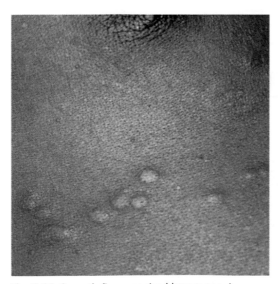

Fig. 2.28 Smooth firm pea-sized brown papules characterize the lenticular form of secondary syphilis.

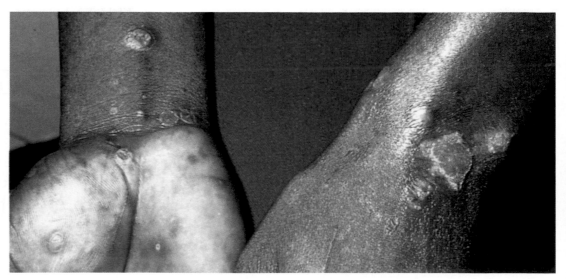

Fig. 2.29 Large and small psoriasiform plaques with thick scale and an irregular shape in late secondary syphilis.

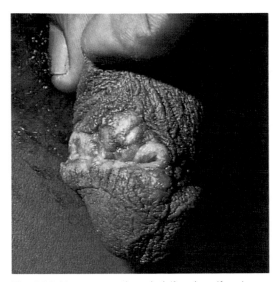

Fig. 2.30 Verrucous and eroded (framboesiform) lesions of late secondary syphilis in the coronal sulcus. Courtesy of Heidi Watts.

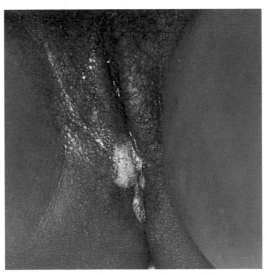

Fig. 2.31 Condylomata lata. Typical condylomata lata on the labia and perineum are moist gray plaques and papules.

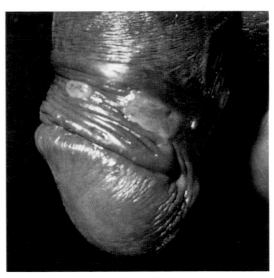

Fig. 2.32 Condylomata lata. Flat, broad-based dark-field positive plaques are seen in the folds of the foreskin.

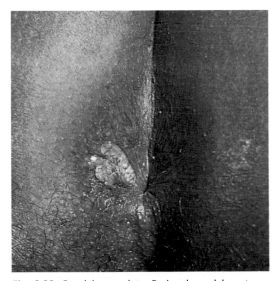

Fig. 2.33 Condylomata lata. Perianal condylomata detected in a patient who sought help because of a palmar rash.

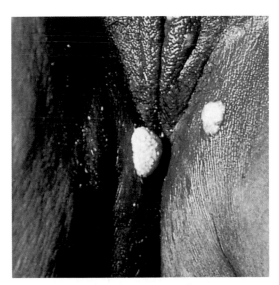

Fig. 2.34 Condylomata lata. Unusually verrucous condylomata lata resembling condylomata acuminata in a patient who presented with a generalized macular eruption.

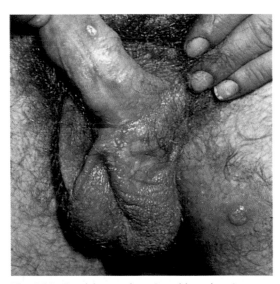

Fig. 2.35 Condylomata lata. Broad-based moist, dark-field-positive condylomata lata on the thigh. Note the other erosive lesions of secondary syphilis on the penile shaft.

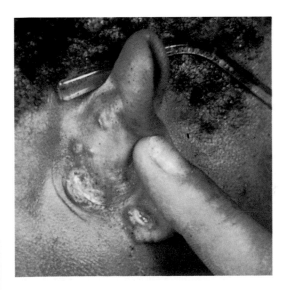

Fig. 2.36 Split papules, seen here on the posterior auricular fold, may also be present at the angles of the mouth. Courtesy of Centers for Disease Control in Atlanta, Georgia.

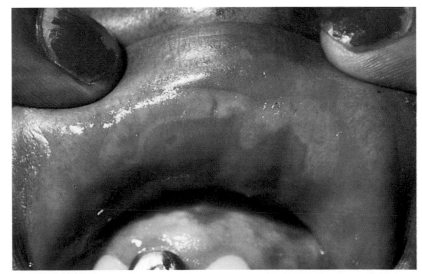

Fig. 2.37 Serpiginous mucous patches on the labial mucosa and tongue were the presenting sign of syphilis in this patient.

areas (*Fig. 2.35*). Condylomata lata are usually covered with a grayish exudate containing numerous spirochetes, making them much more infectious than other secondary syphilids. Another variant of papular syphilis is the so-called split papules found in the postauricular area (*Fig. 2.36*) or in the oral commissures. Nonspecific superficial erosions of the oral or genital mucous membranes, called mucous patches, are another common manifestation of secondary syphilis. These round or oval lesions appear as grayish or denuded patches on the buccal or labial mucosa (*Fig. 2.37*), on the tongue (*Figs 2.38* and *2.39*), or on the palate or tonsils.

Alopecia may occur during secondary syphilis as a patchy thinning (*Fig. 2.40*) or as a more diffuse loss of hair (*Fig. 2.41*). Eyebrows, beard hair, or any other hairy body areas may be involved. The alopecia regrows in both treated and untreated patients.

The signs and symptoms of secondary syphilis usually last only a few weeks. Relapses may occur in the untreated patient, usually within the first year or two after infection, but are rare after adequate penicillin therapy.

Differential Diagnosis

The eruptions of secondary syphilis are almost infinitely varied and mimic many common dermatoses. In this section, examples of common presentations of secondary syphilis are compared to the nonsyphilitic dermatoses that resemble them.

The brown-red hyperpigmentation and fine scale seen in cases of secondary syphilis (*Fig. 2.42*) may closely resemble the characteristically oval, slightly scaly, brown-red eruptions of pityriasis rosea (*Fig. 2.43*). However, generalized adenopathy is notably absent in pityriasis rosea.

The appearance of hyperpigmented oval plaques of secondary syphilis on the upper back (*Fig. 2.44*) resembles a common form of hyperpigmented tinea versicolor. Tinea versicolor is usually found in this location and has adherent KOH-positive scales, which may not be readily visible (*Fig. 2.45*).

The generalized macular and papular eruptions of syphilis (*Fig. 2.46*) may at first glance resemble generalized scabies (*Fig. 2.47*). However, the pruritus in scabies is pronounced, and the lesions are often excoriated. Lack of these signs and symptoms should suggest syphilis in eruptions of this sort.

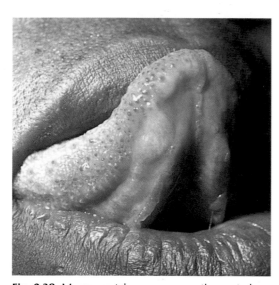

Fig. 2.38 Mucous patches are seen on the ventral tongue.

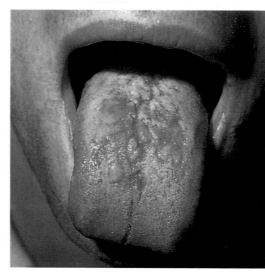

Fig. 2.39 Mucous patches are seen on the dorsum of the tongue.

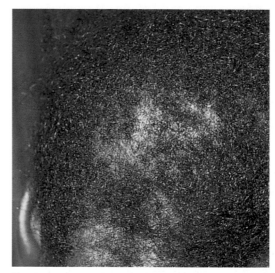

Fig. 2.40 The patchy or 'moth-eaten' alopecia may not be noticed by the patient, but can be found by the alert examiner.

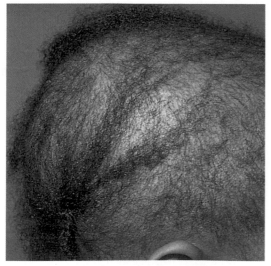

Fig. 2.41 Occasionally a more diffuse alopecia accompanies secondary syphilis.

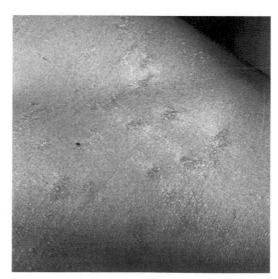

Fig. 2.42 Early papulosquamous form of syphilis.

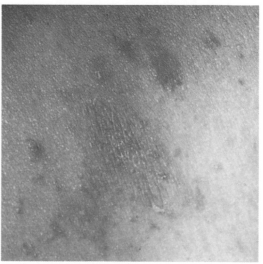

Fig. 2.43 Differential diagnosis in secondary syphilis. Pityriasis rosea (compare with Fig. 2.42).

Occasionally, the scattered papulosquamous eruptions of secondary syphilis (*Fig. 2.48*) resemble the guttate variety of psoriasis (*Fig. 2.49*). However, psoriatic scaling is frequently quite thick and adherent. In addition, involvement of the scalp and extensor surfaces in psoriasis may offer further clues as to the correct diagnosis. Adenopathy and alopecia, common in syphilis, are generally absent in psoriasis. Involvement of the genitals may occur in either disorder (*see Chapter 1*).

Secondary syphilis may be the cause of fairly large erythematous plaques on the penis, which resemble fixed drug eruptions (*Fig. 2.50*). The latter has a predilection for the genitals and hands. The erythematous plaques of early fixed drug eruptions (*Fig. 2.51*), which later become scaly and hyperpigmented, can closely resemble the eruptions of secondary syphilis. Tetracycline, a commonly prescribed antibiotic in the STD clinic, is one of the drugs most frequently implicated as a causative agent of fixed drug eruptions (*see Chapter 1*).

Annular palmar or plantar macules or plaques in some cases of syphilis (*Fig. 2.52*) may resemble the characteristic 'target' or 'iris' lesions of erythema multiforme (*Fig. 2.53*). However, erythema multiforme is usually not scaly and may even become bullous. Bullae do not occur in acquired secondary syphilis.

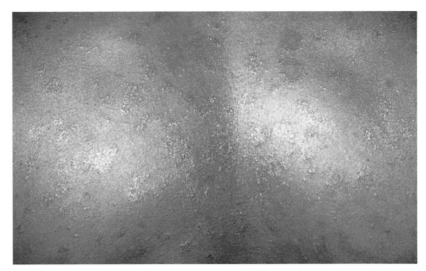

Fig. 2.44 Hyperpigmented oval macules of secondary syphilis.

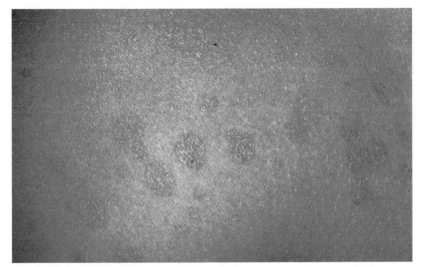

Fig. 2.45 Differential diagnosis in secondary syphilis. Tinea versicolor (compare with Fig. 2.44).

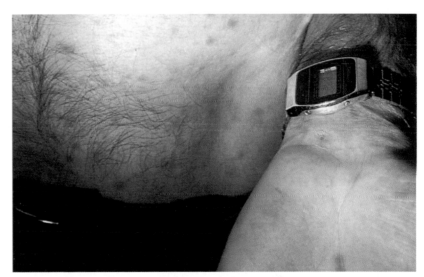

Fig. 2.46 Generalized papular form of secondary syphilis.

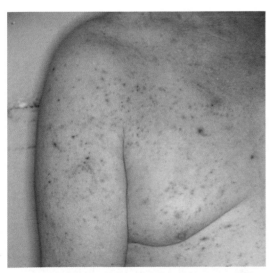

Fig. 2.47 Differential diagnosis in secondary syphilis. Generalized scabies (compare with Fig. 2.46).

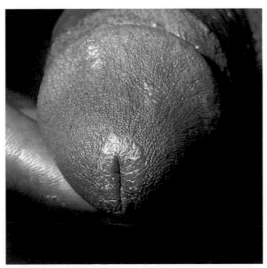

Fig. 2.48 Papulosquamous secondary syphilis of the penis.

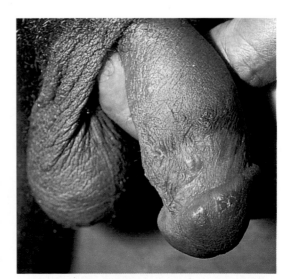

Fig. 2.49 Differential diagnosis in secondary syphilis. Psoriasis involving the genitals (compare with Fig. 2.48).

Plantar or palmar eruptions of syphilis that have developed very little scale (*Fig. 2.54*) may resemble entities such as pityriasis lichenoides chronica (*Fig. 2.55*), a chronic, mildly scaly skin disorder, or even viral exanthems. If serologic testing is not definitive, biopsies may be necessary.

Annular syphilids with central hyperpigmentation on sun-exposed skin (*Fig. 2.56*) resemble discoid lupus erythematosus (*Fig. 2.57*). False-positive syphilis serologies in cases of lupus may confuse the picture. However, rapid plasma reagin titers are generally of high titer in secondary syphilis (1:16 or greater) and low in lupus (1:8 or less).

LATENT SYPHILIS

Latent syphilis is the period of quiescence after completion of the secondary stage of disease, during which there are no clinical manifestations. An exposure history and a reactive serologic test for syphilis is the only way of establishing the diagnosis. Not infrequently, no history of primary or secondary syphilis can be obtained, and, in such a case, a true-positive serology must be distinguished from a false-positive one (*see* laboratory section on interpretation of test results).

Latency is divided into early and late phases according to CDC classification. WHO designates two years after first suspected exposure as the cut-off point for early and late latency.[15] Early latency encompasses the first year after secondary infection. It is during this period that relapses of secondary disease are most apt to occur in the untreated patient. Occasionally, infection of a partner may occur during early latency, and the pregnant woman is at risk of transmitting the disease to her fetus. The patient in late latency (more than 1 year into the latent period) has a decreasing risk of transmission to partner or fetus as latency progresses.

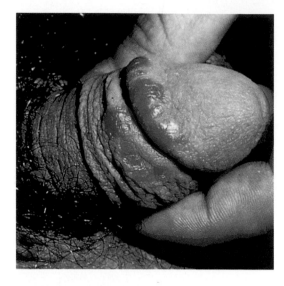

Fig. 2.50 Erythematous penile plaques of secondary syphilis.

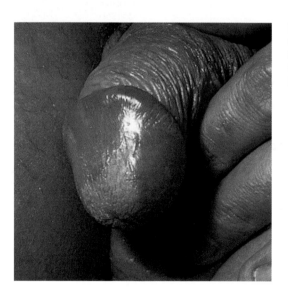

Fig. 2.51 Differential diagnosis in secondary syphilis. Fixed drug eruption (compare with Fig. 2.50).

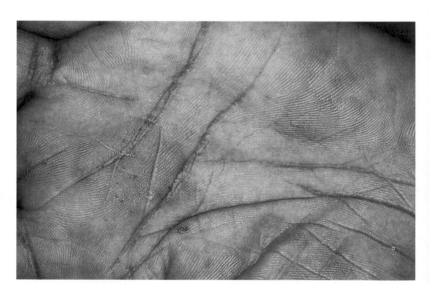

Fig. 2.53 Differential diagnosis in secondary syphilis. Erythema multiforme on the palm of the hand (compare with Fig. 2.52).

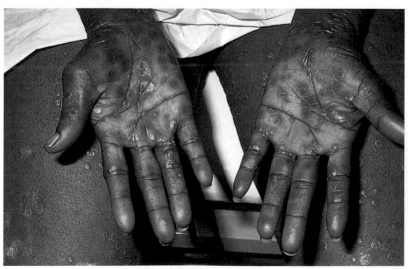

Fig. 2.52 Targetoid annular papulosquamous secondary syphilis of the palms.

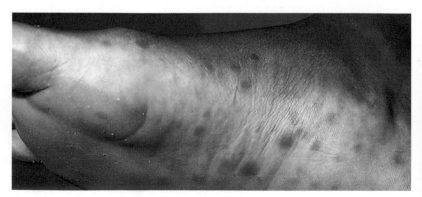

Fig. 2.54 Papular secondary syphilis of the plantar surface of the foot.

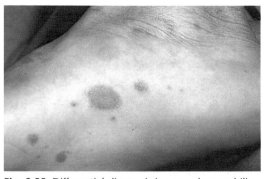

Fig. 2.55 Differential diagnosis in secondary syphilis. Pityriasis lichenoides chronica involving the leg and plantar aspect of the foot (compare with Fig. 2.54).

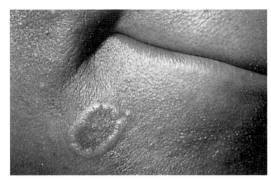

Fig. 2.56 Discoid secondary syphilis of the face.

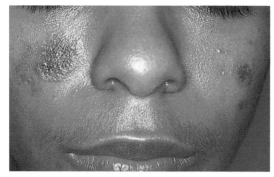

Fig. 2.57 Differential diagnosis in secondary syphilis. Discoid lupus erythematosus (compare with Fig. 2.56).

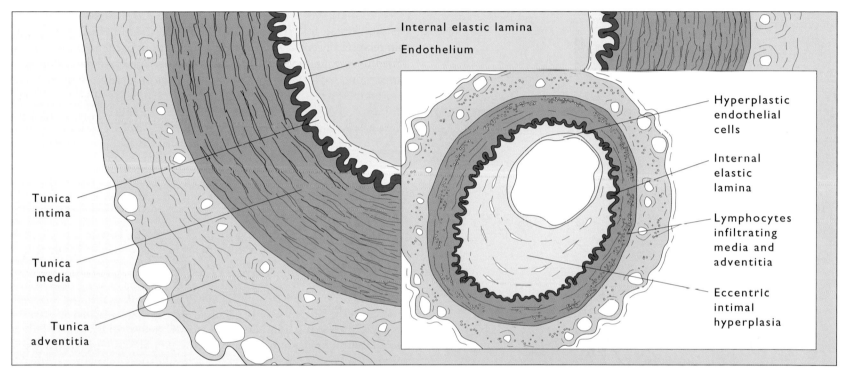

Fig. 2.58 The primary pathologic lesions of neurosyphilis. Schematic diagram showing the endarteritis of cerebral blood vessels, with lymphocytic infiltration and obliteration of the vessel lumen. Courtesy of Karlene Hewan-Lowe, MD (adapted from a drawing).

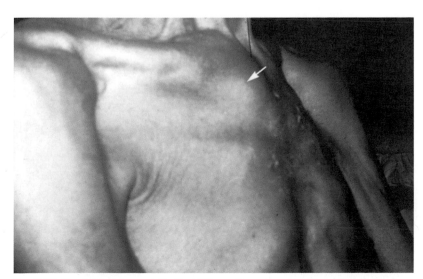

Fig. 2.59 Cardiovascular syphilis. Syphilitic aortic aneurysm with erosion through the chest wall (arrowed). Courtesy of Centers for Disease Control in Atlanta, Georgia.

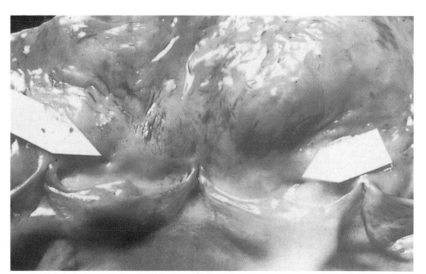

Fig. 2.60 Cardiovascular syphilis. Narrowing of the coronary ostia in syphilitic aortitis. Courtesy of Centers for Disease Control in Atlanta, Georgia.

LATE SYPHILIS

The late manifestations of syphilis fall into three main types: cardio-vascular, gummatous, and meningovascular (neural). In general, these manifestations occur decades after infection, but some of the meningeal and cerebrovascular forms can occur within a year after initial infection.[16] The common underlying pathophysiologic event appears to be an endarteritis and periarteritis of small and medium-sized vessels (*Fig. 2.58*).

Cardiovascular Syphilis

This form of late syphilis is uncommon today, but still needs to be considered in the evaluation of aortic aneurysm and aortic valvular disease (*Fig. 2.59*).[17] Cardiovascular syphilis has been estimated to occur in approximately 10% of cases of untreated syphilis.

The major pathologic changes in cardiovascular syphilis are dilatation of the aortic ring with incompetence of the valve, left ventricular hypertrophy, aortic root dilatation with aneurysm formation, and stenosis of the coronary artery ostia (*Fig. 2.60*).

Benign Gummatous Syphilis

The gummatous lesion probably represents a severe inflammatory response to treponemal antigens, but the exact mechanism of pathogenesis is not known.[18] Microscopically, the active lesions are granulomas. Older lesions show extensive fibrosis and the lesions heal with deep scarring and fibrosis. Treponemes are difficult to detect in gummata.

Virtually any organ system may be affected by this inflammatory process, but the skin and bones are affected most commonly (*Fig. 2.61*). Skin lesions may be nodular, noduloulcerative, or gummatous (*Figs 2.62–2.64*). The nodules appear in groups, and are usually asymmetric in distribution. They are chronic, painless, and slowly progressive, and are found most often on the face, trunk, and extremities. Over time the nodules may break down into ulcers, which heal slowly centrally, leaving a characteristic arciform scar. Gummata of the skin are usually deep in the dermis and are solitary. They evolve into a granulomatous ulcer, with areas of spontaneous healing and scar formation. The most common lesion in bone is an osteitis, usually with periosteal changes. Radiographically, it may be indistinguishable from bacterial osteomyelitis. Characteristic areas of involvement are the hard palate, leading to perforation, and the nasal bones and nasal septum. Any mucous membrane surface may also be affected (*Fig. 2.65*). The digestive system may also be involved, especially the stomach, liver, and esophagus. These lesions are usually misdiagnosed initially as carcinomas.

Neurosyphilis

T. pallidum invades meninges and neural tissue during the secondary stage of the disease.[19,20] Spirochetes may be seen in CSF, and in ocular and middle-ear fluid. There are basically two types of histopathologic lesions found in CNS syphilis:

- A chronic, low-grade meningitis with lymphocytic infiltration of the meninges
- An endarteritis of small vessels of the brain and spinal cord.

Most often, the two lesion types coexist, accounting for the complex constellation of signs and symptoms in the various forms of neurosyphilis. With suitable stains or PCR assays, spirochetes or their nucleic acid may be demonstrated in the neural tissue of patients with neurosyphilis (*Fig. 2.66*). A general classification of neurosyphilis is presented in *Table 2.4*.

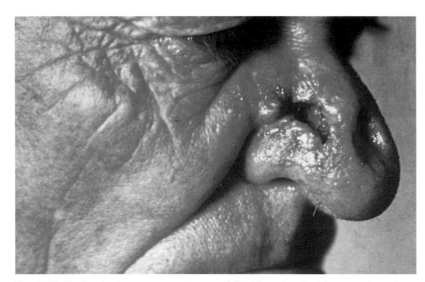

Fig. 2.61 Benign tertiary or gummatous syphilis. Ulcerating facial gummata such as these are now unusual in the USA, though they are still common in other parts of the world.

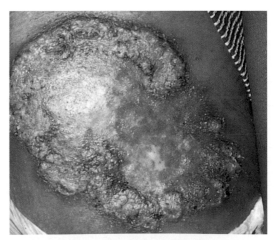

Fig. 2.62 Benign tertiary or gummatous syphilis. The crusted serpinginous border contrasts with the central flatter scarred areas which demonstrate partial spontaneous resolution. Courtesy of Centers for Disease Control in Atlanta, Georgia and Professor Norma Saxe.

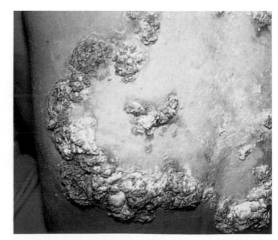

Fig. 2.63 Late nodular syphilis before treatment. Courtesy of Professor Norma Saxe.

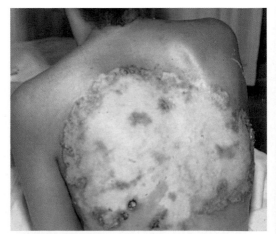

Fig. 2.64 Late nodular syphilis (as seen in Fig. 2.63) after treatment with 10 million units of benzathine penicillin. Courtesy of Professor Norma Saxe.

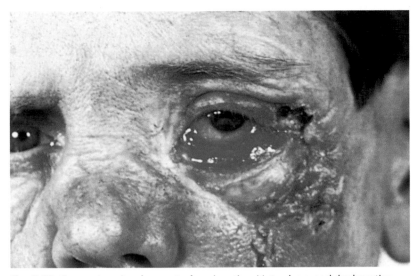

Fig. 2.65 Gummatous involvement of conjunctiva. Note also a noduloulcerative gumma over the right malar surface.

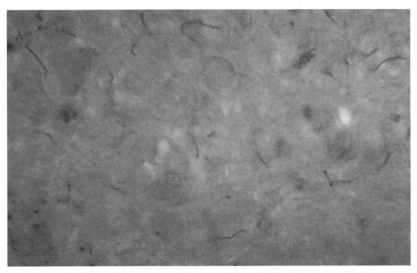

Fig. 2.66 Spirochetes demonstrated in neural tissue (Dieterle's silver stain). Courtesy of Centers for Disease Control in Atlanta, Georgia.

I. MENINGEAL SYPHILIS
  a. Acute syphilitic meningitis
  b. Spinal pachymeningitis

II. MENINGOVASCULAR SYPHILIS
  a. Cerebrovascular syphilis
  b. Meningovascular syphilis of the spinal cord

III. PARENCHYMATOUS NEUROSYPHILIS
  a. General paresis
  b. Tabes dorsalis

IV. CNS GUMMATA

V. ISOLATED NEURAL EVENTS
  a. Optic neuritis/atrophy
  b. Sensorineural hearing loss

VI. CONGENITAL NEUROSYPHILIS

Table 2.4 Neurosyphilitic syndromes.

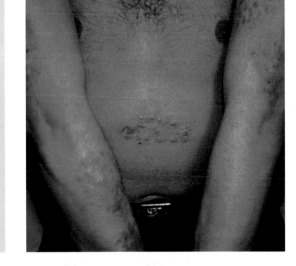

Fig. 2.67 Although an atypically severe rash occurred in this HIV-positive person with secondary syphilis, the serologic results for this individual were typical: VDRL titer of 2048 and a reactive FTA-ABS test result. Courtesy of Jeffrey Gilbert, M.D., Briarcliff Manor, New York.

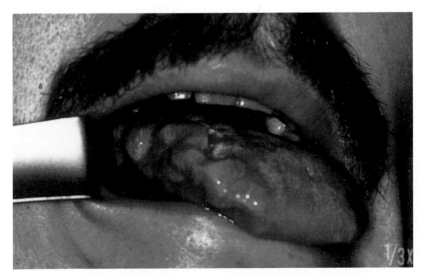

Fig. 2.68 Secondary syphilis resembling hairy leukoplakia. Courtesy of Gregory Mertz, M.D., Department of Medicine, University of New Mexico.

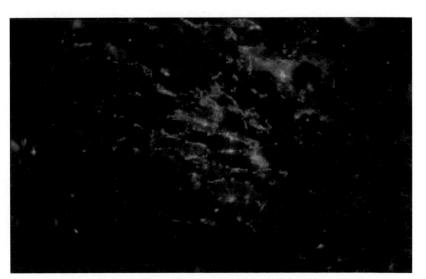

Fig. 2.69 T. pallidum observed in biopsy material of tongue shown in Fig. 2.68, using fluorescein-labeled monoclonal antibody. Courtesy of Gregory Mertz, M.D., Department of Medicine, University of New Mexico.

SYPHILIS AND HUMAN IMMUNODEFICIENCY VIRUS (HIV) COINFECTION

Most HIV-infected persons who also are infected with *T. pallidum* seem to have typical clinical signs and symptoms as well as serologic test results for syphilis. One comparative study[21] found that patients with primary syphilis who had HIV infection were more likely to present with multiple ulcers, and those with secondary syphilis more likely to present with a concomitant genital ulcer than were patients without HIV infection, but that other differences in presentation were small. However, unusual presentations of syphilis in persons with HIV infection have been noted (*Fig. 2.67*). Syphilis, the great imitator, can masquerade in the HIV-seropositive person as hairy leukoplakia (*Figs 2.68* and *2.69*), Kaposi's sarcoma or gastric carcinoma (*Figs 2.70–2.73*). However, most unusual clinical signs and symptoms appear to be associated with a rapid progression to the late stages of syphilis (*Figs 2.74–2.76*), and to neurologic involvement (*Figs 2.77–2.79*) even after treatment of primary or secondary syphilis, though neurologic symptoms may also occur in HIV-seronegative patients with secondary syphilis. Reported aberrant serologic responses in syphilitic patients seem to be related to abnormally low absolute CD4 cell counts and are relatively rare.

The failure of nontreponemal test titers to decline after treatment with standard therapy has been documented for both HIV-seronegative and HIV-seropositive persons treated during latent-stage or late-stage syphilis and in persons treated for reinfection; thus the reported failure of the titer to decline with treatment of the HIV-infected person is probably related to the stage of syphilis rather than to HIV status. A treatment trial for therapy of early syphilis in patients with and without HIV infection[22] demonstrated that patients with HIV infection exhibited a slower serologic response following therapy than patients without HIV infection, but that clinically defined treatment failure was uncommon in both groups.

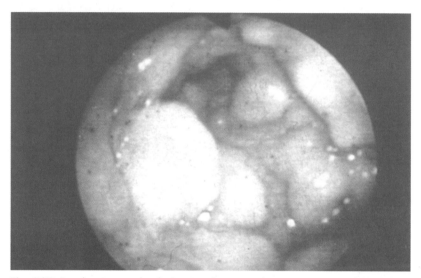

Fig. 2.70 Esophagogastroduodenoscopy demonstrating prominent gastric rugae and multiple polypoid masses with areas of friable mucosa and superficial ulcerations in patient with RPR titer of 512 and a reactive MHA-TP result. Courtesy of John F. Turner, M.D., Dennis B. Weiserbs, M.D., and James B. Francis, M.D., Roanoke Memorial Hospital, Roanoke, Virginia.

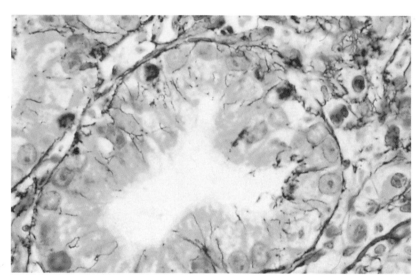

Fig. 2.71 On microscopic examination of gastrointestinal tract biopsy specimen from patient in Fig. 2.70, numerous treponemes were observed (Steiner stain). Courtesy of John F. Turner, M.D., Dennis B. Weiserbs, M.D., and James B. Francis, M.D., Roanoke Memorial Hospital, Roanoke, Virginia.

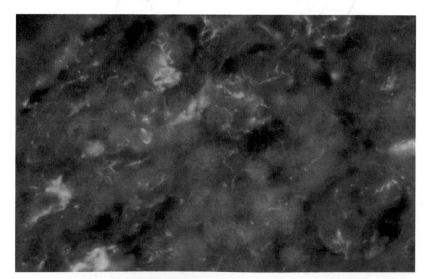

Fig. 2.72 *T. pallidum* observed in gastrointestinal tract biopsy specimen from patient in Fig. 2.70, using fluorescein-labeled monoclonal antibody. Courtesy of John F. Turner, M.D., Dennis B. Weiserbs, M.D., and James B. Francis, M.D., Roanoke Memorial Hospital, Roanoke, Virginia.

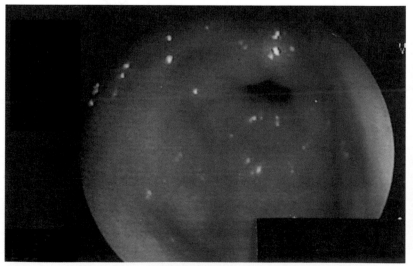

Fig. 2.73 Esophagogastroduodenoscopy of patient in Fig. 2.70 repeated at 3 months following a 10 day course of IV penicillin G, demonstrating normal-appearing gastric mucosa. The patient's RPR titer at 3 months, was 64. Courtesy of John F. Turner, M.D., Dennis B. Weiserbs, M.D., and James B. Francis, M.D., Roanoke Memorial Hospital, Roanoke, Virginia.

TREATMENT

Penicillin remains the mainstay of therapy for all stages of syphilis.[13,23] Although alternative drugs can be used for treatment of men and non-pregnant women, their efficacy is less well documented. The recommendations presented in *Table 2.5* are a synopsis of those provided by the U.S. Public Health Service. Additional treatment recommendations[24,25] are available which differ slightly with respect to duration and alternative treatment choices.

LABORATORY TESTS

COLLECTION OF SPECIMENS

Specimens for dark-field microscopy can be collected from genital lesions or from lymph nodes. In addition, specimens for the direct immunofluorescent antibody test for *T. pallidum* (DFA-TP) can be collected from oral and anal lesions. The ideal specimen for direct examination is serous fluid with minimal red blood cells.[26] To collect serous material from the chancre, any scab or crust should first be gently removed using a scalpel blade, a tongue blade, or a needle. A gauze sponge soaked in 0.9% nonbacteriostatic saline should be used to remove tissue debris and superficial bacteria from the lesion only if necessary. The first few drops of exudate, which may contain blood, are then wiped away. Relatively clear fluid should be collected, either by applying a clean microscope slide or coverslip to the lesion, or by transferring the fluid, using a bacteriologic loop, to the microscope slide. The coverslip is then pressed onto a clean glass slide and examined under dark-field microscopy. The steps for properly collecting

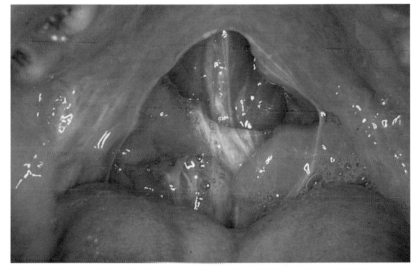

Fig. 2.74 Erosion of hard palate in a patient with a VDRL test titer of 4096. Courtesy of Wesley Wong, Jennifer Flood, M.D., and Joseph Engelman, M.D., San Francisco City Clinic, San Francisco, California.

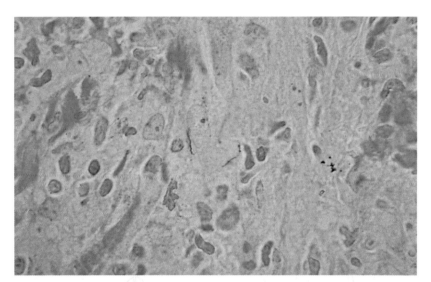

Fig. 2.75 On microscopic examination of erosion in Fig. 2.74, an abscess and intense inflammatory cell infiltrates were observed, as well as abundant ill-defined, confluent granulomas, accompanied by large numbers of plasma cells. The Steiner stain revealed an occasional spirochete. Courtesy of Wesley Wong, Jennifer Flood, M.D., and Joseph Engelman, M.D., San Francisco City Clinic, San Francisco, California.

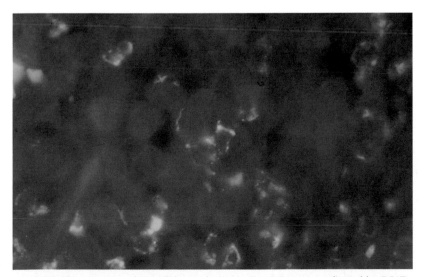

Fig. 2.76 The presence of *T. pallidum* in lesion in Fig. 2.74 was confirmed by DFAT-TP. Five months after treatment with 10 days of IV penicillin, the VDRL titer was 256. Courtesy of Wesley Wong, Jennifer Flood, M.D., and Joseph Engelman, M.D., San Francisco City Clinic, San Francisco, California.

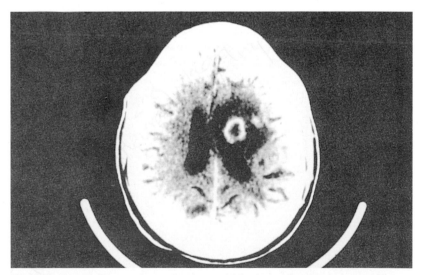

Fig. 2.77 Cranial CT scan demonstrating multiple ring enhancing lesions with a hyperdense nodule in the left centrum semiovale with surrounding edema. Additional lesions were noted in the right parietal area. Patient's serum RPR titer was 8; FTA-ABS results were reactive; CSF showed elevated (11) lymphocytes, increased protein (178 mg/dl), and a titer of 2 in the VDRL CSF test. Courtesy of Harold Horowitz, M.D., New York Medical College, Valhalla, New York, reprinted by permission of the *New England Journal of Medicine* 1884; **331**: 1488–1492.

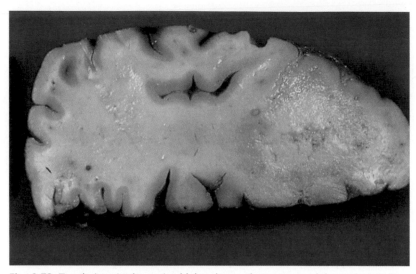

Fig. 2.78 Two lesions in the parietal lobe observed at autopsy of the patient in Fig. 2.77 had rubbery central firm greenish cores surrounded by a darker area. Similar lesions were observed in the white matter, and the presence of treponemes confirmed by PCR. Courtesy of Harold Horowitz, M.D., New York Medical College, Valhalla, New York, reprinted by permission of the *New England Journal of Medicine* 1884; **331**: 1488–1492.

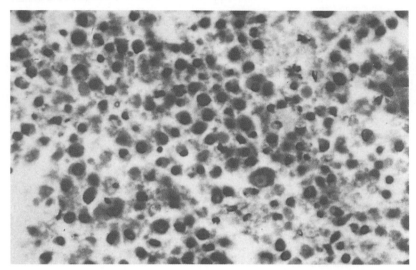

Fig. 2.79 Areas of coagulative necrosis with a marked chronic inflammatory exudate of lymphocytes and plasma cells were observed by microscopic examination (hematoxylin and eosin) of the lesions in Fig. 2.78. Courtesy of Harold Horowitz, M.D., New York Medical College, Valhalla, New York, reprinted by permission of the *New England Journal of Medicine* 1984; **331**: 1488–1492.

A. EARLY SYPHILIS

(primary, secondary, latent <1 year's duration)
1. Benzathine penicillin G: 2.4 million U, IM in a single dose
2. For the penicillin-allergic patient: (a) doxycycline: 100 mg po bid for 14 days, or (b) tetracycline HCl: 500 mg po qid for 14 days.

B. SYPHILIS OF MORE THAN ONE YEAR'S DURATION

(latent syphilis of indeterminate or >1 year's duration, cardiovascular, or late benign syphilis, NOT neurosyphilis
1. Benzathine penicillin G: 2.4 million U, IM once a week for 3 successive weeks (7.2 million U total).
2. Penicillin-allergic patients: Same as early syphilis (A), except the duration of therapy is 28 days.

C. CSF EXAMINATION

Cerebrospinal fluid examination should be done for patients with syphilis who have neurologic or ophthalmic signs of neurosyphilis, evidence of active tertiary syphilis (e.g., arotitis, gumma, or iritis), or evidence of treatment failure, and for patients with latent syphilis or syphilis of unknown duration if they have HIV infection (see F). Other patients with latent syphilis or syphilis of unknown duration may also be considered for this examination, particularly if the nontreponemal titer is elevated (e.g., ≥1:32). Patients who are treated without a CSF examination should be followed closely.

D. NEUROSYPHILIS

1. Aqueous crystalline penicillin G: 18–24 million U a day, administered as 3–4 million U IV every 4 hours or continuous infusion for 10–14 days.
2. Procaine penicillin G: 2.4 million U IM daily plus probenicid 500 mg qid, both for 10–14 days.
3. Benzathine penicillin G 2.4 million U IM weekly for 3 consecutive weeks may be administered following completion of either of the above regimens.
4. Penicillin regimens should be used to treat all cases of neurosyphilis; penicillin-allergic patients may be desensitized before therapy.

E. SYPHILIS DURING PREGNANCY

1. For the nonpenicillin-allergic woman, penicillin prescribed in the doses recommended for nonpregnant patients appropriate for the stage of syphilis should be administered.
2. There are no proven alternatives to penicillin. Pregnant women with a history of penicillin allergy should be treated with penicillin after desensitization, if necessary.
3. Patients should have quantitative nontreponemal serologic tests in the third trimester and at delivery; those at risk for reinfection or who live in areas with high syphilis incidence should be tested monthly for the remainder of pregnancy. Women with a fourfold rise in titer should be treated.

F. SYPHILIS IN HIV-INFECTED PATIENTS

1. When clinical findings suggest that syphilis is present, but serologic tests are nonreactive or confusing, it may be helpful to perform direct fluorescent antibody staining of lesion or biopsy material.
2. Neurosyphilis should be considered in the differential diagnosis of neurologic disease among HIV-infected persons.
3. a) Early syphilis. Treatment as for individuals without HIV infection is recommended. However, some experts recommend additional treatments such as multiple doses of benzathine penicillin G as suggested for late syphilis, or other supplemental antibiotics in addition to benzathine penicillin G 2.4 million units IM.
   b) Latent syphilis. Patients who have late latent syphilis or syphilis of unknown duration and HIV infection should undergo CSF examination before treatment. A patient with latent syphilis, HIV infection, and a normal CSF examination can be treated with benzathine penicillin G 7.2 million U (as 3 weekly doses of 2.4 million U each).
   c) Penicillin regimens should be used to treat all stages of syphilis in HIV-infected patients; penicillin-allergic patients may be desensitized before therapy.

Table 2.5 Treatment schedules for syphilis.

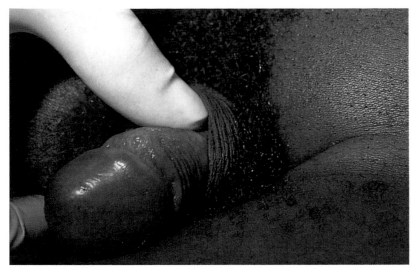

Fig. 2.80 Collection of specimen for dark-field microscopy or DFA-TP test. Penile ulcer after cleaning with gauze.

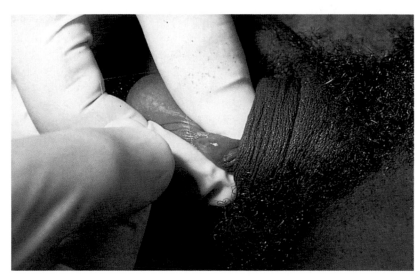

Fig. 2.81 Collection of specimen for dark-field microscopy or DFA-TP test. Squeezing the ulcer to obtain exudate. Coverslip is ready to be pressed onto the ulcer.

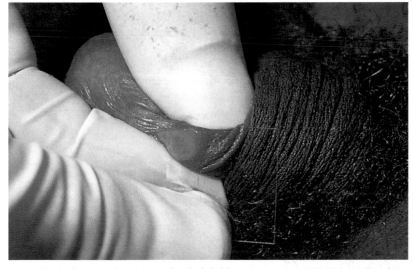

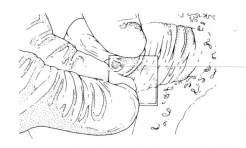

Corner of coverslip touching ulcer

Fig. 2.82 Collection of specimen for dark-field microscopy or DFA-TP test. Touching coverslip to ulcer to obtain fluid for dark-field examination.

this material are demonstrated in *Figs 2.80–2.82*. Specimens collected for dark-field microscopy can also be examined by DFA-TP simply by removing the cover slip and letting the slide air dry, or specimens can be collected in capillary tubes. Material collected from the lesion's depths is more likely to contain motile treponemes than surface material. Healing skin lesions merit examination as well. They should be abraded with a sharp instrument, or fluid may be collected from the lesion by injecting a drop of sterile saline into the base of the lesion and aspirating with a small-gauge needle and syringe.

Collection of lesion material from the cervix or vaginal vault for direct examination follows the same principles, but must always be by direct visualization using a speculum. Aspiration of lymph nodes is performed by injecting 0.2 ml or less of sterile saline into the node through sterilized skin, followed by aspiration of the tissue material. The dark-field examination must be performed immediately after specimen collection; however the specimen for DFA-TP can be held until staining can be conveniently performed. For all serologic tests for syphilis, blood is collected into dry tubes without anticoagulant, allowed to clot, and the serum separated by centrifugation (*Fig. 2.83*). If the test is not to be performed immediately, sera should be removed from the clots and either stored at refrigerator temperature (4°C) or frozen.

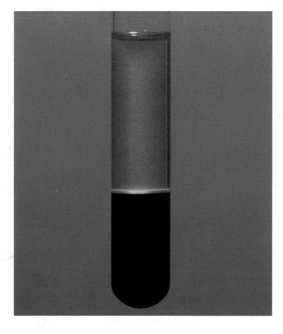

Fig. 2.83 Centrifuged blood clot ready for removal of serum after centrifugation. Serum is collected by venipuncture into a 'red top' vacutainer tube without anticoagulant, centrifuged, and if necessary, separated from clot for storage. Courtesy of Centers for Disease Control in Atlanta, Georgia.

DIRECT DIAGNOSIS

The most specific method for the diagnosis of the early stages of syphilis is direct microscopy of material taken from the lesion or lymph node aspirates. These tests are usually the first to become positive. The demonstration of treponemes with characteristic morphology and motility, or staining with a fluorescent-labeled conjugate specific for *T. pallidum* is diagnostic of primary, secondary, and congenital syphilis, and of relapses during early latent syphilis, provided yaws, bejel, and pinta have been excluded.

Direct microscopy is useful in establishing a diagnosis in cases of reinfection as well. In addition, direct microscopy is often used to rule out syphilis as the cause of lesions associated with other sexually transmitted diseases. When specimens have been properly collected and the patient has not been treated locally or systemically with antimicrobials, direct methods are reasonable.

Dark-field Microscopy

In dark-field microscopy, light rays strike organisms or particles at such an oblique angle that no direct light enters the microscope, except that reflected from the organisms or particles. Thus, anything in the light path appears luminous against a dark background (*Fig. 2.84*). The nonpathogens *T. refringens* and *T. denticola* are usually found in the gastrointestinal tract and are easily confused with *T. pallidum* on dark-field examination.

Direct Fluorescent Antibody Test for T. pallidum

The DFA-TP is an immunofluorescent antibody test in which an anti-*T. pallidum* monoclonal or absorbed polyclonal antibody is labeled with the fluorochrome dye, fluorescein isothiocyanate (FITC) to identify the organism. Motility of the organism is not required in the DFA-TP. As the conjugates used are specific for pathogenic treponemal strains, the DFA-TP is applicable to samples collected from both oral and rectal lesions. Samples collected as for dark-field examination are air-dried, fixed in methanol or acetone, and then stained with the FITC conjugate (*Fig. 2.85*). The use of the DFA-TP test has been extended to include the staining of tissue sections (DFAT-TP) (*Fig. 2.86*). Any tissue can be used (*Figs 2.69–2.76*), but tissue for paraffin-embedded sections are collected most often from the brain, gastrointestinal tract, placenta, umbilical cord, or skin. Often DFAT-TP is used to diagnose late-stage adult syphilis or congenital syphilis, or to distinguish skin lesions of secondary or late syphilis from those of Lyme disease.

Polymerase chain reaction

At the present time, the rabbit infectivity test (RIT) is the gold standard for the direct detection of *T. pallidum* in clinical specimens. This method has a test sensitivity of nearly a single organism when repeated passages in rabbits are used. However, this test is time-consuming (requiring approximately 1 to 2 months to complete), and requires access to an animal facility. As a routine laboratory test, PCR has the potential to replace the RIT for the direct detection of *T. pallidum*.

Several PCR assays have been reported. Each test uses a different target gene, eg, *tpf*-1, *bmp*, *tmp*A, *tmp*B, the 47 kDa protein gene, *polA*, and the 16 S rRNA gene. The analytical sensitivity of these assays varies from 10^{-3} organism equivalents in the reverse transcriptase PCR (RT-PCR), to 10 organisms when the gene encoding the 47-kDa protein is the target.[27] Although RT-PCR is extremely sensitive, the isolation of RNA can be time consuming because great care is required to prevent contamination of the specimen by unrelated organisms and ribonucleases. A multiplex PCR assay has been developed for the simultaneous detection of *T. pallidum*, *Haemophilus ducreyi*, and herpes simplex virus. The *T. pallidum* target in the multiplex PCR is the 47-kDa gene and a capture ELISA is used to detect the amplicons.

A recently developed PCR assay using fluorescent labeled primers for *polA* and an ABI 310 genetic analyzer to detect the amplicons[27] has improved the analytic sensitivity of the assay to approximately one organism per PCR reaction and has improved its specificity permitting visualization of the amplicon and exclusion of bands caused by nonspecific amplification. Thus, this method can be applied to the diagnosis of neurosyphilis and congenital syphilis where the number of organisms is likely to be low.

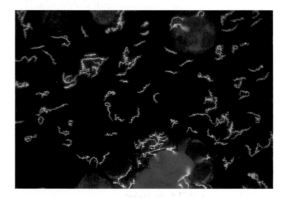

Fig. 2.85 DFA-TP positive smear of ulcer materials.

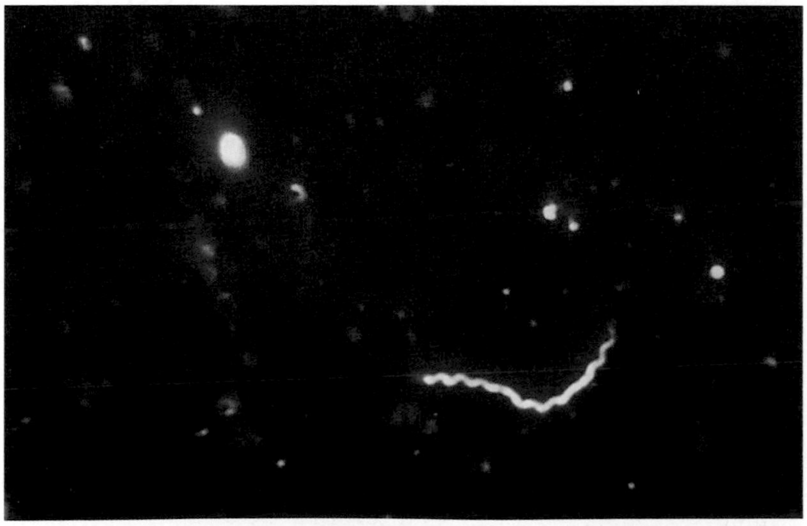

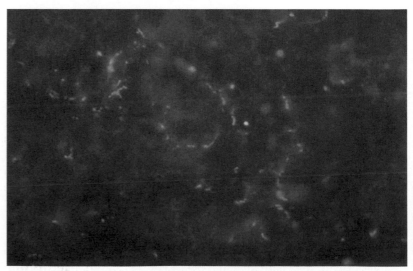

Fig. 2.84 Positive dark-field examination. Treponemes are recognized by their characteristic corkscrew shape and deliberate forward and backward movement with rotation about the longitudinal axis. Courtesy of Ralph Ramsey.

Fig. 2.86 DFA-TP positive tissue section. The DFA-TP has the following advantages over the dark-field examination: motile organisms are not required; pathogenic treponemes can be differentiated from nonpathogenic treponemes in oral lesions; and tissue sections for biopsy can be examined as well as autopsy material. Courtesy of Centers for Disease Control in Atlanta, Georgia.

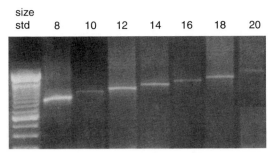

Fig. 2.87 Representative *arp* amplicon sizes (from 8 to 20 repeats). Courtesy of Allan Pillay Ph.D., Centers for Disease Control and Prevention, Atlanta, Georgia.

Representative tpr types

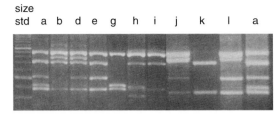

Fig. 2.88 Representative *Mse* I RFLP patterns of *tpr* amplicons (*a* to *l*) Courtesy of Allan Pillay Ph.D., Centers for Disease Control and Prevention, Atlanta, Georgia.

PCR assays have been used successfully with ulcer, CSF or biopsy specimens. Blood has been a problematic specimen due to the presence of PCR inhibitors. Recently, however, a real-time, semi-quantitative PCR assay has been used to show that the number of spirochetes in the blood of patients with syphilis varies with the stage of syphilis and ranges from 200 to 100,000 organisms per ml of blood.[28]

Molecular Subtyping

Recently a molecular method was developed to subtype *T. pallidum* in clinical specimens based upon heterogeneity in a treponemal gene (*arp*) and within a gene family (*tpr*).[29] The *arp* gene encodes for a protein that possesses a region consisting of repeated sequences of 20 amino acids. The number of these repeats varies among strains and can be determined by the size of the amplicon after PCR amplification (*Fig. 2.87*). The second gene target consists of three genes (*tprE, tprG, tprI*) belonging to the *tpr* gene family. These genes are amplified by PCR, the amplicon digested with a restriction endonuclease (*MseI*), and the pattern of the fragments (restriction fragment length polymorphism [RFLP] pattern) determined by agarose gel electrophoresis. The subtype of *T. pallidum* is based on the number of repeats in the *arp* gene, which varies between 4 and 24, and the RFLP pattern of the tpr amplicon (*Fig. 2.88*). For example, the subtype of the Nichols strain of *T. pallidum* is 14*a* (*Table 2.6*).

Based on an analysis of almost 250 strains, 18 *arp* subtypes (alleles), ranging from 4 to 24 repeats (*Fig. 2.89A*) and 12 *tpr* RFLP patterns (*Fig. 2.89B*) designated *a* to *m*, have been identified. Strains with 14 repeats comprise more than 60% of the strains examined to date; however, they can be further subdivided by their tpr RFLP pattern.

Molecular subtyping will be useful in the identification of transmission chains and in determining whether clinical manifestations (e.g., neurosyphilis) are associated with specific subtypes of *T. pallidum*.

INDIRECT DIAGNOSIS USING NONTREPONEMAL SEROLOGIC TESTS

The serologic tests for syphilis are divided into screening tests and confirmation tests, based on the specific antigen used. Nontreponemal (reagin) tests may be used either as qualitative or quantitative tests. Qualitative nontreponemal tests are frequently used as screening tests to measure IgM and IgG antibodies to lipoidal material released from damaged host cells, as well as to lipoprotein-like material released from the treponemes. The antilipoidal antibodies are antibodies that are produced not only as a consequence of syphilis and other treponemal diseases, but also in response to nontreponemal diseases of an acute or chronic nature in which tissue damage occurs.

In primary syphilis, reactivity in these tests does not develop until 1–4 weeks after the chancre first appears. For this reason, patients with suspected lesions and nonreactive nontreponemal tests should have repeat tests performed at 1-week, 1-month, and 3-month intervals from the time of initial testing. Nonreactive tests during the 3-month period exclude the diagnosis of syphilis.

Subtypes	African strains	American strains	Total isolates	Notable strains
4f	0	1	1	
4i	0	1	1	
5f	0	1	1	
6i	1	0	1	
7d	3	0	3	
7k	1	0	1	
8d	1	0	1	
10b	3	0	3	
10d	2	0	2	
11b	1	0	1	
11d	0	1	1	
12a	0	3	3	Bal-9; US-D8531
12d	4	0	4	
12f	0	3	3	
12g	0	1	1	
12h	2	0	2	
13b	2	0	2	
13d	3	1	4	
13k	3	0	3	
14a	15	7	22	Nichols; Ba-73-1; Chicago
14b	15	0	15	
14c	1	0	1	
14d	66	4	70	
14e	4	1	5	
14f	0	28	28	Street 14; Sea81-8
14g	2	0	2	
14i	8	1	9	
14j	1	0	1	
14l	8	0	8	
15a	2	6	8	
15d	10	3	13	
16b	1	0	1	
16d	12	3	15	Mexico A; US-D8502
16e	7	0	7	
16f	0	1	1	US-8520
18a	1	0	1	
20b	5	0	5	
20d	4	0	4	
21b	2	0	2	
24b	4	0	4	
Total isolates	194	66	260	

Table 2.6 Distribution of molecular subtypes of *T. pallidum* strains.

The nontreponemal tests are reactive in secondary syphilis almost without exception, and usually in titers of 16 or greater regardless of the test method used. Less than 2% of sera will exhibit a prozone (*Fig. 2.90*). Nontreponemal test titers in early latent syphilis are similar to those of secondary syphilis. However, as the duration of the latent stage increases the titer decreases.

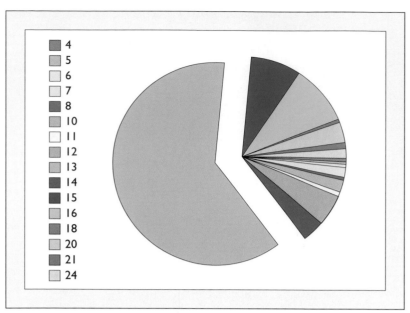

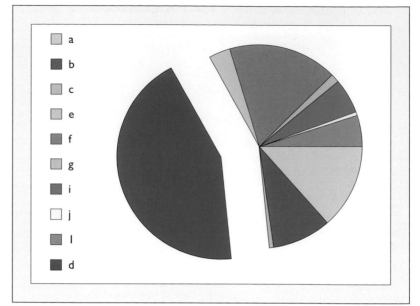

Fig. 2.89 A. Distribution of number of repeats in *arp* amplicons. Strains with 14 repeats are the predominant type and represent >60% of isolates. B. Distribution of *tpr* RFLP patterns among strains with 14 repeats. Subtype 14d accounts for 44% of the strains with 14 repeats.

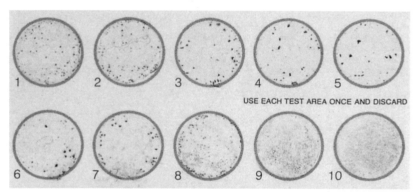

Fig. 2.90 The prozone phenomenon. Some high-titered sera, such as this one at 1:256, when tested undiluted may appear to give rough nonreactive or minimally reactive (circle 1) results. However, upon dilution, the flocculation intensifies (circle 5) and then progressively decreases to become nonreactive (circle 10). The prozone phenomenon may be due not only to an antibody excess, but also to blocking or incomplete antigen–antibody complex formation.

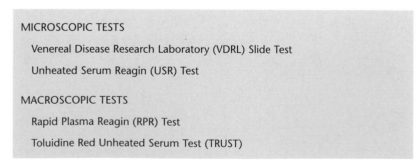

MICROSCOPIC TESTS

Venereal Disease Research Laboratory (VDRL) Slide Test

Unheated Serum Reagin (USR) Test

MACROSCOPIC TESTS

Rapid Plasma Reagin (RPR) Test

Toluidine Red Unheated Serum Test (TRUST)

Table 2.7 Standard nontreponemal tests.

The nontreponemal cerebrospinal fluid veneral disease research laboratory (CSF VDRL) test (*Table 2.7*) is the only serologic test recognized as a standard test for the diagnosis of neurosyphilis. However, asymptomatic neurosyphilis should not be diagnosed by a reactive CSF VDRL alone. CSF criteria for the diagnosis of neurosyphilis are:

- Reactive CSF VDRL
- Reactive serum treponemal test

- Five or more lymphocytes/mm³ CSF
- CSF total protein of ≥ 45 mg/dl.

Symptomatic neurosyphilis is diagnosed by clinical symptoms and signs, supplemented with positive results in the above diagnostic procedures.

Serial quantitative nontreponemal tests can be used to measure the adequacy of therapy. Titers should be obtained at 3-monthly intervals for at least 1 year. A fourfold drop in titer is frequently noted by 3 months, in adequately treated early syphilis.

In congenital syphilis, the role of nontreponemal tests is to monitor the antibody titer. Titers will decrease following treatment; however, a rising titer in monthly tests from an infant over a 6-month period is diagnostic for congenital syphilis. If an infant has not been infected *in utero*, passively transferred nontreponemal antibodies should no longer be detected by 3 months postpartum. All nontreponemal tests will occasionally give false-positive results. In general populations, this occurs in 1–2% of tests. Acute false-positive reactions lasting less than 6 months usually occur after febrile diseases or immunizations, or during pregnancy. However, false-positive rates may exceed 10% in populations with a high prevalence of intravenous drug use. The titers of false-positive reactions are usually less than 8. Since titers are also low in very early and during latency, not all low titers are false positives. In addition, not all high titers are true positives. In intravenous drug users, approximately 12% of false-positive titers are 8 or greater. Chronic false-positive reactions are more often associated with autoimmune disorders, such as rheumatoid arthritis and systemic lupus erythematosus, or with chronic infections such as leprosy. Titers in chronic false-positive reactions also are usually low, with titers less than 8.

Specific Nontreponemal Serologic Tests
The standard nontreponemal tests for syphilis are listed in *Table 2.7*. All four tests use the VDRL antigen (cardiolipin, cholesterol, and lecithin) as the principal component. The VDRL slide test is the only test using an antigen that has not been stabilized by the addition of EDTA, and which does not contain choline chloride to eliminate the need for heat-inactivation of the serum. The rapid plasma reagin (RPR) test is the most widely used test. The CSF VDRL slide test is the only recognized procedure for the serodiagnosis of neurosyphilis. All four tests use similar equipment (*Fig. 2.91*).

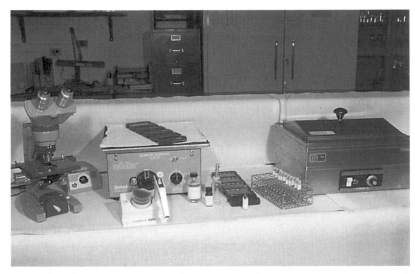

Fig. 2.91 This is an example of equipment required to perform the nontreponemal tests for syphilis. Shown here are a mechanical rotator, a water bath, a microscope, a safety pipetter, and reagents. Courtesy of Centers for Disease Control in Atlanta, Georgia.

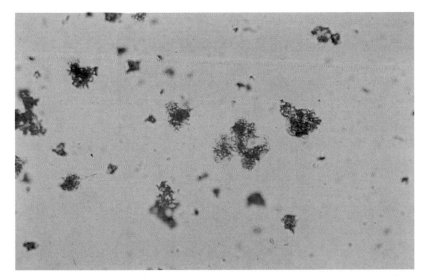

Fig. 2.92 Reactive VDRL or USR result. Specimens exhibiting medium and/or large flocculation particles are reported as reactive (R). Those with small particles are reported as weakly reactive (W), while those with complete dispersion of antigen particles or slight roughness are reported as nonreactive (NR). Sera exhibiting slight roughness should be quantitated to check for the prozone phenomenon. Courtesy of Centers for Disease Control in Atlanta, Georgia.

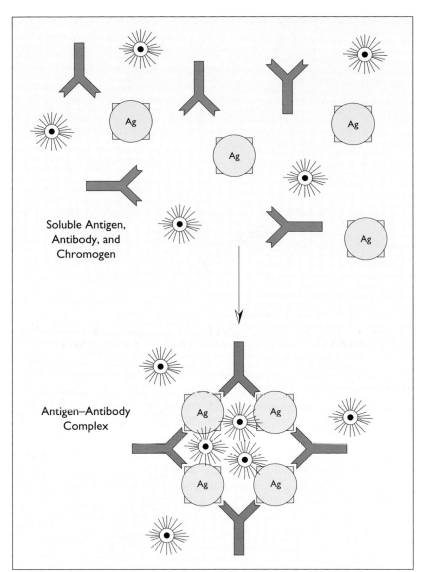

Soluble Antigen, Antibody, and Chromogen

Antigen–Antibody Complex

Fig. 2.93 In the macroscopic nontreponemal tests, sized colored particles become entrapped in the antigen–antibody formation. Results for these card tests are reported as reactive or non-reactive; there is no weakly reactive report.

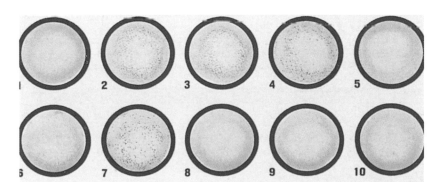

Fig. 2.94 Qualitative RPR card test. Specimens exhibiting medium to large flocculation are reported as reactive (circles 4 and 7). Specimens with definite but small flocculation are read as reactive minimal (Rm) (circle 2 and 3). Specimens with an even dispersion of antigen particles (circles 1, 5, 8, and 10) or specimens that are slightly rough (circle 6) are reported as non-reactive. Courtesy of Centers for Disease Control in Atlanta, Georgia.

VDRL SLIDE TEST   Because of the nature of the VDRL antigen, when the antigen is reacted with antibody, the antigen–antibody complex remains suspended rather than precipitating or agglutinating as in most serologic tests (*Fig. 2.92*). The resulting antigen–antibody complex in the VDRL antigen-based tests results in flocculation, and because the complex particles are usually small, they must be viewed with a microscope.

UNHEATED SERUM REAGIN (USR) TEST is a microscopic test like the VDRL. The principle of the USR is identical to that of the VDRL, although the antigen for the USR has been stabilized. The USR has two advantages over the VDRL: firstly, the antigen is ready for use once it reaches room temperature; and secondly, the sera do not require heating before testing. In all other aspects, the test is performed and read like the VDRL slide test (*see Fig. 2.92*).

RPR CARD TEST AND TRUST   The principle of the TRUST and RPR card tests is the same as that of the VDRL slide test. However, in these two tests, particles of specific sizes (charcoal for the RPR and red paint pigment for the TRUST) are added to the USR antigen to enhance visualization of the antigen–antibody complex (*Fig. 2.93*). The particles become entrapped within the antigen–antibody lattice during a positive reaction, yielding flocculation that is visible to the naked eye (*Figs 2.94* and *2.95*). No microscope is needed, which makes these macroscopic tests more convenient than the VDRL or USR, accounting for their present popularity. The TRUST antigen does not require refrigerated storage conditions.

VDRL-EIA   A new format for a nontreponemal test is the enzyme immunoassay (EIA). In the 'Visuwell' Reagin Test, the wells of the microtiter plate are coated with VDRL antigen. Anticardiolipin antibodies in the patient's serum bind to the antigen in the wells and the bound antibodies are detected following the addition of urease-labeled antihuman IgG and substrate.

INDIRECT DIAGNOSIS USING TREPONEMAL SEROLOGIC TESTS

In contrast to the nontreponemal tests, the treponemal tests should be reserved for confirmatory testing when the clinical signs and/or history disagree with the reactive nontreponemal test results. Treponemal tests are based on the detection of antibodies formed specifically to the antigenic determinants of the treponemes. They are qualitative procedures, which therefore cannot be used to monitor the efficacy of treatment. Like the nontreponemal tests, treponemal tests are almost always reactive in secondary and latent syphilis. For most cases, once the treponemal tests are reactive, they remain so for the patient's lifetime. In fact, in some patients with late syphilis, a reactive treponemal test may be the only means of confirming the suspected diagnosis. Currently, none of the treponemal tests are recommended for use with CSF.

The greatest value of the treponemal tests is to differentiate true-positive nontreponemal test results from false-positive results. However, false-positive treponemal test results do occur with about the same frequency (1%) as false-positive nontreponemal test results. Although some false-positive results in the treponemal tests are transient and of unknown cause, they have been associated with connective tissue diseases. When unexplained reactive tests occur in elderly patients, attempts should be made to rule out acquired or congenital syphilis, or infections with other treponemes, before a diagnosis of false-positive serology is made.

Characteristics of Individual Treponemal Serologic Tests
Standard treponemal tests for syphilis are listed in *Table 2.8*.

FTA-ABS AND FTA-ABS DS   Both of these indirect immunofluorescence tests are based on the same principle (*Fig. 2.96*). The two tests differ in that the double-stain test employs a FITC-labeled conjugate as a direct stain for *T. pallidum* and a tetramethyl rhodamine isothiocyanate (TMRITC)-labeled antihuman IgG conjugate to detect the antibody in the patient's serum. This eliminates the need for first having to use dark-field microscopy on the smear to find treponemes (*Figs 2.97* and *2.98*). Both tests are reported as shown in *Table 2.9*.

TPHA AND TP-PA   Passive hemagglutination of erythrocytes sensitized with antigen is an extremely simple method for the detection of antibody (*Fig. 2.98*). The antigen used in the procedure is formalized, tanned avian erythrocytes sensitized with ultrasonicated material from *T. pallidum* (Nichols strain). Unsensitized cells are used as a control for nonspecific reactivity. This test is still used in many laboratories worldwide. The microhemagglutination assay for antibodies to *T. pallidum* (MHA-TP) is no longer available and has been replaced with the

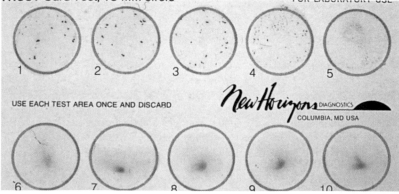

Fig. 2.95 Quantitative TRUST. The reading of the TRUST is identical to that of the RPR card test.

Fluorescent treponemal antibody absorption (FTA-ABS) Test
FTA-ABS double-staining (DS) test (FTA-ABS DS)
T. pallidum hemagglutination assay (TPHA)
T. pallidum particle agglutination (TP-PA)

Table 2.8 Standard treponemal tests.

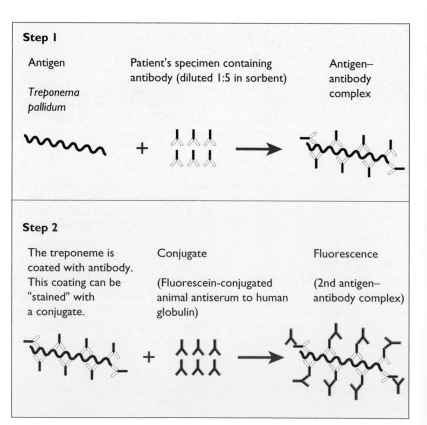

Step 1

Antigen	Patient's specimen containing antibody (diluted 1:5 in sorbent)	Antigen–antibody complex
Treponema pallidum		

Step 2

The treponeme is coated with antibody. This coating can be "stained" with a conjugate.	Conjugate (Fluorescein-conjugated animal antiserum to human globulin)	Fluorescence (2nd antigen–antibody complex)

Fig. 2.96 Theory of FTA test – reactive reaction. To perform the FTA-ABS tests, the patient's serum, which has been diluted with sorbent, is layered on a microscope slide to which *T. pallidum* has been fixed. If the patient's serum contains antibody, it will coat the treponeme. Next fluorochrome-labeled antihuman IgG conjugate is used to detect the initial antigen–antibody reaction.

T. pallidum particle agglutination (TP-PA) test, which uses the same antigen mix attached to red gelatin beads instead of to erythrocytes. The sensitivity and specificity of the latter test is essentially the same as the MHA-TP. Hemagglutination results are read and reported as in *Figs 2.100* and *2.101*.

TREPONEMAL EIA   Several commercial EIA tests have been designed to replace the FTA-ABS tests and MHA-TP as confirmatory tests for syphilis. These tests are relatively similar in that a treponemal antigen, either cloned or sonicated, coats the plate. The patient's serum is added and the mixture is then incubated and washed. An enzyme-labeled antihuman immunoglobulin conjugate and an enzyme substrate are then added to detect the initial antigen–antibody reaction. Initial evaluations of several of these EIA tests have found that they all have sensitivities and specificities similar to those of other treponemal tests, but more extensive evaluation is necessary.

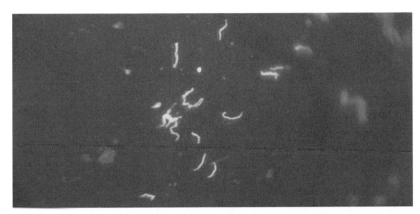

Fig. 2.97 Example of the FTA-ABS DS. In reading the FTA-ABS DS, the treponemes are easily located, since the antigen is counterstained with the direct-staining FITC-labeled antitreponemal globulin component. If the patient's serum does not contain anti-*T. pallidum* antibodies, when the slide is read using the rhodamine filter set, no treponemes will be observed. Courtesy of Centers for Disease Control in Atlanta, Georgia.

	Interpretation of fluorescence	
Initial test	Repeat test	Report
2+ to 4+		Reactive
1+	>1+	Reactive
1+	=1+	Reactive minimal*
<1+		Nonreactive
–		Nonreactive

*In the absence of historical or clinical evidence of treponemal infection, the test result should be considered equivocal. A second specimen should be submitted for serologic testing.

Table 2.9 Interpretation and reporting of FTA-ABS and FTA-ABS DS tests.

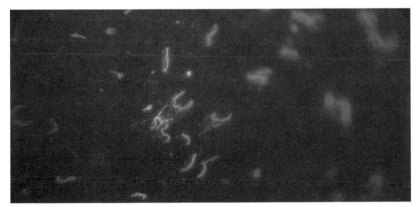

Fig. 2.98 Reactive FTA-ABS DS test. If the patient's serum contains antibodies to *T. pallidum*, the treponemes will appear reddish-orange when the rhodamine filters are used, due to the TMRITC-labeled antihuman IgG globulin used as the indicator stain or indirect component of the system. Courtesy of Centers for Disease Control in Atlanta, Georgia.

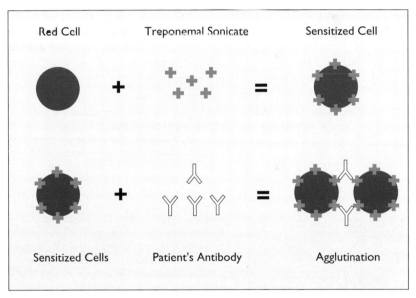

Fig. 2.99 To perform the TPHA, the patient's serum is first mixed with absorbing diluent made from nonpathogenic Reiter treponemes and other absorbents and stabilizers. The serum is then placed in a microtiter plate and sensitized sheep red cells are added. Serum that contains antibodies reacts with these cells to form a smooth mat of agglutinated cells in the microtiter plate.

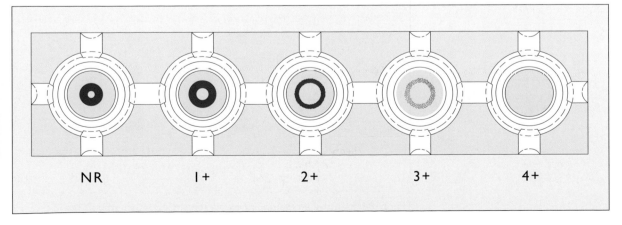

Fig. 2.100 Hemagglutination test results. Results for the TPHA are reported as reactive (1+, 2+, 3+, 4+) or nonreactive (±, –). Completely negative readings vary in pattern from a solid compact button of cells to a circle of cells with a small central hole, as seen in this drawing.

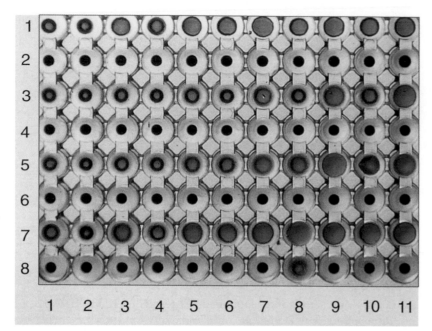

Fig. 2.101 Example of a microhemagglutination test result. (Rows are horizontal and wells are vertical.) Agglutination patterns vary from 1+ (well 5, row 3) to 4+ (well 5, row 1). An example of a 2+ is seen in well 7, row 5, while an example of a 3+ appears in well 7, row 7. A ± reading appears in well 3 of row 3. Heterophile reactions can occur in the TPHA procedure; an example of a heterophile reaction is seen in well 8, row 8. Courtesy of Centers for Disease Control in Atlanta, Georgia.

WESTERN BLOT FOR SYPHILIS Another test format that has been used frequently in the research laboratory is the Western blot for *T. pallidum* (*Fig. 2.102*). The test using IgG conjugate appears to be at least as sensitive and specific as the FTA-ABS tests and efforts have been made to standardize the procedure. To date, many investigators agree that the presence of antibodies to the immunodeterminants with molecular weights of 15.5, 17, 44.5 and 47 kDa appear to be diagnostic for acquired syphilis. Several studies have found the Western blot for *T. pallidum* to have its greatest value as a diagnostic test for congenital syphilis when an IgM-specific conjugate is used.[30]

RAPID TESTS Recently, several companies have developed methods for syphilis screening and conformation tests using immuno-chromatographic strips. Currently, none have been licensed by the FDA for use in the U.S. These tests are targeted for developing country markets although they would also work well for rapid diagnosis in

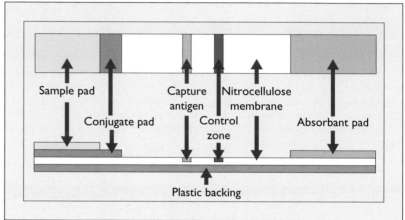

Fig. 2.103 Structural design of an immunochromatographic strip.

Fig. 2.102 The syphilis Western blot test is commercially available. The strips with electrophoresed treponemal antigens are incubated with the patient's serum. If antibody is present, this antigen–antibody reaction is detected using a second antibody, such as in other indirect tests such as EIA. Examples of different reactions are shown in each lane: Lane 14, positive control serum; Lane 15, minimum positive serum; Lane 16, negative serum; Lane 17, positive serum specimen. To be considered reactive in the Westerm blot, the patient's serum must react with bands of 15.5 kDa, 17 kDa, and 47 kDa. Courtesy of Robert George M.S., Centers for Disease Control and Prevention, Atlanta, Georgia.

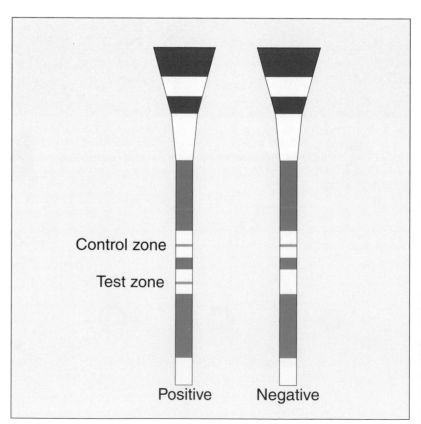

Fig. 2.104 Immunochromatographic strip tests. (Courtesy of Abbott Labs.)

developed countries. Even though the current tests are slightly different, they share common design and principles: (1) they require serum or whole blood; (2) they work on the principle of capillary action; and (3) the physical design of each strip are very similar. Each has a nitrocellulose strip attached to a plastic backing (*Fig. 2.103*). On the nitrocellulose membrane are 3 pads. At one end, a sample pad is on top of a conjugate pad containing a colloidal gold labeled anti-human antibody. An absorbent pad is on the opposite end. Between these two pads are two test zones. The first zone contains a specific capture antigen such as recombinant Tp47 lipoprotein; the second zone is a control containing anti-human antibody.

In practice, a small volume of patient serum or blood is placed in a test tube and the strip is inserted into the tube with the sample pad at the bottom. Capillary action draws the liquid through the sample and conjugate pads where it picks up the colloidal gold labeled anti-human antibody. During this process, the colloidal gold anti-human conjugate binds to the antibody in the serum. The liquid continues to be drawn up the nitrocellulose membrane and flows across the capture antigen and control zones. If the patient sera contains anti-treponemal antibodies, they will bind to the antigen in the capture zone and produce a colored line. As the serum flows across the control zone, some human antibody will be captured and also produce a second colored line. Excess sample that flows past the two test zones will be taken up by the absorbent pad. Thus, if the patient's serum is positive, there will be two colored lines on the strip; and if it is negative, there will only be one at the top (*Fig 2.104*). If the top zone does not produce a colored line, the strip is defective and the results should be disregarded.

Various companies use different capture antigens and slightly modified designs and reagents, but basically they produce the same results. To date, non-treponemal tests have not been adapted to this format. However, several companies and laboratories are exploring the development of a single strip that incorporates both a treponemal and a non-treponemal test. If successful, a dual test strip would revolutionize syphilis diagnosis because: (1) both a screening and confirmatory test would be incorporated into a single assay; (2) the test would be very rapid (10–15 minutes); (3) little equipment would be required and thus it would be very useful in resource-limited clinics and survey environments; (4) it would require very little sample manipulaton and labor; and (5) the results are objective and less prone to technician error or misintrepretation.

SENSITIVITY AND SPECIFICITY OF SEROLOGIC TESTS

While the overall sensitivity of the nontreponemal tests (*Fig. 2.105*) is approximately 90%, up to 28% of patients with early primary syphilis will have nonreactive nontreponemal test results on the initial visit. In addition, patients will present with nonreactive nontreponemal tests in about 30% of cases of late untreated syphilis. Specificity for the nontreponemal tests is 98%. However, the specificity of the test is greatly influenced by the population being tested. In intravenous drug users, the specificity may be as low as 79% for the VDRL slide test and approximately 89% for the RPR test. The VDRL CSF test is 90% sensitive and 100% specific in symptomatic cases of neurosyphilis, but it is only about 10% sensitive in asymptomatic neurosyphilis.

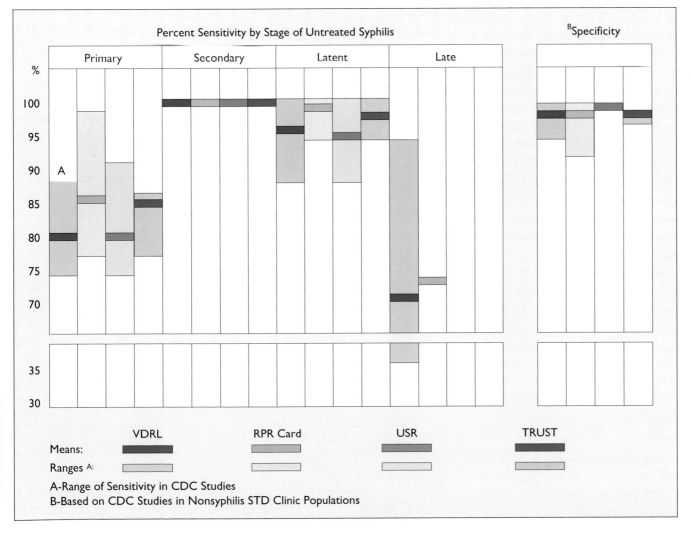

Fig. 2.105 Sensitivity and specificity of nontreponemal tests.

Percent Sensitivity by Stage of Untreated Syphilis

Primary Secondary Latent Late

^BSpecificity

Means:
VDRL   RPR Card   USR   TRUST

Ranges ^A:

A-Range of Sensitivity in CDC Studies
B-Based on CDC Studies in Nonsyphilis STD Clinic Populations

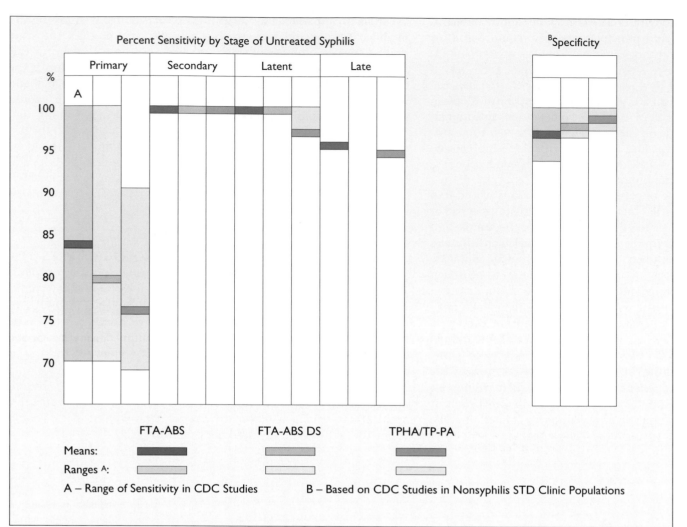

Fig. 2.106 Sensitivity and specificity of treponemal tests.

The overall sensitivity (about 98%) of the FTA-ABS test is greater than that of the other three major treponemal tests (each of which has a sensitivity of approximately 95%) (*Fig. 2.106*). The major difference in the sensitivities of these tests is found in primary syphilis. However, if data are analyzed according to the diagnosis of primary syphilis based on dark-field positive lesions alone, and primary cases are separated into those with reactive nontreponemal test results, then the sensitivities of the four treponemal tests are almost identical and are greater than 99%. False positives can occur in the treponemal tests, but only rarely do false positives occur in both treponemal and nontreponemal tests for the same patient. Individuals with connective tissue diseases may present difficult serodiagnostic problems.

Serologic tests must be interpreted according to the disease stage, possible underlying disease conditions, and the possibility of false-positive test results. Ideally, all sera in suspected cases of syphilis should be tested first with a nontreponemal procedure and reactive results verified with a second specimen and quantification. Cases in which clinical or epidemiologic evidence is counter to the diagnosis of syphilis should be confirmed with a treponemal test. With the proper use of serologic tests, a reactive nontreponemal test with a reactive treponemal test gives a positive predictive value of approximately 97%, or only a 3% error factor. In contrast, if any one test is used, the positive predictive value, regardless of the method, is less than 50% in a low-prevalence setting such as Europe or the U.S.

Misinterpretation of test results for nontreponemal tests most often results from:

- The failure to recognize the variation of plus or minus one dilution inherent in most serologic tests

- The failure to establish the true positivity of test results
- The failure to recognize reactivity due to nonvenereal treponematoses.

In summary, serologic testing often plays a crucial role in making a diagnosis of syphilis. Many tests are commercially available and are of high quality. All tests require rigid standardization with negative and positive control sera before being used to test sera from patients. Finally, the serologic test results should be interpreted carefully, in the light of a thorough history, physical, and, if possible, dark-field examination, before a diagnosis of syphilis is made.

ACKNOWLEDGMENTS

A special thanks to Mr. Arnold Castro for his discussions on rapid diagnostics and Mr. Robert George on Western blot analyses.

References

1. Radolf JD. Role of outer membrane architecture in immune evasion by *Treponema pallidum* and *Borrelia burgdorferi*. *Trends in Microbiol* 1994; **2**:307–311.
2. Radolf JD, Robinson EJ, Bourell KW *et al*. Characterization of outer membranes isolated from *Treponema pallidum*, the syphilis spirochete. *Infect Immun* 1995; **63**:4244–4252.
3. Norris SJ, Cox DL, Weinstock GM. Biology of *Treponema pallidum*: correlation of functional activities with genome sequence data. *J Mol Microbiol Biotechnol* 2001; **3**:37–62.
4. Cox DL, Akins DR, Porcella SF, Norgard MV, Radolf JD. *Treponema pallidum* in gel microdroplets: a novel strategy for investigation of treponemal molecular architecture. *Mol Microbiol* 1995; **15**:1151–1164.

5. Radolf JD, Norgard MV, Schulz WW. Outer membrane ultrastructure explains the limited antigenicity of virulent *Treponema pallidum*. *PNAS* 1989; **86**:2051–2055.

6. Walker EM, Borenstein LA, Blanco DR, Miller JN, Lovett MA. Analysis of outer membrane ultrastructure of pathogenic *Treponema* and *Borrelia* species by freeze-fracture electron microscopy. *J Bacteriol* 1991; **173**:5585–5588.

7. Radolf J.D. *Treponema pallidum* and the quest for outer membrane proteins. *Mol Microbiol* 1995; **16**:1067–1073.

8. Cox DL. Culture of *Treponema pallidum*. *Methods Enzymol* 1994; **236**:390–405.

9. Fraser CM, Norris SJ, Weinstock GM *et al*. Complete genome sequence of *Treponema pallidum*, the syphilis spirochete. *Science* 1998; **281**:375–388.

10. Radolf, J D, Steiner B, Shevchenko D. *Treponema pallidum*: Doing a remarkable job with what it's got. *Trends Microbiol* 1999; **7**:7–9.

11. Gerbase AC, Rowley JT, Mertens TE. Global epidemiology of sexually transmitted diseases. *Lancet* 1998; **351**(suppl III):2–4.

12. Centers for Disease Control and Prevention. *Sexually transmitted disease surveillance, 1999*. Atlanta: Division of STD Prevention, National Center for HIV, STD, and TB Prevention, 2000.

13. Centers for Disease Control and Prevention. Guidelines for treatment of sexually transmitted diseases. *MMWR* 2002; 51:RR6.

14. Clark EG, Dunbolt N. The Oslo study of the natural course of untreated syphilis: An epidemiologic investigation based on a re-study of the Boeck–Bruusgaard material. *Med Clin North Am* 1964; **48**:613.

15. World Health Organization. *Treponemal Infections*. Technical Report Series No. 674. Geneva, WHO, 1982.

16. Kampmeier RH. The late manifestations of syphilis: skeletal, visceral and cardiovascular. *Med Clin North Am* 1964; **48**:667.

17. Heggtveit HA. Syphilis aortitis: A clinicopathologic autopsy study of 100 cases, 1950 to 1960. *Circulation* 1964; **29**:346.

18. Olansky S. Late benign syphilis. *Med Clin North Am* 1964; **48**:653.

19. Bayne LL, Sidley JW, Goodin DS. Acute syphilitic meningitis: Its occurrence after clinical and serologic cure of secondary syphilis with penicillin G. *Arch Neurol* 1986; **43**:137.

20. Hooshmand H, Escobar MR, Kopf SW. Neurosyphilis. A study of 241 patients. *JAMA* 1972; **219**:726.

21. Rompalo AM, Joesoef R, O'Donnell JA *et al*. Clinical manifestations of early syphilis by HIV status and gender: results of the syphilis and HIV study. *Sex Transm Dis* 2001; **28**:158–165.

22. Rolfs RT, Joesoef MR, Hendershot EF *et al*. A randomized trial of enhanced therapy for early syphilis in patients with and without human immunodeficiency virus infection. *N Engl J Med* 1997; **337**:307–314.

23. Augenbraun MH, Rolfs R. Treatment of syphilis: Nonpregnant adults. *Clin Infect Dis* 1998; **28**(Suppl 1):S21–S28.

24. WHO. *Guidelines for the management of sexually transmitted infections*. http://www.who.int/HIV_AIDS/STIcasemanagement/STIManagementguidelines.

25. Clinical Effectiveness Group. National guideline for the management of early syphilis. *Sex Transm Inf* 1999; **75**(Suppl 1):S29–S33.

26. Larsen SA, Pope V, Johnson R, Kennedy Jr E (eds). *A manual of tests for syphilis*, 9th ed. Washington, DC: American Public Health Association, 1998.

27. Liu H, Rodes B, Chen C-Y, Steiner B. New tests for syphilis: Rational design of a PCR method for the detection of *Treponema pallidum* in clinical specimens using unique regions of the DNA polymerase gene. *J Clin Microbiol* 2001; **39**:1941–1946

28. Liu H, McCaustland K, Holloway B. Evaluating the concentration it *Treponema pallidum* in blood and bodily fluid using a semi-guantitative PCR method. *Intd STD AIDS* 2001; **12**:142–143.

29. Pillay A, Liu H, Chen C-Y, Holloway B, Strum AW, Steiner B, Morse S. Molecular subtyping of *Treponema pallidum* ssp. *pallidum*. *Sex Transm Dis* 1998; **25**:408–414.

30. George R, Pope V, Fears M, Morrill B, Larsen S. An analysis of the value of some antigen–antibody interactions used as diagnostic indicators in a treponemal Western blot (TWB) test for syphilis. *J Clin Lab Immunol* 1998; **50**:27–44.

Chancroid

R Ballard and S Morse

3

INTRODUCTION

Chancroid, or soft chancre (ulcus molle), is characterized by one or more genital ulcers and often by painful inguinal lymphadenopathy. The disease was differentiated clinically from syphilis by Bassereau in France in 1852.[1] In 1889, Ducrey in Italy demonstrated the infectious nature of the disease by inoculating the forearm skin of human volunteers with purulent material from their own genital ulcers.[2] At weekly intervals, he inoculated a new site with material from the most recent ulcer and, following the fifth or sixth reinoculation in each patient, he found a single microorganism in the ulcer exudate. The organism described was a short, compact, streptobacillary rod. Ducrey did not, however, isolate the causative bacterium that now bears his name, *Haemophilus ducreyi*. Isolation was accomplished by other workers by 1900.[3]

EPIDEMIOLOGY

Chancroid is particularly common in parts of Africa, Asia, and Latin America where its incidence may exceed that of syphilis as a cause of genital ulceration (*Fig. 3.1*). Data obtained using a polymerase chain reaction assay (PCR), showed that chancroid accounts for between 10 to more than 60% of genital ulcers among STD clinic patients examined in North and Sub-Saharan Africa, India, and the Caribbean (*Fig. 3.2*). The limited data from South America indicate that chancroid is present but

that its magnitude is unknown. Chancroid is presently considered an uncommon sexually transmitted infection in Europe and the United States. Based on data forwarded to the Centers for Disease Control and Prevention (CDC), the reported number of chancroid cases in the US peaked in 1947 at 9515 cases before beginning a decline which lasted until the mid-1980s (*Fig. 3.3*). During the 20-year period between 1965 and 1984, the number of reported cases averaged 925 cases per year. However, beginning in 1985, the number of reported cases of chancroid increased dramatically, with 4986 cases reported in 1987. Since 1987, the number of reported cases of chancroid has decreased steadily, with a 50-year low of 99 cases reported in 2000.

Chancroid cases are not evenly distributed throughout the United States (*Fig. 3.2*). Most cases are reported among minorities living in eastern cities and in the South. Recent data obtained using a multiplex PCR (M-PCR) assay indicate that chancroid remains an under-appreciated cause of genital ulcers in some areas of the United States.[4]

The increase in the incidence of chancroid that occurred in the United States in the mid-1980s occurred at the same time that the incidence of primary and secondary syphilis increased among minority heterosexual men and women (*Fig. 3.4*). The increase in syphilis was associated with cocaine use in both men and women and, among women, with the exchange of drugs or money for sexual favors. It has been postulated that similar factors might also have been responsible for the increase in chancroid.[5]

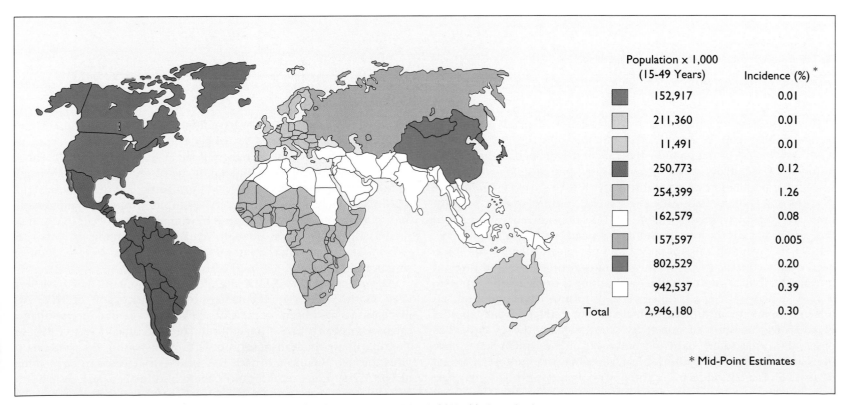

	Population x 1,000 (15-49 Years)	Incidence (%) *
	152,917	0.01
	211,360	0.01
	11,491	0.01
	250,773	0.12
	254,399	1.26
	162,579	0.08
	157,597	0.005
	802,529	0.20
	942,537	0.39
Total	2,946,180	0.30

* Mid-Point Estimates

Fig. 3.1 Estimated incidence of chancroid. Courtesy of the Global Program on AIDS, World Health Organization.

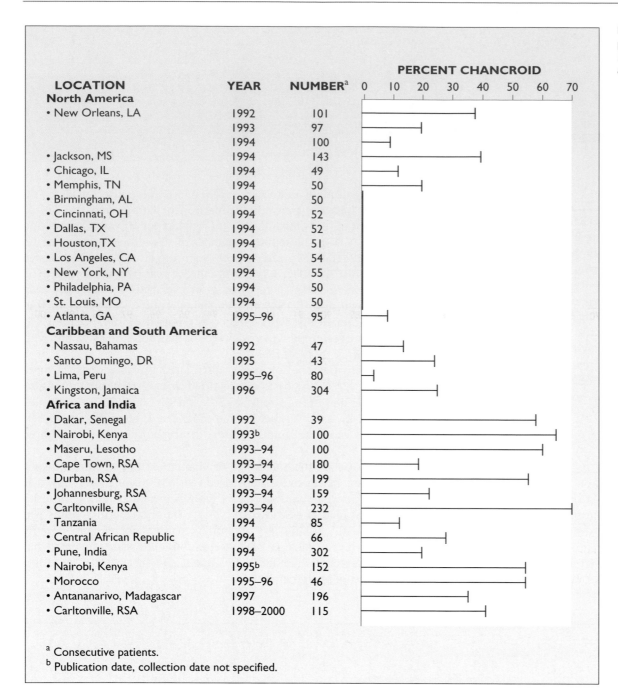

Fig. 3.2 Geographic differences in the proportion of genital ulcers caused by *Haemophilus ducreyi* as determined by nucleic acid amplification assays.

The persistence of chancroid in a population depends on several factors, which can be expressed mathematically by the equation $R_0 = \beta Dc$ where R_0 is the reproductive rate and is defined as the average number of secondary cases generated by one primary case in a susceptible population of defined density; β is the average probability that the infection is transmitted per sexual partner contact per unit time; D is the average duration of infectiousness of an infected individual; and c is the average number of sexual partners per unit time. If $R_0 < 1$ the infection will not persist and no epidemic will occur. It has been estimated that the probability of transmitting chancroid from an infected male to an uninfected female during a single sexual exposure is 0.35, whereas the probability of transmitting chancroid from an infected female to an uninfected male during a single sexual exposure is 0.30.[6] The duration of infectivity is estimated to be 45 days. The observation that some chancroid outbreaks in the United States have been associated with prostitution[7] suggests that the number of sexual partners (c) is a critical factor in the spread of chancroid. This may also help explain the association of chancroid with certain risk factors such as crack cocaine and alcohol use since individuals who abuse cocaine or alcohol have been reported to have more sexual partners and are more likely to engage in high-risk sexual behavior.

The majority of cases of chancroid occur in males (*Fig. 3.4*). This is probably the result of a combination of factors: more easily visible male anatomy; small numbers of infected prostitutes having sexual relations with many men; women with cervical ulcers who are asymptomatic; and spontaneous healing of lesions in women which occur in dry areas such as the inner thighs. Male to female ratios among patients with proven chancroid range from 1.6:1 to has high as 25:1 in outbreak situations.[8]

STDs in general, and genital ulcerative disease in particular, have been cited as risk factors in the heterosexual transmission of HIV. Two mechanisms have been proposed to explain how genital ulcers enhance the transmission of HIV. Chancroid and other genital ulcerative diseases could facilitate the transmission of HIV by increasing the shedding of virus through the ulcer. In fact, HIV has been detected in chancroidal ulcers.[4,9] The presence of an ulcer could also increase susceptibility to HIV infection by disrupting the epithelial barrier and perhaps by increasing the number of HIV-susceptible cells at the point of entry.

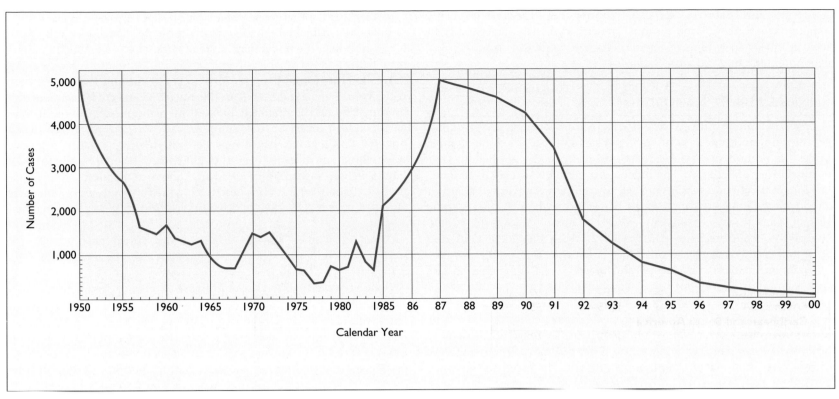

Fig. 3.3 Numbers of reported cases of chancroid in the USA from 1950 to 2000.

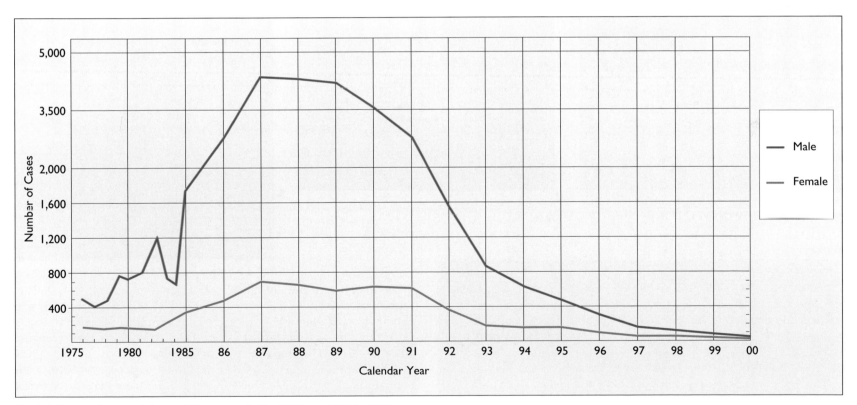

Fig. 3.4 Reported cases of chancroid by gender in the USA from 1976 to 2000.

A dermal infiltrate of CD4 T-lymphocytes, Langerhans cells, macrophages, and polymorphonuclear leukocytes is characteristically seen in biopsy specimens of papular chancroidal lesions from persons experimentally infected with *H. ducreyi*.[10]

CLINICAL MANIFESTATIONS

H. ducreyi naturally infects stratified squamous epithelium including genital and nongenital skin, mucosal surfaces, and regional lymph nodes.[8] It is thought to enter through breaks in the epithelium that occur during intercourse.[8] The incubation period is usually 4–10 days, but longer incubation periods are not uncommon. The lesions begin as a tender, erythematous papule at the site of inoculation (*Fig. 3.5*) within several hours to days of exposure. Over the next 1–2 days, the papule evolves into a pustule. Some patients do not recall a papule but describe an initial erythematous, shallow ulcer. After several days, the pustules ulcerate, and patients develop painful ulcers. Usually, patients do not seek medical attention until they have had ulcers for several weeks.[8] Some ulcers may be quite superficial (*Fig. 3.6*, see also *Fig. 3.20*), but many are deep (*Fig. 3.7–3.10*); the ulcers are excavated into the skin and often have a beefy, granular, or purulent base. The edge of the ulcer is usually irregular, has a red margin, and is not indurated. The tenderness of the ulcer often makes examination difficult. The ulcer is sometimes masked by dried or crusted exudate that, when gently removed by saline-soaked gauze, will reveal the ulceration. In men, ulcers often occur on the prepuce, resulting in phimosis, a painful inability to retract the prepuce (*Figs 3.11* and *3.12*).

As the disease progresses, as many as 50% of cases develop unilateral or bilateral inguinal lymphadenopathy, which is characteristically painful even though the nodes may be small (*Fig. 3.13A*). Adenopathy ranges from being barely palpable — yet quite painful — to quite large. Buboes (large, fluctuant lymph nodes) may occur, a finding that is not seen with syphilis or genital herpes. In the absence of effective treatment and prophylactic needle drainage, buboes often suppurate, leaving fistulas or secondary ulcers at the drainage site (*Fig. 3.13B*). Rarely, both inguinal and femoral glands may become involved creating a groove sign, which has formerly been thought to be pathognomonic for LGV (*Fig. 3.14*). A variant form of ulcer known as chancre mou volant (transient chancre) has been described, which involutes spontaneously after 4–6 days but may be followed by diagnostically puzzling inguinal adenopathy.

Ulcers in women usually occur in the vulval area; carriage of *H. ducreyi* without any sign of infection appears to be uncommon (*Figs 3.15–3.19*).

There are several differences in disease expression between men and women (*Table 3.1*). In about one-half of individuals, there is more than one ulcer. Men are invariably symptomatic, but an occasional woman may not be symptomatic due to the presence of asymptomatic ulcers on the cervix or on the vaginal wall. Anal ulcers in women are thought to be the result of drainage or auto-inoculations and not necessarily anal intercourse. Transient ulcers may frequently be seen on the inner thighs of infected women. The relative infrequency of adenopathy in women is presumably due to differences in lymphatic drainage between males and females.

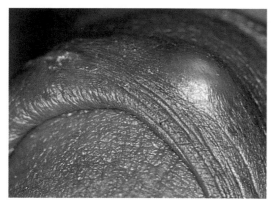

Fig. 3.5 A pustule, the first sign of infection, at the site where an ulcer will appear.

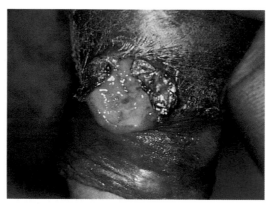

Fig. 3.6 Pustules and a newly erupted ulcer on shaft of penis.

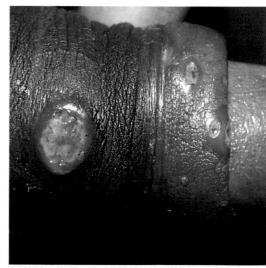

Fig. 3.7 Ulcer on the penile shaft with small ulcers on foreskin.

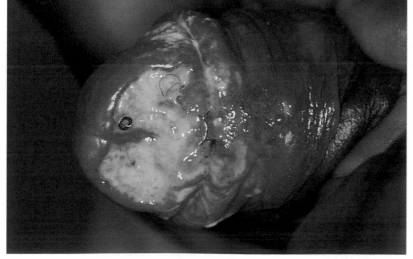

Fig. 3.8 Extensive ulceration may occur. The base of the ulcer is granular and friable.

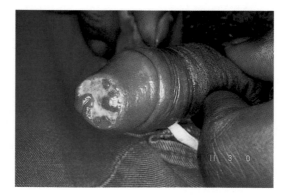

Fig. 3.9 Although most ulcers in men occur on the foreskin or shaft, ulcers can occur on the glans.

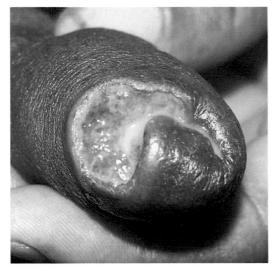

Fig. 3.10 Another example of extensive ulceration, in which the base of the ulcer is granular and friable.

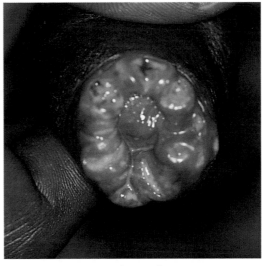

Fig. 3.11 Lesions occurring on the prepuce are commonly associated with swelling of the prepuce, and retraction of the foreskin may be impossible.

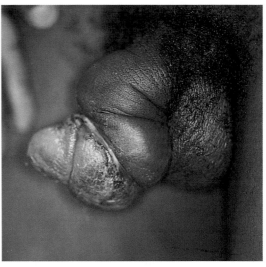

Fig. 3.12 Ulcer on the retracted prepuce with secondary edema.

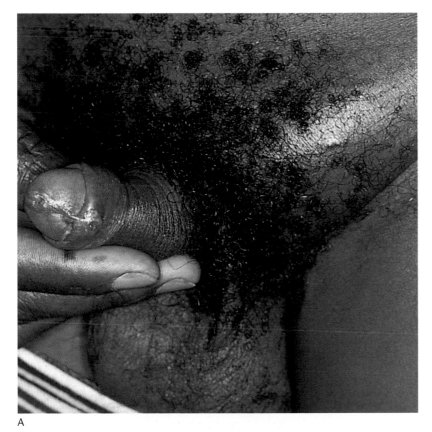

A

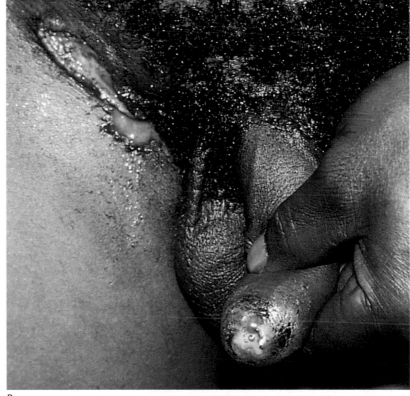

B

Fig. 3.13 (A) Ulcer on the prepuce, with visibly enlarged inguinal lymph nodes showing overlying erythema of the skin. (B) Buboes may spontaneously suppurate and subsequently form draining, chronic fistulas.

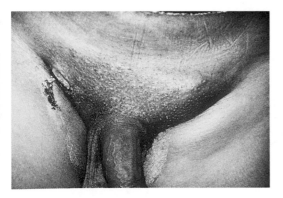

Fig. 3.14 Groove sign associated with chancroid.

Features	Men	Women
Genital ulcers	Multiple ulcers Usually on prepuce (uncircumcised), shaft or coronal sulcus (circumcised) Painful ulcers	Multiple ulcers Usually vulvar, but anal and cervical ulcers may occur Painful ulcers on vulva or anus; cervical ulcers frequently asymptomatic
Regional lymphadenopathy	Up to 50% of cases Painful inguinal and/or femoral glands Large nodes suppurate May be bilateral	Occasionally painful inguinal and/or femoral glands Suppuration not common May be bilateral

Table 3.1 Clinical features of chancroid in men and women.

Lip and mouth ulcers may occur as a result of oral intercourse, and may rarely occur elsewhere on the body as a result of auto-inoculation. Colonization of the mouth, cervix, and penis in the absence of signs or symptoms has been described. Unfortunately, chancroid ulcers often have atypical clinical appearance which results in misdiagnosis and thus failure to provide appropriate therapy. Chancroid can mimic genital herpes (*Fig. 3.20*), gonorrhea (*Fig. 3.21A and B*) and donovanosis (*Fig. 3.22*). The situation is further complicated by changes in clinical presentation, which may occur as a result of concomitant infection with *H. ducreyi* and HIV. Lesions may become less purulent and more closely resemble those of syphilis (*Fig. 3.23A and B*). Alternatively, they may spread locally with large numbers of painful lesions (*Figs 3.24 and 3.25*) or found in association with other STDs, particularly genital warts (*Fig. 3.26*).

DIFFERENTIAL DIAGNOSIS

The two diseases that most commonly have to be differentiated from chancroid are syphilis and genital herpes; one of these diseases coexists with chancroid in about 10% of chancroid cases. In contrast to the

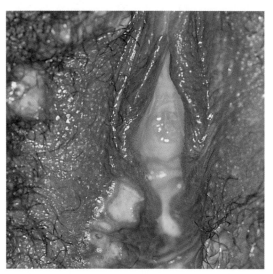

Fig. 3.15 Multiple vulvar lesions.

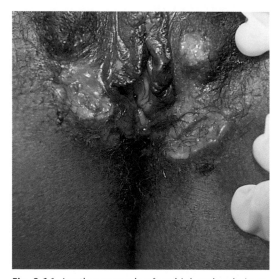

Fig. 3.16 Another example of multiple vulvar lesions.

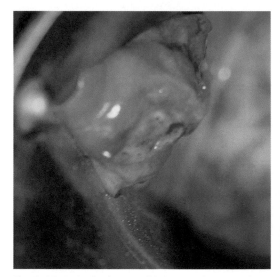

Fig. 3.17 A single chancroid lesion on the vaginal walt.

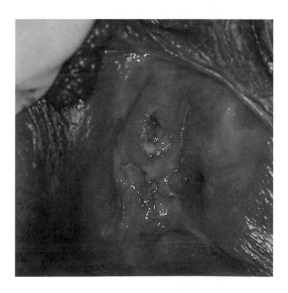

Fig. 3.18 Single periurethral lesion. Courtesy of the American Academy of Dermatology.

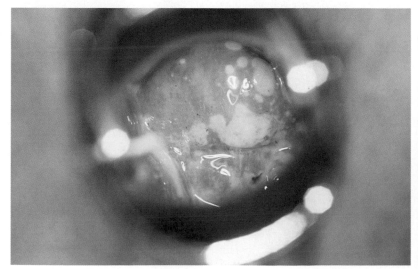

Fig. 3.19 Multiple cervical chancroid lesions.

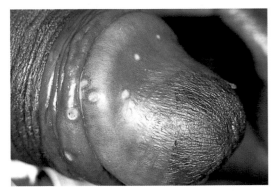

Fig. 3.20 Small lesions which clinically resemble genital herpes lesions.

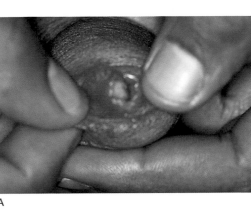

A

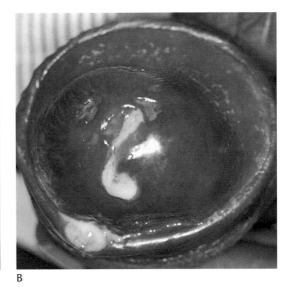

B

Fig. 3.21A and B. Endourethral lesions which may be misdiagnosed as gonorrhea.

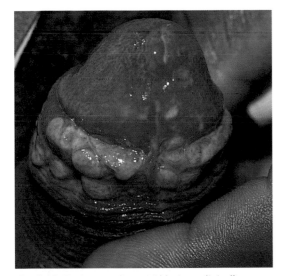

Fig. 3.22 Exuberant chancroid lesions clinically resembling those of donovanosis.

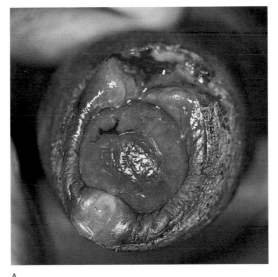

A

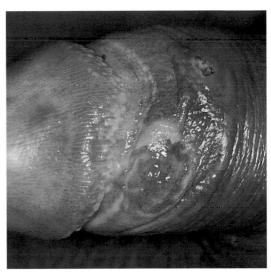

B

Fig. 3.23 A and B. Atypical lesions of chancroid in HIV-positive patients. Lesions are often less purulent in HIV-positive cases.

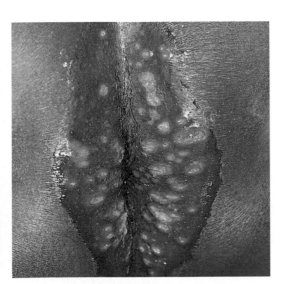

Fig. 3.24 Extensive lesions of chancroid between the buttocks in an HIV-positive patient.

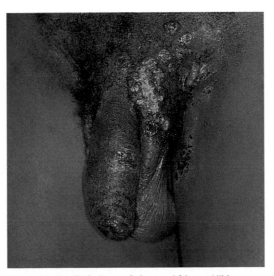

Fig. 3.25 Penile lesions of chancroid in an HIV-positive patient.

Fig. 3.26 Co-existing chancroid and genital warts in an HIV-positive patient.

59

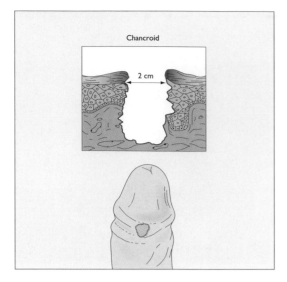
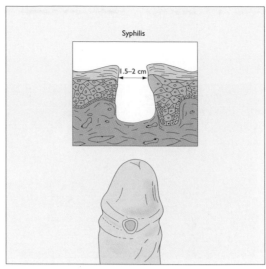
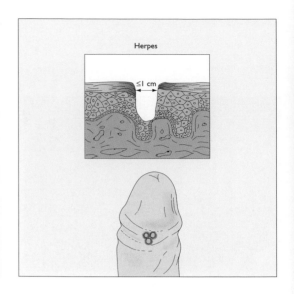

SENSITIVITY AND SPECIFICITY OF SELECTED CLINICAL SIGNS OF CHANCROID[a]		
Clinical signs	Sensitivity (%)	Specificity (%)
Undermined lesion border	85	68
Tenderness, ≥2+	57	52
Purulence, ≥2+	64	75
Classic chancroid (All three signs present)	34	94

SENSITIVITY AND SPECIFICITY OF SELECTED CLINICAL SIGNS OF SYPHILIS[a]		
Clinical signs	Sensitivity (%)	Specificity (%)
Ulcer induration, 3+	47	95
Tenderness, ≤1+	67	58
Purulence, ≤1+	82	53
Classic primary syphilis (All three signs present)	31	98

SENSITIVITY AND SPECIFICITY OF SELECTED CLINICAL SIGNS OF GENITAL HERPES[a]		
Clinical signs	Sensitivity (%)	Specificity (%)
Three or more lesions	63	64
Lesion depth, ≥1+	60	88
Tenderness, ≤2+	60	50
Classic genital herpes (All three signs present)	35	94

A   B   C

Fig. 3.27 Sensitivity and specificity of a clinical diagnosis of genital ulcer disease based on selected clinical signs. (A) Chancroid; (B) Syphilis; and (C) Genital herpes. a Data from DiCarlo RP, Martin DH. *Clin Infect* Dis 1997; **25**:292–8.

ulcers of syphilis, the ulcers of chancroid are more tender and, in contrast to the ulcers of genital herpes, they tend to be deeper and not grouped (*Figs 3.27A, 3.27B,* and *3.27C*). However, the use of clinical signs alone for the diagnosis of chancroid, syphilis, and genital herpes is insensitive as only about one-third of genital ulcers are classical in appearance; however, when the classic signs are present they are highly specific. Even under optimal circumstances, clinical impressions alone should not be used to base treatment, surveillance, or STD control programs.[11]

A dark-field examination of the lesion and a serologic test for syphilis should always be performed. Ideally, a follow-up serologic test for syphilis should be performed, as current therapy for chancroid cannot be relied upon to treat syphilis. Lymphogranuloma venereum (LGV) may occasionally need to be differentiated from chancroid, particularly when lymphadenopathy is the prominent feature of the clinical presentation. The ulcer sometimes associated with LGV, however, is not a prominent part of the illness, is transitory and precedes the appearance of lymphadenopathy. LGV is characterized by a longer incubation period. Donovanosis (granuloma inguinale), though causing destructive lesions in the genital area, is usually not associated with acute, painful ulcerations or lymphadenopathy.

HISTOPATHOLOGY

The biopsy of ulcers, though not extensively evaluated, was formerly described as being diagnostically useful.[12] A 4-mm punch biopsy obtained under local anesthetic from the edge of the ulcer to include adjacent epithelium, is adequate for study. The ulcer is characterized by the presence of a superficial zone of necrotic slough and neutrophils and tissue edema (*Fig. 3.28*).[13] Histological findings consist of a dense perivascular and interstitial inflammatory infiltrate (*Fig. 3.29*). The cellular infiltrate consists predominantly of CD4 and CD8 T lymphocytes and macrophages with areas of granulomatous change. Plasma cells are not prominently represented. Vascular endothelial changes consist of endothelial swelling, endothelial cell proliferation and erythrocyte extravasation. Histologically these changes are consistent with those of a delayed-type hypersensitivity reaction.

PATHOGENESIS

Human inoculation experiments have provided much of our knowledge concerning the initial stages of natural infection.[14] Bacteria are delivered to the epidermis and dermis of the upper arm (*Fig. 3.30A*) by puncture wounds made by the tines of an allergy testing device simulating the presumed natural route of infection. The estimated delivered dose required to initiate papule formation is as few as 1 to 2 colony forming units. The kinetics of papule and pustule formation resemble those of natural infection. Papules form within 24 hours of inoculation and evolve into pustules in 3 to 5 days (*Fig. 3.30B*) or resolve spontaneously. The immune response during these initial stages resembles a delayed-type hypersensitivity reaction, even in volunteers with no prior history of chancroid[15] (*Fig. 3.31*). Few bacteria are microscopically detectable at 24 hours, however; by 48 hours, extracellular bacteria are readily seen in the dermis and epidermis[16] (*Fig. 3.32*). Bacteria are seen in association with phagocytes but appear to survive by resisting phagocytic killing (*Fig. 3.33*). Bacteria do not appear to interact with keratinocytes or fibroblasts throughout experimental infection.[16,17] However, studies using transmission and scanning electron microscopy[18] have shown that *H. ducreyi* attaches to and invades human foreskin epithelial cells cultured *in vitro* (*Fig. 3.34A–D*). Additional studies are needed to resolve these discrepancies.

The human challenge model has been used to identify genes that may be required for the virulence of *H. ducreyi* by comparing the papule and pustule formation rates of the parent strain and an isogenic mutant defective in one or more genes. Results to date have identified several mutants that are attenuated with respect to their ability to produce pustules[19] (*Table 3.2*).

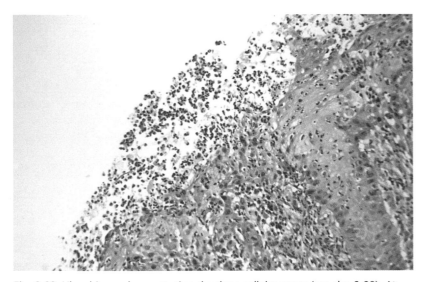

Fig. 3.28 Ulcer biopsy demonstrating the three cellular zones (see also 3.29). At the surface, there is an inflammatory exudate with partial ulceration of the skin (hematoxylin and eosin).

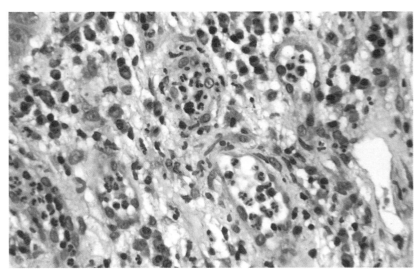

Fig. 3.29 Below the base of the ulcer, there is a wide cellular zone, with proliferating blood vessels (hematoxylin and eosin). Courtesy of Bhagirath Majmudar, MD.

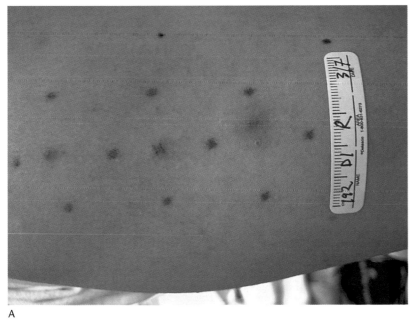

A

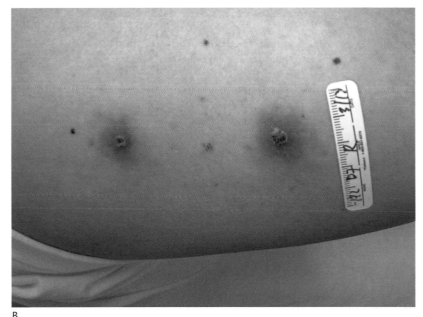

B

Fig. 3.30 Arm of human volunteer after delivery of *H. ducreyi* inoculum with an allergy testing device. Papules (A) form within 24 hours and evolve into (B) pustules in 3 to 5 days. Courtesy of Stanley M. Spinola, MD.

TAXONOMY

The taxonomic position of *H. ducreyi* as a *Haemophilus* species has been questioned for a number of years. *H. ducreyi* was originally placed in the genus *Haemophilus* because of its requirement for hemin (X-factor) and a G + C content that was in the accepted range for *Haemophilus* species. However, more recent studies have demonstrated that *H. ducreyi* was unrelated to the true haemophili such as *H. influenzae*. Sequencing of the 16S rRNA of several strains showed that although *H. ducreyi* was a member of the family *Pasteurellaceae*, it belonged to a different cluster than the true haemophili.

LABORATORY TESTS

SPECIMEN COLLECTION

Before obtaining a clinical specimen, the ulcer base should be exposed and free of pus. If necessary, crusted pus can be removed by gentle soaks

with sterile saline; otherwise, the ulcer does not need cleaning. Gram-stain material should be obtained from the base or margins with a cotton or calcium alginate swab and rolled over the slide to preserve cellular morphology, which might be disturbed by smearing the material. Culture material or specimens for PCR analysis should be obtained from the base or margins of the ulcer with either a swab or a loop (wire or plastic). Although transport media to maintain *H. ducreyi* have been described, it is best to inoculate culture plates directly with the swab or loop. Also, primary isolation plates frequently have only small numbers of colonies. It is conceivable that the dilution effect of liquid transport might cause some cultures to be falsely negative.

GRAM-STAIN CHARACTERISTICS

H. ducreyi is a small, Gram-negative, nonmotile rod, 0.5–0.6 μm in width by 1.6–2.0 μm in length. Examination of Gram-stained smears of human genital lesion material reveals groups or clumps of *H. ducreyi*

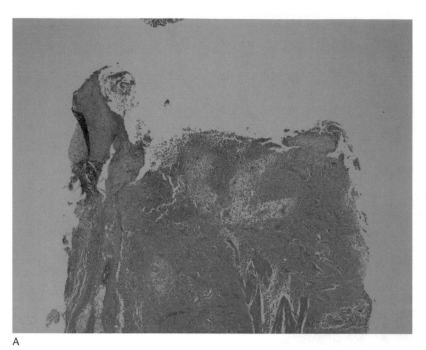

A

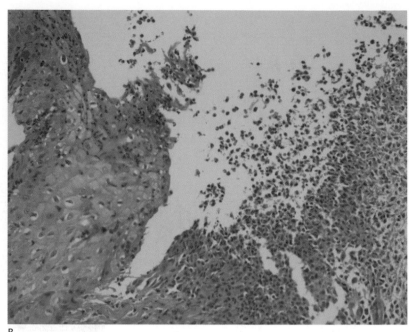

B

Fig. 3.31 (A) Hematoxylin and eosin staining of a biopsy of a pustule obtained 8 days after inoculation of a human volunteer (× 40); (B) Infiltrates of PMNs in the epidermis and mononuclear cells in the dermis can be seen at higher magnification (× 200). Courtesy of Stanley M. Spinola, MD.

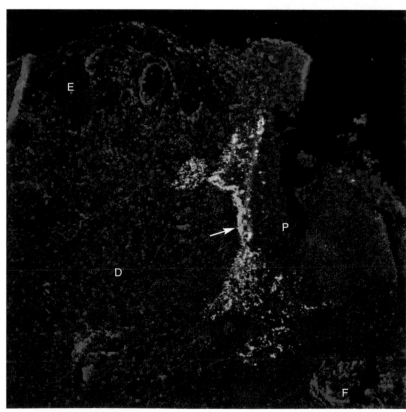

Fig. 3.32 Localization of *H. ducreyi* in a biopsy of a pustule from a human volunteer. Confocal microscopic image of tissue stained with anti-neutrophil elastase monoclonal (red), polyclonal anti-*H. ducreyi* antiserum (green), and Lens culinaris agglutinin (blue) to show tissue architecture. Note that the neutrophil infiltrate of the pustule disrupts the epidermis and that *H. ducreyi* are found primarily at the base of the pustule (indicated by the arrow) and in the dermis below the pustule. D. dermis; E, epidermis; P, pustule. Courtesy of Margaret M. Bauer, MD.

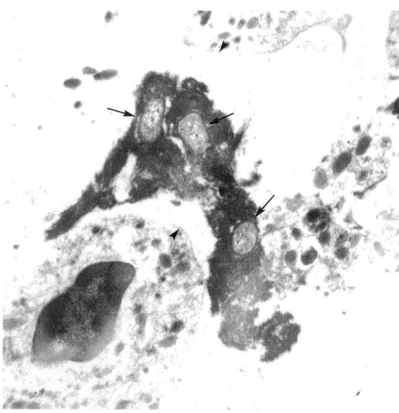

Fig. 3.33 Transmission electron micrograph of *H. ducreyi* (arrows) surrounded by fibrin and near PMNs. Arrowheads point to the membranes of PMNs. Note that the bacteria are between PMNs and near necrotic cellular debris, but have not been engulfed by the PMNs. Courtesy of Margaret M. Bauer, MD.

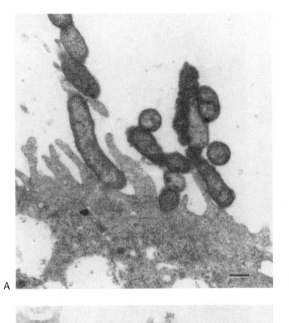
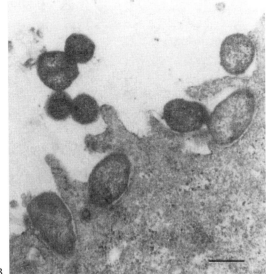
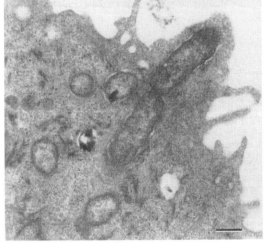
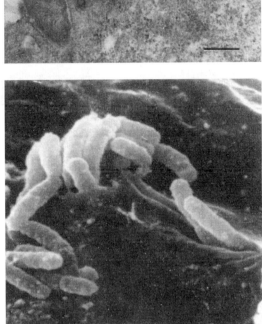

Fig. 3.34 Interaction of cultured human foreskin epithelial cells (HFECs) with *H. ducreyi*. Panels A, B, and C are transmission electron micrographs. (A) Bacteria attached to protrusions from the HFECs. (B) Bacteria engulfed by the cells. (C) Bacteria contained within vacuoles inside the HFECs. (D) Scanning electron micrograph showing bacteria which appear to be entering the HFEC. Bar = 0.5 µm (panels A, B, and C); bar = 1 µm (panel D). Courtesy of Patricia Totten, PhD and the American Society for Microbiology.

Attenuated (Pustule Formation Rate Decreased)
  Hemoglobin receptor
  PAL (outer membrane lipoprotein)
  DsrA (outer membrane protein required for serum resistance)

Virulent (Pustule Formation Rate Unaffected)
  Hemolysin
  CDT (Cytolethal Distending Toxin)
  CDT and Hemolysin
  Glucosyltransferase (lipooligosaccharide biosynthesis)
  Heptosyltransferase (lipooligosaccharide biosynthesis)
  Sialyltransferase
  Fine Tangled Pilus
  MOMP (OmpA homolog)

Data from Spinola SM, Bauer ME, Munson RS. Immunopathogenesis of *Haemophilus ducreyi* infection (chancroid). *Infect Immun* 2002; 70:1667–1676.

Table 3.2 Mutants that are attenuated or virulent in the human challenge model of chancroid.

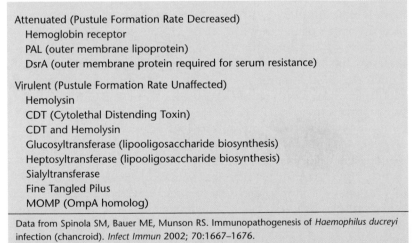

Fig. 3.35 Gram-stained human genital lesion material showing groups of organisms (oil immersion × 1,000). Courtesy of Bhagirath Majmudar, MD.

cells with occasional short streptobacillary chains among the lesion debris (*Fig. 3.35*). Sometimes organisms forming long trails within mucus strands are seen, the so-called 'railroad tracks', which are felt to be characteristic of *H. ducreyi* (*Fig. 3.36*). The utility of the Gram stain in diagnosing chancroid is unclear. A sensitivity of 40–60% versus culture has been generally accepted, but the specificity has not been well defined, as organisms with a similar morphology that might be mistaken for *H. ducreyi* may be found in genital secretions. Thus, the Gram stain from lesion material should be used as a presumptive means of diagnosis only (*Table 3.3*). Gram stains of material aspirated from buboes are more specific, but organisms are difficult to find in such smears.

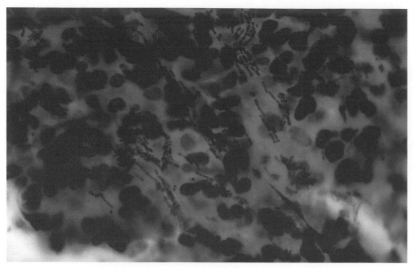

Fig. 3.36 Gram-stained human genital lesion material showing the 'railroad track' appearance of *H. ducreyi* (oil immersion × 1,000).

Presumptive	Diagnostic
Gram stain of material from genital lesion	Culture
	Nucleic acid amplification (e.g., PCR)

Table 3.3 Diagnostic methods in chancroid.

Medium#	Comments	Sensitivity* Culture	PCR
GC agar base (Gibco) + 1 or 2% hemoglobin + 5% fetal bovine serum (FBS) + 1% CVA enrichment (Gibco) (GcHbFBS)	Best medium when only a single medium is used to isolate *H. ducreyi*	60%	–
Mueller Hinton agar (BBL) + 5% chocolatized horse blood + 1% IsoVitaleX (BBL) (MH-HB)	About as sensitive as GcHbFBS. However, some isolates will grow on MH-HB that do not grow on GcHbFBS	60%	–
GcHbFBS and MH-HB	Can be used in a single biplate	72–75%	95–98%
Columbia agar base + 5% FBS + 1% hemoglobin + 1% IsoVitaleX (BBL) + 0.2% activated charcoal	Able to detect strains which grow on GcHbFBS and those which grow on MH-HB	80%	96%

*The sensitivity of culture and PCR was calculated relative to the expanded standard of culture + PCR
#The manufacturer is given where the composition of the medium may vary with the manufacturer. All media contained vancomycin (3 μg/ml).

Table 3.4 Comparative sensitivities of culture and PCR for the diagnosis of chancroid.

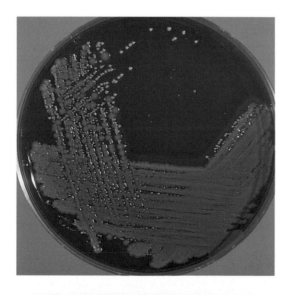

Fig. 3.37 Growth of microorganisms from human genital lesion material on heart infusion agar containing 5% rabbit blood, 1% IsoVitaleX, and 10% fetal bovine serum.

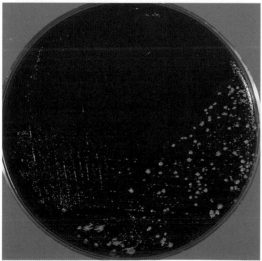

Fig. 3.38 The same medium as described in Fig. 3.37 has been used, but with the addition of vancomycin (3.0 μg/ml). On the left side of this plate, there is almost pure growth of *H. ducreyi*.

GROWTH CHARACTERISTICS

H. ducreyi is a fastidious organism that requires microbiologists experienced with working with this microorganism to obtain optimal isolation rates. The isolation of *H. ducreyi* as the primary means of diagnosis has been a difficult task. Most isolation rates of *H. ducreyi* from patients who have PCR-confirmed chancroid have been 60% or less, though studies in New Orleans[20] and Lesotho[21] reported culture sensitivity rates of 74–75%. Isolation of *H. ducreyi* from buboes, for reasons that are unclear, is even less successful than isolation from ulcers. Growth temperatures of 33–35°C are recommended, although incubation at 33°C may result in higher isolation rates.[22] Inoculated plates are incubated in a water saturated atmosphere with 5% CO_2 or in a microaerophilic atmosphere; these conditions are met by the use of a candle jar with a moist, but not dripping, paper towel in the bottom of the jar, or a commercial anaerobic jar from which the catalyst has been removed plus gas generating packets.

H. ducreyi can be grown on an enriched medium containing supplements such as IsoVitaleX (Becton Dickinson), Vitox (Oxoid), or CVA (Gibco); the organism requires the X (hemin) factor, but not the V (NAD) factor for growth. A variety of media have been devised for the cultivation of *H. ducreyi*, but no single medium appears to be able to support the growth of all strains from clinical material[23] (*Table 3.4*). To increase isolation rates, most workers recommend that two media are used.[23] The addition of vancomycin (3 μg/ml) greatly enhances the ability to recover *H. ducreyi* from clinical specimens by suppressing the growth of other microorganisms, and its effect can be quite dramatic (*Figs 3.37 and 3.38*).

Colonies growing on solid media are semi-opaque, translucent, and yellow-light gray in color and vary in size (*Fig. 3.39*). The colonies are nonmucoid and can easily be pushed intact across the agar surface with an inoculating loop. The removal of colonies may show a slight pitting of the agar surface.

A transport medium, comprising agar, hemin, thioglycolate and balanced salts supplemented with bovine albumin and glutamine, has

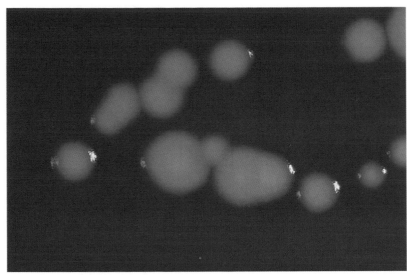

Fig. 3.39 Colonies of *H. ducreyi* growing on heart infusion agar, 5% rabbit blood, 1% IsoVitaleX, and 10% fetal bovine serum.

Methods of preserving *H. ducreyi*
Solutions
Heart infusion broth, trypticase soy broth, or bovine serum albumin, containing 10% glycerol and 10% fetal bovine serum (filter sterilized)
Skim milk, with or without 10% glycerol (filter sterilized)
Defibrinated rabbit blood
Serum-inositol (for lyophilization)
Storage conditions
Liquid nitrogen
−70°C
−35°C
−20°C
Lyophilization

Table 3.5 To preserve *H. ducreyi*, growth is removed from the agar surface, mixed into any one of the listed freezing solutions, and then immediately frozen.

Fig. 3.40 Gram stain of *H. ducreyi* colony removed intact from agar medium.

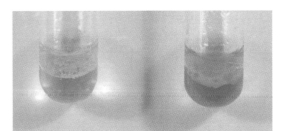

Fig. 3.41 Porphyrin test viewed in room light. A negative result with *H. ducreyi* is shown on the left.

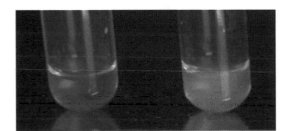

Fig. 3.42 Porphyrin test viewed with a Wood's lamp. A negative result for *H. ducreyi* is shown on the left.

been developed which will maintain the viability of *H. ducreyi* in swabs taken from clinical lesions for up to 1 week, provided the specimens are stored at 4°C.[24]

PRESERVATION

H. ducreyi can be removed from the agar surface with a swab, suspended in one of several freezing solutions, and stored at varying temperatures (*Table 3.5*). The cell suspensions can be stored in liquid nitrogen, at −70°, −35°, or −20°C. The latter two temperatures should be used only for short-term storage because marked losses in viability may occur.

CULTURE CHARACTERIZATION

On primary isolation media, growth may be visible at 24 hours, but identifiable colonies of *H. ducreyi* may not be seen until after 48–72 hours of incubation. Plates should not be discarded as negative, however, until after at least 5 days of incubation.

Colonies of *H. ducreyi* are almost invariably smaller than colonies of other bacteria isolated from the genital tract. A unique characteristic of colonies of *H. ducreyi* is that they can be pushed intact across the agar surface with a wire loop, which is a useful diagnostic clue. A Gram stain

should be performed on smears prepared from colonies suspected of being *H. ducreyi* (*Fig. 3.40*). Various arrangements of Gram-negative bacilli may be present, depending upon the age of the culture and the medium from which a colony is isolated. These include individual organisms, 'school-of-fish' arrangements (cells lined up parallel with one another, suggesting a school of fish swimming in one direction), 'fingerprint' swirls (a variation of the 'school-of-fish' pattern), and short strepto-bacillary chains.

Gram-negative bacilli from colonies compatible with *H. ducreyi* should be biochemically tested. Carbohydrate fermentation tests are not useful in confirming the identity of *H. ducreyi*, and differentiation from other *Haemophilus* species. As *H. ducreyi* requires X factor (hemin) for growth, it is negative in the porphyrin test (*Figs 3.41* and *3.42*). *H. ducreyi* is also negative in the catalase test (*Fig. 3.43*). Positive reactions are generally observed in the alkaline phosphatase (*Fig. 3.44*) and nitrate reductase (*Fig. 3.45*) tests. In the oxidase test, a positive reaction is only observed using tetramethyl-*p*-phenylenediamine; it is important not to use the dimethyl reagent, which will result in a negative result (*Fig. 3.46*).

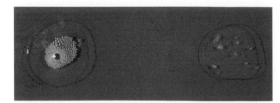

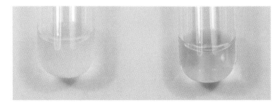

Fig. 3.43 Catalase test. A negative result with *H. ducreyi* is shown on the right.

Fig. 3.44 Alkaline phosphatase test. A positive result with *H. ducreyi* is shown on the right.

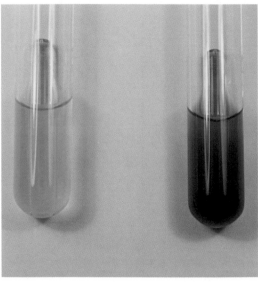

Fig. 3.45 Nitrate reductase test. A positive result with *H. ducreyi* is shown on the right.

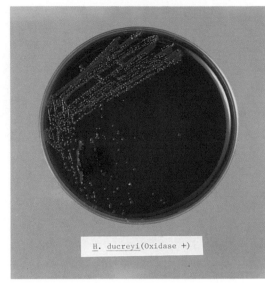

Fig. 3.46 Oxidase test. A positive result with *H. ducreyi*, showing dark colonies where oxidase reagent has been placed.

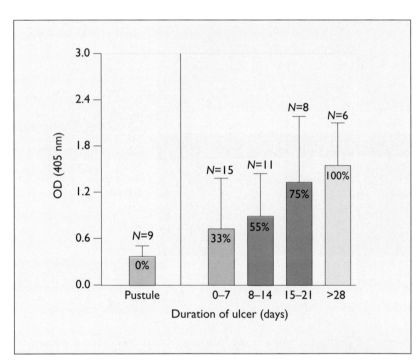

Fig. 3.47 Effect of ulcer duration on IgG response to *H. ducreyi* as measured by adsorption EIA. Initial serum specimens from PCR-confirmed chancroid patients were divided into 4 groups according to reported duration of disease. Pustule group, experimentally infected volunteers (see Fig. 3.30B), was included for comparison. Number of serum specimens in each group is indicated above bar. Proportion of seropositive patients is indicated within bar. Bars represent the mean optical density values ± SD.

Fig. 3.48 Schematic representation of ribotyping using a radiolabeled probe.

Nonculture Diagnostic Tests

There are no commercially available nonculture tests for the diagnosis of chancroid. However, recent studies have indicated that PCR is more sensitive than culture[20,21] or clinical diagnosis.[21] A multiplex PCR assay which will detect *H. ducreyi*, *Treponema pallidum*, and herpes simplex virus in a single specimen has been developed,[20] but is not currently commercially available.

HUMAN IMMUNE RESPONSE AND SEROLOGY

Delayed-type hypersensitivity to *H. ducreyi* antigens and complement fixation were formerly used as aids in the diagnosis of chancroid. However, their poor sensitivity and specificity preclude their current use in diagnosis. Because of a lack of longitudinally collected clinical specimens, the human immune response to *H. ducreyi* is poorly understood. In experimental human infection of ≤14 days' duration and limited to the pustular stage of the disease, the humoral immune response is not a major feature of the host response.[10] However, patients with chancroid usually seek care after several days to weeks of ulcerative symptoms. Recent data suggest that the humoral immune response occurs as the disease progresses into the ulcerative stage[25] (*Fig. 3.47*).

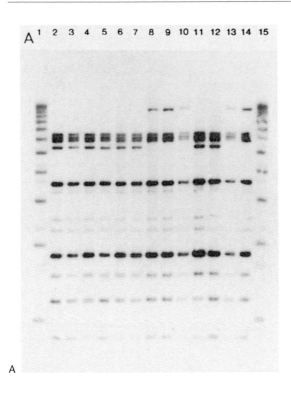

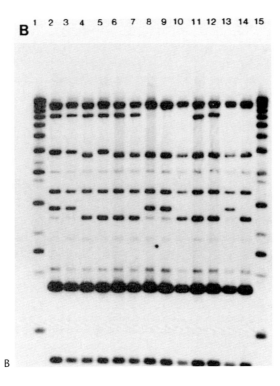

Fig. 3.49 Southern blots of *H. ducreyi* DNA, digested with *Hind*III, separated by agarose gel electrophoresis, and hybridized with ^{32}P-labeled 16S and 23S *E. coli* rRNA. Lanes: 1 and 15, 1-kb DNA ladder labeled with ^{32}P by nick translation; 2 to 14, isolates of *H. ducreyi* from different geographic areas. Courtesy of Sarafian SK, Woods TC, Knapp JS, Swaminathan B, Morse SA. Molecular characterization of *Haemophilus ducreyi* by ribosomal DNA fingerprinting. J Chin Microbiol 1991; 29:1949–1954, and the American Society for Microbiology.

STRAIN TYPING

H. ducreyi has very limited biochemical activities which can be used to characterize individual strains. A typing system with a high degree of discrimination could accomplish the following:

- Address unanswered questions concerning the geographic distribution of strains and mode of transmission
- Discriminate between treatment failure and reinfection
- Identify strains of different virulence
- Provide a means to study the genetic diversity of *H. ducreyi*

Ribotyping, based on restriction fragment length polymorphisms of ribosomal RNA genes, provides a reproducible method to discriminate between different strains of *H. ducreyi*.[26,27] Ribosomal RNA genes are highly conserved and are present in multiple copies on the genome of *H. ducreyi*. DNA isolated from *H. ducreyi* is first digested with an endonuclease such as *Hind*III, *Hinc*II, *Bgl*II, or *Bst*EII;[28,29] the resulting fragments are separated by agarose gel electrophoresis and transferred onto nylon membranes. The ribosomal DNA-containing fragments are visualized following hybridization with either ^{32}P-labeled or digoxigenin-labeled probe prepared from the 16S and 23S ribosomal RNA of *Escherichia coli* (*Fig. 3.48*). Ribotypes obtained using *Hind*III (*Fig. 3.49*) can differentiate between strains isolated from different geographic areas (*Table 3.6*).

Over the past decade, *H. ducreyi* has acquired plasmids encoding resistance to penicillins, sulfonamides, and tetracyclines (*Table 3.7*). Geographic variation in plasmid distribution has been reported (*Table 3.8*). Many strains from East Africa contain a 7.0 MDa plasmid that encodes for β-lactamase. The 3.2 MDa, 5.7 Mda, and 7.0 MDa β-lactamase plasmids are related to one another as well as to the β-lactamase plasmids found in *Neisseria gonorrhoeae*. Plasmid analysis with *H. ducreyi*, as with other organisms, may offer an epidemiological tool for distinguishing similarities among strains in varying geographical areas or during outbreaks of chancroid. Plasmid profiles can be used to differentiate further between strains belonging to a single ribotype.[30]

Source	Year	HindIII ribotype												
		1	2	3	4	5	6	7	8	9	10	11	12	13
Hanoi, Vietnam	1954	1												
Atlanta, USA	1954–1962				2	1								5
Winnipeg, Canada	1976	1												
Seattle, USA	1979			1										
Orange Country, USA	1981–1982				17		1							
Los Angeles, USA	1982						1							
London, UK	1982								1					
Atlanta, USA	1982				2									
Nairobi, Kenya	1982		2											
	1984		5	1	2			5		1				
	1990		4	2	2							1		
West Palm Beach, USA	1984		2											
Bangkok, Thailand	1984		13		11								5	1
Tampa, USA	1989				1									
San Francisco, USA	1989–1990		4		4	13				8	2	1		
New Orleans, USA	1989		4		1									
	1990		2		21									
	1991–1992				5									
Jackson, USA	1994–1995	3	1											1
Total		5	38	3	51	42	6	1	1	9	2	6	1	6

Table 3.6 Geographic source and *Hind*III ribotypes of 171 isolates of *Haemophilus ducreyi*.

Size ((MDa)	Antibiotic	Comments
3.1	Streptomycin and kanamycin	Encodes for two APH; enzyme modifying kanamycin appears to be a type I 3^I, 5^{II}-APH.
3.1	Sulfonamide, streptomycin, and kanamycin	Encodes for type II Su^r dihydropteroate synthase (Su/II) and Sm^r determinant, StA, similar to those found on plasmid RSF1010: Km^r gene similar to that found on Tn 903.
3.2	Ampicillin	Encodes for a TEM-I-type β-lactamase; plasmid is identical to the 3.2-MDa gonococcal Ap^r plasmid and carries about 40% of the TnA sequence.
3.5	Ampicillin	Encodes for ROB-I-type β-lactamase; plasmid is identical to the ROB-I β-lactamase plasmid originally isolated in Actinobacillus pleuropneumoniae.
4.9	Sulfonamide	Plasmid is related to the enteric streptomycin and sulfonamide resistance plasmid RSF1010.
5.7	Ampicillin	Encodes for TEM-I-type β-lactamase; plasmid is homologous to the 3.2-MDa gonococcal Ap^r plasmid and contains the complete TnA sequence; it differs from the 7.0-MDa Ap^r plasmid by the absence of a 1.3-MDa insertion element.
7.0	Ampicillin	Encodes for a TEM-I-type β-lactamase; plasmid is homologous to the 4.4-MDa gonococcal Ap^r plasmid and contains the complete TnA sequence.
30	Tetracycline	A conjugative plasmid; will not mobilize 7.0-MDa Ap^r plasmid; appears to be related to a Tc^r plasmid found in H. influenzae.
34	Tetracycline and chloramphenicol	A conjugative plasmid; can mobilize Ap^r plasmids; 70–80% homologous to pR1234 from H. influenzae; encodes for a type II CAT and possesses a class B Tc^r determinant.
34	Tetracycline	A conjugative plasmid; will not mobilize Ap^r plasmids; carries most, if not all, of the TetM transposon.
23	None	Able to mobilize nonconjugative R plasmids; it can cross species and generic lines.

Ap^r, ampicillin resistant; APH, Aminoglycoside phosphotransferase; CAT, chloramphenicol acetyltransferase, Cm^r, chloramphenicol resistant; Km^r, kanamycin resistant; Sm^r, streptomycin resistant; Su^r, sulfonamide resistant, Tc^r, tetracycline resistant.

Table 3.7 Antibiotic resistance conferred by various plasmids of H. ducreyi.

Location	Year of isolation	Plasmid content (MDa)*						
		N	None	7.0	5.7	4.9/(4.4)5.7	3.2	1.8*
UK	1954–1961	8	8	–	–	–	–	–
New York, NY	1989	1	–	–	1	–	–	–
Chicago, IL	1989–1990	2	–	–	2	–	–	–
Columbus, OH	1988	1	1	–	–	–	–	–
Elkins Park, PA	1989	4	1	–	–	–	–	–
Nashville, TN	1952–1958	8	8	–	–	–	–	–
Atlanta, GA	1980–1989	16	1	4	1	9	1	–
Augusta, GA	1990	1	–	–	1	–	–	–
Jacksonville, FL	1986–1990	4	1	–	3	–	–	–
Belle Glade, FL	1983	3	–	–	3	–	–	–
Fort Meyers, FL	1990	1	1	–	–	–	–	–
Orlando, FL	1985	2	–	–	2	–	–	–
Tampa, FL	1987–1990	159	76	–	83	–	–	–
New Orleans, LA	1989–1992	67	3	–	48	16	–	–
Houston, TX	1989	3	–	–	3	–	–	–
Jackson, MS	1994–1995	5	4	–	1	–	–	–
Orange Country, CA	1981–1982	22	3	–	–	–	19	–
Long Beach, CA	1987	17	2	–	6	–	9	–
Los Angeles, CA	1987	6	1	–	3	–	2	–
San Francisco, CA	1989–1990	32	10	–	2	5	14	1
Winnipeg, Canada	1978	19	16	–	3	–	–	–
Nairobi, Kenya	1980–1982	274	7	157	110	–	–	–
Johannesburg, South Africa	1988	29	–	4	21	4	–	–
Bangkok, Thailand	1984	30	–	–	1	–	–	29
Hanoi, Vietnam	1954	1	1	–	–	–	–	–
Santo Domingo, Dominican Republic	1995	1	–	–	1	–	–	–
Nassau, Bahamas	1992	1	–	–	1	–	–	–

*MDa = megadalton
Combination of the 1.8-, 2.6-, 2.8-, and 3.2-, 5.7- or 7.0-MDa β-lactamase plasmids.

Table 3.8 Plasmid profiles of selected H. ducreyi isolates, worldwide from 1952 to 1990.

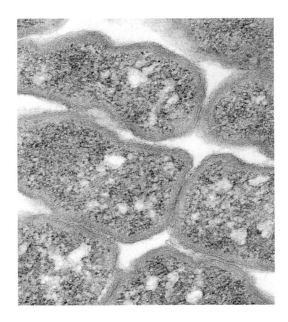

Fig. 3.50 Transmission electron micrograph of a thin-section of *H. ducreyi* grown on agar medium (× 90,000).

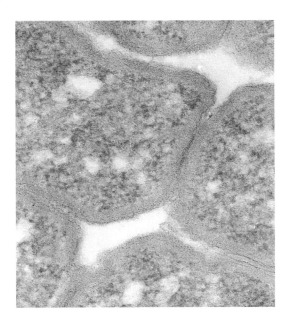

Fig. 3.51 Transmission electron micrograph of a thin-section of *H. ducreyi* grown on agar medium (× 175,000).

| Country | N | Antimicrobial* | |
		Erythromycin	Ceftriaxone/cefotaxime
United States			
Orange County, CA	38	0.004–0.016 (0.004)	≤ 0.001
New York, NY	22	< 0.008–0.064 (< 0.064)	≤ 0.001–0.008 (0.004)
San Francisco, CA	25	0.002–0.25 (0.015)	0.06–0.125 (0.06)
Thailand	100	0.007–0.06 (0.03)	0.0007–0.007 (0.003)
France	29	0.002–0.032 (0.016)	0.004–0.016 (0.008)
South Africa	122	0.002–0.125 (0.06)	0.002–0.008 (0.004)

*Expressed as µg/ml
Figure in parentheses indicates minimum inhibitory concentration of 90% of strains.

Table 3.9 Susceptibility of strains of *H. ducreyi* to clinically useful antimicrobials.

ULTRASTRUCTURE

H. ducreyi ultrastructure viewed by transmission electron microscopy shows the typical streptobacillary chains with cells adhering to each other end-to-end (*Figs 3.50* and *3.51*). Organisms also appear to adhere at the sides or from end to side, which may explain the appearance of clumps of cells that are frequently observed in Gram-stained smears. The cell envelope is typical of Gram-negative bacteria and is bordered on the outside by an outer membrane and on the inside by a cytoplasmic membrane, between which is a layer of medium electron-dense material (peptidoglycan). The outer membrane contains lipopolysaccharide (LPS), which lacks the repeating O-antigens that are characteristic of organisms such as *E. coli*. The *H. ducreyi* LPS is similar in size and structure to other mucosal pathogens and thus is more properly referred to as a lipooligosaccharide (LOS). Like *N. gonorrhoeae*, the *H. ducreyi* LOS is also sialylated.[31]

ANTIMICROBIAL SUSCEPTIBILITIES AND TREATMENT

Little variability in minimum inhibitory concentrations (MIC) to currently recommended antimicrobials occurs in isolates from around the world (*Table 3.9*). Ceftriaxone, cefotaxime, erythromycin, and members of the quinolone family are highly active *in vitro*. *H. ducreyi* resistance to trimethoprim-sulfamethoxazole (TMP-SMX) has been reported in Rwanda where the prevalence of resistant strains has increased dramatically between 1988 and 1991. All of the TMP-SMX-

resistant isolates were resistant to TMP (MIC, >4.0 µg/ml). Strains resistant to TMP-SMX have also been isolated in the United States, South Africa, Thailand, and Kenya. These data suggest that TMP-SMX should no longer be recommended for the treatment of chancroid.

Although animal models for chancroid infection have been described,[32–34] they have not been used routinely for evaluating the efficacy of various treatment regimens. The validity of *in vivo* susceptibility testing of *H. ducreyi* has therefore been confirmed almost exclusively by clinical trials conducted on patients with clinical chancroid. Despite differences between the various techniques used to measure *in vitro* susceptibilities, the results of several studies indicate a good correlation between conventional breakpoint values and clinical outcome.[35–37] Studies conducted in the 1950s and 60s indicated that sulfonamides and tetracycline were appropriate therapeutic agents for the treatment of chancroid.[38] Treatment failures with these antimicrobial agents were subsequently recorded in both the Far East[39] and Africa,[37] and were correlated with the emergence of *in vitro* resistance. However, occasional treatment failures may also occur even when the isolates appear to be fully susceptible to the antibiotic used to treat the disease.

In general, the main criteria which correlate with clinical cure include: sterilization of the ulcer base within 72 hours; a reduction in pain and purulence of the exudate covering the base of the ulcer; and, ultimately the re-epithelialization of the ulcer base, which usually takes less than 10 days.[35] The majority of patients who do not show a significant improvement in these criteria within 7 days should be regarded as treatment failures and retreated with an alternative antimicrobial agent. Factors which may also affect the rate of healing of ulcers include the initial size and site of the ulcerations; with larger ulcers and those found in warm, moist areas such as the introitus and in the coronal sulcus of uncircumcised men taking longer to heal.[40]

In contrast, resolution of inguinal and/or femoral buboes should not be used as a measure of the efficacy of a particular antimicrobial regimen, since buboes may continue to fluctuate and may even ulcerate even though adequate antimicrobial chemotherapy has been initiated. As a result, repeated aspiration of fluctuant buboes may be required in order to prevent spontaneous rupture and formation of inguinal or femoral ulcers.[41] The exudate obtained on aspiration of these glands usually changes from frankly purulent to serous or sero-sanguinous if therapy has been successful.

The emergence of β-lactamase-producing strains of *H. ducreyi*[42] (*see Table 3.7*) has resulted in the abandonment of penicillin and other

US Public Health Service	World Health Organization	UK Clinical Effectiveness Group
RECOMMENDED	RECOMMENDED	RECOMMENDED
Azithromycin, 1 g po in a single dose	*Ciprofloxacin, 500 mg po bid for 3 days	Azithromycin, 1 g po in a single dose
Ceftriaxone, 250 mg im in a single dose	Erythromycin base, 500 mg po qid for 7 days	Ceftriaxone, 250 mg im in a single dose
*Ciprofloxacin, 500 mg po bid for 3 days	Azithromycin, 1 g po in a single dose	*Ciprofloxacin, 500 mg po bid for 3 days
Erythromycin base, 500 mg po tid for 7 days		Erythromycin base, 500 mg po qid for 7 days
	ALTERNATIVES	ALTERNATIVES
	Ceftriaxone, 250 mg im as a single dose	Norfloxacin, 800 mg po in a single dose
		Spectinomycin, 2 g im in a single dose

*Ciprofloxacin is contraindicated for pregnant and lactating women, and for persons ≤ 18 years of age.

Table 3.10 Therapeutic regimens recommended by the US Public Health Service, the World Health Organization, and the United Kingdom Clinical Effectiveness Group.

β-lactamase-susceptible antibiotics for the treatment of chancroid. However, treatment of chancroid with amoxicillin plus clavulanic acid has yielded cure rates in excess of 90% in patients seen in Nairobi, Kenya.[43] The tetracycline antibiotics have been used extensively for the treatment of sexually transmitted infections world wide. However, high rates of treatment failure have been observed when patients with proven chancroid were treated with either tetracycline or doxycycline. In a trial conducted in Johannesburg, South Africa significantly higher cure rates were obtained following treatment with minocycline than with doxycycline given at the same dosage and duration. In that study, treatment outcome was correlated with *in vitro* susceptibilities of the isolates to the two tetracyclines.[44] However, significantly higher rates of treatment failure have recently been observed among chancroid patients receiving minocycline, and were correlated with an increase in high-level tetracycline resistance resulting from the presence of a plasmid encoding TetM (see Table 3.7). Although rifampicin has been shown to be effective in the treatment of chancroid,[45] the high likelihood of the emergence of resistance and the fact that this very active drug should probably be reserved to treat patients with tuberculosis mitigate against its acceptance for use in the treatment of chancroid.

After extensive clinical trials,[46–49] multidose therapy with erythromycin is regarded as the treatment of choice for chancroid by the US Public Health Service,[50] the World Health Organization (WHO),[51] and the UK Clinical Effectiveness Group[52] (*Table 3.10*). However, single-dose therapies with antimicrobial agents exhibiting good *in vitro* activity against *H. ducreyi* and appropriate pharmacokinetics have resulted in cure rates in excess of 90% in clinical trials conducted more recently.

The efficacy of these single-dose therapies for the treatment of chancroid in HIV-infected individuals has, for some time, remained a contentious issue.[40,53] Early reports from studies undertaken in Nairobi, Kenya indicated that treatment of chancroid with single doses of either fleroxacin, ciprofloxacin, ceftriaxone, spectinomycin, or azithromycin were less effective than multidose regimens, particularly in those patients co-infected with HIV. However, recent studies[54–56] have suggested that some of these single-dose regimens may be more effective than was initially thought. Differences in methodology and the increased frequency of co-infection with HSV-2 in HIV-positive patients presenting with chancroid could explain the apparent differences in response.[56,57] The regimens listed in *Table 3.10* have proved to be effective in over 95% of proven cases of chancroid in both HIV-positive and HIV-negative individuals.

Unfortunately, establishment of a definitive diagnosis of chancroid is impossible in individual cases of disease seen in endemic areas owing to the lack of laboratory facilities and the need to provide treatment at the initial visit to the clinical service. As a result, the WHO has advocated syndromic case management of genital ulcerations.[51] In areas where chancroid and syphilis are commonly encountered, combination therapy employing benzathine penicillin (2.4 mU) as a single intramuscular injection should be accompanied by appropriate treatment for chancroid to achieve cure rates of more than 95% in cases of GUD.

References

1. Bassereau PI. *Traite de affections de la peau symptomatiques de la syphilis*. Paris: JB Balliere, 1852.
2. Ducrey A. Experimentelle untersuchungen uber den ansteckungsstof des weichen schankers und uber die bubonen. *Montash fur Prakt Dermatol* 1889; **9**:387–405.
3. Bezancon F, Griffon V, Le Sourd L. Culture du bacille du chancre mou. *CR Soc Biol* 1900; **11**:1048–1051.
4. Mertz KJ, Weiss JB, Webb RM, et al. An investigation of genital ulcers in Jackson, Mississippi, with use of a multiplex polymerase chain reaction assay: high prevalence of chancroid and human immunodeficiency virus infection. *J Infect Dis* 1998; **178**:1060–1066.
5. DiCarlo RP, Armentor BS, Martin DH. Chancroid epidemiology in New Orleans men. *J Infect Dis* 1995; **172**:446–452.
6. Over M, Piot P. *HIV infection and sexually transmitted diseases: health sector priorities review HSPR-26*. 1991. Washington, DC; The World Bank.
7. Blackmore CA, Limpakarnjanarat K, Rigau-Perez JG, Albritton WL, Greenwood JR. An outbreak of chancroid in Orange County, California: descriptive epidemiology and disease control measures. *J Infect Dis* 1985; **151**:840–844.
8. Morse SA. Chancroid and *Haemophilus ducreyi*. *Clin Micro Rev* 1989; **2**:137–157.
9. Kreiss JK, Coombs R, Plummer F, et al. Isolation of human immunodeficiency virus from genital ulcers in Nairobi prostitutes. *J Infect Dis* 1989; **160**:380–384.
10. Spinola SM, Orazi A, Arno JN, et al. *Haemophilus ducreyi* elicits a cutaneous infiltrate of CD4 cells during experimental human infection. *J Infect Dis* 1996; **173**:394–402.
11. Ronald A. Genital ulceration and clinical acumen. *Clin Infect Dis* 1997; **25**:299–300.
12. Freinkel AL. Histological aspects of sexually transmitted genital lesions. *Histopathology* 1987; **11**:819–831.
13. King R, Gough J, Ronald A, Nasio J, Ndinya-Achola JO, Plummer F, Wilkins JA. An immunohistochemical analysis of naturally occurring chancroid. *J Infect Dis* 1996; **174**:427–430.
14. Al-Tawfiq JA, Thornton AC, Katz BP, et al. Standardization of the experimental model of *Haemophilus ducreyi* infection in human subjects. *J Infect Dis* 1998; **178**:1684–1687.
15. Palmer KL, Schnizlein-Bick CT, Orazi A, et al. The immune response to *Haemophilus ducreyi* resembles a delayed-type hypersensitivity reaction throughout experimental infection of human subjects. *J Infect Dis* 1998; **178**:1688–1697.
16. Bauer ME, Goheen MP, Townsend CA, Spinola SM. *Haemophilus ducreyi* associates with phagocytes, collagen, and fibrin and remains extracellular throughout infection of human volunteers. *Infect Immun* 2001; **69**:2549–2557.
17. Bauer ME, Spinola SM. Localization of *Haemophilus ducreyi* at the pustular stage of disease in the human model of infection. *Infect Immun* 2000; **68**:2309–2314.
18. Totten PA, Lara JC, Norn DV, Stamm WE. *Haemophilus ducreyi* attaches to and invades human epithelial cells in vitro. *Infect Immun* 1994; **62**:5632–5640.
19. Spinola SM, Bauer ME, Munson RS. Immunopathogenesis of *Haemophilus ducreyi* infection. *Infect Immun* 2002; **70**:1667–1676.

20. Orle KA, Gates CA, Martin DH, Body BA, Weiss JB. Simultaneous PCR detection of *Haemophilus ducreyi*, *Treponema pallidum*, and herpes simplex virus types 1 and 2 from genital ulcers. *J Clin Microbiol* 1996; **34**:49–54.

21. Morse SA, Trees DL, Htun Y, *et al*. Comparison of clinical diagnosis, standard laboratory and molecular methods for the diagnosis of genital ulcer disease in Lesotho: association with HIV infection. *J Infect Dis* 1997; **175**:583–589.

22. Schmid GP, Faur YC, Valu JA, Sikandar SA, McLaughlin MM. Enhanced recovery of *Haemophilus ducreyi* from clinical specimens by incubation at 33 versus 35°C. *J Clin Microbiol* 1995; **33**:3257–3259.

23. Pillay A, Hoosen AA, Loykissoonlal D, Glock C, Odhav C, Sturm AW. Comparison of culture media for the laboratory diagnosis of chancroid. *J Med Microbiol* 1998; **47**:1023–1026.

24. Dangor Y, Radebe F, Ballard RC. Transport medium for *Haemophilus ducreyi*. *Sex Transm Dis* 1993; **20**:5–9.

25. Chen CY, Mertz KJ, Spinola SM, Morse SA. Comparison of enzyme immunoassays for antibodies to *Haemophilus ducreyi* in a community outbreak in the United States. *J Infect Dis* 1997; **175**:1390–1395.

26. Sarafian SK, Woods TC, Knapp JS, Swaminathan B, Morse SA. Molecular characterization of *Haemophilus ducreyi* by ribosomal DNA fingerprinting. *J Clin Microbiol* 1991; **29**:1949–1954.

27. Flood JM, Sarafian SK, Bolan GA, *et al*. Multistrain outbreak of chancroid in San Francisco, 1989–1991. *J Infect Dis* 1993; **167**:1106–1111.

28. Brown TJ, Ison CA. Non-radioactive ribotyping of *Haemophilus ducreyi* using a digoxigenin labelled cDNA probe. *Epidemiol Infect* 1993; **110**:289–295.

29. Pillay A, Hoosen AA, Kiepiela P, Sturm AW. Ribosomal DNA typing of *Haemophilus ducreyi* strains: proposal for a novel typing scheme. *J Clin Microbiol* 1996; **34**:1613–1615.

30. Haydock AK, Martin DH, Morse SA, Cammarata C, Mertz KJ, Totten PA. Molecular characterization of *Haemophilus ducreyi* strains from Jackson, Mississippi, and New Orleans, Louisiana. *J Infect Dis* 1999; **179**:1423–1432.

31. Trees DL, Morse SA. Chancroid and *Haemophilus ducreyi*: an update. *Clin Microbiol Rev* 1995; **8**:357–375.

32. Reestierna J. Experimental soft chancre in rabbits. *Urol Cut Rev* 1921; **25**:332–333.

33. Tuffrey M, Abeck D, Alexander F, Johnson AP, Ballard RC, Taylor-Robinson D. A mouse model of *Haemophilus ducreyi* infections (chancroid). *FEMS Microbiol Lett* 1988; **50**:207–209.

34. Purcell BK, Richardson JA, Radolf JD, Hansen EJ. A temperature-dependent rabbit model for production of dermal lesions by *Haemophilus ducreyi*. *J Infect Dis* 1991; **164**:359–367.

35. Bowmer MI, Nsanze H, D'Costa LJ, *et al*. Single-dose ceftriaxone for chancroid. *Antimicrob Ag Chemother* 1987; **31**:67–69.

36. D'Costa LJ, Plummer F, Nsanze H, *et al*. Therapy of genital ulcer disease: a comparison of rosaramicin and erythromycin. In Periti P, Grassi GG (ed). *Current chemotherapy and immunotherapy*. Proceedings of the 12th International Congress of Chemotherapy, vol 2. Washington, DC: American Society for Microbiology, p 903–904.

37. Fast MV, Nsanze H, D'Costa LJ, *et al*. Antimicrobial therapy of chancroid: an evaluation of five treatment regimens correlated with in vitro sensitivity. *Sex Transm Dis* 1983; **10**:1–6.

38. Willcox RR. The treatment of chancroid. *Br J Clin Pract* 1963; **17**:455–460.

39. Marmar JL. The management of resistant chancroid in Viet Nam. *J Urol* 1972; **107**:807–808.

40. Tyndall MW, Agoki E, Plummer F, Malisa W, Ndinya-Achola JO, Ronald AR. Single dose azithromycin for the treatment of chancroid: a randomized comparison with erythromycin. *Sex Transm Dis* 1994; **21**:231–234.

41. Dangor Y, Ballard RC, Miller SD, Koornhof HJ. Treatment of chancroid. *Antimicrob Ag Chemother* 1990; **34**:1308–1311.

42. Hammond GW, Lian CJ, Wilt JC, Ronald AR. Antimicrobial susceptibility of *Haemophilus ducreyi*. *Antimicrob Ag Chemother* 1978; **13**:608–612.

43. Ndinya-Achola JO, Nsanze H, *et al*. Three day oral course of Augmentin to treat chancroid. *Genitourin Med* 1986; **62**:202–204.

44. Ballard RC, Duncan MO, Fehler HG, Dangor Y, Exposto F da L, Latif AS. Treating chancroid: summaries of studies in southern Africa. *Genitourin Med* 1989; **65**:54–57.

45. Plummer FA, Nsanze H, D'Costa LJ, *et al*. Short course and single dose antimicrobial therapy for chancroid in Kenya: studies with rifampin alone and in combination with trimethoprim. *Rev Infect Dis* 1983; **5**(Suppl): S565–S572.

46. Carpenter JL, Back A, Gehle D, Oberhoffer T. Treatment of chancroid with erythromycin. *Sex Transm Dis* 1981; **26**:192–197.

47. Duncan MO, Bilgeri YR, Fehler HG, Ballard RC. Treatment of chancroid with erythromycin: clinical and microbiological appraisal. *Br J Vener Dis* 1983; **59**:265–268.

48. Kraus SJ, Kaufman HW, Albritton WL, Thornesberry C, Biddle JW. Chancroid therapy: a review of cases confirmed by culture. *Rev Infect Dis* 1982; **4**(Suppl): S848–S856.

49. Plummer FA, D'Costa LJ, Nsanze H, et al. Antimicrobial therapy of chancroid: effectiveness of erythromycin. *J Infect Dis* 1983; **148**:726–731.

50. Sexually transmitted diseases treatment guidelines 2002. Centres for Disease Conton and Prevention. *MMWR Recomm Rep.* 2002; **51**:1–78.

51. World Health Organzation. 2001 Guidelines for the management of sexually transmitted infections. Http://www.who.int/HIV_AIDS/

52. Clinical Effectiveness Group. National guideline for the management of chancroid. *Sex Transm Inf* 1999; **75**(Suppl 1):S43–S45.

53. Tyndall MW, Malisa M, Plummer FA, Ombetti J, Ndinya-Achola JO, Ronald AR. Ceftriaxone no longer predictably cures chancroid in Kenya. *J Infect Dis* 1993; **167**:469–471.

54. Guzman M, Guzman J, Bernal M. Treatment of chancroid with a single dose of spectinomycin. *Sex Transm Dis* 1992; **19**:291–294.

55. Martin DH, Sargent SJ, Wendel GD, McCormack WM, Spier NA, Johnson RB. Comparison of azithromycin and ceftriaxone for the treatment of chancroid. *Clin Infect Dis* 1995; **21**:409–414.

56. Malonza IM, Tyndall MW, Ndinya-Achola JO, et al. A randomized, double blind, placebo-controlled trial of single-dose ciprofloxacin versus erythromycin for the treatment of chancroid in Nairobi, Kenya. *J Infect Dis* 1999; **180**:1886–1893.

57. Ballard RC, Htun Y, Matta A, Dangor Y, Radebe F. Treatment of chancroid with azithromycin. *Int J STD & AIDS* 1996; **7**(Suppl 1):9–12.

Infections Caused by *Chlamydia trachomatis*

J Schachter and R Stephens

INTRODUCTION

Chlamydia trachomatis is a bacterium with a limited metabolic capability that restricts its growth to within the intracellular environment of parasitized host cells.[1] The organism is distributed worldwide. Similar organisms are found in some other mammals, but those infecting humans are apparently restricted to human hosts, unlike the distantly related *Chlamydia psittaci*, which has a broad host range among non-human vertebrates, but can also infect humans. The first recognition that *Chlamydia* organisms were responsible for STDs occurred before 1910 when the association with inclusion conjunctivitis of the newborn and nongonococcal urethritis (NGU) and cervicitis was described.[2,3] Then, a relationship between *Chlamydia* and LGV was noted in the 1930s. LGV is rare in the USA (*Fig. 4.1*) but occurs frequently in the tropics. The pathogenic role of *C. trachomatis* in STDs other than LGV has been widely recognized only within the past three decades. The organisms causing LGV and these other conditions are easily distinguished in the laboratory and are placed in different biovars (trachoma and LGV)

within *C. trachomatis*. *C. psittaci* is responsible for the zoonotic disease ornithosis ('psittacosis'), which is characterized by respiratory disease in humans who become accidental hosts for avian strains of the organism. Recently, respiratory illness in humans has been associated with the so-called TWAR organism, now recognized as a separate species, *Chlamydia pneumoniae*.[4,5] This organism appears to be found worldwide, and is a very common pathogen with seroprevalence rates often exceeding 50% in adult populations.

Chlamydiae have been successfully propagated in the laboratory only within embryonated chickens' eggs, or in cell or tissue culture. This impeded the study of both the biology and clinical manifestations of infection. The technically complex cell culture methods for the isolation and identification of *Chlamydia* limited the use of isolation as a diagnostic test.

As a result of their small size and obligate intracellular parasitism, *Chlamydia* were considered viruses until the 1960s. However, they possess a characteristic bacterial cell wall, ribosomes, both DNA and RNA, and metabolic functions that confirm their bacterial nature (*Table 4.1*).

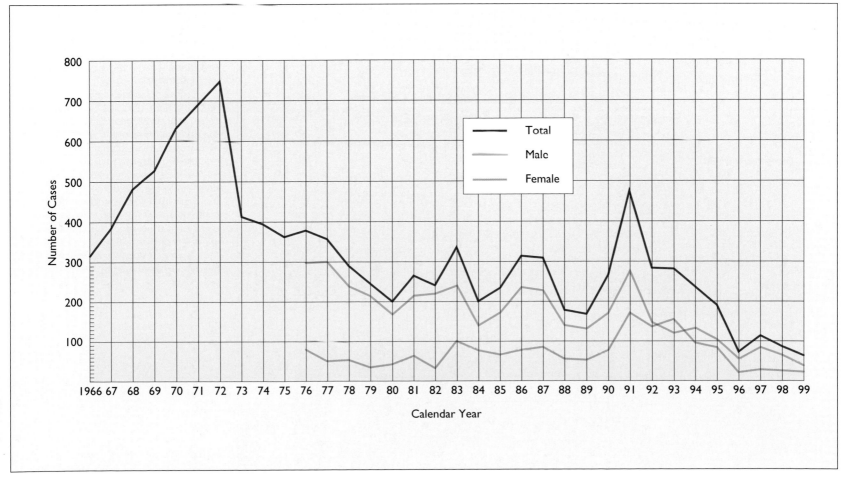

Fig. 4.1 Reported cases of lymphogranuloma venereum (LGV) by year in the USA. The accuracy of such reporting is not known.

Knowledge of the distinctive intracellular development cycle of the chlamydial organism is important in understanding the parasite–host interaction (*Fig. 4.2*). Much of what is known has been obtained through studies of chlamydiae grown in mammalian cell culture.[1] These studies expanded information generated earlier through observation of the growth cycle of the organism as interpreted from microscopic examination of conjunctival scrapings obtained from individuals with trachoma or inclusion conjunctivitis of the newborn, or experimentally infected nonhuman primates. The organism is dimorphic. The infectious form, the elementary body (EB), is a condensed, spore-like spheroid with a diameter of 200–400 nm (*Figs 4.3* and *4.4*). It is metabolically inactive, and contains a tightly compacted chromosome or nucleoid and an outer membrane composed primarily of lipopolysaccharide and proteins that are highly disulfide cross-linked. Upon contact with a

suitable host cell, the EB appears to induce its own entry by a process of receptor-mediated endocytosis; however, the host cell receptor is unknown. The ingested EB resides within a membrane-limited endosome, which is able to avoid fusion and destruction by the primary lysosomes of the parasitized cell by an unknown mechanism.

Several hours following invasion of the host cell, the EB undergoes conversion to the vegetative form, the reticulate body (RB). The RB is metabolically active, and competes with the host cell for metabolic precursors. It is less electron-dense, suggesting relaxation of the condensed DNA, and has a diameter of 500–900 nm (*Fig. 4.5*). Approximately 6 hours following invasion of the host cell, the RB begins to replicate by binary fission. By 24 hours, the RBs form visible 'inclusions' within the membrane-limited endosome (*Fig. 4.6*), each inclusion ultimately containing up to several hundred organisms. During the next 24–36 hours, the RBs both divide and condense into EBs, such that by 60–72 hours the inclusion contains primarily EBs.

After 48–60 hours of development, polysaccharide components within the inclusion may be seen following iodine staining. This staining distinguishes *C. trachomatis* from *C. psittaci* and *C. pneumoniae*, which do not produce large quantities of glycogen or glycogen-like deposits and thus do not stain with iodine. Other biologic properties that distinguish these species are illustrated in *Table 4.2*. The processes by which EBs egress from the host cell are unclear, and may include both lysis of the host cell and extrusion of intact inclusions without the immediate death of the host cell. The trachoma biovar of *C. trachomatis* is unable to establish multiple cycles of infection in vitro in cell monolayers, greatly limiting its ability to propagate to high concentrations.

The infectious EB possesses a distinct outer membrane containing protein and lipopolysaccharide components. The major outer mem-

---

Obligate intracellular parasitism

Deficient in endogenous ATP production

Contain DNA, RNA, and typical prokaryotic ribosomes

Outer membrane similar to other Gram-negative bacteria

Dimorphic developmental cycle which takes place in an intracellular cytoplasmic inclusion

Small genome size (1.1–1.2 million nucleotides)

Phylogenetically distantly related to other bacteria

Table 4.1 Distinguishing features of chlamydiae.

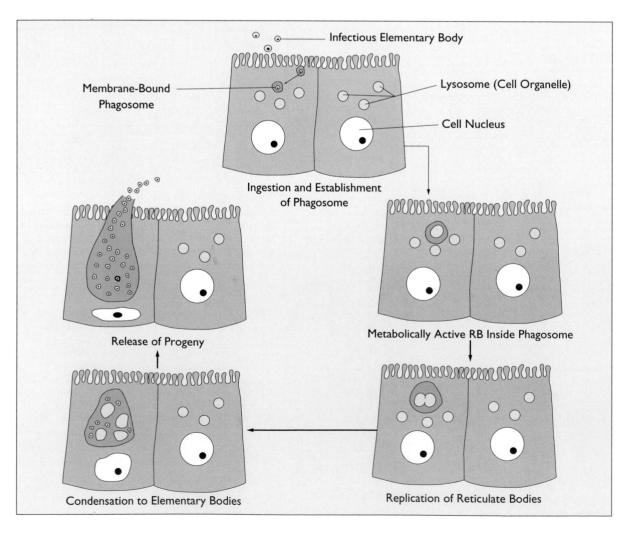

Fig. 4.2 Chlamydial development cycle. The infectious elementary body (EB) attaches to the host cell and is ingested by a process that is poorly understood. The EB resides within a membrane-bound endosome. The normal process of fusion with lysosomes is aborted, and transformation to the metabolically active reticulate body (RB) begins. Synthesis of chlamydial constituents and replication of the RB through binary fission occurs next. A chlamydial inclusion body containing numerous replicative forms can be seen 24–48 hours following infection. At 48–72 hours following infection, RBs condense to the spore-like EB. The inclusion body contains several hundred infectious particles at the peak of its maturation. The infectious progeny EBs are released from the infected host cell by extrusion of the inclusion body and/or by lysis of the host cell.

brane protein (MOMP) is a porin and comprises the bulk of the outer membrane protein.[1] The MOMP has an approximate subunit mass of 40 kDa, though the mass differs among the various serovars of *C. trachomatis*. Structural rigidity of the EB appears to be maintained by disulfide bonds among three cysteine-rich proteins (MOMP, OmpB and OmpA). Another protein of approximately 60 kDa is not structurally important, but is related to common heat-shock proteins and may have an immunopathogenic role. The MOMP is exposed on the surface of chlamydiae and has genus, species, subspecies, and serovar-specific epitopes. Other surface proteins are represented by members of a high molecular weight polymorphic membrane protein (Pmp) consisting of 9 distinct but related proteins with unknown function. The most prominent genus-specific antigen is the chlamydial lipopolysaccharide that resembles the rough lipopolysaccharide of Re ('deep rough') mutants of *Salmonella minnesota*.

C. trachomatis strains can be grouped by antiserum or monoclonal antibodies into 18 readily distinguished serovars. Endemic trachoma is usually associated with infection by serovars A, B, Ba, and C, while genital infection is usually caused by serovars B and D–K. Lymphogranuloma venereum infections (see Clinical Manifestations) are caused by the invasive LGV biovar which includes serovars L1–L3 (*Table 4.3*). Chlamydial genital infection by multiple serovars has been reported, and can be replaced *in vitro* (*Fig. 4.7*).

	C. trachomatis	*C. psittaci*	*C. pneumoniae*
HOST RANGE	Humans, mice	Non-human vertebrates	Humans
INCLUSION MORPHOLOGY	Granular, vacuolar	Lucent, dense	Dense
INCLUSION STAINING	Iodine +	Iodine –	Iodine –
ELEMENTARY BODY SHAPE	Coccoid	Coccoid	Pear-shaped
FOLATE ANTAGONISTS	Sensitive	Resistant	Resistant

Table 4.2 Distinguishing characteristics of *C. trachomatis*, *C. psittaci*, and *C. pneumoniae*.

Serovar	Disease
A, B, Ba, C	Endemic trachoma
B, D–K	Genitourinary disease
L1, L2, L3	LGV

Table 4.3 Diseases commonly associated with serovars of *C. trachomatis*.

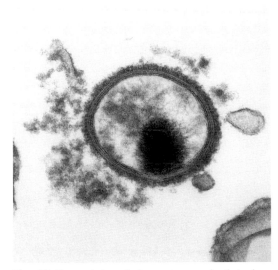

Fig. 4.3 Transmission electron micrograph of single *C. trachomatis* elementary body (× 120,000). Courtesy of Elizabeth H. White.

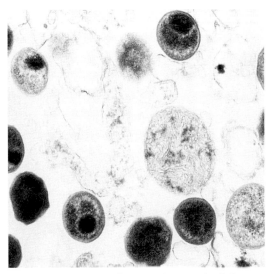

Fig. 4.4 Transmission electron micrograph of *C. trachomatis* elementary bodies outside the host cell. A single, electron-lucent reticulate body and a mitochondrion are also seen (× 67,500). Courtesy of Elizabeth H. White.

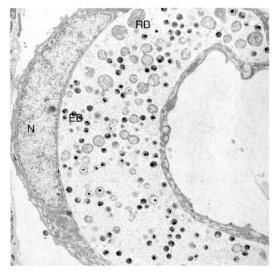

Fig. 4.5 A mature *C. trachomatis* inclusion displaces the host cell nucleus and includes various chlamydial developmental forms. N, nucleus; EB, elementary bodies; RB, dividing reticulate bodies. Courtesy of Wyrick PB, Gutman LT, Hodinka RL. Chlamydiae, in Joklik W *et al.* (eds): *Zinsser Microbiology*, ed. 19. New York: Appleton-Lange, 1983, pp 609–616.

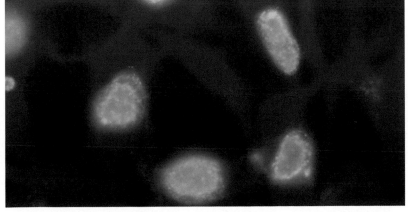

Fig. 4.6 Chlamydial inclusions in cell monolayer stained with fluorescein-labeled monoclonal antibody specific for *C. trachomatis*.

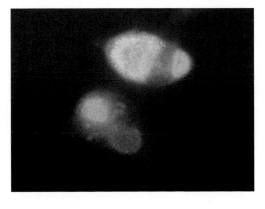

Fig. 4.7 HeLa cells infected simultaneously with two serovars of *C. trachomatis* and stained with two type-specific monoclonal antibodies, each labeled with a different fluorochrome. The upper cell shows two inclusions, one containing both serovars, illustrating that multiple serovars can coexist within the same host cell. Clinical examples of chlamydial infection by two serovars have been reported.

C. trachomatis EBs contain a plasmid that exhibits considerable similarity between serovars. This plasmid is approximately 7,500 base pairs in size, and has 8 open reading frames capable of encoding polypeptide products. Although the ubiquitous nature of this cryptic plasmid suggests that it may be functionally important, no virulence functions have been ascribed to it, and rare plasmid-free strains have been isolated from humans. The genome of *C. trachomatis* has been sequenced and encodes 894 proteins[6] (see STD Sequence Databases at http://www.stdgen.lanl.gov). Thus, chlamydiae have about 1/4 the coding capacity of a free-living organism such as *Escherichia coli*. Although the function of many of the proteins cannot yet be inferred, functions have been predicted for most of the encoded proteins which has enhanced our understanding of the physiology, molecular genetics and intracellular biology of chlamydiae (*Fig. 4.8*). Underrepresented in the chlamydial genome are capacities for amino acid biosynthesis and

nucleotide metabolism, precursors of which are obtained from the host cell. The identification of novel outer membrane proteins, virulence-associated proteins that were not anticipated, and regulatory mechanisms provides the basis for new research in infection and disease intervention strategies.

EPIDEMIOLOGY

Chlamydial infections are the most frequently occurring bacterial STDs in the USA (*Figs 4.9* and *4.10A,B*), and probably in most developed countries.[7,8] As testing is not uniform, and under-reporting is common, only crude estimates of the incidence of these infections are available, based on extrapolation of data from individual clinics. The US Public Health Service estimates about 3 million cases occur each year (*Table 4.4*). Data from private health care reports suggest that although cases of urethritis due to *Neisseria gonorrhoeae* have been decreasing, office visits by men with NGU — due in large part to *C. trachomatis* infection — have remained high (*Fig. 4.11*). Risk factors for chlamydial genitourinary infection are shown in *Table 4.5*.

The classic venereal disease caused by *Chlamydia* is lymphogranuloma venereum, or LGV.[2] This disease is rare in the USA but common in many developing countries, especially in Africa. *Figure 4.1* illustrates the number of cases of LGV reported to the CDC between 1966 and 1999. Most cases are imported, many from Central America.

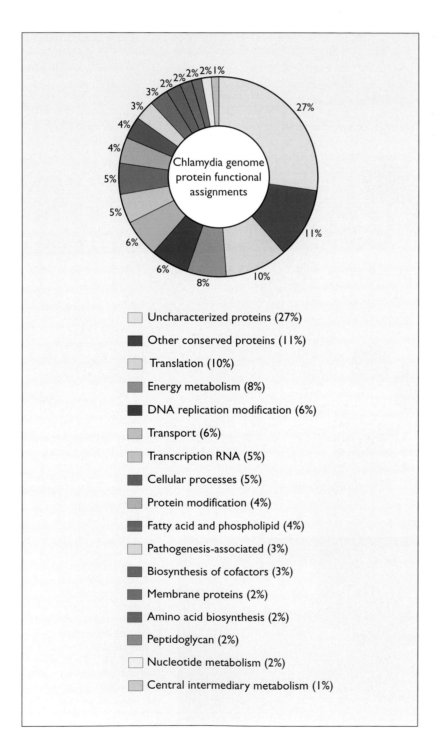

Uncharacterized proteins (27%)

Other conserved proteins (11%)

Translation (10%)

Energy metabolism (8%)

DNA replication modification (6%)

Transport (6%)

Transcription RNA (5%)

Cellular processes (5%)

Protein modification (4%)

Fatty acid and phospholipid (4%)

Pathogenesis-associated (3%)

Biosynthesis of cofactors (3%)

Membrane proteins (2%)

Amino acid biosynthesis (2%)

Peptidoglycan (2%)

Nucleotide metabolism (2%)

Central intermediary metabolism (1%)

Fig. 4.8 Functional attributes inferred from the *C. trachomatis* genome sequence.

Infection	Incidence
MALE	
Nongonoccal urethritis	1,550,000
Epididymitis	250,000
FEMALE	
Asymptomatic cervical infection	700,000
Symptomatic cervical infection	300,000
Pelvic inflammatory disease	300,000
NEONATAL	
Total infections	247,000
Conjunctivitis	74,000
Pneumonia	37,000

Table 4.4 Estimated annual incidence of *C. trachomatis* infections in the USA. Courtesy of NIH, NIAID Study Group of Sexually Transmitted Disease: 1980. Status report. Summaries and panel recommendations. Washington D.C.: U.S. Government Printing Office 1981: 215–264; and courtesy of Washington AE, Johnson RE, Sanders LL, Barnes RC, Alexander ER: Incidence of *Chlamydia trachomatis* in the United States: Using reported *Neisseria gonorrhoeae* as a surrogate, in Oriel D, Ridgway G, Schachter J, Taylor-Robinson D, Ward M (eds): *Chlamydial Infections*. Cambridge: Cambridge University Press, 1986, pp 487–490.

Patients with other STDs

Patients with chlamydia-associated syndromes

Sexual partners of patients with gonorrhea or chlamydia-associated syndromes

Younger patients

Patients with multiple sexual partners

Neonates born to infected mothers

Table 4.5 Patient groups at high risk for chlamydial STDs. Courtesy of Centers for Disease Control.

Genital infection with the trachoma biovar occurs in adults as a result of sexual transmission. In the 1980s, the USA witnessed substantial increases in hospitalizations of women for ectopic pregnancy (*Fig. 4.12*) (changes in management of ectopic pregnancy make more recent statistics less reliable) and involuntary infertility, particularly among populations at high risk for prior chlamydial infection. Studies of antibody prevalence to *Chlamydia* have shown that chlamydial exposure is approximately three times more common among women with tubal factor infertility or women having ectopic pregnancies as compared to control populations. *C. trachomatis* is recognized as a major cause of pelvic inflammatory disease (PID) (see Chapter 8). It is likely that these conditions result from tubal damage caused by chlamydial salpingitis. Many of the women suffering from tubal factor infertility or ectopic pregnancy have no prior history of PID. It is therefore likely that they have had a silent episode of salpingitis.

Ocular infection may accompany genital infection. In neonates, infection most commonly occurs during birth, by exposure to chlamydial organisms in the birth canal. Although infection of the genitals and conjunctivae are common, the mucosal surfaces of the pharynx, urethra, and rectum are also sites of chlamydial colonization. *C. trachomatis* infection may persist for years within the genital tracts of infected patients who have not been treated with antimicrobials. Some infants born to infected mothers may also have a clinically inapparent infection for years following birth.

As the causative agent of endemic trachoma, *C. trachomatis* is considered the world's leading cause of preventable blindness.[2]

CLINICAL MANIFESTATIONS

Infection by *C. trachomatis* can occur at several anatomic locations and cause a variety of distinct disease syndromes.[2,9] Several animal models of *C. trachomatis* genital infection have been used to explore the pathophysiology of chlamydial infection. Several models of pneumonitis have been developed in the mouse. Models of upper and lower genital tract infection have been developed using mice, guinea pigs, and nonhuman primates (*Figs 4.13–4.17*). The latter have also been used as an animal model for *C. trachomatis* rectal infections.

LYMPHOGRANULOMA VENEREUM

After genital inoculation, there is apparently systemic spread of the organism until localization in the genital or rectal lymph node tissues occurs. This infection of the lymphatics becomes locally invasive, and

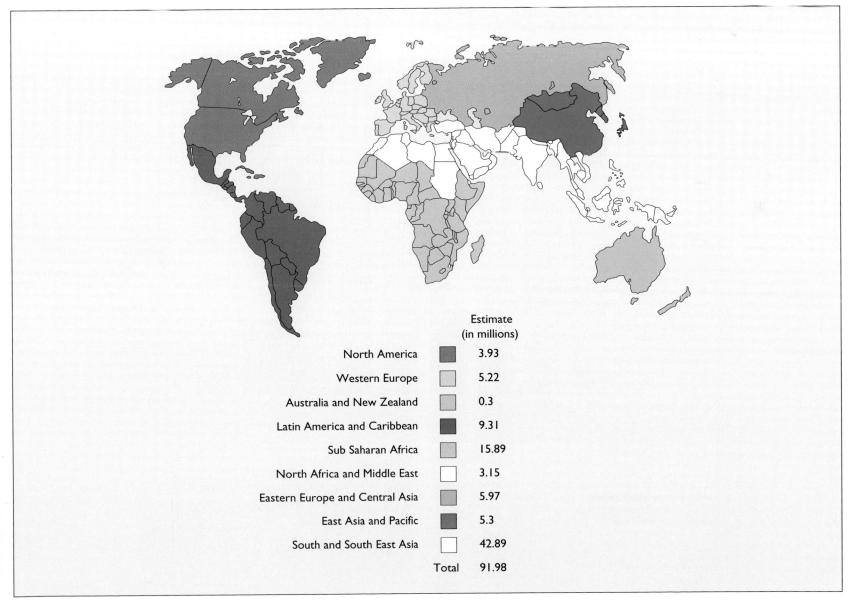

	Estimate (in millions)
North America	3.93
Western Europe	5.22
Australia and New Zealand	0.3
Latin America and Caribbean	9.31
Sub Saharan Africa	15.89
North Africa and Middle East	3.15
Eastern Europe and Central Asia	5.97
East Asia and Pacific	5.3
South and South East Asia	42.89
Total	91.98

Fig. 4.9 Estimated new cases of genital chlamydial infections by region among adults, 1999. Data are probably underestimates due to the relative insensitivity of most diagnostic tests used. Courtesy of JPA, WHO. Source: http://www.who.int/hiv_aids/stiglobalreport

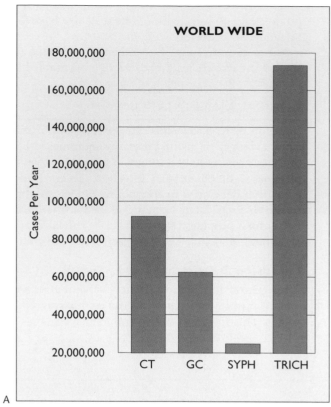

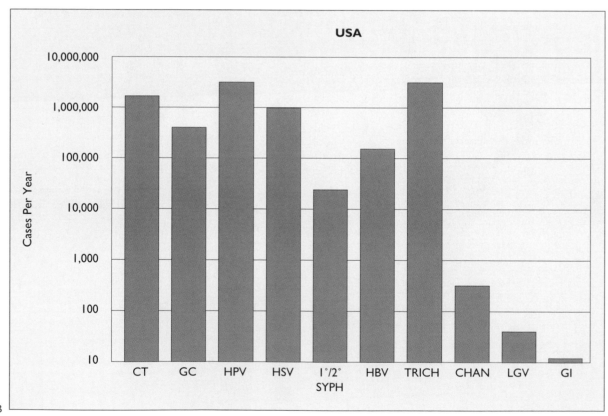

Fig. 4.10 (A) Estimated incidence of non-HIV STDs world-wide and (B) in the USA. Note the logarithmic scale.
Source
*Cates W Jr. Estimates of the incidence and prevalence of sexually transmitted diseases in the United States. Sex. Trarum Dis 1999; 26(suppl):S1–S7.
†Centers for Disease Control STD Surveillance, 1999
**http://www.WHO.INT/HIV_AIDS/STIGLOBALREPORT

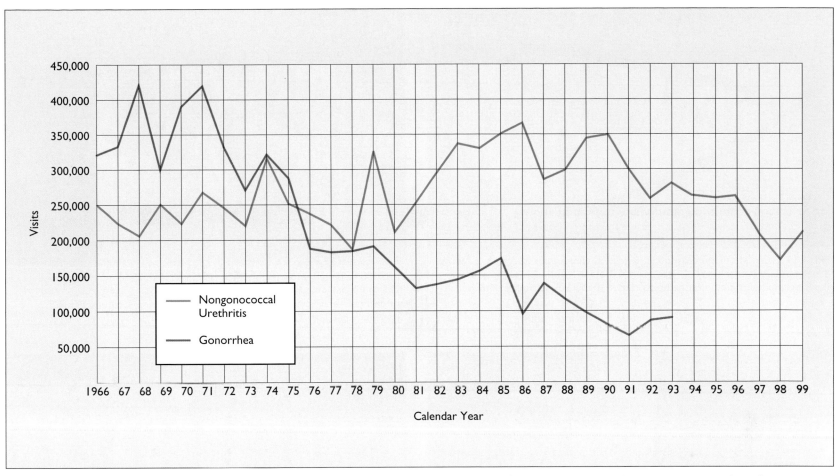

Fig. 4.11 Number of physicians' office visits for urethritis in the USA, from 1966 to 1999. Although visits by men with urethritis due to *Neisseria gonorrhoeae* have decreased, there has been a substantial increase in the number of visits for nongonococcal urethritis. These data suggest that chlamydial genitourinary infection may be increasing. Courtesy of Centers for Disease Control.

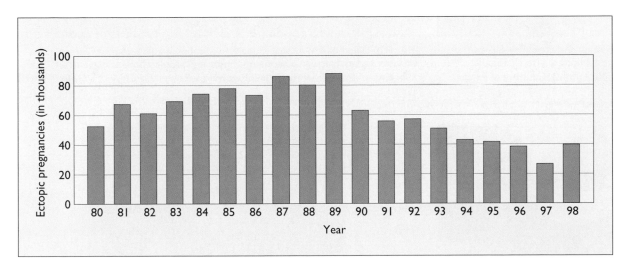

Fig. 4.12 Hospitalizations for ectopic pregnancy in the USA, 1980–1998. Courtesy of Centers for Disease Control.

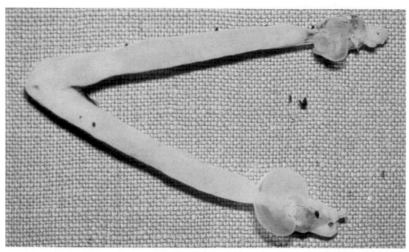

Fig. 4.13 Salpingitis in animal models. Resected reproductive tract from a mouse experimentally infected with *C. trachomatis*. Bilateral hydrosalpinx is seen at the distal extremities of both uterine horns. Courtesy of Julius Schachter, PhD.

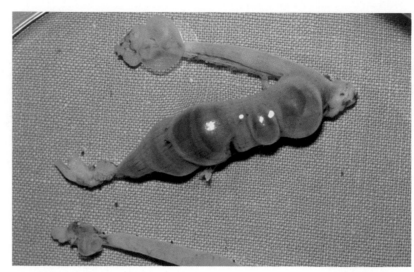

Fig. 4.14 Salpingitis in animal models. Specimen from a mouse impregnated following unilateral hydrosalpinx development. Embryos are implanted in the normal horn, while the hydrosalpinx side is unimplanted. Courtesy of Julius Schachter, PhD.

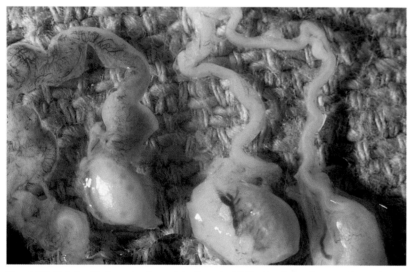

Fig. 4.15 Salpingitis in animal models. Resected fallopian tubes from guinea pigs, showing tubes inflamed and swollen with acute salpingitis due to chlamydial infection (left) compared with the uninfected control (right). Courtesy of Julius Schachter, PhD.

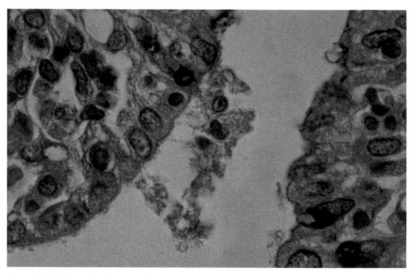

Fig. 4.16 Salpingitis in animal models. Immunoperoxidase stain of *C. trachomatis* inclusions (dark black) in a segment of monkey fallopian tube transplanted subcutaneously and stained 5 days following infection. Courtesy of Dorothy Patton, PhD.

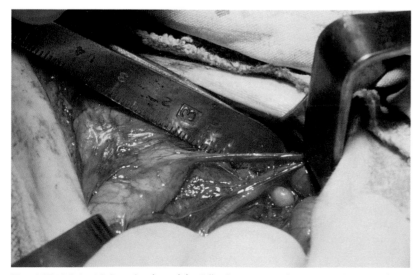

Fig. 4.17 Salpingitis in animal models. Adhesions seen at laparotomy in a monkey following experimentally induced *C. trachomatis* salpingitis. Such experimental animal models provide knowledge regarding mechanisms of scarring following salpingitis. Courtesy of Dorothy Patton, PhD.

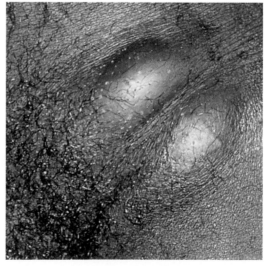

Fig. 4.18 'Groove sign' in a man with lymphogranuloma venereum (LGV). Although often said to be pathognomonic for LGV, this sign is seen infrequently in LGV patients and may be produced by other conditions. Courtesy of P. Morel, Hôpital Saint-Louis, Paris. See also Fig. 3.14.

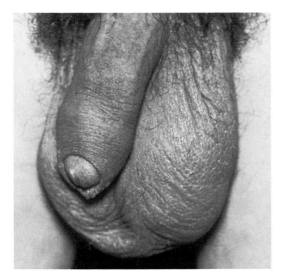

Fig. 4.19 Red, swollen scrotum of a man with chlamydial epididymitis. Courtesy of Richard E. Berger, MD, University of Washington.

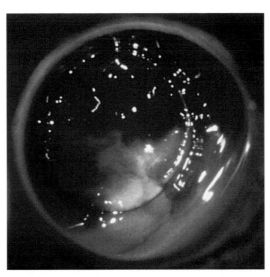

Fig. 4.20 Anoscopic view of rectal mucosa with area of focal purulence in a man with chlamydial proctitis. Courtesy of Walter E. Stamm, MD, University of Washington.

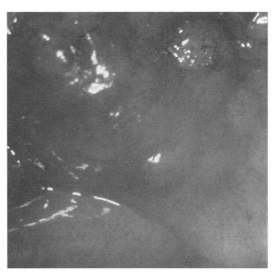

Fig. 4.21 Lymphoid follicular proctitis seen in a case of *C. trachomatis* rectal infection. Courtesy of Bingham JS: *Pocket Picture Guide to Clinical Medicine. Sexually Transmitted Diseases*. London, Gower Medical Publishing Ltd., 1984.

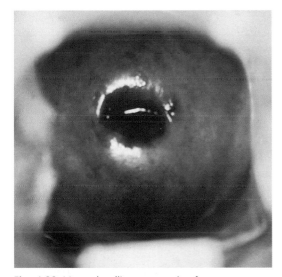

Fig. 4.22 Normal nulliparous cervix of a postmenarchal female, showing no cervical ectopy.

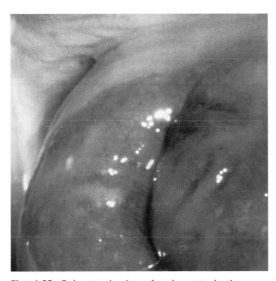

Fig. 4.23 Colposcopic view of early metaplastic changes in the cervical epithelium. This is a normal finding with sexual maturity. Courtesy of Fernando Guijon, MD.

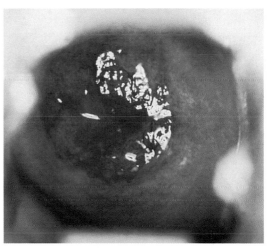

Fig. 4.24 Cervix showing effacement of the transitional zone (squamocolumnar junction) as might be observed in a young patient or in an oral contraceptive user. Courtesy of Paul Weisner, MD.

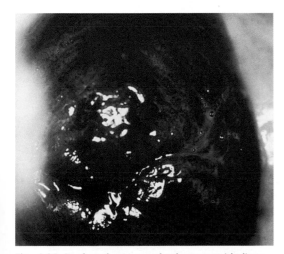

Fig. 4.25 Beefy red mucosa of columnar epithelium in chlamydial infection. Courtesy of Paul Weisner, MD.

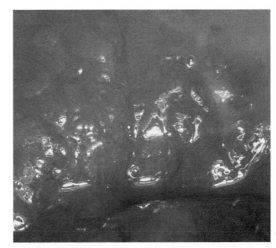

Fig. 4.26 Columnar epithelium cobblestoned by follicular changes of chlamydial infection. Courtesy of Bingham JS: *Pocket Picture Guide to Clinical Medicine. Sexually Transmitted Diseases*. London, Gower Medical Publishing Ltd., 1984.

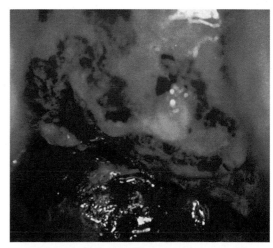

Fig. 4.27 Cervicitis showing purulent discharge from the os. Focal bleeding at areas previously touched during external cleansing of the cervix is evidence of friability.

is characterized by induration, multifocal suppuration, and fistula formation. Involvement of both femoral and inguinal lymph node groups, more frequent among infected men than women, can produce swelling on both sides of the inguinal ligament. The resulting 'groove sign' (*Fig. 4.18*) has been said to be pathognomonic of LGV, but occurs in only 10–15% of infected patients and has been described in a minority of patients with chancroid (see Chapter 3). LGV can produce chronic scarring and lymphedema, particularly if the rectum is infected. Scarring can produce long fibrotic narrowings of the colonic lumen.

URETHRITIS AND PROCTITIS IN MEN

Chlamydia causes about a third to a half of the infections in men presenting to STD clinics with urethral inflammation from which *N. gonorrhoeae* cannot be identified. The majority of men with chlamydial infection of the urethra have symptoms of urethral discharge, dysuria, or pruritus of the urethra. Up to 25% of men found upon culture screening to have urethral infection by *C. trachomatis* are asymptomatic. *Chlamydia* may cause acute epididymitis (*Fig. 4.19*), apparently due to infection ascending from the urethra. *Chlamydia* causes the majority of cases of epididymitis in young heterosexual men without anatomic anomalies of the genitourinary system.

In homosexual men, infection of the rectal mucosa by *C. trachomatis* can result in proctocolitis (*Figs 4.20* and *4.21*). Although infection is usually asymptomatic, infection by organisms of the more invasive LGV biovar can produce a more severe symptomatic form.

CERVICITIS AND URETHRITIS IN WOMEN

In women, *C. trachomatis* has been isolated from the cervix, the urethra, Bartholin's ducts, the fallopian tubes, the uterus, and the rectal mucosa. However, up to 70% of genital infections in women are asymptomatic. When symptoms of cervicitis and urethritis are described in association with proven infection of the cervix, they are nonspecific, and may include dysuria, vaginal discharge, or vaginal pruritus. Many studies have failed to associate specific symptoms with endocervical chlamydial infection. Upon examination of the infected patient, a mucopurulent cervical discharge and/or easily induced bleeding of the cervix (*Figs 4.22–4.28*) may be noted, though these signs are also neither sensitive nor specific for chlamydial infection. Sampling from the endocervical canal can produce gross evidence of purulent inflammation (*Figs 4.29–4.31*). *C. trachomatis* has been isolated from the urethra of women presenting with dysuria; it is also responsible for a proportion of abacteriuric pyuria in sexually active young women — the 'acute urethral syndrome.'

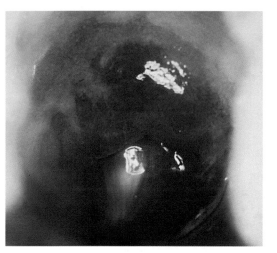

Fig. 4.28 Mucopurulent discharge seen coming from the cervical os following removal of ectocervical mucus. Endocervical swab from this patient was culture-positive for *C. trachomatis*. Courtesy of Lourdes Frau, MD.

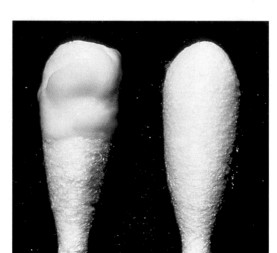

Fig. 4.29 Swab from the endocervical canal of a *Chlamydia*-infected woman (left) compared with fresh swab. The yellow–green exudate may reflect infection of the endocervix or endometrium. Courtesy of George Schmid, MD.

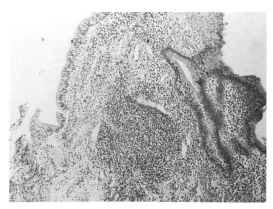
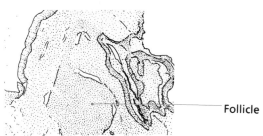

Fig. 4.30 Histologic image of *Chlamydia*-infected human cervix on biopsy, showing an intense follicular inflammatory infiltrate. Courtesy of Robert Brunham, MD (Kunimoto *et al.*) *Rev Infect Dis* 1985; **7**(5): 666.

Follicle

Fig. 4.31 Transmission electron micrograph, showing both a chlamydial inclusion and microabscess. Courtesy of John Swanson, MD. *J Infect Dis* 1975; **3**: 678–687.

Microabscess

Inclusion

SALPINGITIS AND PERIHEPATITIS

The most serious complication of chlamydial genital infection in women is acute salpingitis, presumably caused by ascent of the organism from the lower genital tract to the endometrium and fallopian tubes (*Fig. 4.32*) (see also Chapter 8). The clinical manifestations of upper reproductive tract infection by *C. trachomatis* are nonspecific, but can be severe, with fever, lower abdominal pain, prostration, and tenderness of the uterus and adnexae. Silent salpingitis may also be a result of chlamydial infection. A severe inflammatory response can be observed on laparoscopy involving the fallopian tubes and peritoneum (*Figs 4.33* and *4.34*). Peritoneal inflammation can result in hepatic capsular adhesions, which may produce the Fitz–Hugh–Curtis syndrome: pain, tenderness in the right upper quadrant, and occasionally a hepatic friction rub on auscultation (*Fig. 4.35*). In addition to the acute morbidity of PID, scarring of the tubal transport system following chlamydial salpingitis may lead to infertility and/or ectopic pregnancy (*Figs 4.36* and *4.37*).

PERINATAL INFECTIONS

Exposure to *C. trachomatis* during passage through an infected birth canal can cause infection in newborns (see Chapter 16).[8] The most common symptomatic illness of these children is a self-limited purulent conjunctivitis (*Fig. 4.38*), which usually occurs within three weeks following birth. About 20–30% of children born to infected mothers develop this infection. Approximately 10–20% of exposed children develop a distinctive pneumonitis syndrome.

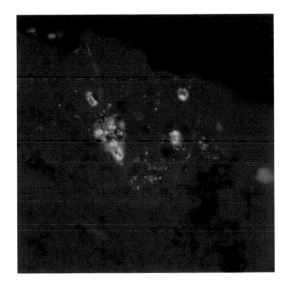

Fig. 4.32 Fluorescence micrograph showing chlamydial inclusions developing in an experimentally infected monkey fallopian tube. Chlamydial infection may ascend from the endocervix to the endometrium and fallopian tube epithelium. Courtesy of Dorothy Patton, PhD.

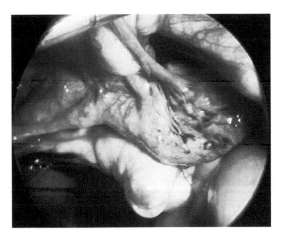

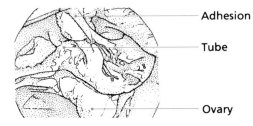

Fig. 4.33 Acute salpingitis. The fallopian tube is congested and swollen. A dense adhesion has formed between the ampulla of the tube and the pelvic sidewall.

Adhesion

Tube

Ovary

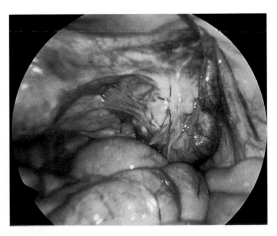

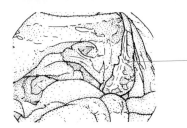

Swollen dye-filled tube

Fig. 4.34 Acute salpingitis. Hydrosalpinx with adhesions. Dye has been instilled into the grossly swollen fallopian tube on the right. Dense adhesions obscure the ovary.

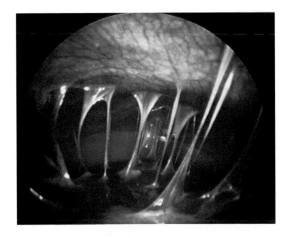

Fig. 4.35 Acute salpingitis. Laparoscopic view of 'violin-string' adhesions in a patient with perihepatitis (Fitz–Hugh–Curtis syndrome). Courtesy of Richard Sweet, MD, University of California.

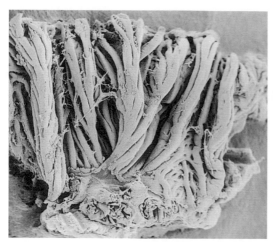

Fig. 4.36 Scanning electron micrograph of a monkey fallopian tube ampulla following experimental infection with *C. trachomatis*. Adhesions such as seen on both low power and magnified (Fig. 4.37) images are presumably responsible for the development of tubal obstruction with infertility and/or ectopic pregnancy. Courtesy of Dorothy Patton, PhD.

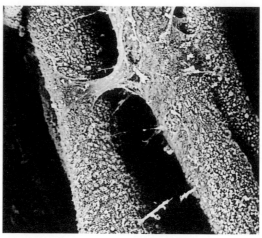

Fig. 4.37 Scanning electron micrograph of a monkey fallopian tube ampulla following experimental infection with *C. trachomatis* (see also Fig. 4.36). Courtesy of Dorothy Patton, PhD.

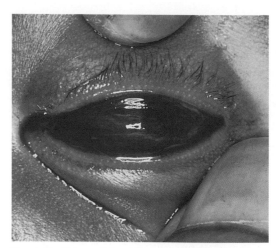

Fig. 4.38 Chlamydial ophthalmia neonatorum. Erythematous conjunctiva is seen in this infant.

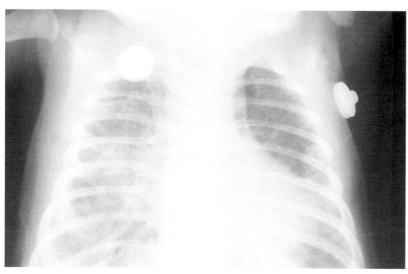

Fig. 4.39 Chlamydial pneumonitis. X-ray of a neonate showing the generalized patchy infiltrates. Courtesy of E.R. Alexander, MD.

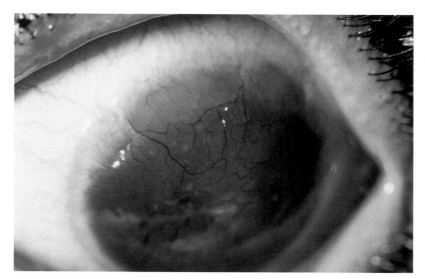

Fig. 4.40 Inflammatory infiltration and neovascularization of the cornea (pannus). Similar destructive lesions are infrequently observed in ocular infection by genital strains of *C. trachomatis* (paratrachoma). Courtesy of Spalton DJ, Hitchings RA, Hunter PA: *Atlas of Clinical Ophthalmology*. London, Gower Medical Publishing Ltd, 1984.

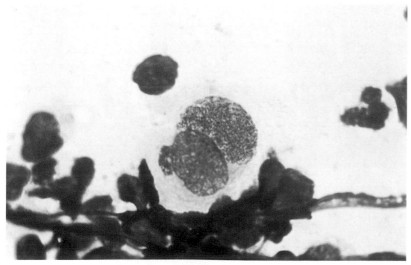

Fig. 4.41 Giemsa stain of an ocular scraping from a patient with trachoma, showing a *C. trachomatis* intracellular inclusion. Courtesy of Julius Schachter, PhD.

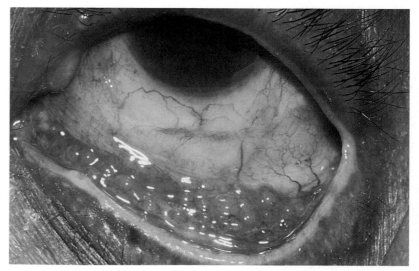

Fig. 4.42 Follicular conjunctivitis. Infection of the palpebral conjunctiva with lymphocytic follicle formation by *C. trachomatis*. Courtesy of George Waring, MD, Emory University.

The incubation period of the pneumonitis is variable, ranging from 2 weeks to 3 months. Infants generally show failure to thrive. Respiratory disease has an insidious onset, is afebrile and is characterized by a hacking nonproductive cough. The radiographic picture is not distinctive, but frequently shows hyperaeration and generalized interstitial changes (*Fig. 4.39*). *C. trachomatis* is the most commonly identified cause of infant pneumonitis in the first 6 months of life in the US.

OTHER CHLAMYDIAL INFECTIONS IN ADULTS

Ocular infection by *C. trachomatis* is not limited to perinatally acquired infection. Although not an STD, endemic trachoma is one of the most common causes of visual impairment in the developing world, causing millions of cases of blindness (*Figs 4.40* and *4.41*). Similarly, ocular infection in sexually active adults can occur frequently, probably as a consequence of genital–ocular autoinoculation. This infection is usually self-limiting and without severe sequelae, though a distinctive follicular conjunctivitis can result (*Fig. 4.42*).

Genital infection by *C. trachomatis* has been associated in serologic studies with the development of reactive arthropathy in Reiter's syndrome, which consists of conjunctivitis, urethritis, and arthritis (*Fig. 4.43*). Chlamydial particles and nucleic acids have been detected in joint aspirates from patients with this postinfectious arthropathy, suggesting that direct infection of the joint space may produce this complication. Reiter's syndrome is a chronic, fluctuating disease that may have striking rheumatologic and dermatologic presentations (*Figs 4.44* and *4.45*). See also Figs 1.59 and 1.60.

In humans, uncomplicated genital infection by *C. trachomatis* produces few diagnostic symptoms and signs. Similarly, a number of organisms can be responsible for PID. The lack of specific clinical criteria in the diagnosis of chlamydial infection mandates laboratory diagnosis in almost all cases of infection.

EFFECTS OF *CHLAMYDIA* CONTROL PROGRAMS

Where *Chlamydia* control programs have been in effect for a number of years there has been a reduction in prevalence of *Chlamydia* and the percentage of the different diseases that could be attributed to *Chlamydia* may be markedly reduced.[8] For example, nongonoccocal urethritis in heterosexual men typically has chlamydial infection rates of 25–35%. But recovery of *C. trachomatis* may be as low as 10–15% when control programs are in effect and predictably over time could reach figures that are even lower. Infant infections are largely preventable through programs that screen pregnant women and treat those found to be infected.[10]

PATHOLOGY

Histopathology

Histopathologic characteristics of chlamydial infection include chronic inflammation and fibrotic changes with granulation. In many sites, the response to infection includes follicle formation. Left untreated, these processes lead to morbid complications regardless of location of the infection. In LGV, there is local acute and granulomatous inflammation in involved lymph nodes, often with formation of stellate abscesses (*Fig. 4.46*). One underlying basis for pathology is the response of cells infected with chlamydiae to produce and persistently secrete potent mediators of inflammation that are amplified by the host immune response network.[14] Infected cells also secrete growth factors that likely promote fibrotic changes and tissue remodeling (e.g., scarring).

LABORATORY TESTS

The diagnosis of endemic trachoma can usually be made by an experienced clinician on the basis of patient history and physical examination. The diagnosis of *C. trachomatis* genital infection, however, is dependent upon specific laboratory identification.[11] Infection is asymptomatic in the majority of infected women, and a substantial proportion of infected men. In addition, the symptoms and signs of infection are highly variable when present, and may be caused by other infectious agents or by noninfectious processes. The medical history and physical examination, while necessary in every instance, are neither sensitive nor specific enough to identify infected patients.

Isolation of *Chlamydia* in eggs or cell culture was originally the only practical method for detection of infection. Thereafter, the development of monoclonal antibodies directed against the organism and increased knowledge about the components of the EB resulted in new tests capable of detecting the presence of chlamydial antigen in clinical specimens. The introduction of antigen detection methods in the early 1980s was followed by a nucleic acid hybridization test. These tests were

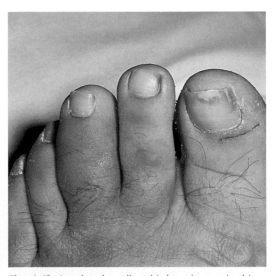

Fig. 4.43 A red and swollen third toe is seen in this photograph of the foot of a man presenting with Reiter's syndrome arthritis. Courtesy of Robert Wilkens, MD.

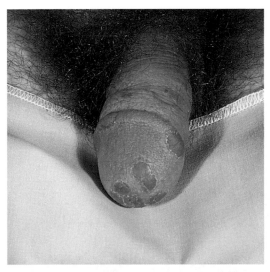

Fig. 4.44 Scaling erythematous plaques on the penis. Circinate balanitis of Reiter's syndrome. This is one of the infrequent but distinctive cutaneous findings associated with this syndrome. Courtesy of Robert Wilkens, MD.

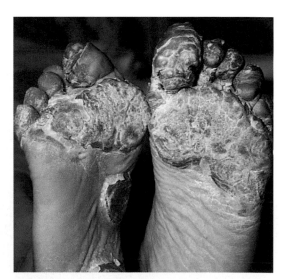

Fig. 4.45 Keratoderma blenorrhagica in Reiter's syndrome. Note the thick scales and crusts on the feet of this patient. Courtesy of Dorothy Patton, PhD.

widely accepted and made diagnosis of *C. trachomatis* genital infection a part of the routine clinical laboratory armamentarium.[12] In the mid 1990s, nucleic acid amplification tests (NAATs) were introduced. These were far more sensitive than any previously existing technology and provided tools for the screening of asymptomatic individuals because the tests could be applied to specimens that were collected on a non-invasive basis.[13] These included first catch urine specimens and vaginal swabs from women.

SPECIMEN COLLECTION

Proper collection of a specimen for culture is essential for successful results. A fiber-tipped swab is the most commonly used instrument for collection of a clinical specimen. Swab shafts should be made of inert material, preferably plastic or metal. Soluble components eluting from wooden shafts may be cytotoxic for chlamydial cell culture systems.

Swab tips made of cotton or dacron appear to be less inhibitory to propagation than tips of nylon or alginate; however, individual lots of swabs should be tested to assure a lack of toxicity to cell monolayers and of chlamydial growth. Collection devices resembling biopsy brushes have been developed to improve the sensitivity of sample collection from the endocervix. For enzyme immunoassays and DNA detection tests, it is imperative that manufacturers' instructions concerning appropriate collection methods are followed. There may be specific requirements for swab types to assure optimal performance of the tests. Typical sample collection instruments are shown in *Figure 4.47*.

Transport media for chlamydial culture may contain buffered salt solution, sucrose, and antibiotics that do not inhibit *Chlamydia* such as vancomycin, gentamicin, and nystatin. Many laboratories add fetal bovine serum to the media to enhance specimen recovery.

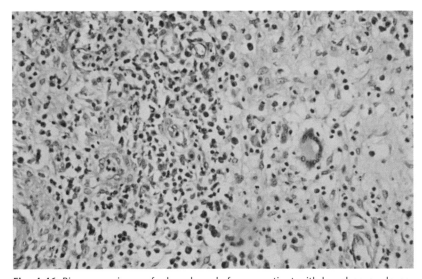

Fig. 4.46 Biopsy specimen of a lymph node from a patient with lymphogranuloma venereum showing acute and chronic inflammation with occasional multinucleate giant cells.

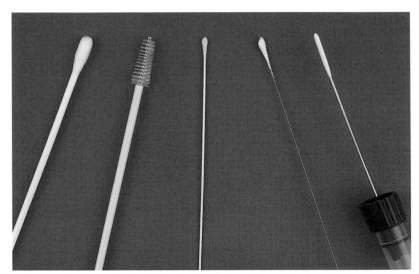

Fig. 4.47 Various instruments available for sampling for *Chlamydia* from the genitourinary tract. Left to right: The large-diameter cotton or dacron swab on a nontoxic plastic shaft and the brushlike device are satisfactory for endocervical sampling, though the latter is more traumatic. Urethral specimens may be obtained with the rigid aluminum-shafted swab or a flexible, steel, cotton-tipped device. An example of a swab for urethral enzyme immunoassay is seen on the far right.

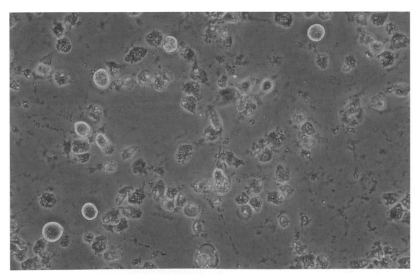

Fig. 4.48 Cytotoxicity in cell culture. Cells exhibit a round morphology and have sloughed from the cover slip, resulting in a diffuse cytopathic effect.

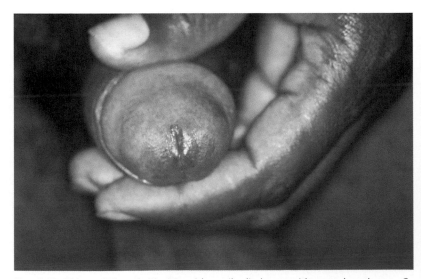

Fig. 4.49 Chlamydial urethritis. Mucoid, penile discharge with meatal erythema. *C. trachomatis* was isolated whereas *N. gonorrhoeae* was not. Courtesy of Woodruff JD, Parmley TH: Atlas of Gynecologic Pathology. New York, Gower Medical Publishing, 1988.

The organism may be difficult to isolate from specimens containing excess mucus or inflammatory cells, such as from bubo aspirates in patients with LGV. Likewise, components in semen are toxic to cell culture systems (*Fig. 4.48*). *C. trachomatis* can exhibit direct cytotoxicity to cell monolayers when inoculated at high multiplicities of infection. Cytopathic effects seen in clinical specimens are unlikely to be due to *Chlamydia*, as the number of organisms in clinical samples is probably never sufficient to produce this effect. Cytotoxicity, due to collection or transport system components, or to semen components, inflammatory cells, or genital microorganisms other than *Chlamydia*, may interfere with cell culture identification of *Chlamydia* in up to 5% of specimens from STD clinics. Dilution of such specimens prior to attempting cell culture has improved organism recovery.

Once collected, specimens should be refrigerated at 4°C and inoculated into cell culture within 48 hours. If specimens must be stored for longer periods prior to culture, they should be frozen at temperatures below –70°C.

GRAM STAIN
The diagnosis of NGU in men is usually based on the clinical presentation of scanty urethral discharge (*Fig. 4.49*) and a Gram stain of urethral exudate. The Gram stain is sensitive and specific for the diagnosis of gonorrhea (*Fig. 4.50*). Many men with gonococcal urethritis also have chlamydial infection. Thus only the absence of intracellular Gram-negative diplococci in the presence of an inflammatory exudate (*Fig. 4.51*) is useful in microscopically distinguishing NGU from gonorrhea.

CELL CULTURE
The typical procedure for isolation of *C. trachomatis* by cell culture is seen in *Figure 4.52*. If frozen, specimens to be cultured are thawed at 37°C and mixed. The specimen is inoculated onto the surface of confluent monolayers of susceptible cells. Commonly used cells include McCoy, HeLa 229, and BHK lines. The inoculated cell monolayers are centrifuged at room temperature at 2,000–3,000 g to improve the sensitivity of the culture. Following inoculation and centrifugation, the monolayer is overlaid with pre-warmed growth medium. Cycloheximide is included to increase the number and size of chlamydial inclusions by inhibiting host cell protein synthesis.

After incubation of the inoculated cell monolayer for 48–72 hours, characteristic inclusions may be observed. The inclusion of *C. trachomatis* is surrounded by a distinct membrane and is visible under direct microscopic examination, particularly when using phase microscopy. The inclusions may be visualized by staining with iodine, Giemsa, acridine orange, fluorescein-conjugated monoclonal or polyclonal antibody preparations, or with immunochemical stains using enzyme-conjugated antichlamydial monoclonal antibodies (*Figs 4.53–4.60*). The most common stains used are iodine and fluorescein-labeled antibodies. Staining with fluorescein-labeled monoclonal antibodies to the MOMP of *C. trachomatis* is more sensitive and specific than iodine staining. Iodine stains intracellular glycogen, which is maximal at 40–60 hours following infection with the trachoma biovar. Although inexpensive and easily performed, iodine stains are more subject to artifact due to aberrant staining of nonchlamydial material.

Isolation of *Chlamydia* in cell culture is relatively insensitive. Studies using multiple sampling in the same patient or repeated passage of inoculated host cells have suggested that a single endocervical swab may detect infection in only 70% of infected women. Additional sampling of women using a urethral swab has been shown to improve the sensitivity substantially. More recently, comparative studies with NAATs have shown that culture typically has a sensitivity of 50% to 70%.

DIRECT FLUORESCENT ANTIBODY DETECTION
Detection of *C. trachomatis* infection by nonculture methods (antigen detection) became feasible with the development of immunologic reagents specific for chlamydial outer membrane components. Direct fluorescent antibody (DFA) detection uses one or more monoclonal antibodies (MAbs) conjugated to fluorescent molecules as shown in *Figure 4.61*. Monoclonal antibodies directed against species, subspecies, and genus (lipopolysaccharide) specific antigens have been developed for this method. Data to date suggest that monoclonal antibodies reacting to the chlamydial MOMP produce superior staining and characteristic morphology compared with anti-lipopolysaccharide antibodies. As with chlamydial cultures, proper technique in the collection of the clinical specimen is necessary to ensure adequate test performance. Upon addition to a specimen smear, these reagents bind to chlamydial EBs, producing brightly fluorescing and morphologically distinctive dots. Several to several hundred organisms may be seen in any smear (*Fig. 4.62*). The sensitivity of the DFA method in comparison with cell culture has varied in published studies, but averages 80–90% in women and symptomatic men. When a cutoff value for positive test results of 10 EB is used, the test specificity will be approximately 97–98% in experienced, expert laboratories.

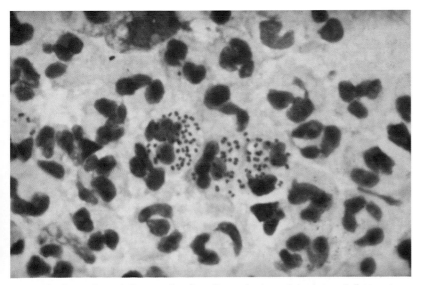

Fig. 4.50 Gonorrhea. A Gram stain of penile urethral exudate shows inflammatory cells containing gonococci.

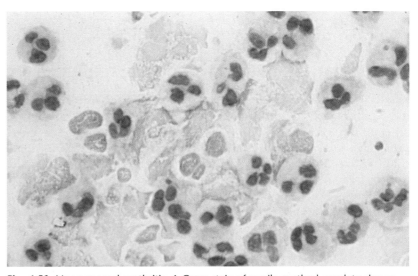

Fig. 4.51 Nongonoccal urethritis. A Gram stain of penile urethral exudate shows inflammatory cells without visible gonococci. Courtesy of Francisco J. Candal.

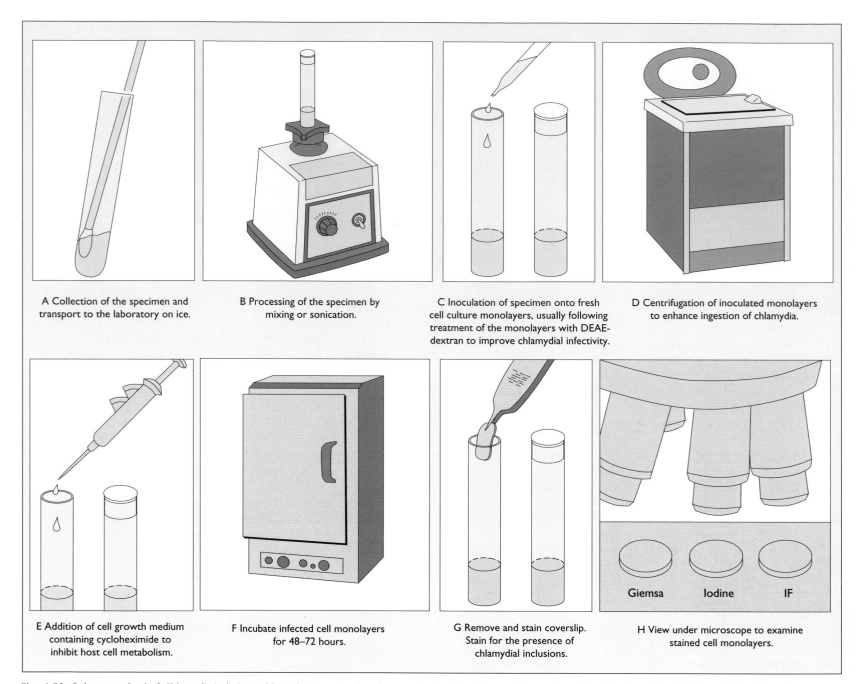

Fig. 4.52 Culture method of *Chlamydia* isolation. Although recognized as the standard method for sensitive and specific laboratory identification of *C. trachomatis* organisms, the required skill and laboratory resources, coupled with the 2–7 days' turnaround for results, has made less demanding techniques generally more acceptable for routine clinical diagnosis.

A significant advantage of the DFA method is the lack of necessity for rapid transportation of specimens to the laboratory and maintenance of a cold chain, since slides can be fixed and mailed to a central laboratory for staining and interpretation. In addition, the cellular background observed on the smear allows microscopists to reject slides without sufficient cellular material from the endocervix (*Figs 4.63–4.65*). Some studies have shown that up to 10% of all specimens are inadequate for the DFA method, suggesting that inadequate specimen collection contributes significantly to the insensitive nature of all *Chlamydia* detection methods. Disadvantages of the DFA method include the need for a trained microscopist, who must devote several minutes to the interpretation of each specimen, and the need for a fluorescence microscope. Some artifacts have been noted to occur as a result of cross-reactivity of reagents with nonchlamydial organisms (*Figs 4.66* and *4.67*), but an experienced microscopist is rarely confused by these.

ENZYME IMMUNOASSAY

Other methods for the detection of chlamydial components use *Chlamydia*-specific or second antibodies labeled with an enzyme. Following incubation of a specimen with the antibody preparation, an enzyme substrate is added to generate a colored product, which can be detected visually or photometrically (*Figs 4.68* and *4.69*). These enzyme immunoassay (EIA) tests can be designed to allow testing of numerous specimens for chlamydial antigen. EIA tests, like the DFA method, are less sensitive than culture methods; they are also somewhat less specific than the DFA method. The advantages of EIAs include the high-throughput capability for screening large numbers of patients, and due to the objective nature of the test results, the lack of requirement for highly skilled personnel to interpret the information. The reagents for EIAs are expensive, costing $3–$7 per test. Tests based upon the reactivity of polyvalent antisera with chlamydial lipopolysaccharide

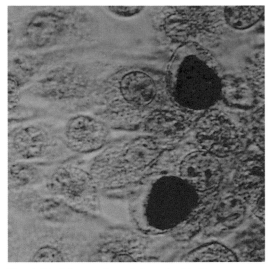

Fig. 4.53 Cell monolayer infected with *C. trachomatis*. Dark-red inclusions are positive in this specimen stained with Jones' iodine.

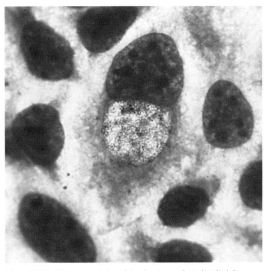

Fig. 4.54 Giemsa-stained inclusions (bright-field) showing the open, granular nature of an intracellular inclusion of *C. trachomatis*. Compare this with the dense inclusions seen with TWAR and *C. psittaci* (Fig. 4.56). Courtesy of Billie R. Bird.

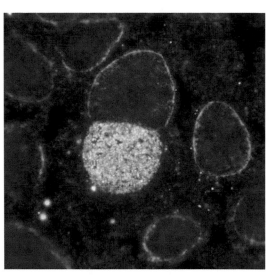

Fig. 4.55 Giemsa-stained inclusions (dark-field) showing the open, granular nature of an intracellular inclusion of *C. trachomatis*. Compare this with the dense inclusions with TWAR and *C. psittaci* (Fig. 4.56). Courtesy of Billie R. Bied.

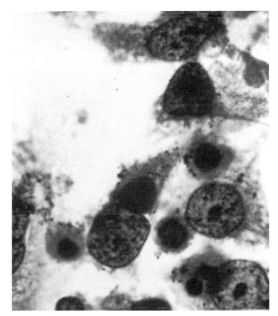

Fig. 4.56 Giemsa-stained inclusions (bright-field) showing the dense inclusion seen in TWAR and *C. psittaci* following staining. Courtesy of Billie R. Bird.

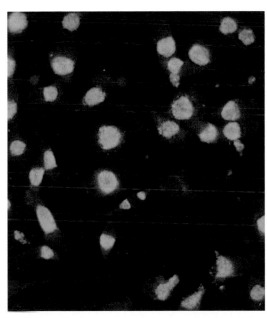

Fig. 4.57 Chlamydial inclusions in cycloheximide-treated McCoy cell monolayers stained with a fluorescein-labeled genus-specific monoclonal antibody. *C. trachomatis* inclusions occur individually. Courtesy of Shannon Mitchell and Janice C. Bullard.

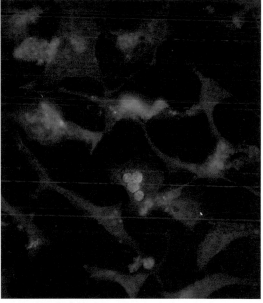

Fig. 4.58 Chlamydial inclusions in cycloheximide-treated McCoy cell monolayers stained with a fluorescein-labeled genus-specific monoclonal antibody. *C. psittaci* or TWAR may produce multiple or multilobed inclusions within a single infected cell. Courtesy of Shannon Mitchell and Janice C. Bullard.

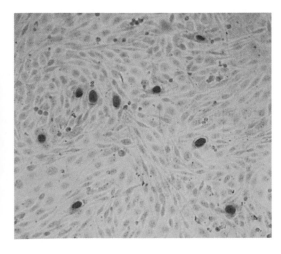

Fig. 4.59 Distinct red chlamydial inclusions detected using an alkaline-phosphatase monoclonal antibody method with naphthol-AS chromogenic substrate (original magnification × 250). Courtesy of James Mahoney, PhD.

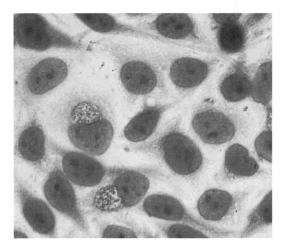

Fig. 4.60 Black, granular *C. trachomatis* inclusion produced using peroxidase-labeled monoclonal antibody and 1-chloro-4-naphthol chromogenic substrate (original magnification × 400). Courtesy of Robert Suchland.

Fig. 4.61 Direct fluorescent antibody detection of *C. trachomatis*.

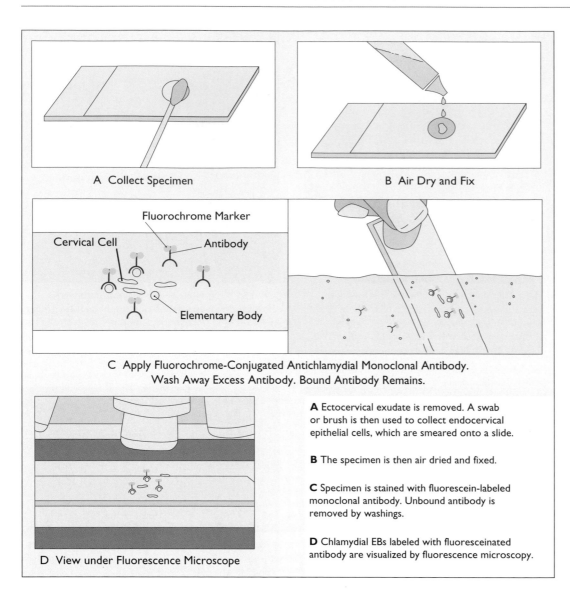

A Collect Specimen

B Air Dry and Fix

Fluorochrome Marker

Cervical Cell

Antibody

Elementary Body

C Apply Fluorochrome-Conjugated Antichlamydial Monoclonal Antibody.
Wash Away Excess Antibody. Bound Antibody Remains.

D View under Fluorescence Microscope

A Ectocervical exudate is removed. A swab or brush is then used to collect endocervical epithelial cells, which are smeared onto a slide.

B The specimen is then air dried and fixed.

C Specimen is stained with fluorescein-labeled monoclonal antibody. Unbound antibody is removed by washings.

D Chlamydial EBs labeled with fluoresceinated antibody are visualized by fluorescence microscopy.

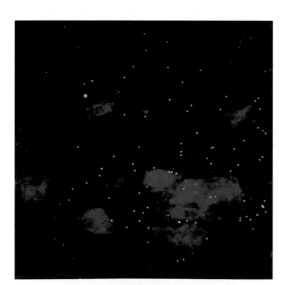

Fig. 4.62 Direct fluorescent antibody stain of chlamydia elementary bodies from a smear of cervical exudate (× 630). Courtesy of Howard Soule, PhD, Kallestad Diagnostics.

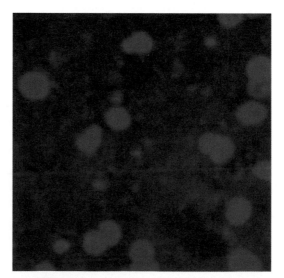

Fig. 4.63 Normal endocervical epithelial cells stained with a commercial chlamydial DFA reagent. The presence of such cells indicates the satisfactory quality of the sample collection to the microscopist (× 630). Courtesy of Janice C. Bullard, Centers for Disease Control.

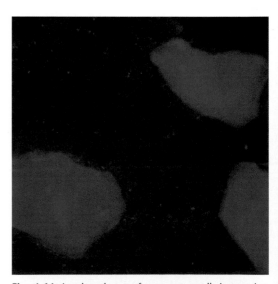

Fig. 4.64 An abundance of squamous cells is seen in this genital specimen from a women. This indicates that specimen collection has been unsatisfactory (× 630). Courtesy of Janice C. Bullard, Centers for Disease Control.

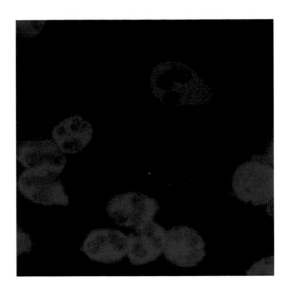

Fig. 4.65 Inflammatory cells stained as in Fig. 4.63 (× 630).

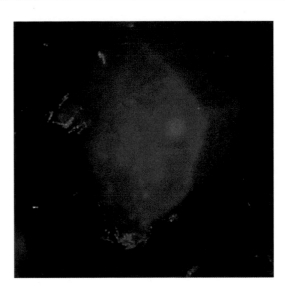

Fig. 4.66 Example of cross-reacting microorganisms seen in a clinical specimen stained with a chlamydial MOMP-specific monoclonal antibody. Such artifacts are uncommon and are not confusing to an experienced microscopist. Courtesy of Janice C. Bullard, Centers for Disease Control.

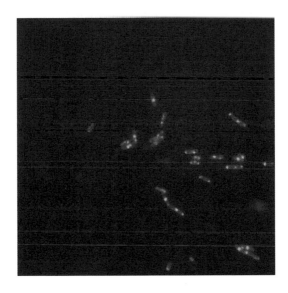

Fig. 4.67 Another artifactual example of cross-reacting microorganisms in a clinical specimen stained with a chlamydial MOMP-specific monoclonal antibody. Courtesy of Linda Cles.

may cross-react with those bacteria of the gastrointestinal tract that share common lipopolysaccharide antigenic determinants. For this reason, these tests are limited to those sites not potentially contaminated by gastrointestinal flora. The specificity of the EIA tests has been improved by the introduction of confirmatory blocking tests. In these procedures, all positive results are repeated in the presence of antibodies that will inhibit the specific anti-chlamydial reaction. If the EIA test result is adequately reduced, the initial positive result is confirmed.

Rapid or 'point-of-care' tests

Rapid tests are performed in physician's offices, do not require sophisticated equipment, and can yield results in about 30 minutes. Some of these tests are lateral flow immunoassays that employ membrane capture technology (*Fig. 4.70*). Like some EIAs, the first-generation rapid tests use antibodies against lipopolysaccharide antigens that detect all chlamydial species and are subject to the same potential for false-positive results due to cross-reactivity with lipopolysaccharide antigens of other microorganisms. In general, rapid tests are less sensitive and specific than laboratory-performed EIAs. Since the rapid tests are designed to be performed by non-laboratory personnel, quality assurance is essential. Rapid tests should not be used in low-prevalence populations, for asymptomatic individuals, or for general screening due to the potential for both false-positive and false-negative results.

According to current guidelines, positive nonculture EIA and DFA test results in high-risk populations, such as in STD clinics, are acceptable. In all other settings, confirmatory tests (either blocking tests or use of other tests aimed at a different antigen or molecule) are needed. Thus, all positive results are considered presumptive until confirmed in low- to moderate-prevalence screening situations. In cases where there are legal ramifications, such as child abuse, incest, rape, etc., the use of culture is mandated and nonculture tests should not be used.

SEROLOGY

Although not occurring in every case of uncomplicated genital infection, antibody to *C. trachomatis* usually occurs following infection and persists for years. IgM responses can be seen in first episodes of infection. These antibody responses have been used for decades to diagnose chlamydial infection.

Complement Fixation

With the availability of high-quality antigen in the 1940s, the chlamydial group complement fixation (CF) test was developed. The CF test uses the chlamydial 'group' antigen to detect serum antibody to any of the members of this genus. This test is still used in the diagnosis of LGV, in which a negative single-serum test rules out the disease, and in ornithosis, in which a change in titer between acute and convalescent sera can be diagnostic.

Microimmunofluorescence

The limited sensitivity and genus specificity of the CF test limits its use in seroepidemiologic studies. The development of the microimmunofluorescence (MIF) test in the 1970s allowed studies of the clinical epidemiology of chlamydial infection.[15] The MIF uses fixed, purified chlamydial antigens, which are dotted onto a glass slide and reacted with the patient serum (*Figs 4.71* and *4.72*). The test is sensitive, and usually provides information regarding the infecting serotype in *C. trachomatis* infections. It is also capable of determining IgM responses characteristic of acute infection, and is of particular use in the diagnosis of infant chlamydial pneumonia. However, the technique is laborious and technically demanding, and interpretation requires extensive experience. Less demanding ELISA tests or inclusion–indirect immunofluorescence tests using a single serovar have been described or are available commercially, but have not been critically examined in large clinical trials. Several studies have indicated the association of local antibody in acute chlamydial disease, and serum IgA has been suggested to predict infection; however, these tests have not been sufficiently researched to be recommended. Due primarily to the background prevalence of

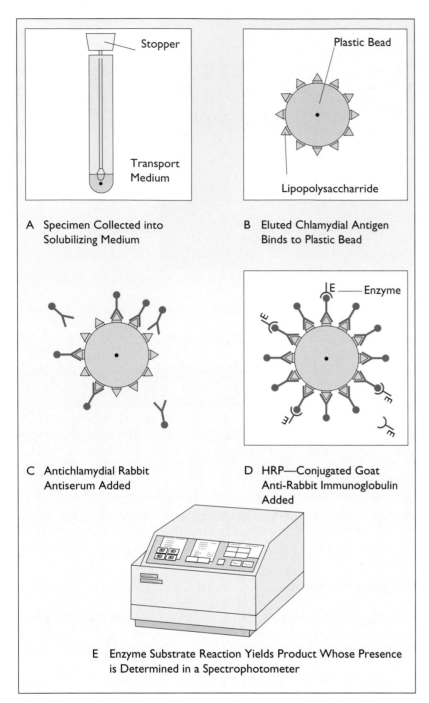

Fig. 4.68 Detection of *Chlamydia* by enzyme immunoassay (EIA), using direct antigen capture technique.

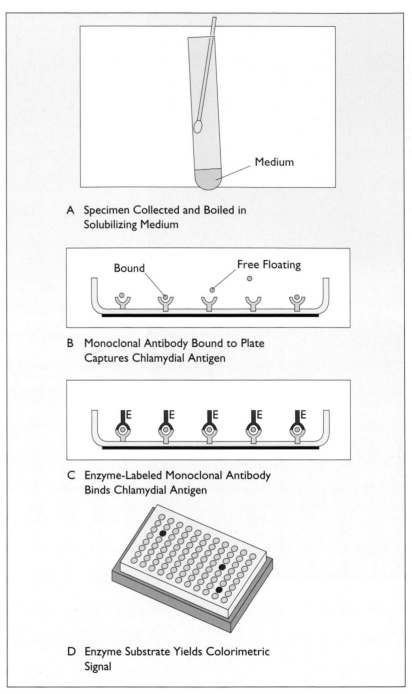

Fig. 4.69 Detection of *Chlamydia* by enzyme immunoassay (EIA), using the MAb sandwich antigen capture technique.

chlamydial infections, serologic diagnosis of *C. trachomatis* infection has limited utility (*Table 4.6*).

PAPANICOLAOU SMEAR

Another method advocated by some for the laboratory diagnosis of chlamydial infection is examination of Papanicolaou-stained cervical smears (Pap smear). The detection of intact chlamydial inclusions in the Pap smear is insensitive. In addition, the cytologic changes that accompany *C. trachomatis* cervical infection are nonspecific. For these reasons, the Pap smear cannot be used to diagnose chlamydial endocervical infection; however, the finding of inflammatory cells may indicate the need for specific chlamydial testing.

NUCLEIC ACID PROBE AND AMPLIFICATION TESTS

Straightforward detection of nonamplified chlamydial nucleic acid, including commercially available probes, which detect ribosomal RNA,

Test	Diagnostic use	Performance
Complement fixation	LGV Ornithosis	Sensitive but not specific. Can rule out LGV if negative.
Microimmunofluorescence	LGV Infant pneumonia	Sensitive but not specific. IgM responses in majority of cases.
ELISA	Unknown	Sensitivity and specificity undefined. Various methods not standardized.

Table 4.6 Uses of serology in *Chlamydia* diagnosis.

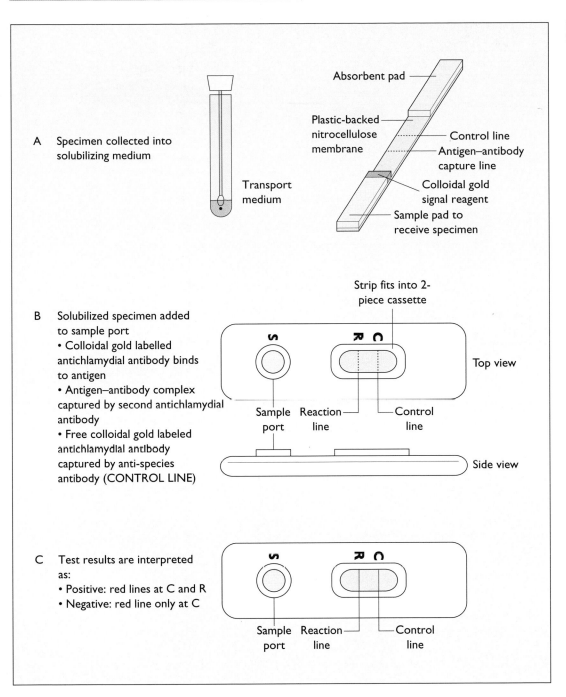

Fig. 4.70 Detection of *Chlamydia* by a lateral flow immunoassay.

A Specimen collected into solubilizing medium

Transport medium

Absorbent pad

Plastic-backed nitrocellulose membrane

Control line

Antigen–antibody capture line

Colloidal gold signal reagent

Sample pad to receive specimen

B Solubilized specimen added to sample port
• Colloidal gold labelled antichlamydial antibody binds to antigen
• Antigen–antibody complex captured by second antichlamydial antibody
• Free colloidal gold labeled antichlamydial antibody captured by anti-species antibody (CONTROL LINE)

Strip fits into 2-piece cassette

Top view

Sample port Reaction line Control line

Side view

C Test results are interpreted as:
• Positive: red lines at C and R
• Negative: red line only at C

Sample port Reaction line Control line

is less sensitive than culture. These tests (see Appendix 4) appear to have a sensitivity of the same order as the modern EIAs. In contrast, the amplified DNA tests are more sensitive than culture for detection of urethral *C. trachomatis* infection in men and cervical infection in women (see Appendix 4). These tests (*Table 4.7*) involve detection of specific chlamydial DNA or RNA sequences using either target, probe, or signal amplification technologies. These NAATs are theoretically capable of detecting one chlamydial particle. It is important that manufacturers' instructions be followed when collecting, transporting and processing specimens. There are four commercially available nucleic acid target amplification tests, one probe amplification test, and one signal amplification test. All of these tests can be applied to urines and vaginal swabs. They are all more sensitive than culture and more sensitive than the previously existing technologies including antigen detection and direct nucleic acid hybridization.[13]

Noninvasively Collected Specimens

The use of urine as a specimen for chlamydial diagnosis has been explored. Chlamydial lipopolysaccharide antigens can be detected by

Category	Technology	Company
Target amplification	Polymerase chain reaction (PCR)	Roche Molecular Systems
	Strand displacement amplification (SDA)	Becton Dickinson
	Transcription mediated amplification (TMA)	Gen-Probe
	Nucleic acid sequence based amplification (NASBA)	Organon Teknika
Probe amplification	Ligase chain reaction (LCR)	Abbott Laboratories
Signal amplification	Hybrid capture (HC)	Digene

Table 4.7 Commercially available NAATs for the detection of *C. trachomatis*.

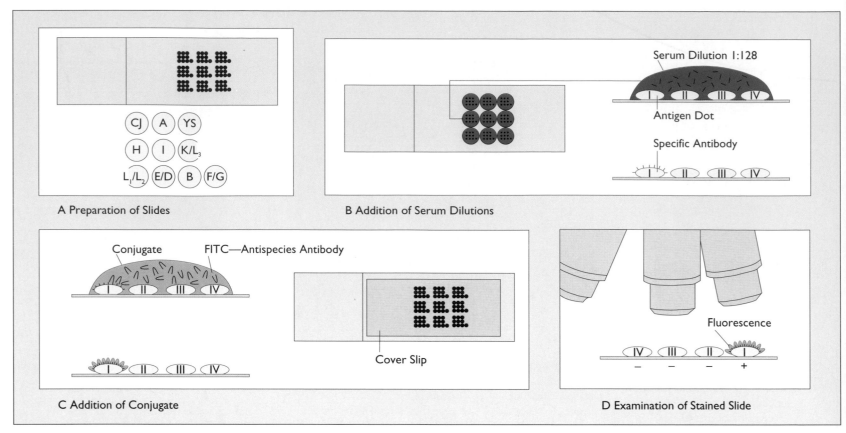

Fig. 4.71 Microimmunofluoresence assay. Courtesy of Janice C. Bullard, Centers for Disease Control.

Fig. 4.72 Fluorescent chlamydial EBs suspended in egg yolk sac material as viewed by the micro-immunofluorescence method. The laborious nature of this test and the degree of skill required for proper interpretation have limited its acceptance outside research laboratories.

Antimicrobial	MIC (μg/ml)
Tetracycline	0.03–0.50
Doxycycline	0.02–0.03
Azithromycin	0.25–1.0
Erythromycin	0.50–2.0
Clindamycin	2.0–16.0
Rifampicin	0.005–0.25
Sulfamethoxazole	0.50–4.0

Variability of strains and methods used in the determination of chlamydial susceptibilities limits the clinical utility of these in vitro data.

Table 4.9 Representative values of *C. trachomatis* MICs. Adapted from (1) Schachter J: Chlamydial Infection. *N Engl J Med* 1978; **298**:428, 490, 540, (2) Bowie WR, Shaw CE, Chan DGW, Black WA: *AAC* 1987; **31**:470–472, (3) Walsh M, Kappus EW, Quinn TC: *AAC* 1987; **31**:811–812.

Men	Women
Urethral swabs*	Cervical swabs*
First-catch urine*	Urethral swabs*
	First-catch urine*
	Vaginal swabs
	Vulvar swabs
	Tampons

Types of specimens that have been extensively evaluated for use in NAATs.

Table 4.8 Specimens that have been used successfully for the detection of *C. trachomatis* with NAATs.

EIA in urine sediment from men with symptomatic urethritis; however, these assays are relatively insensitive for detecting infection in asymptomatic men and may give false-positive results with urine specimens from women. Protocols have been developed by the manufacturers of NAATs for use with urine specimens (*Table 4.8*). Urine sediments can be used to diagnose chlamydial infection in men with an efficiency that is equal to or greater than the use of urethral swabs. While urine testing for women is probably less sensitive than doing a pelvic examination and then performing tests on cervical and urethral swabs, the noninvasive nature of the specimen collection makes it likely that urine (or vaginal swabs) will ultimately become the specimen of choice for screening purposes. Vaginal swabs have also been used, and

Patient	Condition	Therapy	Comments
Adults	Uncomplicated urethral, endocervical, or rectal infections	Doxycycline 100 mg po bid for 7 days[a,b,c] or Azithromycin I g po in a single dose[a,b,c]	Alternatives: Erythromycin base 500 mg po qid for 7 days[a,b,c] or Erythromycin ethylsuccinate 800 mg po qid for 7 days[a] or Ofloxacin 300 mg bid for 7 days[a,b] or Levofloxacin 500 mg po for 7 days or Amoxycillin 500 mg po tid for 7 days[b] or Tetracycline 500 mg po qid for 7 days[b,c] or Erythromycin base 500 mg po bid for 14 days[c] or Ofloxacin 200 mg bid or 400 mg once a day for 7 days[c]
Pregnant women	Urogenital infection	Erythromycin base 500 mg po qid for 7 days[a,b,c] or Amoxycillin 500 mg po tid of 7 days[b,c]	If 2 g daily dose not tolerated decrease to 250 mg po qid for 14 days; or erythromycin ethylsuccinate either 800 mg po qid for 7 days or 400 mg qid for 14 days. If the patient cannot tolerate erythromycin, use amoxicillin[a,b,c] Azithromycin 1 g po in a single dose
Neonates or infants	Conjunctivitis or pneumonitis	Erythromycin syrup 12.5 mg/kg po qid for 10–14 days[a,b]	Concurrent gonococcal conjunctival infection must be ruled out in conjunctivitis. Topical therapy not beneficial. Alternative: Trimethoprim 40 mg with sulfamethoxazole 200 mg po bid for 14 days (conjunctivitis) or 21 days (pneumonitis)[b]
Young men	Epididymitis (in presence of urethritis and absence of bacteriuria)	Doxycycline 100 mg po bid for 10 days[a,c] or Ofloxacin 300 mg po bid for 10 days[a]	Given in conjunction with effective antigonococcal therapy. Ofloxacin is contraindicated in persons ≤17 years of age
Women	PID*	*	*
Adults	LGV	Doxycycline 100 mg po bid for 21 days[a,c] (14 days)[b] or Erythromycin 500 mg po qid for 21 days[a,c] (14 days)[b]	Alternative: Tetracycline 500 mg po qid for 14 days[b]

*See Chapter 8 (PID)
[a]CDC. Sexually transmitted diseases: treatment guidelines. MMWR 2002; 51:82.
[b]WHO Guidelines for the Management of Sexually Transmitted Infections http://www.who.int/HIV_AIDS/STIcasemanagement/STIManagementguidelines/who_hiv_aids_2001.01/index.htm
[c]UK national guidelines on sexually transmitted infections and closely related conditions. Sexually Transmitted Infections 1999; 75(S1):S1–S88.

Table 4.10 Treatment regimens for chlamydial infections and chlamydial-associated conditions.

while the experience is less, the data are convincing. Sensitivities of clinician-collected, and patient-collected vaginal swabs are similar, and consistent with results from cervical swabs. The ability to test for chlamydial infection, without performing a pelvic examination, will reduce cost and improve access to diagnostic testing.[16]

TREATMENT

Treatment of chlamydial infection in the acute stages of disease is straightforward; chlamydiae are susceptible to many antibiotics, and acquired resistance to antimicrobials has not yet been recognized (*Table 4.9*).[8] As the cell wall differs from that of many bacteria, β-lactam antibiotics such as penicillin lack bactericidal activity against these organisms. Azithromycin, tetracyclines and macrolides of the erythromycin class are the currently recommended choices for proven or suspected chlamydial infection. Sulfonamides have activity against *C. trachomatis*, as does rifampin and its derivatives. Quinolones have variable activity in vitro against *C. trachomatis*. Resistance is easily induced *in vitro* to rifamyoins and quinolones. The currently recommended therapies are presented in *Table 4.10*.

References

1. Stephens RS. *Chlamydia: Intracellular Biology, Pathogenesis, and Immunity.* Washington, DC: American Society for Microbiology; 1999.

2. Schachter J, Dawson CR. *Human Chlamydial Infections.* Littleton, MA: Publishing Sciences Group; 1978.

3. Schachter J. Chlamydial infections (in three parts). *N Engl J Med* 1978; **298**:428–435; 490–495; 540–549.

4. Grayston JT, Kuo C-C, Campbell LA, Wang S-P. *Chlamydia pneumoniae* sp. nov. for *Chlamydia* sp. strain TWAR. *Int J Syst Bacteriol* 1989; **39**:88–90.

5. Grayston JT. *Chlamydia pneumoniae,* strain TWAR. *Chest* 1989; **95**:664–669.

6. Stephens RS, Kalman S, Lammel C *et al.* Genome sequence of an obligate intracellular pathogen of humans: *Chlamydia trachomatis. Science* 1998; **282**:754–759.

7. Gerbase AC, Rowley JT, Mertens TE. Global epidemiology of sexually transmitted diseases. *Lancet* 1998; **351**(Suppl 3):2–4.

8. Centers for Disease Control and Prevention (CDC). Recommendations for the prevention and management of *Chlamydia trachomatis* infections, 1993. *MMWR* 1993; 42:1–39.

9. Schachter J. Infection and disease epidemiology. In: Stephen RS, ed. *Chlamydia: Intracellular Biology, Pathogenesis, and Immunity.* Washington, DC: ASM Press, 1999: 139–169.

10. Schachter J, Sweet RL, Grossman M, Landers D, Robbie M, Bishop E. Experience with the routine use of erythromycin for chlamydial infections in pregnancy. *N Engl J Med* 1986; **314**:276–279.

11. Schachter J, Stamm WE. *Chlamydia.* In: Murray PR, Baron EJ, Pfaller MA, Tenover FC, Yolken RH, eds. *Manual of Clinical Microbiology.* 7th ed. Washington, DC: American Society for Microbiology, 1999: 795–806.

12. Stamm WE. Diagnosis of *Chlamydia trachomatis* genitourinary infections. *Ann Intern Med* 1988; **108**:710–717.

13. Schachter J. Nucleic acid amplification tests to diagnose *Chlamydia trachomatis* genital infection. A promise still unfulfilled. *Expert Review of Molecular Diagnostics* 2001; 1:137–144.

14. Rasmussen SJ, Eckmann L, Quayle AJ *et al.* Secretion of proinflammatory cytokines by epithelial cells in response to *Chlamydia* infection suggests a central role for epithelial cells in chlamydial pathogenesis. *J Clin Invest* 1997; **99**:77–87.

15. Wang SP, Grayston JT. Immunologic relationship between genital TRIC, lymphogranuloma venereum, and related organisms in a new microtiter indirect immunofluorescence test. *Am J Ophthalmol* 1970; **70**:367–374.

16. Shafer MA, Pantell RH, Schachter J. Is the routine pelvic examination needed with the advent of urine-based screening for sexually transmitted diseases? *Arch Pediatr Adolesc Med* 1999; **153**:119–125.

Donovanosis

F Bowden

INTRODUCTION

Donovanosis is a bacterial infection that predominantly causes genito-ulcerative disease. It occurs in geographical clusters in all continents except Europe and North America but is now generally considered a 'tropical' disease. In 1905, Donovan described organisms in tissue taken from the mouth of an Indian boy with 'ulcerating granuloma of the pudenda'.[1] In 1913, Aragao and Vianna believed a Gram-negative bacillus that they identified in patients with donovanosis was the causative agent of the disease and named it *Calymmatobacterium granulomatis* (from *calymma* Greek for sheath and *bakterion* for small rod).[1] Although the claims to have isolated the causative agent were subsequently retracted by Aragao, the genus name persisted.

Since its first description, the disease has been referred to as 'granuloma inguinale/venereum/tropicum/contagiosa,' 'ulcerating/sclerosing granuloma' and 'donovanosis.' As the disease does not just affect the inguinal region, and the term is easily confused with lymphogranuloma venereum (LGV), 'granuloma inguinale' should be replaced by 'donovanosis.'

Although donovanosis is usually confined to the genitals and can be treated with a wide range of antibiotics, it is associated with significant morbidity. Patients often present late and extensive tissue destruction may have occurred by the time of diagnosis.

It has been estimated that there were 10,000 prevalent cases in the United States in the 1940s, but 10 years after the introduction of antibiotics it was difficult to find enough patients to undertake any further work on the disease.[1] As a result, research interest waned and the disease came to be regarded as a tropical oddity. More recently, culture of the organism,[2,3] insights into its molecular biology[4] and its potential to facilitate HIV transmission[5] have renewed interest in the condition.

EPIDEMIOLOGY

Donovanosis occurs in isolated clusters throughout the world.[6] Donovanosis is a disease of poverty and disadvantage and its geographical distribution reflects this fact (*Fig. 5.1*). It is endemic in parts of Papua New Guinea, the Caribbean, South America, India, southern Africa, Vietnam and Central and Northern Australia. Surveillance of donovanosis is incomplete and it is likely that the condition exists in many other parts of Africa, Indonesia and South East Asia. Isolated, imported cases have been reported in several non-

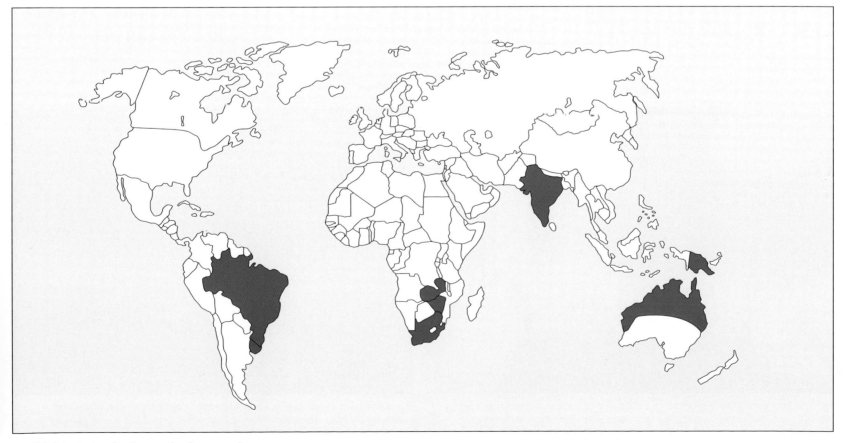

Fig. 5.1 Principal endemic areas for donovanosis.

endemic areas (e.g., Japan, Holland and Canada). Even in endemic areas donovanosis is a relatively rare condition, usually representing less than 10% of genito-ulcerative diagnoses.

The peak incidence of infections is the third decade of life with more than 70% of cases occurring between the ages of 20 and 40.[7] Markedly different male-to-female incidence ratios have been reported and it is likely that different surveillance and sampling methodologies are responsible for these discrepancies.[7]

Is donovanosis a sexually transmitted disease?

Of all the sexually transmitted infections, the criteria for sexual transmission have been least adequately fulfilled for donovanosis. In favor of sexual transmission are the following:

- Most lesions occur in the genital region;
- Most patients are sexually active when the diagnosis is made;

- The age of peak incidence of donovanosis correlates with other STIs;
- Many patients have concurrent STIs;
- Most male patients with anal lesions admit to receptive anal sex;
- Donovanosis has developed after ritual sexual practices and rape.

In support of non-venereal transmission are the following:

- Donovanosis occurs in sexually inactive individuals and the very young;
- Primary extra-genital donovanosis is well recognized;
- Low incidence among prostitutes and sexual contacts of infected patients.

It is generally agreed that donovanosis has a low transmission rate although there are no universally agreed upon figures and estimates range from 0.4% to 54%.[7] Although never reproduced, the causative

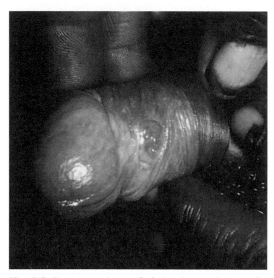

Fig. 5.2 Donovanosis, penile lesion in a male. A well-punched-out, clean, and shallow ulcer is seen upon retraction of the foreskin. Courtesy of the Centers for Disease Control and Prevention.

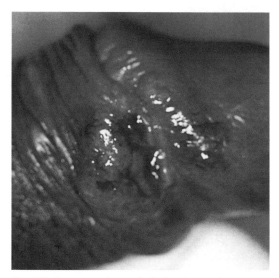

Fig. 5.3 Donovanosis, penile lesion in a male. Occasionally the ulcer can be large but with an elevated appearance. Courtesy of Adele Moreland, MD.

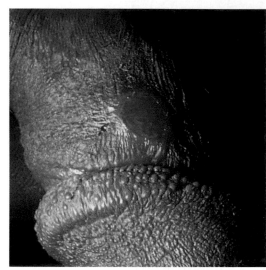

Fig. 5.4 Donovanosis, penile lesion in a male. An ulcer exhibiting red granulation tissue in the ulcer base. Courtesy of Adele Moreland, MD.

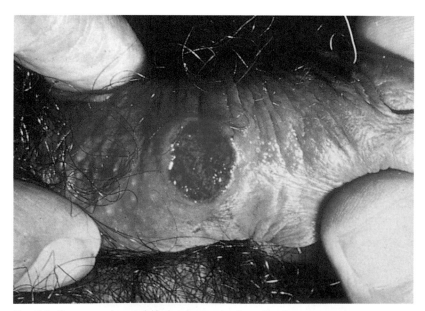

Fig. 5.5 Donovanosis, penile lesion in a male. A penile ulcer, as seen here, can mimic a hard chancre of syphilis. The latter can be diagnosed by dark-field examination, revealing spirochetes. Donovanosis will show the characteristic intracellular *C. granulomatis*. Courtesy of American Academy of Dermatology.

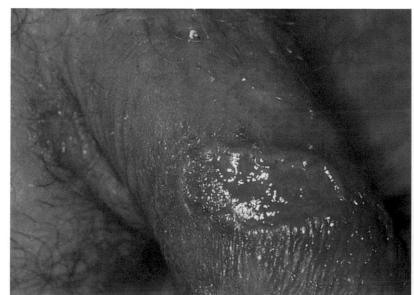

Fig. 5.6 Donovanosis, penile lesion in a male. A large ulcer with raised and indurated margins. The floor of the ulcer is granular and red due to granulation tissue. Courtesy of American Academy of Dermatology.

organism was cultured in 1962 from a stool specimen,[8] and it is possible that fecal soiling of the perineum is responsible for the initial infection in some cases. Congenital infection, presumably due to intrapartum transmission, is uncommon but well recognized.[9] Thus, it may be concluded that donovanosis is predominantly sexually transmitted but that other means of transmission exist.

CLINICAL FEATURES

Donovanosis is unusual among the bacterial STIs in that the primary manifestations of the disease are the commonest and most important morbidities. The incubation period of donovanosis is 1–4 weeks but incubation periods of up to 1 year have been reported.[7]

Lesions have been grouped into four main clinical variants (but it should be noted that there is considerable overlap between the types described below):

Ulcerogranulomatous: this is the commonest form and refers to beefy-red, fleshy lesions, with exuberant granulomatous tissue (*Figs 5.2–5.8*). The disease begins as single or multiple subcutaneous nodules that soon erode through the skin and slowly enlarge. The lesions are soft, bleed easily on contact and are relatively (but not completely) painless. They can extend by contiguous spread (*Figs 5.9–5.10*) and 'kissing' lesions are common. Auto-inoculation can lead to local spread to the thighs, scrotum, perineum and abdominal wall. However, simple lesions can become secondarily infected and present atypically (*Figs 5.11–5.13*).

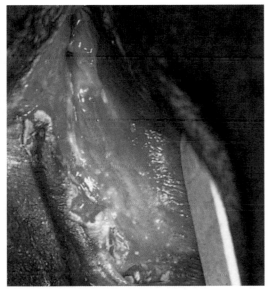

Fig. 5.7 Donovanosis lesion in a female. The morphology of the ulcers is similar in males and females. Retraction of the left labium shows a shallow, clean ulcer. Courtesy of the Centers for Disease Control and Prevention.

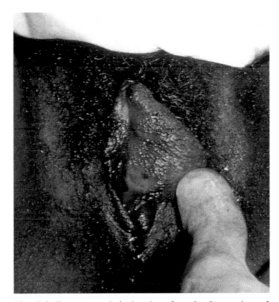

Fig. 5.8 Donovanosis lesion in a female. Retraction of the left edematous labium partially reveals a beefy red, ulcerating lesion.

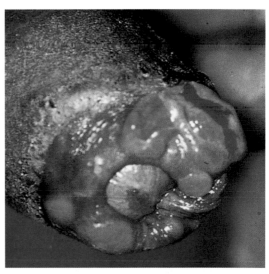

Fig. 5.9 The disease spreads by formation of satellite lesions in adjacent skin. Courtesy of Ron Ballard, PhD.

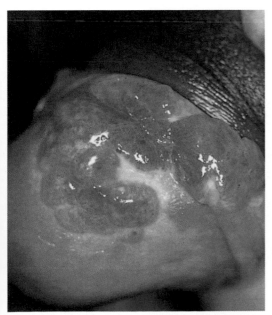

Fig. 5.10 Similar lesions to those in Fig. 5.9 undergoing spread on the glans penis. Courtesy of Ron Ballard, PhD.

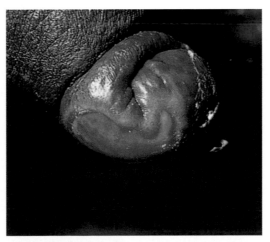

Fig. 5.11 Secondary infection in donovanosis. An irregular penile ulcer with an angry-red border and purulent floor suggesting a secondary infection. The lesion of donovanosis becomes painful when infected. Also note the marked edema of the surrounding skin. Courtesy of Adele Moreland, MD.

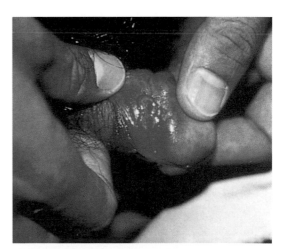

Fig. 5.12 Secondary infection of penile donovanosis makes the lesion painful, red, and vascular. Courtesy of Adele Moreland, MD.

Hypertrophic or verrucose: an ulcer or growth with a raised or irregular edge, usually dry with a walnut-like or cauliflower-like appearance (*Figs 5.14–5.16*).

Necrotic: a deep ulcer associated with tissue destruction. A profuse, foul-smelling exudate (caused by bacterial superinfection) is commonly encountered and is a distinctive feature of this type (*Fig. 5.17*).

Sclerotic or cicatricial: these lesions are characterized by the formation of fibrous and scar tissue as a result of chronic untreated infection (*Figs 5.18–5.20*). This is now the least common form and the diagnosis of donovanosis may be delayed.

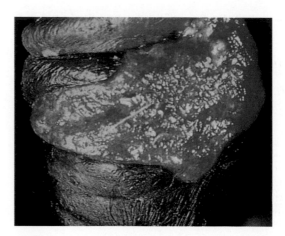

Fig. 5.17 Destructive donovanosis penile lesion in a male. A large and necrotic ulcer mimicking carcinoma. Note that the floor of the ulcer is clean, shallow, and smooth, unlike what one expects to see in a malignant ulcer.

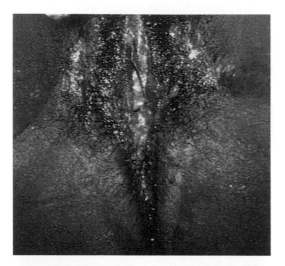

Fig. 5.13 Multiple, shallow ulcers seen on the vulvar skin. Secondary infection made them painful. Multiple lesions are usually caused by autoinoculation.

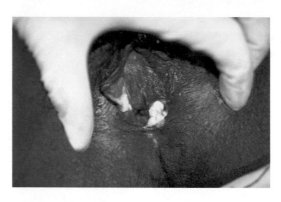

Fig. 5.18 Donovanosis: sclerotic variant; lesions present for many years; confusion with neoplasia is common; biopsy should be performed on presentation.

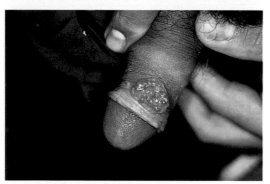

Fig. 5.14 Donovanosis: hypertrophic variant; lesion only visible when foreskin retracted.

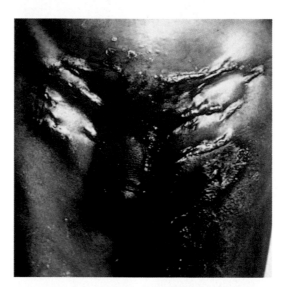

Fig. 5.19 Destructive donovanosis penile lesion in a male. Severe donovanosis with extensive scarring in the inguinal region. Courtesy of Ron Ballard, PhD.

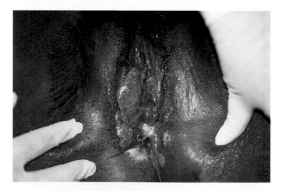

Fig. 5.15 Donovanosis: ulcerogranulomatous/ hypertrophic lesions in young woman.

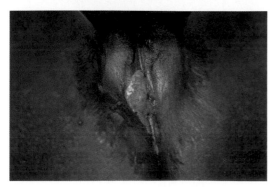

Fig. 5.16 Donovanosis: hypertrophic variant affecting right labium.

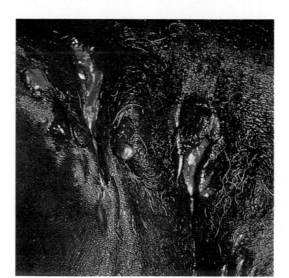

Fig. 5.20 Destructive donovanosis lesion in a female. Extensive scarring of the vulva and inner thighs associated with progressive disease. Courtesy of Ron Ballard, PhD.

The inguinal swellings seen in donovanosis are called 'pseudo-buboes' and are subcutaneous granulomata, not affected lymph nodes (*Fig. 5.21*). The disease can lead to severe, recalcitrant edema of the glans penis and labia (*Figs 5.22–5.26*) which has been described as 'pseudoelephantiasis.'

The genitals and perineum are the usual sites of lesions. Primary infection of, or local extension to, the cervix is common and the disease may extend to pelvic structures and disseminate (*Fig. 5.27*).

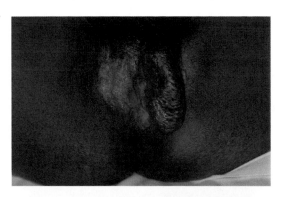

Fig. 5.24 Donovanosis: pseudo-elephantiasis of the left labium majora with healing lesions visible on right side of vulva.

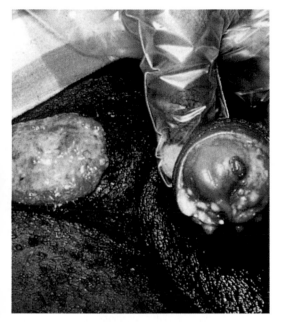

Fig. 5.21 Pseudobuboes. Penile donovanosis seen as an ulcerating, nodular lesion with marked tissue destruction. There is a large, inguinal ulcer indicating soft tissue breakdown in the area secondary to donovanosis. This is known as a 'pseudobubo.' Courtesy of American Academy of Dermatology and Bingham JS: *Pocket Picture Guide to Sexually Transmitted Diseases*, London, Gower Medical Publishing, 1984.

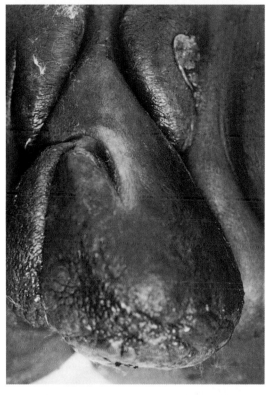

Fig. 5.25 Swelling of the labia minora resulting in elephantiasis (pseudo-elephantiasis) in a patient who presented with longstanding donovanosis.

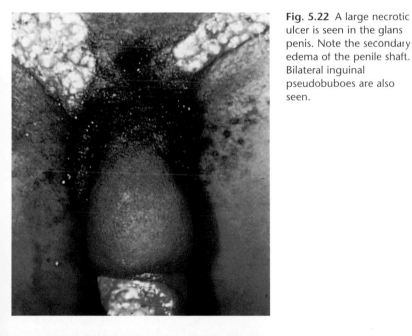

Fig. 5.22 A large necrotic ulcer is seen in the glans penis. Note the secondary edema of the penile shaft. Bilateral inguinal pseudobuboes are also seen.

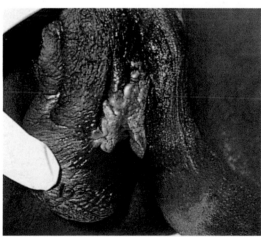

Fig. 5.26 A clearer view of the same lesion in Fig. 5.25. Many effective antibiotics are contraindicated in pregnancy – see text for list of suitable agents.

Fig. 5.23 Donovanosis: ulcero-granulomatous variant with pseudo-elephantiasis of right labium majora; note 3 small punch biopsies have been performed.

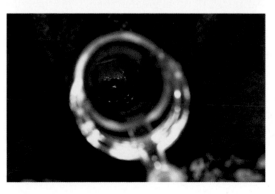

Fig. 5.27 Donovanosis: primary involvement of the cervix; young women who presented for investigation of infertility; friable lesions visible on cervix that bled on contact.

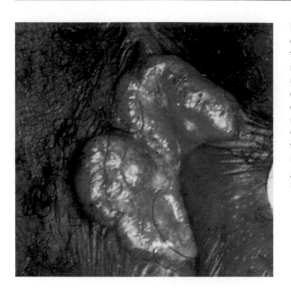

Fig. 5.28 Destructive donovanosis lesion in a female. There is an irregular, large vulvar ulcer with indurated, edematous, and partly everted margins mimicking carcinoma. Courtesy of the Centers for Disease Control and Prevention and the Journal of Reproductive Medicine.

The commonest non-genital site is the mouth, accounting for up to 6% of cases.[10] Primary non-genital lesions can occur in the upper arms and chest, scalp, legs and arms. The disease can affect bones (usually the tibia) and systemic symptoms of fever, sweats, weight loss and anorexia are common when there is bony involvement but less common when other sites are involved. Rare sites of dissemination include the abdominal cavity, psoas muscle, bowel, spleen, liver, lung, uterus, ear and ovaries.

In endemic areas, extragenital presentations of donovanosis are often missed until discovered during surgery or at post-mortem examination. A high index of suspicion should be maintained to avoid missing this treatable condition.

DIFFERENTIAL DIAGNOSIS

The differential diagnosis of donovanosis includes primary and secondary syphilis, chancroid, lymphogranuloma venereum, condylomata acuminata, rhinoscleroma, leishmaniasis, amebiasis, histoplasmosis and cancer (*Fig. 5.28*).

The misclassification of donovanosis as an anogenital cancer has been recognized for at least 50 years and the disease is still misdiagnosed in the first instance as a carcinoma, especially of the cervix and the vulva.

The diagnosis of donovanosis is often overlooked because several genital infections are similar clinically, prior antibiotic therapy alters presentation, and there may be a failure to consider it as a diagnosis because of its low incidence.

Syphilis: The chancre of early syphilis may be confused with early lesions of donovanosis. Its exclusion is usually made by negative serology and by failure to demonstrate spirochetes in lesions (*refer to Chapter 2*).

Lymphogranuloma venereum: The disease is characterized by bilateral tender, inguinal nodes (buboes) that often become suppurative. Elephantiasis of the external genitalia may be seen. Exclusion is aided by serology with chlamydial micro-IF titers greater than 1:256 (*refer to Chapter 4*).

Chancroid: Chancroid is manifested by shallow, painful, exudate-filled ulcers and tender inguinal adenopathy. The causative agent (*Haemophilus ducreyi*) can be cultured on a selective agar medium (*refer to Chapter 3*).

Genital herpes: The disease is characterized by symptomatic initial vesicles that quickly break down to form shallow, clean-based ulcers. Local edema and enlargement of inguinal lymph nodes may be present. Exclusion is by failure to detect intranuclear inclusions and multinucleated giant cells in smears or to detect herpes simplex virus by culture or nucleic acid amplification (e.g. PCR) (*refer to Chapter 11*).

Genital cancers: These conditions are usually excluded by biopsy. Exophytic lesions or large necrotic ulcers of donovanosis may closely simulate carcinoma on clinical examination. Parametrial involvement may add to this confusion.

Donovanosis can coexist with other sexually transmitted infections. It should always be considered when genital lesions have a history of considerable duration and slow progression (weeks to months).

DONOVANOSIS AND HIV INFECTION

An association between donovanosis and HIV infection has been reported in Africa.[11] There are no prospective studies showing that donovanosis increases the risk of HIV acquisition, but since donovanosis causes relatively painless genital ulcers which bleed on contact, it is a reasonable hypothesis. One study has suggested that patients with donovanosis who are HIV infected have more extensive disease and respond slowly to treatment[12] but a study in pregnant women did not confirm this.[13]

DONOVANOSIS AND CANCER

Although there are no formal studies that established a relationship between longstanding donovanosis and the subsequent development of genital cancers. Rajam and Rangiah[10] observed only 5 cases of cancer in 2,000 cases of donovanosis. Using a rudimentary antibody assay, Goldberg and Annamunthodo[14] found that serum from 9 of 62 patients with penile cancer had reactivity against 'Donovania' antigens; however, this study was never repeated. Regardless of the causal relationship, a biopsy should be performed in any case of suspected donovanosis if there are features suggestive of neoplasia.

TAXONOMY

The causative organism of donovanosis has undergone many name changes since its first description: these include *C. granulomatis*, *Encapsulatus inguinalis*, *Klebsiella granulomatis* and *Donovania granulomatis*. The similarities between *C. granulomatis* and *Klebsiella* species were first noted on the basis of serologic cross-reactivity[8] and subsequently on ultrastructural grounds.[15] A detailed description of the phylogeny of *C. granulomatis* based on molecular studies has been published[4] and, although some uncertainty remains,[16] the name *Klebsiella granulomatis* comb. nov. has been recently proposed.

GENOTYPIC ANALYSIS

The *pho*E genes (encodes for an outer membrane protein involved in phosphate transport) of Australian isolates of *C. granulomatis* have a 99.7–99.8% nucleotide similarity with those of *Klebsiella pneumoniae* and *Klebsiella rhinoscleromatis*.[17] The 16s rRNA genes of these organisms are 98.8–99.8% homologous.[4] Two base changes in the *pho*E gene sequence eliminate *Hae*III restriction sites, a feature which has been exploited in the development of a diagnostic PCR.[18] A total of 2089 base pairs of the *pho*E and 16s rRNA genes were sequenced in these studies. Slightly divergent results have been reported by others where only 95% homology between African isolates of *C. granulomatis* and *K. pneumoniae* was observed.[16]

LABORATORY TESTS

HISTOPATHOLOGY, CYTOLOGY AND MICROSCOPY

A combination of biopsy and cytologic smears are the most reliable of the traditional diagnostic tools for donovanosis, but their sensitivity is considerably less than 100%. The diagnostic yield will depend on the technique of the clinician who collects the specimen and the patience and skill of the histo/cytopathologist who reads the slides.

After gently cleaning the area with normal saline, one to three punch biopsies (3–5 mm diameter) or snip biopsies (approximately the size of a match head) should be taken from the periphery of the lesion. One or two of the entire biopsy specimens should be fixed in 10% formalin/saline solution for histology, and an air dried smear can be prepared at the bedside from the other specimen. Smear the underside of the specimen over the surface of a glass slide. Do not re-spread any area and stop when the specimen starts to dry. The smear is air-dried, fixed in 95% ethanol for 5 minutes and then stained. A more convenient but less than optimum specimen can be obtained by carefully, but firmly, pressing a glass slide directly onto the lesion. A hematoxylin and eosin-stained specimen will demonstrate the acute and chronic inflammation with granulation tissue formation, but will not demonstrate the organisms unless they are present in large numbers.

There are four basic histopathological features consistently observed in donovanosis:[19] a massive cellular infiltrate, principally of polymorphonuclear cells; large mononuclear cells; epithelial proliferation; and a paucity of lymphocytes (Fig. 5.29). The epithelial border of the lesion frequently shows acanthosis, epidermal microabcesses, elongation and intercommunication of the rete pegs and pseudo-epitheliomatous hyperplasia. Caseation, suppuration and epithelioid giant cells are uncommon. Inclusions of C. granulomatis (Donovan bodies) within macrophages result in pathognomonic cells (Fig. 5.30). These enlarged cells (20–90 μm) have an eccentric nucleus and contain individual or groups of organisms in capsular or cyst-like compartments within the cytoplasm. Confusion with neoplasia may occur if pseudoepitheliomatous hyperplasia is present.

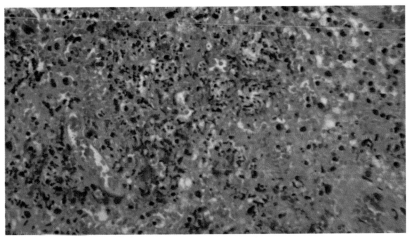

Fig. 5.29 Microscopic section of the ulcer in Fig. 5.28 to show acute inflammation with microabscess formation and granulation tissue (hematoxylin and eosin ×50).

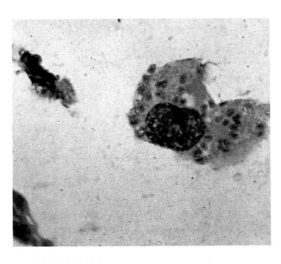

Fig. 5.30 A fragmented mononuclear cell containing Donovan bodies. Bipolar staining creating a closed safety pin appearance is seen (Wright-Giemsa ×1,000). Courtesy of American Academy of Dermatology.

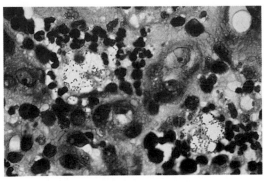

Fig. 5.31 Donovanosis: punch biopsy specimen of donovanosis lesion (overnight Giemsa stain, ×100); Donovan bodies are visible inside large monocytes

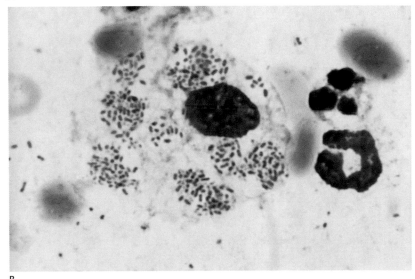

Fig. 5.32 (A) Light micrograph of an impression smear of granulation tissue from genital lesion stained by RapiDiff showing large vacuolated mononuclear cells filled with numerous Donovan bodies in the cytoplasm. (B) Light micrograph of an impression smear of granulation tissue stained by RapiDiff stain showing numerous Donovan bodies in pockets of vacuoles within the cytoplasm of the mononuclear cell.

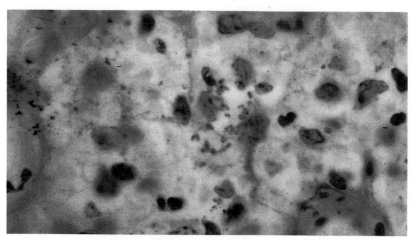

Fig. 5.33 Warthin-Starry stain in tissue to show intracellular Donovan bodies (×320).

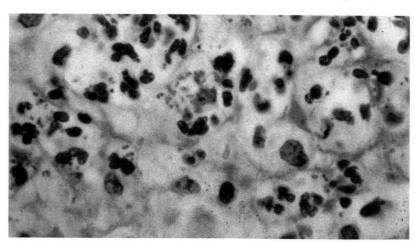

Fig. 5.34 Intracellular Donovan bodies. Another view of the same tissue as in Fig. 5.46 (×320). Courtesy of the Centers for Disease Control and Prevention.

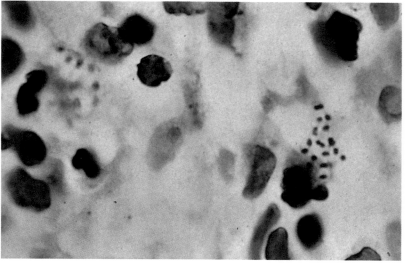

Fig. 5.35 Intracellular Donovan bodies. Higher magnification of same tissue as in Fig. 5.46 (×1,000 approximately).

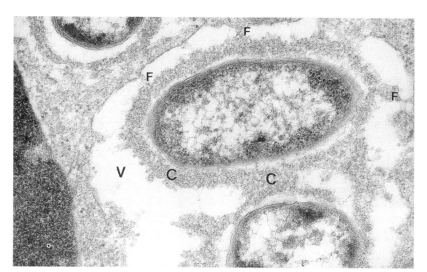

Fig. 5.36A Electron micrograph of *C. granulomatis* within a phagocytic vacuole (V). Capsular material (C) between adjacent bacilli seen to be continuous with each other. The fine fibrillar (F) strands are evident at intervals attaching the capsule to the limiting membrane of the vacuole (×30,000).

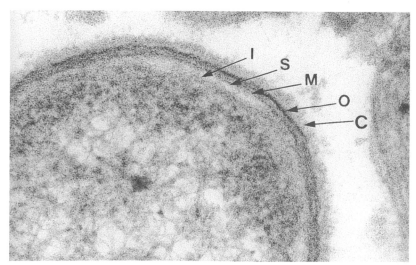

Fig. 5.36B Electron micrograph showing the details of the cell wall structure consisting of an outer membrane (O), middle electron opaque layer (M), inner plasma membrane (I), with periplasmic space (S). Note the narrow electron dense capsule (C) (×120,000).

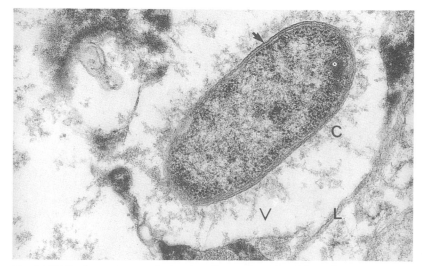

Fig. 5.36C Electron micrograph showing *C. granulomatis* within a phagocytic vacuole (V) surrounded by a limiting membrane (L). The trilaminar cell wall structure is evident (arrow). Note the fibrous nature of capsular material (C) (×30,000).

Fig. 5.36 (A–C) Transmission electron microscopy of *C. granulomatis* in tissue biopsy specimen. Courtesy of Ayesha Kharsany, PhD.

Overnight Giemsa stain is extremely sensitive[20] (*Fig. 5.31*) although a modified Giemsa stain (Rapidiff) appears to have similar sensitivity and is less time consuming[21] (*Fig. 5.32*). A silver stain such as Warthin-Starry may be the most sensitive method, especially when there are few Donovan bodies present (*Figs 5.33–5.35*). Other stains that have been used include Leishman's and Wright's.[7]

C. granulomatis is a Gram-negative, intracellular, pleomorphic, encapsulated bacillus. Histologically, *C. granulomatis* appears as dark, bipolar staining bodies ('closed safety pins') within macrophages — the so-called Donovan bodies (*see Fig. 5.30*). These are pathognomonic for donovanosis. Cells of *C. granulomatis* often appear ovoid or bean-shaped and range from 1–1.5 μm in size. However, cells may also appear coccoid, diplococcoid or bacillary and vary in size from 0.6–1.0 μm. Electron microscopy reveals a prominent capsule surrounding the organism (*Fig. 5.36A–C*).[15] The cell envelope is similar to that of other Gram-negative bacteria. The nucleoplasm is located centrally and there are prominent electron dense granules located in the periphery of the cell.

CULTURE AND GROWTH CONDITIONS

C. granulomatis is found in the cytoplasm of large mononuclear cells and, less commonly, in polymorphonuclear leukocytes.[15] When inoculated into the yolk sac of chicken embryos, the organisms were shown to grow within epithelial cells.[22] *In vitro* culture has been difficult; however, successful cultivation using a variety of semi-solid and liquid media was reported in the 1940s and 1950s.[6] Optimum growth occurred at 37°C. More recently, two new methods for the culture of *C. granulomatis* have been developed: co-culture in fresh human monocytes[23] and in a human epithelial cell line (HEp-2 cells), using a modified chlamydial culture technique (*Fig. 5.37*).[2]

DIAGNOSIS

Confirmation of the diagnosis is currently based on the demonstration of typical Donovan bodies within large mononuclear cells.

NUCLEIC ACID AMPLIFICATION

A polymerase chain reaction (PCR) assay that can be used on simple swab or biopsy specimens has been used in Australia for diagnostic purposes,[18] but there is currently no commercial kit available. Further development and validation of nucleic acid amplification tests is an important priority for research.

SEROLOGICAL TESTS

A number of skin tests and complement fixation tests were used in the 1940s and 50s but none have been introduced into routine practice.[6] More recently, an indirect immunofluorescent test has been developed with reportedly high sensitivity and specificity[24] but, again, the test has not been widely adopted.

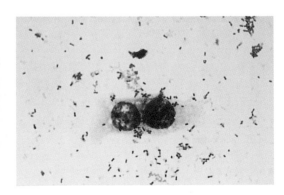

Fig. 5.37 Culture of *C. Granulomatis* in HEp-2 cells using modified chlamydial culture techniques.

TREATMENT

Arragao and Vianna demonstrated the efficacy of tartar emetic (potassium antimony tartrate) for the treatment of donovanosis in 1913,[6] although it was of limited use if relapse occurred. Nevertheless, this was one of the earliest examples of an effective therapy against a bacterial pathogen.[1] Penicillin was tried unsuccessfully soon after it became available but streptomycin was subsequently shown to be effective. Since then a wide range of antibiotics with Gram-negative activity have demonstrated clinical utility although most recommendations are based upon observational studies only.

GENERAL PRINCIPLES OF TREATMENT

Donovanosis is usually a chronic disease and patients may have received many incomplete courses of antibiotics with little benefit. Treatment should therefore be supervised and, in some cases, hospital admission may be required to ensure adherence to antibiotic regimens. Provision of successful treatment usually results in healing from the periphery towards the center of the lesions (*Figs 5.38–5.52*). It is usually recommended that treatment be continued at least until all lesions are completely epithelialized and some texts suggest that it should continue for a further period after healing to reduce the rate of relapse.

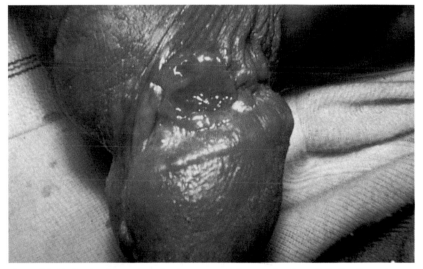

Fig. 5.38 Earlier healing stages In donovanosis in a male. A partially healing ulcer seen at the coronal sulcus.

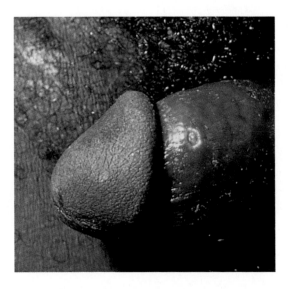

Fig. 5.39 Later healing stages in donovanosis in a male. Penile ulcer at an advanced stage of healing. Courtesy of the *Journal of Reproductive Medicine.*

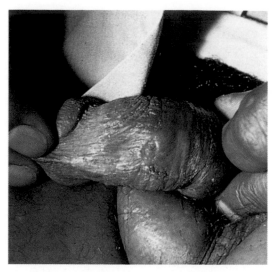

Fig. 5.40 Later healing stages in donovanosis in a male. Penile ulcer at an advanced stage of healing. Courtesy of the *Journal of Reproductive Medicine.*

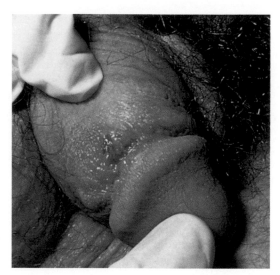

Fig. 5.41 Later healing stages in donovanosis in a male. This lesion is almost completely healed, leaving behind a small, red area. Courtesy of the *Journal of Reproductive Medicine.*

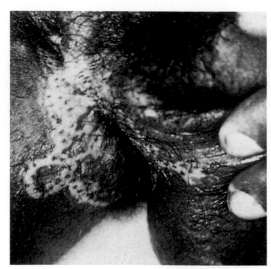

Fig. 5.42 Healing stages in donovanosis in a female. Fibrosis and re-epithelialization of a healed lesion.

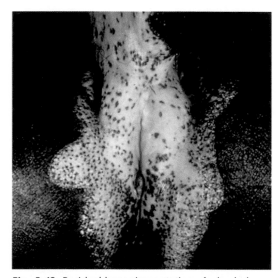

Fig. 5.43 Residual hypopigmentation of a healed lesion. Courtesy of the Centers for Disease Control and Prevention.

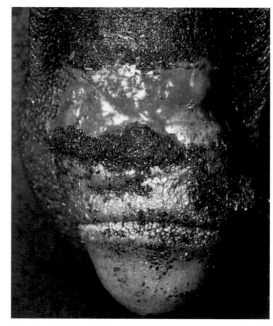

Fig. 5.44 Active donovanosis in a male prior to initiation of therapy. Courtesy of Ron Ballard, PhD.

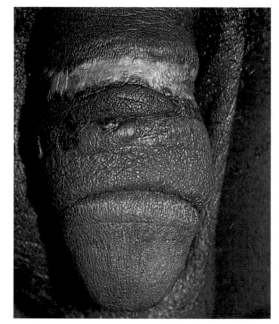

Fig. 5.45 The same patient as in Fig. 5.44, following complete healing as a result of tetracycline therapy. There is marked depigmentation. Courtesy of Ron Ballard, PhD.

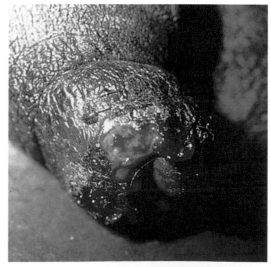

Fig. 5.46 Fibrosis and edema causing a marked penile deformity. The patient had a large, long-standing lesion, which healed after antibiotic therapy. Courtesy of Adele Moreland, MD.

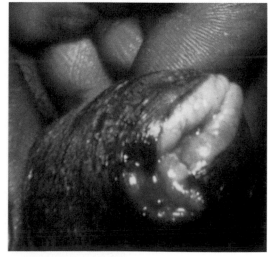

Fig. 5.47 Urethral stenosis in a case of healed donovanosis. Courtesy of Adele Moreland, MD.

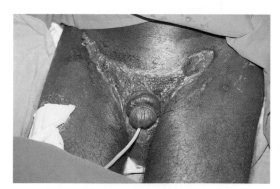

Fig. 5.48 Donovanosis: extensive ulcero-granulomatous disease with destruction of penile tissue.

CHOICE OF ANTIBIOTICS

The lack of a routine culture system has meant that there have been no *in vitro* antibiotic susceptibility studies performed since the 1950s. It is therefore difficult to determine if the relatively common problem of treatment failure is related to antimicrobial resistance, sub-optimal bio-availability or poor compliance; treatment failure is rare if the patient is admitted to hospital for supervised therapy, suggesting that adherence to therapy is the most important factor. Nevertheless, antibiotic treatment will inevitably produce a selective pressure on the organism and the emergence of antibiotic resistance is to be expected. A summary of antibiotic choices is shown in *Table 5.1*.

Ampicillin. There are conflicting reports of the efficacy of ampicillin and it therefore cannot be recommended as first-line therapy.[7]

Chloramphenicol has been used with success in Papua New Guinea, and is inexpensive and well tolerated. Despite the rarity of irreversible bone marrow suppression in this context, it is generally not recommended because of the availability of other agents which are perceived to be safer.

Ceftriaxone, a third generation cephalosporin, requires daily parenteral administration but is curative if given until lesions have healed.[25] Single dose therapy is ineffective.[26]

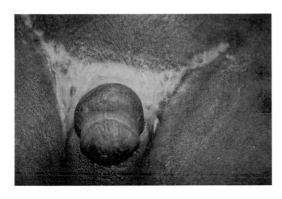

Fig. 5.49 Donovanosis: same patient as in Fig. 5.48; 8 weeks after commencement of supervised doxycycline treatment; note loss of penile tissue, depigmentation and scarring.

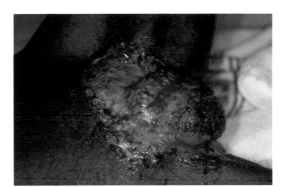

Fig. 5.50 Donovanosis: necrotic variant; patient presented after lesion had been present for many years; Donovan bodies only seen after 3rd biopsy; associated with offensive odor due to secondary bacterial infection.

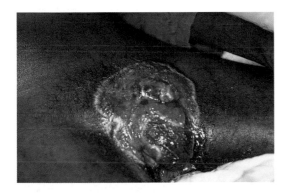

Fig. 5.51 Donovanosis; same patient as in Fig. 5.50; 14 days after patient received azithromycin 500 mg orally for 7 days; note lesion is clean and epithelialization is visible at margins of the ulcer.

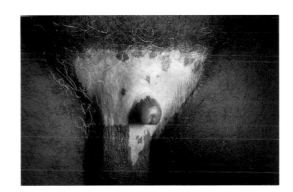

Fig. 5.52 Donovanosis: same patient as in Figs 5.50 and 5.51; 3 months after presentation; ulcers have completely healed but depigmented scar tissue and penile deformity persist.

Antibiotic	Route (dosage)	Comments
Ampicillin	Oral, 500 mg q6h	Conflicting results from small number of patients in case reports; not recommended.
Ceftriaxone	Intramuscular, 1 g daily	Requires prolonged parenteral administration.
Trimethoprim/sulfamethoxazole	Oral, 1 double strength tablet (160/800 mg) q12h	Non-randomized study[27] comparing TMP/SMZ with streptomycin/tetracycline showed 100% efficacy in both groups.
Erythromycin	Oral, 500 mg q6h	Effective, safe in pregnancy. Compliance poor due to GI side effects.
Chloramphenicol	Oral, 500 mg q8h	Highly effective but concerns about bone marrow toxicity usually preclude its use except in life-threatening illness
Doxycycline	Oral, 100 mg q12h	Effective and well tolerated; contraindicated in pregnancy and children
Streptomycin	Intramuscular, 1 g q12h	Parenteral therapy only, sometimes used in combination with other oral therapy
Gentamicin	Intramuscular, 1 mg/kg q12h	Limited experience but appears effective; parenteral only
Norfloxacin	Oral, 400 mg q12h	Effective and well tolerated; contraindicated in pregnancy and children
Ciprofloxacin	Oral, 500 mg q12h	Effective and well tolerated; contraindicated in pregnancy and children
Azithromycin	Oral, 500 mg daily for 7 days or 1.0 g once weekly for 4–6 weeks	Effective and long tissue half-life allows flexible dosing regimen and short course therapy; can be used in pregnancy and children

Table 5.1 Antibiotic regimens used for treating donovanosis.

Erythromycin is relatively inexpensive and has been especially useful for treatment during pregnancy. However, the requirement of multiple daily doses, prolonged therapy and the commonly associated gastro-intestinal side effects make this a less than optimal first line agent.

Tetracyclines. Short-acting tetracyclines and the longer-acting doxycycline are effective but they are contraindicated in pregnancy or in breast-feeding mothers, thus limiting their usefulness.

Trimethoprim/sulfamethoxazole (cotrimoxazole) is inexpensive, effective and well tolerated but requires prolonged therapy to ensure a cure.[27]

Miscellaneous. Ciprofloxacin, norfloxacin, lincomycin and gentamicin have all been reported to be clinically effective.

Azithromycin, a long-acting azalide compound, is effective either as a daily therapy (500 mg daily for 7 days) or as an intermittent treatment course (1.0 g once weekly for 4 weeks).[28,29] The drug is well tolerated, has high oral bioavailability and long tissue half-life. It also appears to be effective when other antibiotic regimens have failed. In view of the chronic nature of the illness in many patients and the need to continue therapy until complete healing has occurred with other antimicrobial agents, it has been suggested that azithromycin may be the most cost-effective way to manage extensive ulcers.[5]

SURGICAL TREATMENT

Persistent pseudo-elephantiasis of the vulva can occur even after adequate antibiotic treatment has been completed. Rarely, surgical excision of these lesions may be required.

PUBLIC HEALTH

Diseases with a low reproductive number (R_0), such as donovanosis, are likely to be eradicable with the implementation of targeted screening and appropriate management protocols. Donovanosis has a low transmissibility and there is no evidence for the existence of a carrier state. In areas where appropriate antibiotics have become available in the context of an organized health care system (e.g. southern USA in the 1950s), the disease has effectively disappeared. The incidence of donovanosis in some endemic populations in Australia fell dramatically in the late 1990s as a result of the introduction of clinician education, active case finding, the development of molecular based diagnostic tests and the availability of short course azithromycin therapy.[30]

Public health action should include improved passive and active surveillance, the establishment of centralized diagnostic expertise and the application of consistent treatment protocols using agents with proved efficacy.

ACKNOWLEDGMENTS

The author gratefully acknowledges the helpful comments of John Richens and Ivan Bastian.

References

1. Richens J. Donovanosis. In: Cox FEG, ed. Wellcome Trust History of Tropical Diseases: Trustees of the Wellcome Trust, 1996.
2. Carter J, Hutton S, Sriprakesh S, *et al.* Culture of the causative organism of donovanosis (*Calymmatobacterium granulomatis*) in HEp-2 cells. *J Clin Micro* 1997; **35**:487–489.
3. Kharsany AB, Hoosen AA, Kiepiela P, Naicker T, Sturm AW. Culture of *Calymmatobacterium granulomatis*. *Clin Infect Dis* 1996; **22**(2):391.
4. Carter JS, Bowden FJ, Bastian I, Myers GM, Sriprakash KS, Kemp DJ. Phylogenetic evidence for reclassification of *Calymmatobacterium granulomatis* as *Klebsiella granulomatis* comb. nov. *Int J Syst Bacteriol* 1999; **49**:1695–1700.
5. O'Farrell N. Donovanosis. In: Holmes KK SP, Mardh PA, Lemon SA, Stamm WE, Piot P, Wasserheit JN., ed. *Sexually Transmitted Diseases*. McGraw-Hill, 1999; pp. 525–531.
6. Richens J. The diagnosis and treatment of donovanosis (granuloma inguinale). *Genitourin Med* 1991; **67**(6):441–452.
7. Hart G. Donovanosis. *Clinical Infectious Diseases* 1997; **25**:24–32.
8. Goldberg J. Studies on granuloma inguinale V. Isolation of a bacterium resembling *Donovania granulomatis* from the faeces of a patient with granuloma inguinale. *Br J Vener Dis* 1962; **38**:99–102.
9. Richens J. Sexually transmitted diseases in children in developing countries. *Genitourin Med* 1994; **70**(4):278–283.
10. Rajam RV, Rangiah PN. Donovanosis (granuloma inguinale, granuloma venereum). Geneva: World Health Organisation, 1954.
11. O'Farrell N. Global eradication of donovanosis: an opportunity for limiting the spread of HIV-1 infection. *Genitourin Med* 1995; **71**(1):27–31.
12. Jamkhedkar PP, Hira SK, Shroff HJ, Lanjewar DN. Clinico-epidemiologic features of granuloma inguinale in the era of acquired immune deficiency syndrome. *Sex Transm Dis* 1998; **25**(4):196–200.
13. Hoosen AA, Mphatsoe M, Kharsany AB, Moodley J, Bassa A, Bramdev A. Granuloma inguinale in association with pregnancy and HIV infection. *Int J Gynaecol Obstet* 1996; **53**(2):133–138.
14. Goldberg J, Annamunthodo H. Studies on granuloma inguinale: VIII. Serological reactivity of sera from patients with carcinoma of the penis when tested with Donovania antigens. *Brit J Venereal Dis* 1966; **45**:205–209.
15. Kuberski T, Papadimitriou JM, Phillips P. Ultrastructure of *Calymmatobacterium granulomatis* in lesions of granuloma inguinale. *J Infect Dis* 1980; **142**(5):744–749.
16. Kharsany AB, Hoosen AA, Kiepiela P, Kirby R, Sturm AW. Phylogenetic analysis of *Calymmatobacterium granulomatis* based on 16S rRNA gene sequences. *J Med Microbiol* 1999; **48**(9):841–847.
17. Bastian I, Bowden FJ. Amplification of *Klebsiella*-like sequences from biopsy samples from patients with donovanosis. *Clin Infect Dis* 1996; **23**(6):1328–1330.
18. Carter J, Bowden FJ, Sriprakash KS, Bastian I, Kemp DJ. Diagnostic polymerase chain reaction for donovanosis. *Clin Infect Dis* 1999; **28**(5):1168–1169.
19. Sehgal VN, Shyamprasad AL, Beohar PC. The histopathological diagnosis of donovanosis. *Br J Vener Dis* 1984; **60**(1):45–47.
20. Sehgal VN, Jain MK. Tissue section Donovan bodies — identification through slow-Giemsa (overnight) technique. *Dermatologica* 1987; **174**(5):228–231.
21. O'Farrell N, Hoosen AA, Coetzee K, van den Ende J. A rapid stain for the diagnosis of granuloma inguinale. *Genitourin Med* 1990; **66**(3):200–201.
22. Anderson K. The cultivation from granuloma inguinale of a microorganism having the characteristics of Donovan bodies in the yolk sac of chick embryos. *Science* 1943; **97**:560–561.
23. Kharsany AB, Hoosen AA, Kiepiela P, Naicker T, Sturm AW. Growth and cultural characteristics of *Calymmatobacterium granulomatis* — the aetiological agent of granuloma inguinale (Donovanosis). *J Med Microbiol* 1997; **46**(7):579–585.
24. Freinkel AL, Dangor Y, Koornhof HJ, Ballard RC. A serological test for granuloma inguinale. *Genitourin Med* 1992; **68**(4):269–272.
25. Merianos A, Gilles M, Chuah J. Ceftriaxone in the treatment of chronic donovanosis in central Australia. *Genitourin Med* 1994; **70**(2):84–89.
26. O'Farrell N. Failure of single dose ceftriaxone in donovanosis (granuloma inguinale). *Genitourin Med* 1991; **67**:269–270.
27. Latif AS, Mason PR, Paraiwa E. The treatment of donovanosis (granuloma inguinale). *Sex Transm Dis* 1988; **15**:27–29.
28. Bowden FJ. Azithromycin for the treatment of donovanosis. *Sexually Transmitted Infections* 1998; **74**:78–79.
29. Bowden FJ, Mein J, Plunkett C, Bastian I. Pilot study of azithromycin in the treatment of genital donovanosis. *Genitourin Med* 1996; **72**(1):17–19.
30. Miller PJ, Torzillo PJ, Hateley W. Impact of improved diagnosis and treatment on prevalence of gonorrhoea and chlamydial infection in remote aboriginal communities on Anangu Pitjantjatjara Lands. *Med J Aust* 1999; **170**(9):429–432.

Gonorrhea

C Ison and D Martin

INTRODUCTION

The clinical syndrome of gonorrhea was described by biblical authors, but the etiologic agent, *Neisseria gonorrhoeae*, was not described until 1879, when Albert Neisser observed the organism in smears of purulent exudates from urethritis, cervicitis, and ophthalmia neonatorum. The genus *Neisseria* includes the pathogenic species *N. gonorrhoeae* and *N. meningitidis*, as well as species that are normal flora of the oropharynx and nasopharynx. *N. gonorrhoeae* colonizes primarily the mucosa of the lower genital tract and occasionally ascends to colonize the normally sterile upper genital tract or invade into the blood to cause disseminated infection. The cell envelope of *N. gonorrhoeae* consists of a cytoplasmic membrane, a thin peptidoglycan layer and an outer membrane. Colonization of the mucosal surface by the organism occurs by attachment to the epithelial cell surface, which is mediated by pili and opacity proteins, followed by internalization and transcytosis, mediated by opacity proteins and porins, to establish an infection in the subepithelial space. An immune response is elicited resulting in a polymorphonuclear infiltrate (*Fig 6.1*). Sialylation of the lipo-oligosaccharide results in resistance to the bactericidal action of serum, an attribute necessary for dissemination into the blood to occur.

N. gonorrhoeae is always considered a pathogen that requires treatment and is not considered part of the normal flora. However, strains of commensal *Neisseria* spp. may occasionally be isolated in clinical specimens from anogenital sites and observed intracellularly in polymorphonuclear leukocytes, and are morphologically indistinguishable from the pathogenic *Neisseriae*. Thus, accurate laboratory identification of the gonococcus is essential because of the social and medicolegal consequences of misidentifying strains of nonpathogenic *Neisseria* spp. as *N. gonorrhoeae*.

Because of the fastidious growth requirements of *N. gonorrhoeae*, it was difficult to culture the organism until the development of chocolatized blood agar supplemented with growth factors. In the 1960s, the development of selective media containing antimicrobial and antifungal agents (such as Thayer–Martin medium), which enhanced the isolation of the gonococcus by inhibiting not only Gram-positive bacteria but also the closely related *Neisseria* spp., further simplified the laboratory diagnosis of gonorrhea. Rapid biochemical and serologic tests are available, allowing identification of the gonococcus within a few hours of its isolation. More recently, DNA amplification technology has been brought to bear on the problem of diagnosing gonococcal infections in asymptomatic patients. All of these innovations have advanced our knowledge of this common pathogen, its epidemiology and the diseases it causes. The goal of this chapter is to put this new knowledge into the context of what we already know about *N. gonorrhoeae*.

EPIDEMIOLOGY

Gonorrhea is a disease of worldwide importance (*Fig. 6.2*). In the USA the gonorrhea rate per 100,000 population dropped steadily until 1995 at which point the rate leveled off and in the past few years has even increased slightly (*Fig. 6.3*). These data probably reflect the fact that the extensive screening programs for asymptomatic gonorrhea infections in women attending prenatal, family planning, sexually transmitted disease clinics, and other clinics have achieved maximal effect in shortening the average duration of gonococcal infection in that country's population. Further reductions in annual infection rates will require extending female screening programs to unconventional sites

Fig. 6.1 Pathogenesis of gonococcal infection.

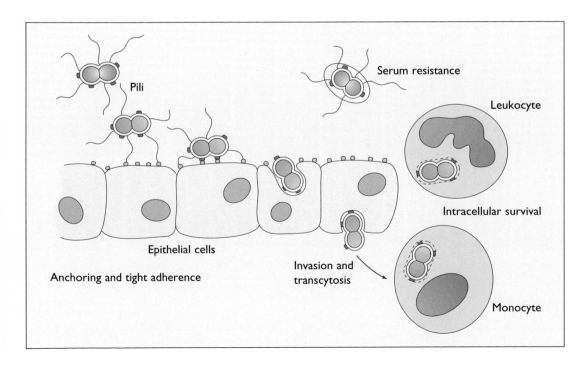

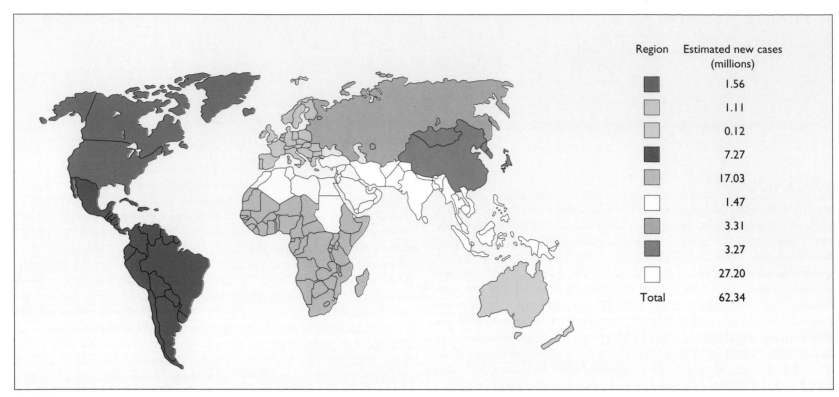

Fig. 6.2 Estimated new cases of gonorrhea (in millions) in adults, 1999. Courtesy WHD, 2001.

Region	Estimated new cases (millions)
	1.56
	1.11
	0.12
	7.27
	17.03
	1.47
	3.31
	3.27
	27.20
Total	62.34

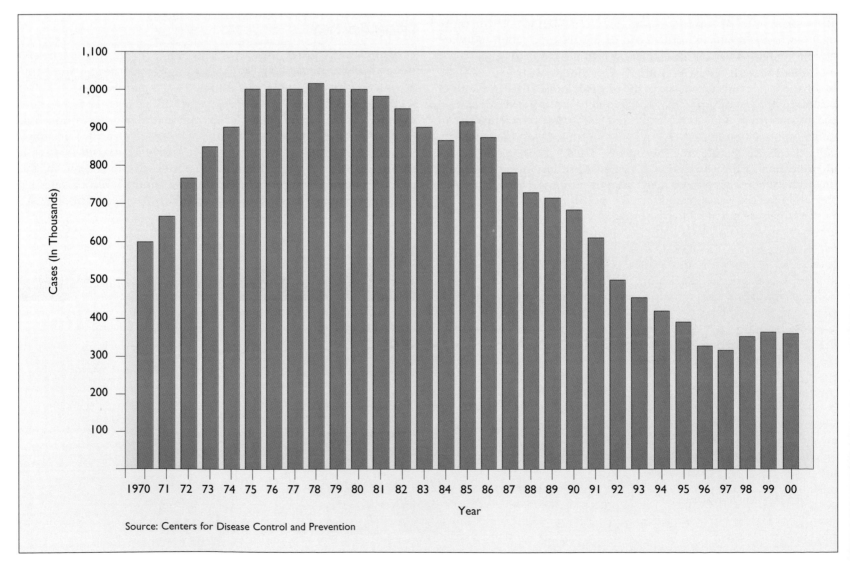

Fig. 6.3 Reported cases of gonorrhea in the USA, 1970–2000.

Source: Centers for Disease Control and Prevention

such as schools and including men in the search for asymptomatic cases. In the UK the decline in the number of cases of gonorrhea seen in the 1980s and early 1990s has now been reversed with the diagnoses of gonorrhea reaching a 10-year high in 2000 (*Fig. 6.4*).

Gonorrhea is transmitted almost exclusively by sexual contact. Persons under 25 years of age who have multiple sexual partners are at highest risk. Rates of clinical gonococcal infection are higher in men and, overall, infection prevalence is higher in minority and inner-city populations.

As noted above, gonorrhea is often acquired from a sexual partner who is either asymptomatic or who has only minimal symptoms. Transmission efficiency (a measure of transmission through one sexual exposure) is estimated to be 50–60% from an infected man to an uninfected woman and 20% from an infected woman to an uninfected man. More than 90% of men with urethral gonorrhea will develop symptoms within 5 days of infection. Most men with symptomatic urethritis will seek health care because of the relative severity of the symptoms. Infections at other anatomic sites in men and infections in women are far less likely to produce early symptoms and, therefore, are less likely to be diagnosed and treated. The rationale for public health measures, such as screening and contact tracing, is to identify and treat patients with asymptomatic or minimally symptomatic infections, thus shortening the duration of infection and preventing further transmission of the disease. Additionally, because all women with lower genital tract gonococcal infection regardless of the presence or absence of symptoms are at risk for PID, the early identification and treatment of infected women is important.

The epidemiology of gonorrhoea has been studied extensively using phenotypic methods, auxotyping (*Fig. 6.5*) and serotyping, to monitor temporal changes and movement of antibiotic resistant strains. Phenotyping has been useful in identifying potential clusters but isolates of the same phenotype may not necessarily reflect the same genotype. *N. gonorrhoeae* exhibit a high degree of genetic variation due to their competence for horizontal gene exchange and are non-clonal in nature. In vivo mixed infections are thought to occur frequently, particularly in individuals with multiple partners or a high rate of partner change, contributing to genetic variation. The rate of genetic variation is unknown but it is possible, depending on the gene and method chosen, that each isolate can appear distinct unless part of a short transmission chain. While this questions the validity of using typing for long-term studies it has the potential for a greater level of discrimination that can distinguish between isolates of the same serovar, determine the genetic relatedness of antibiotic-resistant isolates and can identify isolates from sexual contacts. A variety of genotyping methods have been used with differing levels of discrimination; restriction endonuclease finger-printing, ribotyping and amplification by polymerase chain reaction using arbitrary or repetitive element sequence-based primers are the least discriminatory while pulsed field gel electrophoresis, *opa*-typing (*Fig. 6.6*) and *por* sequencing give the greatest discrimination.[1] All of these methods show discrimination equal to or greater than pheno-typing and therefore it is essential that the question to be addressed is considered carefully before the genotypic method is chosen. Highly discriminatory methods have now been shown to identify isolates from a common source but this may only be true for short chains of trans-mission. The definition of a short transmission chain will be dependent on the potential for genetic diversity, presumably through mixed infec-tion, and hence may reflect the level of sexual activity of the individuals infected. Phenotyping maintains its role as an epidemiological tool because it is quick and simple to perform and can identify potential clusters for further analysis by genotyping. The most informative data will be obtained when microbiological and epidemiological approaches are combined.

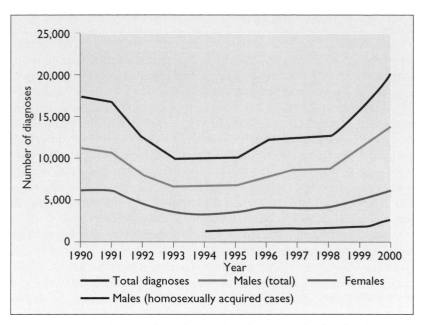

Fig 6.4 Diagnoses of uncomplicated gonorrhoea by sex: England and Wales 1990–2000.

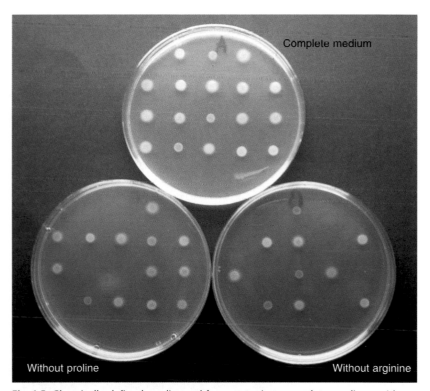

Fig 6.5 Chemically defined media used for auxotyping: complete medium, without proline and without arginine. Absence of growth indicates requirement for the specific amino acid.

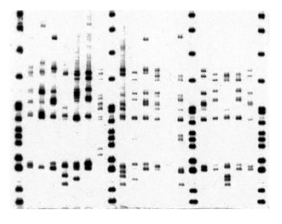

Fig 6.6 Polyacrylamide gel showing different *opa*-types of *N. gonorrhoeae*. Molecular weight markers in lanes 1, 9, 16 and 22, all other tracks different strains of gonococci.

ANTIMICROBIAL RESISTANCE

The evolution of antimicrobial resistance in *N. gonorrhoeae* has, in both developed and developing countries,[2,3] potential negative implications for the control of gonorrhea (*Table 6.1*). Resistance to new therapeutic agents has generally developed within a few years of the introduction of a new agent (*Table 6.2*). Strains with chromosomal resistance to penicillin, tetracycline, erythromycin, and cefoxitin, as well as decreased susceptibility to ceftriaxone, have been identified in the USA and most of the world, especially Southeast Asia. Sporadic high-level resistance to spectinomycin has also been reported. Decreased susceptibility and high-level chromosomal resistance to the fluoroquinolones has now been widely reported and presents a considerable problem in some areas, such as the Western Pacific. Strains with MICs of ≥1 µg/ml to ciprofloxacin and ofloxacin are classed as resistant and are unlikely to be treated successfully with a fluoroquinolone, with some strains showing MICs of 64 µg/ml or higher. Therapeutic failure has also been noted with strains exhibiting decreased susceptibility, with MICs of 0.12–0.5 µg/ml, albeit at a lower level. The mechanisms of fluoro-quinolone resistance has been found to be due to mutations in the DNA gyrase gene, *gyrA*, and/or the topoisomerase IV gene, *parC*. It seems probable that strains exhibiting high-levels of resistance also have changes in membrane permeability that may be associated with an efflux system.[4]

Penicillinase-producing *N. gonorrhoeae* (PPNG) strains, which inactivate penicillins and other β-lactams, were first described in 1976. Four β-lactamase plasmids have been identified in PPNG strains, 3.2 MDa 'African', 4.4 MDa 'Asian', 3.05 MDa 'Toronto' and 4.0 MDa 'Nimes' plasmids. The 2.9 MDa 'Rio' plasmid has been found to be identical to the Toronto plasmid. All of these encode for the TEM-1-type β-lactamase but differ in size due to deletions in the non-functional part of the plasmid. The highest prevalence of PPNG strains is found in parts of Africa and Asia, but they have been endemic in the USA and Europe since 1981. PPNG exhibit high levels of resistance that make the penicillins inappropriate agents for gonococcal therapy.

Plasmid-mediated, high-level resistance to tetracycline was reported in *N. gonorrhoeae* (TRNG) in 1985. It has resulted from the insertion of

Type of resistance	Antimicrobial agent
Chromosomal (genes located on the chromosome)	Penicillin
	Tetracycline
	Spectinomycin
	Fluoroquinolones
	Broad spectrum cephalosporins (decreased susceptibility)
Plasmid-mediated (genes located on plasmids)	Penicillin (β-lactam antibiotics) — PPNG
	Tetracycline — TRNG

Table 6.1 Types of antimicrobial resistance in *N. gonorrhoeae*.

- PPNG – Penicillinase-producing *N. gonorrhoeae*, tetracycline MIC <16 µg/ml
- TRNG – nonPPNG, tetracycline MIC ≥16 µg/ml
- PP/TRNG – PPNG, tetracycline MIC ≥16 µg/ml
- CMRNG – penicillin MIC ≥2 µg/ml (≥1 µg/ml*), tetracycline MIC 2–8 µg/ml
- QRNG – PPNG, nonPPNG, TRNG, PP/TRNG, or CMRNG with ciprofloxacin MIC ≥1 µg/ml.

MIC varies with medium used;
≥2 µg/ml (GC agar) and ≥1 µg/ml (DST agar and Isosensitest agar).

Table 6.2 Categories for resistant isolates of *N. gonorrhoeae*.

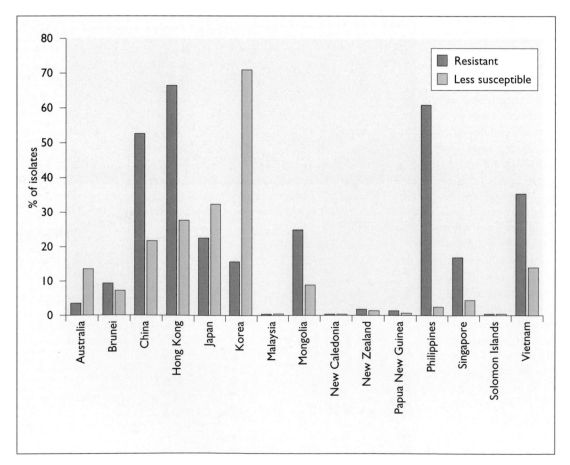

Fig. 6.7 WHO Western Pacific Surveillance Programme: quinolone resistance in 15 countries in 1999.

the TetM determinant into the 24.5 MDa conjugal plasmid resulting in a plasmid of 25.2 MDa. Based on restriction analysis, Two TetM plasmids have been identified in *N. gonorrhoeae*, which have been designated 'US' and 'Dutch'. These plasmids can mobilize themselves between both gonococcal isolates and different species and have been reported in *Neisseria meningitidis* and *Kingella denitrificans*. They also have the ability to mobilize β-lactamase plasmids and isolates with plasmid-mediated resistance to penicillin and tetracycline (PP/TRNG) are commonly found. Like the penicillins, tetracyclines are inappropriate sole therapies for gonococcal infections.

Current alternative therapies for resistant strains include broad-spectrum cephalosporins and azithromycin. Resistance to the newer cephalosporins has not been described in *N. gonorrhoeae* although isolates with decreased susceptibility to azithromycin were identified by the Gonococcal Isolate Surveillance Project (GISP) in 1999.[5]

The continued emergence of resistance to antimicrobial agents used for the treatment of gonorrhea is a concern and requires effective surveillance programs to monitor susceptibility patterns, detect drifts in susceptibility and emergence of resistance. There are established surveillance programs in the USA, Canada, Australia and The Netherlands which have produced valuable temporal data in these individual countries. The gonococcal antimicrobial susceptibility program (GASP) was established to provide a global surveillance network. GASP is co-ordinated by the World Health Organization and the aim was to create a series of networks based on WHO regions. Important elements of GASP are that data should be comparable between laboratories and this requires the development of training and quality assurance programs. Currently GASP is most active in the Americas and the Caribbean, the western Pacific region and the southeast Asian region. The problem of quinolone resistance has been recently highlighted by data collected by the western Pacific Region in 1999[6] where resistance was monitored in 15 countries with levels of 16% or greater in eight of the countries, the highest being 66.6% in Hong Kong (*Fig. 6.7*).

CLINICAL MANIFESTATIONS

In the majority of cases, gonococcal infections are limited to mucosal surfaces.[7] Infection occurs in areas of columnar epithelium including the cervix, urethra, rectum, pharynx, and conjunctiva. Squamous epithelium is not susceptible to infection by the gonococcus. However, the prepubertal vaginal epithelium which has not been keratinized under the influence of estrogen, may be infected. Hence, gonorrhea may present in a young girl as a vulvovaginitis. In mucosal infections, there is usually a brisk, local neutrophilic response manifested clinically as a purulent discharge (*Table 6.3*).

Site of infection	Uncomplicated	Complicated

Urethra	Symptomatic
	  Scant, clear discharge
	  Copious purulent discharge
	Asymptomatic
		(Epididymitis)*
		
		(Penile edema)
		(Abscess of Cowper's, Tyson's glands)
		(Seminal vesiculitis)
		DGI
		  Bacteremia
		  Fever
		  Skin lesions: macular, erythematous, pustular, necrotic, hemorrhagic
		  Tenosynovitis
		  Joints; septic arthritis
		  Endocarditis
		  Meningitis

Cervix	Symptomatic
	  Red, friable cervical os
	  Purulent discharge from os
	  Bilitarel or unilateral lower abdominal tenderness
	
	Asymptomatic
		PID
		  Endometritis
		  Salpingitis
		  Tubo-ovarian abscess
		  Ectopic pregnancy
		  Infertility
		DGI

Rectum	Symptomatic
	  Copious, purulent discharge
	  Burning/stinging pain
	  Tenesmus
	  Blood in stoods
	Asymptomatic
		DGI

Pharynx	Symptomatic
	  Mild pharyngitis
	  Mild sore throat
	  Erythema
	Asymptomatic
		DGI

Conjunctiva	Symptomatic Copous purulent discharge	Keratitis and corneal ulceration; perforation, extrusion of lens Scarring; opacification of lens Blindness

Syndromes listed in parenthesis occur infrequently.

Table 6.3 Clinical manifestations of gonococcal infections.

In women, untreated cervical infection may lead to endometritis and salpingitis, a sign–symptom complex more commonly known as pelvic inflammatory disease, or PID (see also Ch. 8). It has been estimated that in approximately 1–3% of patients with mucosal infection, hematogenous spread occurs, causing disseminated gonococcal infection (DGI). However, the risk may be much lower in populations with a low prevalence of the gonococcal auxotypes that have been shown to be associated with dissemination.

GONORRHEA

The most common symptom of gonorrhea in men is urethral discharge that may range from a scanty, clear, or cloudy fluid to one that is copious and purulent (*Figs 6.8* and *6.9*). Dysuria is usually present. However,

men with asymptomatic urethritis may be an important reservoir for transmission. Although most men with gonorrhea develop symptoms, those who ignore their symptoms or have asymptomatic infection are at increased risk of developing complications (*see Table 6.3*).

Endocervical infection is the most common type of uncomplicated gonorrhea in women (*Figs 6.10* and *6.11*). At least one-half of infected women are asymptomatic or have symptoms that are mild to non-specific. Cervical infections may be accompanied by vaginal discharge, abnormal vaginal bleeding, or dysuria. Local complications include abscesses in Bartholin's and Skene's glands (*Fig. 6.12*). Asymptomatic infections are found most often in women who are screened for gonorrhea in routine gynecologic examinations or who are seen as sexual contacts of men with gonorrhea. On examination, the cervical os

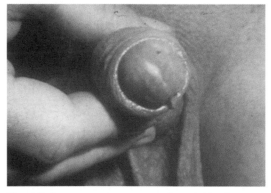

Fig. 6.8 Symptomatic gonococcal urethritis. Scanty urethral discharge obtained after urethral stripping.

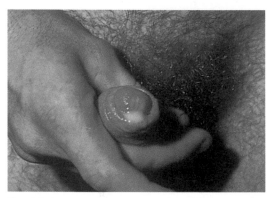

Fig. 6.9 Symptomatic gonococcal urethritis. Copious spontaneous urethral discharge.

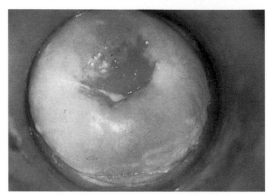

Fig. 6.10 Endocervical gonorrhea. A small amount of purulent discharge is visible in the endocervical canal.

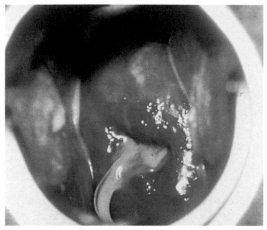

Fig. 6.11 Signs of endocervical gonorrhea: cervical edema and erythema as well as discharge.

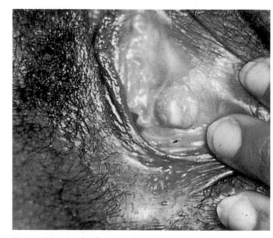

Fig. 6.12 Urethral gonorrhea in the female. Purulent discharge is visible, with involvement of Bartholin's gland.

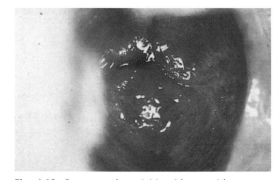

Fig. 6.13 Gonococcal cervicitis with mucoid discharge and marked cervical erythema and edema. This is indistinguishable clinically from chlamydial cervicitis.

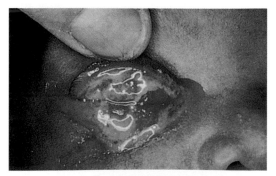

Fig. 6.14 Gonococcal ophthalmia neonatorum. Lid edema, erythema, and marked purulent discharge are seen. The Gram-stained smear was loaded with Gram-negative diplococci within neutrophils.

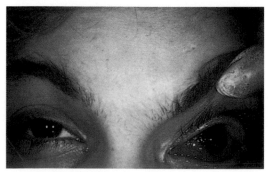

Fig. 6.15 Early gonococcal ophthalmia in an adult showing marked chemosis and tearing with no discharge.

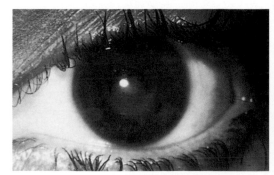

Fig. 6.16 Corneal clouding following gonococcal ophthalmia in an adult.

may be erythematous and friable, with a purulent exudate (*Figs 6.11* and *6.13*), or may be normal.

Rectal infections, which occur in 30% of women with cervical gonorrhea, probably represent secondary colonization from a primary cervical infection and are symptomatic in less than 5% of women. Infections in homosexual men, however, result from anal intercourse and are more often symptomatic (18–34%). Symptoms and signs range from mild burning on defecation to itching to severe tenesmus, and from mucopurulent discharge to frank blood in the stools.

Pharyngeal 'infections' are diagnosed most often in women and homosexual men with a history of fellatio. There has never been a convincing demonstration of a relationship between pharyngeal infection (or colonization, as some would put it) and the signs and symptoms of a sore throat or tonsillitis.

Ocular infections occur in newborns who are exposed to infected secretions in the birth canal of an infected mother (*Fig. 6.14*). Occasionally, keratoconjunctivitis is seen in adults (*Fig. 6.15*). Conjunctival infection, tearing, and lid edema occur early, followed rapidly by the appearance of a frankly purulent exudate. Prompt diagnosis and treatment are important because corneal scarring or perforation may result (*Fig. 6.16*).

DISSEMINATED GONOCOCCAL INFECTION

Disseminated gonococcal infection (DGI) is the result of gonococcal bacteremia. The sources of infection are primarily asymptomatic infections of the pharynx, urethra, or cervix. In describing this disease, it is useful to divide patients into two groups: those with suppurative arthritis and those without. The term tenosynovitis-dermatitis syndrome often is applied to the latter group of patients, because the majority present with, or give a history of, one or both of these signs. Only a minority of patients with suppurative gonococcal arthritis have tenosynovitis and/or skin lesions at the time of presentation. Some experts feel that these two syndromes are part of a disease continuum, with the tenosynovitis-dermatitis syndrome representing the initial stage which then progresses to a frank septic arthritis. However others feel that the two syndromes represent separate clinical entities. Regardless of which hypothesis is correct, the DGI cases reported in the literature have been divided nearly equally between those with and those without suppurative arthritis.

Fever and chills occur more frequently in patients who present with the tenosynovitis-dermatitis syndrome than in those who present with suppurative arthritis, which may explain why the former patients tend to come to medical attention sooner than the latter group. In some cases all symptoms begin at the same time. Positive blood cultures are found almost exclusively in this group of patients, although even here, less than half of cultures will be positive. The majority of tenosynovitis-dermatitis syndrome cases will have skin lesions which begin as small erythematous maculopapular petechial lesions and then usually develop a central pustule which may then progress to a lesion with central necrosis (*Figs 6.17–6.19*). These lesions may be indistinguishable from those caused by staphylococcal endocarditis. Early on the lesions of meningococcemia and DGI may be indistinguishable though the former usually progress to confluent petechial and then hemorrhagic lesions.

Additionally, patients with DGI usually have less than 20 lesions, whereas patients with meningococcemia usually have hundreds or thousands. DGI lesions are located peripherally, with the wrists and ankles being the most common locations. Polyarthralgia is a common presenting symptom of DGI regardless of the clinical classification of the patient. It is seen in approximately 60% to 75% of patients with the tenosynovitis-dermatitis syndrome. Tenosynovitis is characterized as erythema, swelling, and direct tenderness upon palpation of the affected tendon group (*Fig. 6.20*). It is found most commonly around the wrist and dorsum of the hand, with the ankle, including the Achilles tendon, and dorsum of the foot involved somewhat less commonly.

Patients with gonococcal suppurative arthritis also may present with fever although the majority are afebrile. As noted previously, blood cultures are rarely positive in these patients. Roughly one third of these patients also will have skin lesions as described above and a similar proportion will have tenosynovitis in addition to purulent joint effusions. A history of migratory polyarthralgia is obtained from the majority of these patients about half of whom will have symptoms in only one joint at the time of presentation. The most commonly affected joints are the wrists, small joints of the hands and knees.

Left untreated, many cases of DGI eventually resolve without specific therapy, but a significant proportion will suffer serious morbidity including endocarditis, meningitis, and osteomyelitis. Since the introduction of penicillin, these complications have been observed only rarely.

DGI must be distinguished from Reiter's syndrome, meningococcemia, acute rheumatoid arthritis, other forms of septic arthritis, and the immune complex-mediated arthritides caused by hepatitis B virus and HIV (*Tables 6.4* and *6.5*). A diagnosis of DGI may be based on the identification of gonococci in synovial fluid, blood, or CSF. Gonococci are rarely isolated from skin lesions, but a Gram-stained smear of purulent material taken from an unroofed lesion should be examined whenever possible. When present, Gram-negative diplococci within

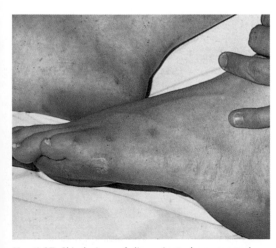

Fig. 6.17 Skin lesions of disseminated gonococcal infection. Papular and pustular lesions on the foot.

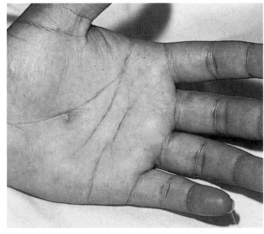

Fig. 6.18 Skin lesions of disseminated gonococcal infection. Small painful midpalmar lesion on an erythematous base.

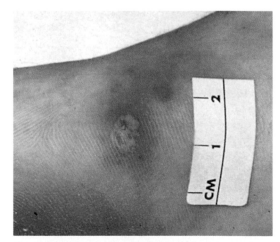

Fig. 6.19 Skin lesions of disseminated gonococcal infection. Classic large lesions with a necrotic, grayish central lesion on an erythematous base.

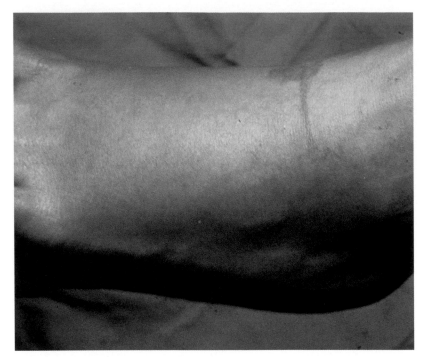

Fig 6.20 Disseminated gonococcal infection. Tenosynovitis of the dorsal foot. (Courtesy of Dr Charles V Sanders, LSU Medical School and Williams & Williams publishers).

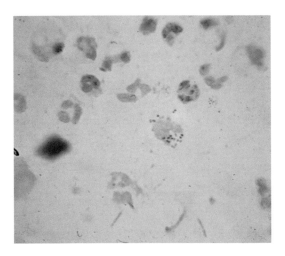

Fig. 6.21 Gram-negative diplococci visible in one neutrophil in a smear of a pustular skin lesion from a patient with disseminated gonococcal infection. Meningococci cannot be distinguished from gonococci with this method.

Meningococcemia
Staphylococcal sepsis or endocarditis
Other bacterial septicemias (rare)
HIV infection: Acute thrombocytopenia and arthritis
Hepatitis B prodrome
Acute Reiter's syndrome
Juvenile rheumatoid arthritis
Lyme disease

Table 6.4 Differential diagnosis of disseminated gonococcal infection. Dermatitis-tenosynovitis syndrome.

Infectious	Noninfectious
Bacterial	Gout, pseudogout*
Adults	Rheumatoid arthritis (especially juvenile
Gonococcus*	rheumatoid arthritis)
Staphylococcus	Trauma
Pneumococcus	Tumors
Streptococcus	Hemarthrosis
Children	Osteochondritis
Staphylococcus	Psoriatic arthritis
Streptococcus	Pigmented/villonodular synovitis
Pneumococcus	
Haemophilus influenzae	
Gram-negative rods	
Tuberculosis	
Fungal	

Most common.

Table 6.5 Differential diagnosis of disseminated gonococcal infection. Monarticular arthritis.

Gonococci are demonstrated in synovial fluid, blood, cerebrospinal fluid, or skin lesions by culture

Observation of diplococci in Gram- or methylene blue-stained smear

Clinical diagnosis of DGI may be based on two of the following three criteria:
  Isolation of gonococci from urogenital, rectal, pharyngeal, or conjunctival sites of the patient or the patient's sexual partner
  Infection is manifested as pustular, hemorrhagic, or necrotic skin lesions distributed on the extremities
  Patient responds rapidly to appropriate antimicrobial therapy

Table 6.6 Criteria supporting a clinical diagnosis of disseminated infection.

polymorphonuclear leukocytes (*Fig. 6.21*) assist in making the diagnosis and, even more importantly, may reveal Gram-positive cocci in clusters thus suggesting the diagnosis of staphylococcal endocarditis. In one-half of cases, gonococci cannot be isolated from blood, CSF, or synovial fluid, even with the best laboratory techniques.[8] It must be stressed that asymptomatic genitourinary, pharyngeal, and/or rectal *N. gonorrhoeae* infections are the rule rather than the exception in this disease. Mucosal surface cultures are by far most likely to demonstrate the organism thus providing objective evidence in support of the diagnosis. Such cultures should be obtained before antibiotics are started in all patients in whom DGI enters into the differential diagnosis. In the absence of positive blood or synovial fluid cultures, a presumptive diagnosis of DGI can be made based upon a combination of two of the following three criteria, provided other diagnoses have been eliminated:

- Isolation of gonococci from a mucosal site of the patient or the patient's sexual partner (in the case of an infant, isolation from the conjunctiva or a nasogastric specimen)
- The presence of pustular, hemorrhagic, or necrotic skin lesions on the extremities

- Rapid resolution of joint signs and symptoms on appropriate antimicrobial therapy (*Table 6.6*).

PELVIC INFLAMMATORY DISEASE (PID, SALPINGITIS)

As is the case with chlamydia, the gonococcus may ascend from the endocervical canal through the endometrium to the fallopian tubes and ultimately to the pelvic peritoneum (*Fig. 6.22*), resulting in endometritis, salpingitis, and finally peritonitis (see also Chapter 8). Patients may report pelvic and abdominal pain, fever, and chills. Adnexal, fundal, and cervical motion tenderness are found on examination. Acute pyogenic complications of PID include tubo-ovarian abscesses,

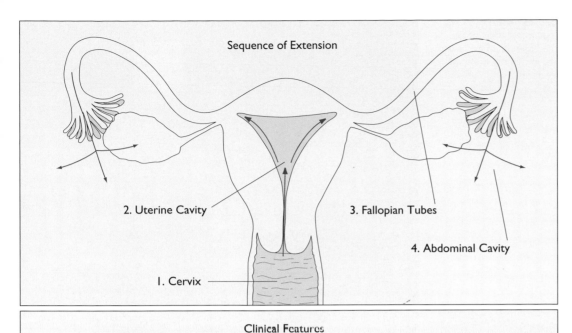

Fig. 6.22 The evolution of gonococcal pelvic inflammatory disease.

Sequence of Extension

2. Uterine Cavity

3. Fallopian Tubes

4. Abdominal Cavity

I. Cervix

Clinical Features

Endocervicitis

May be asymptomatic; vaginal discharge, cervical inflammation, or infection; local tenderness.

Endometritis

Menstrual irregularity.

Endosalpingitis

Constant bilateral lower quadrant abdominal pain aggravated by body motion. Tenderness in one or both adnexal areas. Abscess formation may occur.

Peritonitis

Nausea, emesis, abdominal distention, rigidity, tenderness. Pelvic or abdominal cavity abscess formation may follow.

Neisseria gonorrhoeae	*Bacteroides* spp.
Chlamydia trachomatis	*Peptococcus* spp.
Group B streptococci	*Peptostreptococcus* spp.
Escherichia coli and other enterobacteria	Genital mycoplasmas (?)
Gardnerella vaginalis	*Actnomyces israelii*
Haemophilus spp.	(only with IUD-associated disease)
Fusobacterium spp.	

Table 6.7 Etiologic agents of primary and recurrent pelvic inflammatory disease.

pelvic peritonitis (often mimicking appendicitis), or the Fitz–Hugh–Curtis syndrome, which is an inflammation of Glisson's capsule of the liver. PID may also be caused by many nonsexually transmitted bacteria and these are frequently the same organisms that are associated with the bacterial vaginosis syndrome.[9] The proportion of PID cases caused by *N. gonorrhoeae*, based on the recovery of the organism from laparoscopic specimens, varies from 8 to 70% depending on geographic location. The proportion of women with cervical gonococcal infection who will develop upper tract disease is uncertain. PID is the most common and costly consequence of gonorrhea, and recurrent episodes of PID are common. Initial PID infections are more likely to be gonococcal or chlamydial, while other bacteria are isolated more frequently from recurrent episodes (*Table 6.7*). The consequences of PID include an increased probability of infertility (tubal factor infertility), ectopic pregnancy, and chronic pelvic pain.

The clinical diagnosis of PID is imprecise. The disease should be considered in a woman with lower abdominal pain and adnexal tenderness,

or midline tenderness indicative of endometritis. Abnormally painful menses and metromenorrhagia are common. PID has been associated with the use of intrauterine contraceptive devices (IUDs). Pelvic actinomycosis, a rare cause of PID, is seen exclusively in women using IUDs. Laparoscopy is the best method for confirming the clinical diagnosis; however, especially in early PID, the inflammation may not have extended to the tubal surface, and the peritoneal mucosa may appear normal despite inflammation within the tubes (*Figs 6.23* and *6.24*). Endometrial biopsy represents a less invasive alternative to laparoscopic examination. Abnormalities are seen in as many as 90% of endometrial biopsies from women with laparoscopic evidence of salpingitis. Additionally, as many as one-third of women with examination findings suggestive of PID and negative laparoscopic findings will have histopathologic findings that suggest endometritis. Histopathologic findings consistent with endometritis include the presence of plasma cells in stromal tissue and the presence of neutrophils within the epithelium. Misdiagnosis based on clinical criteria alone is common; ectopic pregnancy and acute appendicitis may be mistaken for PID and vice versa (*Tables 6.8 and 6.9*). As yet laparoscopy and endometrial biopsy are not recommended procedures for all women suspected of having PID due to the invasive nature of these tests and their expense. Therefore their use is a matter of the individual physician's judgment and the availability of the tests. Endocervical specimens for *N. gonorrhoeae* and *C. trachomatis* testing are recommended but not essential in that all recommended empiric treatment regimens must be effective against both pathogens and treatment should be started prior to the availability of test results. However, confirmation of the diagnosis is useful in determining the patient's prognosis and may assist in ensuring that the male partner is also treated.

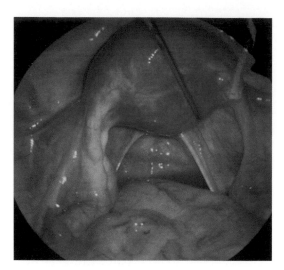

Fig. 6.23 Normal laparoscopic view of the female genital tract: view from above the dome of the uterus.

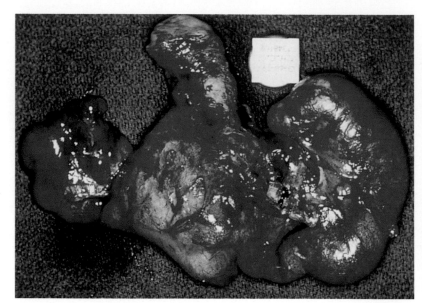

Fig. 6.24 Uterus and fallopian tubes of a patient with advanced recurrent pelvic inflammatory disease, showing so-called 'retort' tubes.

Preoperative diagnosis	
Ovarian tumor	20
Acute appendicitis	18
Ectopic pregnancy	16
Chronic PID	10
Acute peritonitis	6
Pelvic endometriosis	5
Uterine myoma	5
Uncharacteristic pelvic pain	5
Miscellaneous	6
	91

Modified after Jacobson L and Westrom L Am J Obstet Gynecol 1969; 105:1088.

Table 6.8 Erroneous diagnoses among women with lower abdominal pain confirmed laparoscopically to have PID.

Visual findings	
Acute appendicitis	24
Pelvic endometriosis	16
Corpus luteum hematoma	12
Ectopic pregnancy	11
Ovarian tumor	7
Chronic PID	6
Mesenteric lymphadenitis	6
Miscellaneous	16
	98

Modified after Jacobson L and Westrom L Am J Obstet Gynecol 1969; 105:1088.

Table 6.9 Laparoscopy findings among women with lower abdominal pain erroneously diagnosed as PID.

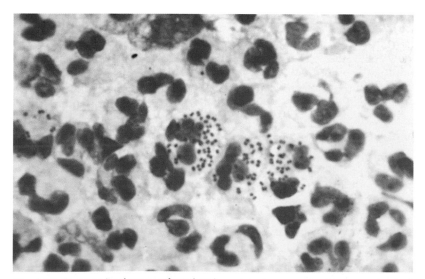

Fig. 6.25 Gram-stained smear of uretheral exudate from a male showing a sheet of neutrophils (PMNs) and many Gram-negative diplococci within PMNs. This finding is sufficient for a presumptive diagnosis of gonorrhea in the male.

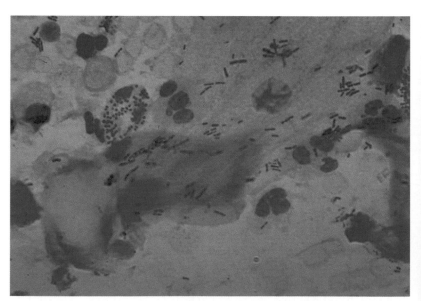

Fig. 6.26 Gram-stained smear of endocervical exudate showing scattered neutrophils and squamous epithelial cells. Gram-negative diplococci are present in one neutrophil. This finding supports a presumptive diagnosis of gonorrhea in the female, but should be confirmed by culture.

LABORATORY TESTS

The laboratory diagnosis of gonorrhea has been classically performed by examination of a Gram-stained smear for the presence of intracellular Gram-negative cocci as a presumptive diagnosis, followed by confirmation by growth of the causative agent, *N. gonorrhoeae*. Presumptive diagnosis can be performed easily even in parts of the world where laboratory facilities are limited.[10] Culture of *N. gonorrhoeae* is standard practice in the industrialized world but requires access to reasonable laboratory facilities to give good isolation rates. Detection of gonococci, without necessity for culture, has become more widely available as commercial kits have become more sensitive, specific and reliable. This has followed the increasing use of molecular detection methods for chlamydial infection, which are now accepted as the gold standard, and in some instances *N. gonorrhoeae* and *C. trachomatis* can be detected simultaneously. Nonculture detection methods avoid the need for a viable organism and are probably less sensitive to problems with transportation to the testing laboratories and hence should be useful in many situations in different parts of the world. The disadvantages are the increased cost compared to culture and the lack of a viable organism for susceptibility testing.

PRESUMPTIVE LABORATORY DIAGNOSIS

Microscopical examination of a Gram-stained smear from the urethra and cervix are considered positive for the presumptive diagnosis of gonorrhoea if Gram-negative diplococci are observed intracellularly in polymorphonuclear leukocytes (*Figs 6.25* and *6.26*). A positive smear is 95% sensitive in men with symptomatic urethritis but is less sensitive in cervical specimens from women (30–50%). This probably reflects the greater number of asymptomatic infections in women and the lower numbers of organisms present. It is common practice to examine rectal smears but the sensitivity is likely to be less (40–60%) in blindly obtained rectal specimens. A rectal smear is most useful if taken with a proctoscope from patients with evidence of infection. Diagnosis of pharyngeal infection cannot be based on the Gram stain because of the frequent presence of other *Neisseria* and related spp. in the oropharynx. In some parts of the world smears are stained with methylene blue which is simple and rapid and particularly useful where laboratory facilities are not well developed (Fig. 6.27). It does, however, lack specificity and is best used to screen for negative smears and then any smears showing intracellular diplococci stained by Gram's method as confirmation of the presumptive diagnosis. (*Fig 6.25*)

CULTURE FOR *N. GONORRHOEAE*

SPECIMEN COLLECTION AND TRANSPORTATION

Specimens for gonorrhea culture should always be collected before treatment is administered. *N. gonorrhoeae* is most successfully isolated when the specimen is inoculated onto media directly from the patient and incubated at 35–36.5°C in a CO_2-enriched atmosphere immediately after collection. Where possible incubation should be in an appropriate incubator but if this is not available it is important to place the media into the presence of a CO_2-enriched atmosphere as soon as possible. Thus, streaked plates should be immediately placed in a CO_2 candle-extinction jar held at room temperature until they can be transported to the laboratory incubator. Specimens may be kept at room temperature for up to 5 hours without loss of viability. For small numbers of specimens CO_2 envelopes designed for individual plates are commercially available.

Specimens for culture may be collected from the urethra, cervix, rectum, and pharynx as well as from the endometrium, fallopian tubes, joint fluid or blood, if PID or DGI is suspected. The precise choice of anatomic sites from which to collect specimens is made on the basis of the patient's potential for sexual exposure and presenting symptoms (*Table 6.10*). Specimens are collected with cotton, polyester, or calcium alginate swabs. Normally, only urethral specimens are collected from heterosexual men, while urethral, rectal, and pharyngeal specimens are collected from homosexual men. Cervical and rectal specimens are routinely collected from women; specimens may also be collected from the urethra and from Bartholin's and Skene's glands when appropriate. In men, *N. gonorrhoeae* may also be isolated from the culture of urine sediment. Blood cultures should be collected from patients with suspected disseminated infection. In patients with septic arthritis, synovial fluid should be cultured.

If specimens must be transported a significant distance from the clinical facility to the laboratory, they should be inoculated onto an isolation medium (Jembec or Transgrow) and incubated overnight before shipment. The transport medium should be shipped by courier or an express delivery service to insure delivery of the inoculated medium within 24–48 hours. Transport of specimens in Amies' or Stuart's medium is only appropriate for transportation when inoculation of the medium will take place within 4–8 hours.

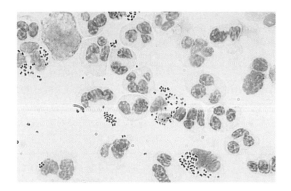

Fig 6.27 Methylene blue-stained smear of urethral exudate from a man showing neutrophils and intracellular organisms.

Patient	Sites
Heterosexual men	Urethra
	Oropharynx
Homosexual men	Urethra
	Rectum
	Oropharynx
Women	Cervix
	Rectum
	Oropharynx

Table 6.10 Sites for usual collection of specimens for the laboratory diagnosis of uncomplicated gonorrhea.

Selective agent	Concentrations used	Organisms inhibited
Vancomycin	2–4 mg/l	Gram-positive bacteria
Lincomycin	1 mg/l	Gram-positive bacteria
Colistin	7.5 mg/l	Gram-negative bacteria (other than *Neisseria*)
Trimethoprim	5 mg/l	Gram-negative bacteria (other than *Neisseria*)
Nystatin	12,500 IU/l	*Candida* spp.
Amphotericin	1–1.5 mg/l	*Candida* spp.

Table 6.11 Antimicrobial agents used in selective media for isolation of *N. gonorrhoeae*.

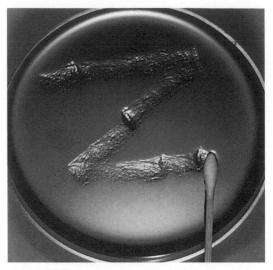

Fig. 6.28 'Z' streak method of inoculation to obtain isolated colonies for the identification of *Neisseria*.

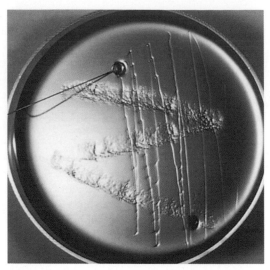

Fig. 6.29 Cross-streaking of 'Z' inoculated plate to insure separation of colonies.

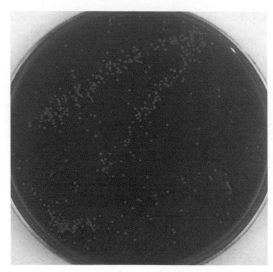

Fig. 6.30 Inoculated plate after 24 hours of incubation.

ISOLATION METHODS

Specimens should be inoculated onto selective media such as Thayer–Martin (TM) medium, modified Thayer–Martin medium (MTM), Martin–Lewis (ML) medium, New York City (NYC) medium, or GC–Lect (GC–L) medium, which are composed of GC base or equivalent media supplemented with growth factors and antimicrobial and antifungal agents (*Table 6.11*); some media contain hemoglobin. If the specimen is obtained from a site that is normally sterile (e.g. blood, synovial fluid, conjunctiva), it may be inoculated on a nonselective medium such as chocolate agar. It should be remembered that other *Neisseria* and related spp. may grow on nonselective media and therefore confirmation procedures should be scrupulously followed. Vancomycin-susceptible strains of *N. gonorrhoeae* occasionally occur and may not grow on selective media containing 4 µg vancomycin/ml, which is routinely used for the isolation of the gonococcus. Selective media have been modified to contain 2 µg or 3 µg vancomycin/ml in order to overcome this problem. Lincomycin has also been used as an alternative but is less inhibitory than vancomycin and overgrowth, particularly from rectal specimens, can occur. Vancomycin-susceptible gonococci should be suspected in a community when false-negative cultures are obtained, as evidenced by a discrepancy between Gram-stain positivity and culture-positivity rates for urethral gonorrhea in men; these should agree for at least 95% of cases.

The specimen should be inoculated over the entire surface of the plate in a 'Z' pattern, followed by streak inoculation of the plate (*Figs 6.28–6.29*). This inoculation technique yields isolated colonies that can be more easily processed, particularly in pharyngeal specimens, from which strains of *N. meningitidis*, *N. lactamica*, and *K. denitrificans* may also be isolated.

Inoculated plates should be incubated immediately at 35–36.5°C in a CO_2-enriched, humid atmosphere. Gonococci require CO_2 for primary isolation; the supplemental CO_2 can be provided in a CO_2 incubator, a container with a CO_2-generating tablet, or a candle-extinction jar with white, unscented, nontoxic candles.

IDENTIFICATION OF *N. GONORRHOEAE*

PRESUMPTIVE IDENTIFICATION

Plates are examined for growth after incubation for 24 hours; those that show no growth at this time are reincubated for 24–48 hours before being discarded and before a report of negative for *N. gonorrhoeae* is issued. Translucent, nonpigmented-to-brownish colonies measuring

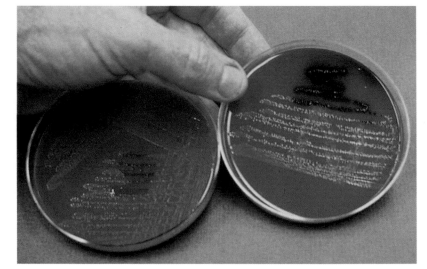

Fig. 6.31 Positive oxidase reaction on culture of *N. gonorrhoeae*.

0.5–1.0 mm in diameter on isolation media should be further characterized (*Fig. 6.30*). Representative colonies are Gram stained and examined for oxidase production. Smears prepared from suspect colonies should be examined microscopically for the presence of Gram-negative diplococci. Cells of *Neisseria* spp. occur as diplococci composed of kidney-shaped cells (0.8 µm × 0.6 µm) with adjacent sides flattened (*see Fig. 6.25*). Oxidase is detected either by placing a drop of oxidase reagent (tetramethyl-paraphenylenediamine-dihydrochloride) on a few representative colonies or by rubbing representative colonies on filter paper moistened with oxidase reagent with a platinum loop; nichrome loops may react with the oxidase reagent, giving a false-positive reaction. In a positive test, the colonies will turn purple within 10 seconds (*Fig. 6.31*). The oxidase reagent should not be placed on all suspect colonies. If few suspect colonies are available, they must be subcultured to chocolate agar immediately after the application of the oxidase reagent because of the toxicity of the reagent to the cells. Thin smears of suspect colonies are Gram stained as described above. If the suspect colonies are oxidase-positive, Gram-negative diplococci, a report of presumptive *N. gonorrhoeae* may be made for cervical, urethral, or rectal specimens.

CONFIRMATION OF IDENTIFICATION

Ideally, all isolates should be confirmed as *N. gonorrhoeae*, although this is not always possible in parts of the world with limited laboratory facilities and resources. Certainly, pharyngeal isolates must be confirmed because other *Neisseria* and related spp. may frequently be isolated on gonococcal selective media. The aim of identification tests is to distinguish between *N. gonorrheae* and other species of *Neisseria* particularly *N. meningitidis* and *N. lactamica*[11,12] (*Tables 6.12* and *6.13*). This is particularly important for organisms isolated from sexual or child abuse cases.

Traditionally, *Neisseria* and related spp. have been identified by a series of biochemical tests, including acid production from glucose, maltose, sucrose, and lactose; reduction of nitrate; and the production of polysaccharide. Traditional biochemical tests must be incubated for 24–48 hours before results can be interpreted (*Figs 6.32* and *6.33*). Acid production tests should be incubated at 35–36.5°C without CO_2, which will produce an acid reaction in the media. Rapid tests have been developed that permit identification of strains from the primary isolation plate or within several hours of the isolation of a pure subculture. The rapid confirmation tests may be divided into three categories: carbohydrate, enzyme substrate and serologic.

Rapid Carbohydrate Tests

Rapid carbohydrate tests permit the detection of acid production from glucose, maltose, lactose, and sucrose. Strains of *N. gonorrhoeae* are distinguished by their ability to produce acid only from glucose; most other *Neisseria* spp. produce acid from maltose and thus are easily differentiated from *N. gonorrhoeae*. However, because strains of other *Neisseria* and related spp. may also provide strong or weak acid reactions from glucose, additional tests may be required to differentiate between them. Strains of several species (maltose-negative *N. meningitidis*, *N. cinerea*, *B. catarrhalis*, and *K. denitrificans*) may be misidentified as *N. gonorrhoeae*. In addition, some strains of *N. gonorrhoeae* produce very weak reactions in glucose tests and may appear to be glucose-negative. Supplemental tests that can be used to distinguish *N. gonorrhoeae* from these species are listed in *Tables 6.12* and *6.13*.

Enzyme Substrate Tests

Strains of *Neisseria* spp. produce enzymes that may be used to differentiate between them. *N. gonorrhoeae* strains produce hydroxyprolyl aminopeptidase, *N. meningitidis* strains produce γ-glutamyl aminopeptidase, and *N. lactamica* strains produce β-galactosidase; strains of *B. catarrhalis* produce none of these enzymes. The use of enzyme substrate tests is

Species	Extra CO_2 needed[a]	Growth on MTM ML, or NYC medium	Growth on Chocolate or blood agar at 22°C	Growth on Nutrient agar at 35°C
N. gonorrhoeae	VI	+[b]	–	–
N. meningitidis	I	+	–	+
N. lactamica	D	+	–	+
N. cinerea	D	–[c]	–	+
N. polysaccharea	D	+	–	+
N. flavescens	I	+	–	+
N. sicca	No	–	+	+
N. subflava biovar *perflava*	No	–[d]	+	+
B. catarrhalis	No	D	+	+
K. denitrificans	I	+	–	–

MTM = modified Thayer–Martin medium; ML = Martin–Lewis medium; NYC = New York City medium; + = Most strains (≥ 90%) positive; – = Most strains (≥ 90%) negative; D = Some strains positive, some strains negative.
[a] Extra CO_2; VI, very important for growth; I, important for growth; No, not needed for growth; D, some strains require extra CO_2.
[b] ≥ 90% of vancomycin-susceptible strains of N. gonorrhoeae *may not grow on TM or MTM media.*
[c] Some strains of N. cinerea *have been isolated on gonococcal selective medium but are colistin-susceptible and will not grow when subcultured on selective media.*
[d] Some strains of N. subflava *biovar* perflava *grow on gonococcal selective media in primary culture, are colistin-resistant, and grow on selective media on subculture.*

Table 6.12 Growth on selective and nonselective media, requirement for supplemental CO_2.

Species	Pigment[a]	Superoxol[b]	Acid produced from Glucose	Acid produced from Maltose	Acid produced from Fructose	Acid produced from Sucrose	Lactose (ONPG)	Polysaccharide from 1% SUCROSE[c]	NO$_3^-$	NO$_2^{-d}$	DNase
N. gonorrhoeae	–	+	+	–	–	–	–	–	–	–	–
N. meningitidis	–	–	+	+	–	–	–	–	–	D	–
N. lactamica	–	–	+	+	–	–	+	–	–	D	–
N. cinerea	–	–	–[e]	–	–	–	–	–	–	+	–
N. polysaccharea	–	–	+	+	–	–	–	+	–	D	–
N. flavescens	+	–	–	–	–	–	–	+	–	–	–
N. sicca	–	–	+	+	+	+	–	+	–	+	–
N. subflava biovar *perflava*	+	–	+	+	+	+	–	+	–	+	–
B. catarrhalis	–	–	–	–	–	–	–	–	+	–	–
K. denitrificans	–	–	+	–	–	–	–	–	+	–	–

ONPG = o-nitrophenyl-β-D-galactopyranoside; DNase = deoxyribonuclease; – = Most strains (≥ 90%) negative; + = Most strains (≥ 90%) positive; D = Some strains positive, some strains negative.
[a] Pigment observed in colonies on nutrient agar. Strains of N. cinerea *and* N. lactamica *are yellow-brown and yellow pigmented when growth is harvested on a cotton applicator or smeared on filter paper.*
[b] All Neisseria *spp. and* B. catarrhalis *give a positive catalase test using 3% H_2O_2;* N. gonorrhoeae *strains give strong reactions with 30% H_2O_2 (superoxol) on chocolatized blood media, whereas other species are usually negative. This test should be used only in conjunction with other tests.*
[c] Some strains may be inhibited by 5% sucrose; reactions may be obtained on a starch-free medium containing 1% sucrose. Strains of N. gonorrhoeae *and* N. meningitidis *do not grow on this medium.*
[d] Results for tests in 0.1% (w/v) potassium nitrite; N. gonorrhoeae *strains and strains of some other species that are negative in 0.1% nitrite can reduce 0.01% (w/v) nitrite.*
[e] Some strains of N. cinerea *may give a weak reaction in glucose in some rapid tests for the detection of acid from carbohydrates.*

Table 6.13 Differential biochemical reactions.

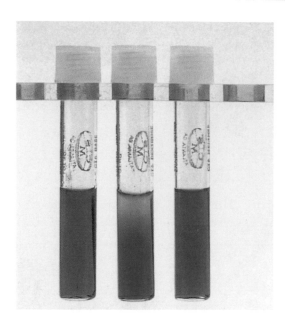

Fig. 6.32 Acid production from carbohydrates in Cystine Trypticase Soy (CTA) medium. Tubes from left to right are CTA base medium containing no carbohydrate, CTA medium containing 1% glucose and CTA medium containing 1% maltose. The organism is *N. gonorrhoeae*.

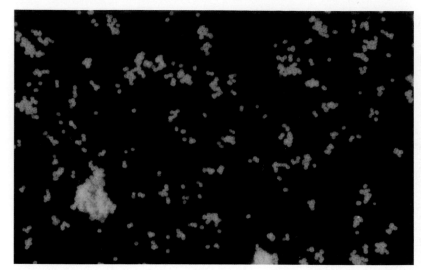

Fig. 6.34 Monoclonal FA stain.

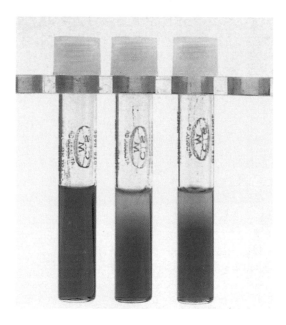

Fig. 6.33 Acid production from carbohydrates in CTA medium (see Fig. 6.32 for further details). The organism is *N. meningitidis*.

Cross-reaction with nongonococcal species has not been observed with monoclonal reagents. Occasionally, some gonococcal strains do not react in this test (false negative). FA confirmation with polyvalent antibodies is not recommended because the reagent may react with other *Neisseria* spp. (false positive).

Coagglutination tests consist of cocktails of monoclonal antibodies directed toward the major gonococcal porin, Por, which have been adsorbed to protein A-producing *Staphylococcus aureus* cells. Suspect colonies are suspended in buffer or saline and heated in a boiling-water bath. A drop of the cooled suspension is mixed with a drop each of the antigonococcal reagents and a negative control. After rotation for 1–2 minutes, the reactions are interpreted. If a suspension gives a positive reaction with the antigonococcal reagent and a negative reaction with the control, the isolate is identified as *N. gonorrhoeae* (Fig. 6.35). Cross-reactions between nongonococcal *Neisseria* and related spp. and the coagglutination reagents have been reported, and some gonococcal strains have not reacted with the reagents.

PRESERVATION

Isolates of *N. gonorrhoeae* must be subcultured every 24–48 hours or suspended in a solution of trypticase soy broth containing 15% glycerol and frozen at –70°C. Strains cannot be stored at –20°C for long periods but can be stored at this temperature for a short time (approximately 2 months).

MOLECULAR DETECTION OF *N. GONORRHOEAE*

Four methods for the molecular detection of gonococci in patient's specimens are available commercially, by DNA probe (Gen-Probe PACE 2) or amplification by polymerase chain reaction (Amplicor PCR, Roche), ligase chain reaction (Abbott LCx), and strand displacement (BDProbTec ET system). These tests have not been used as widely as the equivalent tests for chlamydial infections primarily because culture for *N. gonorrhoeae* is relatively inexpensive and considered to be highly sensitive when appropriate isolation procedures are used. However, molecular detection has proved to be as sensitive as culture and in many instances has increased sensitivity with good specificity. This may reflect the inadequacies of isolation procedures but probably results from the enhanced sensitivity achievable with molecular detection, particularly of non-viable organisms.

In parallel with diagnosis of chlamydial infection, the greater sensitivity has allowed the screening of non-invasive samples such as urine or self-taken swabs. In men, detection of *N. gonorrhoeae* in urine has been found to be as sensitive as urethral swabs but in women the results are

limited to the identification of strains isolated on gonococcal-selective media because strains of the commensal *Neisseria* spp. may produce hydroxyprolyl aminopeptidase and would be identified as *N. gonorrhoeae* without supplemental tests. In addition, strains of *K. denitrificans* and some strains of *N. subflava* biovar *perflava* and *N. cinerea* have also been isolated on gonococcal-selective media and will be misidentified as *N. gonorrhoeae* without additional characterization. Thus using a combination of enzyme substrate and other biochemical tests, strains isolated on selective media can be identified by a process of elimination (*Table 6.13*).

Products that combine acid production, enzyme substrate, and other biochemical tests are also commercially available. These tests provide a more detailed characterization of isolates that will permit the laboratory technician to distinguish *N. gonorrhoeae* from related species. Pure cultures of clinical isolates are required to inoculate all rapid biochemical tests.

Serologic Tests

There are currently no available tests that permit the detection of gonococcal antibodies in serum. Serologic tests for the identification of *N. gonorrhoeae* in primary cultures are commercially available as FA tests or as coagglutination tests. Thin smears may be stained with a monoclonal FA reagent (*Fig. 6.34*) to confirm the identification of *N. gonorrhoeae*.

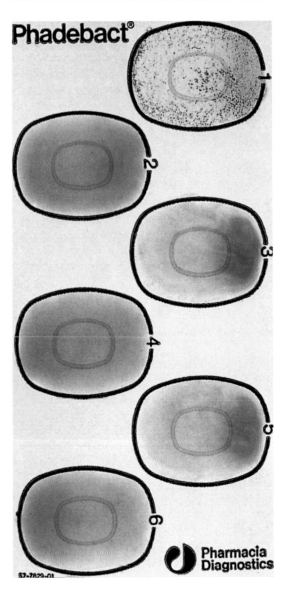

Fig. 6.35 Reactions of *N. gonorrhoeae, N. meningitidis,* and related spp. in the Phadebact coagglutination test:
1. *N. gonorrhoeae.*
2. Negative control.
3. *N. meningitidis.*
4. *N. cinerea.*
5. *N. lactamica.*
6. Negative control.

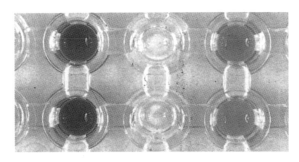

Fig. 6.36 Reactions of β-lactamase-positive (left) and negative (right) strains of *N. gonorrhoeae* in a nitrocefin test.

the substrate. β-lactamase-positive and β-lactamase-negative strains should be included as controls with each batch of clinical isolates.

DETERMINATION OF ANTIMICROBIAL SUSCEPTIBILITY

With the exception of specific β-lactamase tests, resistance in *N. gonorrhoeae* must be detected by measuring the level of susceptibility of strains to an antimicrobial agent. Two methods, the agar-dilution and disk-diffusion procedures, may be used to measure the susceptibilities of isolates.

Agar-Dilution Susceptibility Testing

Agar-dilution susceptibility testing is the reference method for measuring the antimicrobial susceptibilities of strains of *N. gonorrhoeae*. Resistance to antimicrobial agents is measured as the minimal inhibitory concentration (MIC) of the agent that inhibits growth of an isolate. Determination of susceptibilities to antimicrobial agents used for therapy should be tested and may include penicillin, broad-spectrum cephalosporins and fluoroquinolones. The methodology for susceptibility testing of *N. gonorrhoeae* can vary between countries, differing primarily in the base medium used; GC agar base[13] (NCCLS, North America), Isosensitest[14] (Australia) and Diagnostic Sensitivity Agar[15] (Europe). For therapeutic antimicrobial agents this is most important for the concentration of penicillin considered resistant; ≥ 2 μg/ml (GC base agar) and ≥ 1 μg/ml (Isosensitest and DST agar). Other antimicrobials agents are largely unaffected.

Susceptibility testing is performed on the base medium of choice containing 1% (vol/vol) IsoVitaleX or an equivalent supplement; antimicrobial agents are incorporated into the base medium in serial twofold dilutions. Isolates to be tested are grown overnight on chocolate agar and suspended in Mueller–Hinton broth (or equivalent) to an optical density equivalent to a 0.5 McFarland standard, containing approximately 10^8 colony-forming units (CFU)/ml. The suspensions are diluted 1:10 in Mueller–Hinton broth, and 10^4 CFU/ml are inoculated onto the surface of the antibiotic-containing media and an antibiotic-free control medium with a Steer's replicator, multipoint inoculator or a calibrated loop. Plates are incubated at 35–36°C in a CO_2-enriched atmosphere for 24 hours and then examined for growth. The MIC of the antimicrobial agent for an isolate is the lowest concentration that inhibits its growth (*Fig. 6.37*). A modification of the full MIC is the use of breakpoints which uses a similar method but with medium containing one or two concentrations of antibiotic that can be used to categorize isolates as being resistant or having decreased susceptibility. This is useful for screening isolates, particularly for high-level resistance.

Disk-Diffusion Susceptibility Testing

Agar-dilution susceptibility testing of *N. gonorrhoeae* isolates is not routinely performed in clinical microbiology laboratories. Instead, disk-diffusion susceptibility testing is most frequently used to measure the antimicrobial resistance of isolates of *N. gonorrhoeae*. The results of disk-diffusion susceptibility testing can be correlated with treatment outcome (*Table 6.14*).

more variable between studies and it is possible that self-taken vaginal swabs or tampons may be the most appropriate specimen. Prior to the availability of molecular detection, screening for gonorrhea was limited mainly to specialized clinics or to patients presenting with symptoms, but the use of non-invasive samples combined with a highly sensitive test has the potential for screening asymptomatic populations. The evolution of these tests to detect both *N. gonorrhoeae* and *C. trachomatis* simultaneously (BDProbTec, Gen-Probe, PACE-2 System) will give the most information with the least inconvenience to the individual. This is particularly important at this time when rates of gonococcal and chlamydial infection are increasing in many countries and detection of the asymptomatic reservoir is an essential control measure.

ANTIMICROBIAL SUSCEPTIBILITY TESTING

β-LACTAMASE TESTS

All gonococcal isolates should be tested for β-lactamase, which can be detected in colonies on primary isolation medium or after subculture. Several tests for β-lactamase are available commercially; these include chromogenic cephalosporin (*Fig. 6.36*), acidometric, and iodometric tests. The chromogenic cephalosporin (nitrocefin) tests are preferred because the substrate is stable and the reactions are specific and highly sensitive for β-lactamase. The specificity and sensitivity of the acidometric and iodometric tests may be affected by several factors, including incorrect storage of the product, which may result in nonspecific hydrolysis of

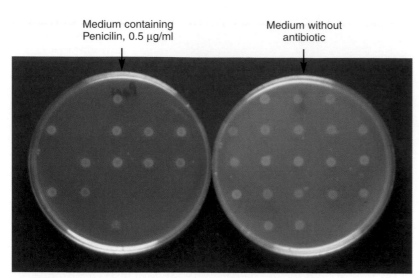

Fig 6.37 Susceptibility of *N. gonorrhoeae* to penicillin determined by the agar dilution method. Medium containing 0.5 µg/ml penicillin showing inhibition of some strains compared to the control medium without antibiotic.

SUSCEPTIBLE	Less than 5% likelihood of treatment failure
INTERMEDIATE	Predictable failure rates of 5 to 15% if the patient is treated with the tested antibiotic in the standard dosage (in most cases of intermediate susceptibility, a higher dose or prolonged therapy results in greater than 95% cure rates)
RESISTANT	May be associated with treatment failure rates of greater than 15%

Table 6.14 Correlates of disk-diffusion susceptibility results with clinical outcome.

Recommended therapy

Cefixime: 400 mg po in a single dose
or
Ceftriaxone: 125 mg IM in a single dose
Ciprofloxacin: 500 mg po in a single dose
or
Ofloxacin: 400 mg po in a single dose
or
Levofloxacin: 250 mg po in a single dose
plus
A regimen effective against possible co-infection with *C. trachomatis* such as doxycycline 100 mg po bid for 7 days or azithromycin one gram po as a single dose

Table 6.15 CDC Recommended guidelines for antimicrobial therapy for uncomplicated gonorrhea.

INTERPRETATION OF ANTIMICROBIAL SUSCEPTIBILITY TEST RESULTS

An antimicrobial susceptibility result determined in the laboratory is only a measure of the in vitro susceptibility of an isolate. A patient may have a positive test-of-cure culture for a variety of reasons:

- Failure of therapy because of infection with a resistant isolate
- Failure of therapy even when the patient is infected with a strain that is susceptible by in vitro measurements because of noncompliance with treatment.
- Reinfection.

Recommended therapy

Ciprofloxacin, 500 mg orally, as a single dose
or
Ceftriaxone: 125 mg by intramuscular injection in a single dose
or
Cefixime: 400 mg orally, as a single dose
or
Spectinomycin: 2 g intramuscular injection, as a single dose
or
Azithromycin, 2 g orally, as a single dose

Table 6.16 WHO Recommended guidelines for antimicrobial therapy for uncomplicated gonorrhea.

Recommended therapy

Ciprofloxacin, 500 mg orally, as in a single dose
or
Ofloxacin: 400 mg orally as in a single dose
or
Ampicillin 2 g or 3 g plus probenecid 1 g orally as a single dose, where regional prevalence of penicillin resistant *N. gonorrhoeae* <5%

Alternative regimens (not usually used as first line therapy in UK)

Ceftriaxone: 250 mg intramuscular injection as a single dose
or
Cefotaxime: 500 mg intramuscular injection as a single dose
or
Spectinomycin: 2 g intramuscular injection as a single dose

All patients with gonorrhoea should be screened for genital infection with C. trachomatis *or receive presumptive treatment for this infection.*

Table 6.17 UK Recommended guidelines for antimicrobial therapy for uncomplicated gonorrhoea.

Thus, antimicrobial susceptibilities must be used as an adjunct to, but cannot be substituted for, clinical findings.

Antimicrobial Therapy

In response to the continued emergence of resistant strains in the USA, the current CDC STD Treatment Guidelines[16] recommend treatment of all gonococcal infections presumptively with antibiotic regimens effective against strains resistant to penicillin and/or tetracycline (*Table 6.15*). In addition to the five recommended regimens for uncomplicated gonococcal infections, other broad-spectrum cephalosporins such as cefotaxime, cefotetan and cefuroxime axetil, are acceptable alternatives. Spectinomycin, 2 g intramuscularly, is a useful regimen for the treatment of patients who can tolerate neither cephalosporins nor fluoroquinolones. An important recent change in the recommendations is that quinolones should not be used for empiric treatment of infections acquired in Asia or the Pacific, including Hawaii because of high rates of resistance. The WHO treatment guidelines[17] (*Table 6.16*) are very similar to those put out by the CDC although WHO recommend the two gram single dose of azithromycin as a first-line therapy and CDC recommended this regimen as an alternative treatment for uncomplicated gonorrhea. The UK guidelines[18] recommend a quinolone or ampicillin as first-line therapy, if the strain is known to be sensitive, with ceftriaxone, cefotaxime or spectinomycin as alternative regimens (*Table 6.17*). It should be noted that treatment recommendations for complicated gonococcal infections (*Table 6.18*) are based on expert opinion, not on therapeutic trials.

Syndrome	Recommended therapy	
Disseminated gonococcal infection	Ceftriaxone*: 1 g, im or iv, every 24 hours	
	All regimens should be continued for 24–48 hours after improvement begins; therapy may then be switched to cefixime 400 mg po bid or ciprofloxacin 500 mg po bid to complete 7 days of therapy	
Meningitis/endocarditis	Consultation with an expert is vital. Ceftriaxone 1–2 g iv every 12 hours. Patients with meningitis should be treated for 10–14 days; those with endocarditis should be treated for at least 1 month	
Ophthalmia		
Neonatal	Ceftriaxone:	25–50 mg/kg body weight, im or iv, in a single dose, not to exceed 125 mg
Adult	Ceftriaxone:	1 g im, 1 dose†

*Or cefotaxime 1 g iv every 8 hours, or ceftizoxime 1 g iv every 8 hours, or spectinomycin 2 g im every 12 hours.
†Infected eye should be lavaged with saline solution.

Table 6.18 Recommended therapy for patients with complicated gonococcal infections.

References

1. Ison CA. Genotyping of *Neisseria gonorrheae*. *Current Opinion in Infectious Diseases* 1998; **11**:43–46.
2. Ison CA, Dillon JR, Tapsall JW. The epidemiology of global antibiotic resistance among *Neisseria gonorrhoeae* and *Haemophilus ducreyi*. *Lancet* 1998; **351**(suppl lll):8–11.
3. Tapsall J. Antimicrobial resistance in *Neisseria gonorrhoeae*. http://www.who.int/emc-documents/antimicrobial_resistance/whocdscsrdrs20013c.html (accessed 11.27.01).
4. DiCarlo RP, Martin DH. Use of the quinolones in sexually transmitted diseases. In: Andriole VT, ed. *The Quinolones*. 3rd Edition. San Diego: Academic Press; 2000:228–254.
5. Center for Disease Control and Prevention. Fluoroquinolone-resistance in *Neisseria gonorrhoeae*, Hawaii, 1999, and decreased susceptibility to azithromycin in *Neisseria gonorrhoeae*, Missouri, 1999. *MMWR Weekly* 2000; **49**:833–837. http://www.cdc.gov/mmwr/preview/mmwrhtml/mm4937a1.htm (accessed 11.27.01).
6. WHO Western Pacific Region Gonococcal Antimicrobial Surveillance Programme. Surveillance of antibiotic resistance in *Neisseria gonorrhoeae* in the WHO Pacific Region, 1999. *Commun Dis Intell* 2000; **24**:1–4.
7. Hook EW, Handsfield HH. Gonococcal infections in the adult. In: Holmes KK, Mardh PA, Sparling PF *et al* eds. *Sexually Transmitted Diseases*. 3rd Edition. New York: McGraw Hill; 1999:451–466.
8. Liebling MR, Arkfeld DG, Michelini GA *et al*. Identification of *Neisseria gonorrhoeae* in synovial fluid using the polymerase chain reaction. *Arthritis and Rheum* 1994; **37**(5):702–709.
9. Walker CK, Workowski KA, Washington EA *et al*. Anaerobes in pelvic inflammatory disease: Implications for the Centers for Disease Control and Prevention's guidelines for treatment of sexually transmitted diseases. *Clin Infect Dis* 1999; **28**(suppl 1):s29–36.
10. Dyck van E, Meheus AZ, Piot P. *Laboratory Diagnosis of Sexually Transmitted Infections*. 1999 World Health Organization. http://www.who.int/HIV_AIDS/index.html (updated 10/29/01, accessed 11.27.01).
11. Knapp JS, Rice RJ. Neisseria and Brahamella. In: Murray PR, Baron EJ, Pfaller MA, Tenover FC, Yolken RH (eds). *Manual of Clinical Microbiology*, 6th ed. Washington, DC, American Society for Microbiology, pp. 324–340, 1995.
12. Division of AIDS, STD and TB Laboratory Research, Center for Disease Control and Prevention. *Identification of Neisseria and related species*. http://www.cdc.gov/ncidod/dastlr/gcdir/NeIdent/Index.html (updated 02/10/00, accessed 11.27.01).
13. National Committee for Clinical Laboratory Standards. *Approved Standard: Performance Standards for Antimicrobial Disk Susceptibility Tests*, 5th ed. Document M2-A5. National Committee for Clinical Laboratory Standards, Villanova, Pa.
14. Members of the Australian Gononococcal Surveillance Programme. Penicillin sensitivity of gonococci in Australia: development of Australian gonococcal surveillance programme. *Br J Vener Dis* 1984; **60**:226–230.
15. Ison CA, Martin IMC and the London Gonococcal Working Group. Susceptibility of gonococci isolated in London to therapeutic antibiotics: establishment of a London surveillance programme. *Sex Transm Inf* 1999; **75**:107–111.
16. Sexually transmitted diseases treatment guidelines 2002. Centers for Disease Control and Prevention. *MMWR Recomm Rep.* 2002; **51**:1–78.
17. World Health Organization. *Guidelines for the management of Sexually Transmitted Infections*. 2001 http://www.who.int/HIV_AIDS/index.html (updated 10/29/01, accessed 11.27.01).
18. Clinical Effectiveness Group, MSSVD. National guidelines for the management of gonorrhoea in adults. *Sex Transm Infect* 1999; **75**(Suppl):S13–15.

Genital Mycoplasmas

7

D Tayor-Robinson, K Waites and G Cassell

INTRODUCTION

Mycoplasmas are the smallest known free-living micro-organisms, intermediate in size between bacteria and viruses (*Fig. 7.1*). They are unique among prokaryotes, differing by one or more characteristics from all other major groups of human pathogens, including viruses (*Table 7.1*). The absence of a rigid cell wall (*Fig. 7.2*) is the single most distinguishing feature of mycoplasmas[1] and is responsible for their being in a separate class, the Mollicutes ('soft skin'). Many of the biologic properties of mycoplasmas are due to the absence of a rigid cell wall, including resistance to all β-lactam antibiotics and marked pleomorphism among individual cells. In contrast to L-phase variants of bacteria, mycoplasmas are unable to synthesize cell-wall precursors under any conditions. The mycoplasmal cell membrane contains phospholipids, glycolipids, cholesterol, and various proteins. The extremely small genome size of mycoplasmas (approximately one-sixth the size of that of *Escherichia coli*) (*Table 7.2*) severely limits their biosynthetic capabilities, helps to explain their complex nutritional requirements for cultivation, and necessitates a parasitic or saprophytic existence for most species.

Mycoplasmas usually reside on the mucosal surfaces of the respiratory and genitourinary tracts and rarely penetrate the submucosa (*Fig. 7.3*). However, although mycoplasmas are found extracellularly, some, like *Mycoplasma pneumoniae*, *M. genitalium*, *M. hominis* (*Fig. 7.4*), *M. fermentans* and *M. penetrans*,[2] also become intracellular.

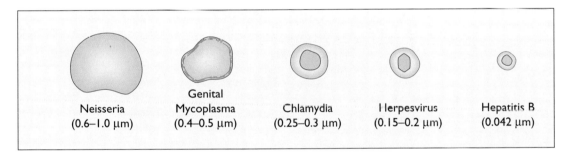

Fig. 7.1 Relative size of mycoplasma in comparison with other sexually transmitted micro-organisms. An individual mycoplasmal cell may be as small as 300 nm in diameter.

Neisseria (0.6–1.0 μm) — Genital Mycoplasma (0.4–0.5 μm) — Chlamydia (0.25–0.3 μm) — Herpesvirus (0.15–0.2 μm) — Hepatitis B (0.042 μm)

Characteristic	Mycoplasmas	Bacteria	Chlamydiae	Rickettsiae	Viruses
Growth in/on cell-free media	+	+	–	–	–
Generation of metabolic energy	+	+	–	+	–
Independent protein synthesis	+	+	+	+	–
Contain both DNA and RNA	+	+	+	+	–
Reproduce by binary fission	+	+	+	+	–
Contain cell wall	–	+	+	+	–
Require sterol for growth	+*	–	–	–	–

Except for the genus Acholeplasma.

Table 7.1 Comparison of mycoplasmas with other microbial agents.

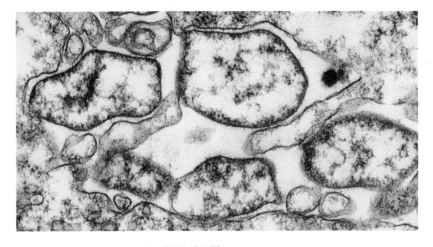

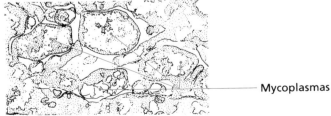
Mycoplasmas

Fig. 7.2 Transmission electron micrograph showing mycoplasmas between two epithelial cells. Unlike other bacteria, mycoplasmas lack a rigid cell wall.

127

The species of mycoplasmas isolated from the genitourinary tract of humans[3–5] are listed in *Table 7.3*. *M. genitalium* (*Fig. 7.5*) has been detected in the urethra of a significantly larger proportion of men (about 25%) with acute non-chlamydial NGU than in those without this disease (about 5%). This, together with the urethral inflammation occurring after intraurethral inoculation of nonhuman primates, especially chimpanzees, with *M. genitalium* indicates that it is a cause of urethritis. *M. genitalium* has also been associated with cervicitis. In addition, serologic studies in humans and experimental studies in nonhuman primates suggest that it may be a cause of PID. The existence of *M. genitalium* in the female genital tract suggests that its role in disease during pregnancy needs to be evaluated, as does its potential impact on the outcome of pregnancy.

Over nearly 50 years, *M. fermentans* has been isolated sporadically from the upper as well as the lower genitourinary and respiratory tracts, bone marrow, and other anatomic sites. In the last 10 years it has been found in patients with AIDS,[6] although there is no substantial evidence to indicate that it contributes to the disease. However, it has been implicated in an acute fatal respiratory disease of non-AIDS patients. *M. fermentans* has also been detected in amniotic fluid collected at the

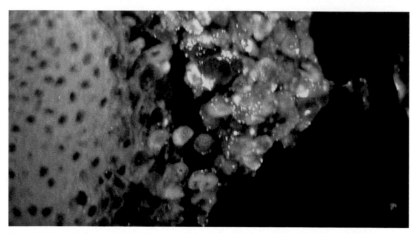

Fig. 7.3 Mycoplasmas attach to epithelial cell surfaces but rarely penetrate the submucosa. Unlike chlamydial organisms, they are mainly extracellular, not requiring an intracellular existence for propagation. However, some are known to penetrate epithelial cells. In this immunofluorescence micrograph, mycoplasmas are seen attached to the surface of inflammatory cells in the cervix. Note that neither *U. urealyticum* nor *M. hominis* has been shown to be a cause of cervicitis.

Organism	Genome size (base pairs)	Predicted protein coding regions
Mycoplasma genitalium	580,070	470
Mycoplasma pneumoniae	816,394	677
Ureaplasma urealyticum	751,719	613
Escherichia coli	4,639,221	4,288

Table 7.2 Mycoplasmas have small genomes.

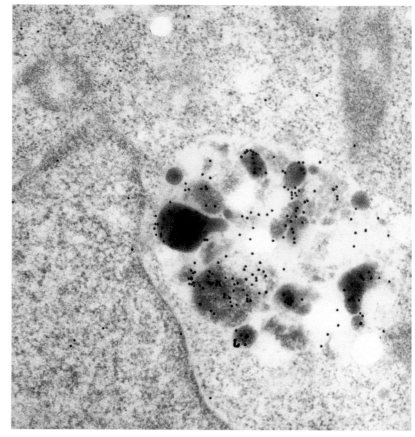

Fig. 7.4 Electron micrograph of immunogold-labelled *M. hominis* organisms within a vacuole in the cytoplasm of a Hela cell.

Mycoplasma	Kidney	Bladder urine	Voided urine	Urethral swab	Seminal fluid	Fallopian tube	Cervix/vagina	Amniotic fluid
Myoplasma hominis	+	+	+	+	+	+	+	+
Ureaplasma urealyticum	+	+	+	+	+	+	+	+
Mycoplasma genitalium			+	+			+	
Mycoplasma fermentans			+	+			+	+
Mycoplasma penetrans			+	+				
Mycoplasma primatum			+					
Mycoplasma salivarium	+							
Mycoplasma spermatophilum					+			
Acholeplasma laidlawii							+	
Acholeplasma oculi								+

Table 7.3 Mycoplasmas isolated from or detected in the genitourinary tract of humans.

time of cesarean section from a small proportion of women with intact membranes. Some of the mycoplasma-positive women had chorio-amnionitis, suggesting that *M. fermentans* should be investigated further as a cause of maternal and fetal infection. In the last 5 years, *M. fermentans* has been detected by PCR technology in the joints of about 20% of patients with idiopathic chronic inflammatory arthritides, including rheumatoid arthritis, but not in those with degenerative or metabolic arthritis, findings that need pursuing.

Of the mycoplasmas occurring in the genitourinary tract, *Ureaplasma urealyticum* (ureaplasmas) and *M. hominis* are probably found most commonly, so that the remainder of this chapter will focus mainly on these two micro-organisms.[3–5]

EPIDEMIOLOGY

The isolation rates of *U. urealyticum* and *M. hominis* in various populations are given in *Table 7.4*. *U. urealyticum* can be found in the cervix or vagina of 40–80% of sexually mature, asymptomatic women, and *M. hominis* in 20–50%. The incidence of each is somewhat lower in the urethra of normal males. In women, colonization is linked to younger age, lower socioeconomic status, sexual activity with multiple partners, Black ethnic group, and oral contraceptive use. *U. urealyticum* and *M. hominis* may be transmitted to about 40% of babies born to infected mothers. The colonization of most infants appears to be transient, with a sharp decline in the rate of isolation after 3 months of age. Less than 10% of older children and sexually inexperienced adults are colonized. Colonization after puberty increases with sexual activity.

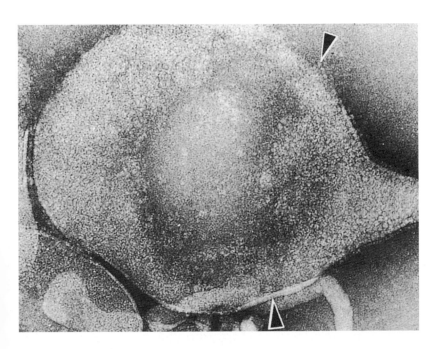

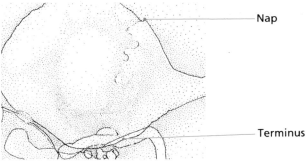

Fig. 7.5 Transmission electron micrograph of *M. genitalium* showing an intact mycoplasma cell negatively stained with ammonium molybdate. The terminus is covered with a nap extending peripherally to the tip.

CLINICAL MANIFESTATIONS

U. urealyticum and *M. hominis* are most often commensals in the lower genital tract of women. Their involvement in bacterial vaginosis is mentioned later. Genitourinary diseases in which these micro-organisms are suspected of having an etiologic role are listed in *Table 7.5*, and are diseases either of the female upper genitourinary tract or of the male tract. Difficulty in accepting these mycoplasmas as the cause of disease has usually arisen because they can be recovered sometimes as often from asymptomatic as from symptomatic individuals, or because samples cannot be obtained easily from the affected site for testing.

The results of some clinical studies and of experimental infection of laboratory animals have confirmed the disease-producing potential of both *U. urealyticum* and *M. hominis*. However, even in diseases in which Koch's postulates have been fulfilled (for example, *M. hominis* and PID), attempts to link inflammatory lesions of the upper tract with isolation of organisms from the lower tract have delayed recognition of the etiologic significance of these micro-organisms. A major principle is that

Population	Isolation rates	
	U. urealyticum	*M. hominis*
Sexually mature, asymptomatic females (cervix or vagina)	40–80%	20–50%
Babies born to infected mothers	ca. 40%	ca. 40%
Older children	< 10%	< 10%
Sexually inexperienced adults	< 10%	< 10%
Normal males	20–40%	10–20%

Table 7.4 Epidemiology of *U. urealyticum* and *M. hominis*.

Disease	Causative agent	
	U. urealyticum	*M. hominis*
Urethritis of males*	+	–
Prostatitis (chronic)	–	–
Epididymitis	±	–
Urinary calculi	±	–
Pyelonephritis	±	+
Bacterial vaginosis	±	±
Cervicitis**	–	–
Pelvic inflammatory disease	–	+
Infertility	±	–
Chorioamnionitis	+	±
Spontaneous abortion	±	±
Prematurity/low birth weight	±	–
Intrauterine growth retardation	±	–
Postpartum and postabortal fever	+	+
Congenital pneumonia	+	+
Pneumonia in newborns	+	+
Meningitis in newborns	+	+
Abscesses in newborns	+	+
Extragenital disease in adults (including septic arthritis)	+	+

– = No association or causal role demonstrated; + = causal role; ± = significant association and/or strong suggestive evidence but causal role not proven.
* M. genitalium *shown to be a cause;* ** M. genitalium *significantly associated*

Table 7.5 Relationship of *U. urealyticum* and *M. hominis* to diseases of the genitourinary tract of humans.

organisms only reach the upper tract in a subpopulation of individuals infected in the lower genitourinary tract, and that disease then develops in only a few of these individuals. There has been no instance in which the factors predisposing to upper tract colonization or the development of disease have been delineated, but it seems that in this situation *U. urealyticum* and *M. hominis* behave primarily as opportunists. In contrast, these mycoplasmas are increasingly being recognized as common causes of extragenital disease in immunocompromised patients and in newborn infants, particularly preterm infants.

Urethritis in Men

The results of human and animal inoculation studies, together with those of controlled antibiotic and serologic investigations, support a causal role for *U. urealyticum* organisms in NGU, particularly chronic disease, although they lag behind *Chlamydia trachomatis* and *M. genitalium* in importance. Furthermore, the exact proportion of cases for which ureaplasmas are responsible has not been established (*Fig. 7.6*). The common occurrence of ureaplasmas in the urethra of asymptomatic men suggests that only certain biovars or serovars are pathogenic and/or that predisposing factors, such as a lack of mucosal immunity, exist in individuals who develop disease. There is no evidence supporting a role for *M. hominis* as a cause of urethritis.

Prostatitis

A number of studies suggest that the prostate can be infected by ureaplasmas during the course of an acute ureaplasmal infection of the urethra. Ureaplasmas have been isolated more often and in greater numbers from specimens from patients with acute prostatitis than from controls and men with more than 10^4 organisms have been reported to respond to tetracycline therapy, unlike those with fewer organisms.

However, unequivocal evidence for a causal role in acute disease does not exist. *U. urealyticum* has not been found in prostatic biopsies from patients with chronic abacterial prostatitis, and *M. hominis* has not been associated with prostatitis of any kind in most studies.

Epididymitis

U. urealyticum has been recovered from the urethra and directly from epididymal aspirate fluid, accompanied by a specific antibody response, in a patient with acute non-gonococcal, non-chlamydial epididymitis. Further studies are required to establish a causal role.

Urinary Calculi

Urinary calculi composed of magnesium ammonium phosphate (struvite) and carbonate–apatite account for 20% of all urinary tract stones (*Fig. 7.7*), and may be the most deleterious variety in terms of urologic complications. These so-called infection stones are induced by the enzymatic breakdown of urea by bacterial urease (*Fig. 7.8*). *Proteus* and to a lesser extent *Klebsiella, Pseudomonas, Providencia, Staphylococcus,* and other bacterial species are the usual causes in humans. However, *U. urealyticum* also produces urease and has been shown experimentally in vitro to induce crystallization of struvite and calcium phosphates in urine and to produce calculi in animal models. However, there is little evidence that it does so under natural conditions in humans, in the absence of other urease-producing organisms. The frequency with which ureaplasmas reach the kidney, the predisposing factors that allow this to occur, and the relative frequency of renal calculi which might be induced by ureaplasmas compared with those induced by other bacteria, remain unanswered.

Pyelonephritis

Despite the high incidence of *M. hominis* in the lower genitourinary tract, this micro-organism has been isolated from the upper urinary tract only in patients with symptoms of acute infection and is often accompanied by a significant antibody response. Overall, *M. hominis* is thought to be involved in about 5% of cases of acute pyelonephritis. Predisposing factors, including obstruction or instrumentation of the urinary tract, are found in about half the cases in which *M. hominis* is thought to be the cause.

REPRODUCTIVE TRACT

Bacterial Vaginosis

M. hominis organisms and, to a lesser extent, ureaplasmas, are found often in much larger numbers in the vagina of women who have bacterial vaginosis than in healthy women; there may be a 1000- to

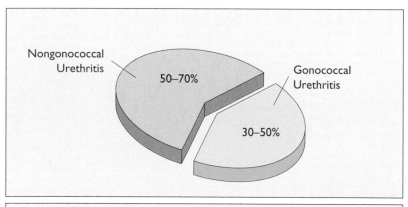

Nongonococcal Urethritis — 50–70%
Gonococcal Urethritis — 30–50%

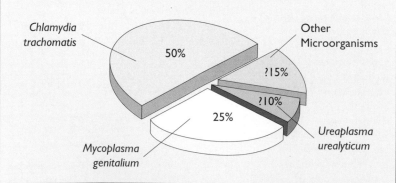

Chlamydia trachomatis — 50%
Other Microorganisms — ?15%
?10%
Mycoplasma genitalium — 25%
Ureaplasma urealyticum

Fig. 7.6 The incidence and causes of nongonococcal urethritis (NGU). (**Top**) Approximate incidence of NGU versus gonococcal urethritis (GU) in the USA. The exact incidence is unknown; however, it is likely that NGU outnumbers GU by as much as 2:1. (**Bottom**) Causes of NGU. It is well established that up to approximately one-half of NGU cases are due to *C. trachomatis*, about 25% due to *M. genitalium,* with the remainder caused by either *U. urealyticum* or other microorganisms (perhaps those involved in bacterial vaginosis), the precise contributions of which have yet to be determined.

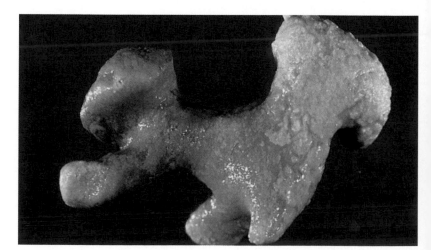

Fig. 7.7 Staghorn renal calculus typically associated with urinary tract infections due to urease-producing bacteria.

10,000-fold more organisms in bacterial vaginosis. However, the mycoplasmas exist with a variety of other bacteria, also in large numbers, so that the contribution of the former, if any, to the symptoms and sequelae of bacterial vaginosis is unknown.

Pelvic Inflammatory Disease

This is an increasingly common disease of multifactorial etiology (*see also Ch. 8*). It can be caused iatrogenically or can occur naturally from infections with various bacteria, the most common of which are *C. trachomatis* and, to a lesser extent, *Neisseria gonorrhoeae*. *M. hominis*, but probably not *U. urealyticum*, is also a likely cause of PID, although the exact contribution of bacterial vaginosis, in which *M. hominis* proliferates together with many other bacterial species, is unknown. *M. hominis* has been isolated apparently in pure culture from the fallopian tubes of almost 10% of women with salpingitis diagnosed by laparoscopy, but not at all from women without lesions. The organisms have also been isolated from the endometrium. In addition, a role for *M. hominis* in cases of PID not associated with either *C. trachomatis* or *N. gonorrhoeae* is supported by significant increases in specific antibody. PID allegedly due to *M. hominis* is clinically indistinguishable from similar disease caused by other micro-organisms, and so antimicrobial coverage for *M. hominis* should always be included in the therapy.

While *U. urealyticum* has been isolated directly from affected fallopian tubes, it is found usually in the presence of other known pathogens. Furthermore, the results of serologic studies in humans and of inoculating subhuman primates and fallopian tube organ cultures do not support a causal role.

Disorders of Reproduction

Given that *M. hominis* is a likely cause of salpingitis, it is reasonable to assume that severe tubal infection with this micro-organism could lead to occlusion and infertility. However, this has not been proven. Although the possibility that ureaplasmas may play a role in involuntary infertility in humans was first raised over 20 years ago, the association remains speculative. Prospective studies based on the isolation of *U. urealyticum* and *M. hominis* from the endometrium or placenta, but not studies based only on vaginal–cervical isolation, show a consistent association with spontaneous abortion, but whether the organisms are responsible is unclear.

Chorioamnionitis and Pregnancy Outcome

In a subpopulation of women colonized in the lower genital tract, both *M. hominis* and *U. urealyticum* may colonize the endometrium (*Fig. 7.9*), with or without evidence of inflammation. Attachment of the organisms to sperm (*Fig. 7.10*) has been suggested as one mechanism by which the organisms are introduced into the upper tract. Both micro-organisms can invade the amniotic sac before 20 weeks of gestation in the presence of intact fetal membranes and apparently in the absence of other micro-organisms. Mycoplasmas have been isolated from the endometrium of 20% and from the placenta of about 10% of unselected women with intact fetal membranes at the time of cesarean section. Isolation from fetal membranes increases with the onset of labor, membrane rupture, and the number of vaginal examinations.

The isolation of *M. hominis* from amniotic fluid is almost always associated with clinical symptoms (maternal fever, uterine tenderness, foul vaginal discharge) and a specific serologic response. *U. urealyticum*, on the other hand, has been known to persist in amniotic fluid for as long as 2 months, in the presence of an intense inflammatory response, yet without discernible clinical signs or symptoms of amnionitis. Although the role of bacterial vaginosis, with its attendant plethora of bacteria, has to be considered in any adverse outcome of pregnancy, an argument in favor of ureaplasmas alone producing chorioamnionitis is provided by the following (*Figs 7.11–7.14*):

- The demonstration of inflammatory cells and ureaplasmas in amniotic fluid over a 2-month period in the absence of other demonstrable micro-organisms
- The direct demonstration of ureaplasmas alone in inflammatory infiltrates in the fetal membranes at the time of premature delivery.

The isolation of *U. urealyticum* from the placenta is significantly associated with histologic chorioamnionitis and funisitis, stillbirth, and perinatal morbidity and mortality. Individual case reports indicate that, at least sometimes, the infection is causal. Isolation of ureaplasmas from the placenta is inversely related to gestational age and birth weight.

PERIPARTUM INFECTIONS

M. hominis and *U. urealyticum* are a cause of postpartum fever as a consequence of inducing postpartum endometritis. Furthermore, they

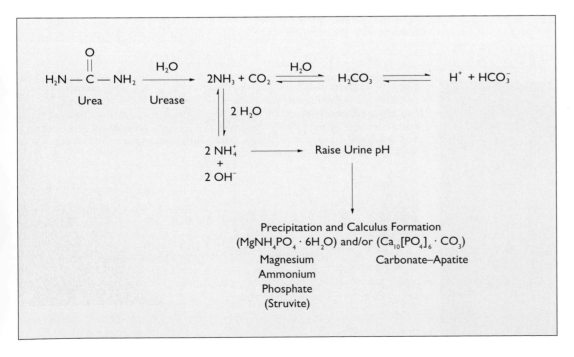

Fig. 7.8 Biochemical reactions leading to the formation of urinary calculi by urease-producing bacteria such as *U. urealyticum*.

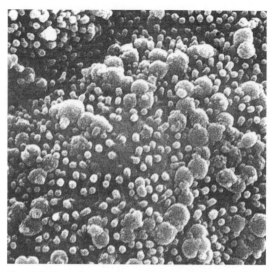

Fig. 7.9 Scanning electron micrograph showing *U. urealyticum* attached to the endometrium; note the organisms (large) and the cellular microvilli (small). Both *U. urealyticum* and *M. hominis* can be isolated from the endometrium with or without evidence of inflammation. The presence of this micro-organism was demonstrated also by culture and by immunofluorescence.

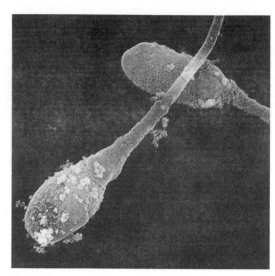

Fig. 7.10 *U. urealyticum* attached to human sperm. The ureaplasmas were cultured and identified specifically by immunofluorescence.

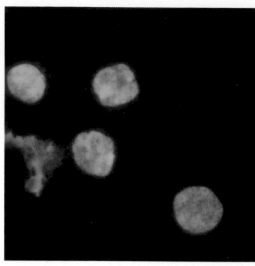

Fig. 7.11 DNA-fluorochrome-stained cytocentrifuged preparation of amniotic fluid collected at 20 weeks' gestation showing amnion cells and the absence of micro-organisms. The fluid was shown subsequently to be culturally negative (× 750).

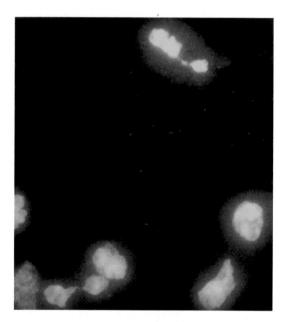

Fig. 7.12 DNA-fluorochrome-stained cytocentrifuged preparation of amniotic fluid collected at 20 weeks' gestation showing large numbers of ureaplasmas (identified by culture) and large numbers of polymorphonuclear leukocytes (× 750). The fluid was culturally negative for other bacteria, viruses, and chlamydiae.

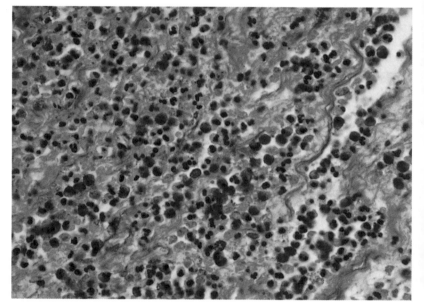

Fig. 7.13 Placenta at 26 weeks' gestation (hematoxylin and eosin × 250). *U. urealyticum* was isolated in pure culture from amniotic fluid 6 weeks prior to delivery. Note the extensive inflammation in the amnion and chorion.

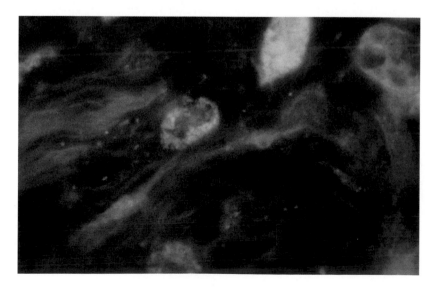

Fig. 7.14 Adjacent section of placenta shown in Fig. 7.13 (× 750) stained with rabbit anti-*U. urealyticum* serovar I serum and reacted with affinity-purified, fluorescein-labeled, goat anti-rabbit IgG. Ureaplasmas are present in the most intense areas of inflammation. Adjacent sections treated with normal rabbit serum and conjugate were negative. Brown and Bren-stained adjacent sections of placenta were negative for other bacteria.

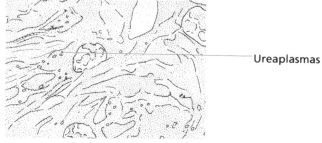

Ureaplasmas

are both known to cause postabortal fever. These infections are often self-limited and do not require treatment. However, *M. hominis* septicemia results in a longer hospital stay, and in some cases results in septic arthritis and post-cesarean wound infection.

M. hominis has been isolated also from the joints of women who developed acute, suppurative arthritis following normal childbirth, with the onset of arthritis occurring from 6 hours to 3 weeks after delivery. In most cases, the organisms were isolated not only from affected joints but also from blood.

DISEASES OF THE NEWBORN

Respiratory Disease

There is evidence that *U. urealyticum* and *M. hominis* sometimes cause congenital pneumonia and respiratory disease in the newborn[7] (*Fig. 7.15*). In particular, *U. urealyticum* has been associated significantly with respiratory disease in very-low-birth-weight infants. Infants whose birth weights are less than 1,000 g, and in whom ureaplasmas have been isolated from the lower respiratory tract within 24 hours of birth, have been found to be twice as likely to develop chronic lung disease and twice as likely to die as infants of similar birth weights, who are uninfected, or infants weighing more than 1,000 g. Also, pneumonia and sepsis due to *U. urealyticum* can be associated with persistent pulmonary hypertension of the newborn. Evidence indicates that many ureaplasmal and *M. hominis* respiratory infections are acquired in utero.

U. urealyticum and *M. hominis* isolated from tracheal aspirates are likely to represent true infections of the lower respiratory tract, particularly if they are isolated in pure culture and are isolated concomitantly from blood, as often occurs. It is not thought that the tracheal isolates are merely due to contamination from the nasopharynx, because of the discrepancy in the isolation rates between the two sites; *U. urealyticum* has been isolated more often from endotracheal aspirates than from nasopharyngeal swabs. Furthermore, *M. hominis* has been isolated from almost 10% of endotracheal aspirates from infants weighing less than 2,500 g with respiratory disease, but rarely from the nasopharynx of these infants. Further evidence that tracheal isolates represent true infection of the lower respiratory tract includes the occurrence of large numbers of organisms, sometimes more than 10^6 colony-forming units, in the aspirates, and repeated isolation over several months. The CSF of infants with respiratory disease is sometimes found to be positive for *U. urealyticum* and *M. hominis*, again indicating the invasive nature of these micro-organisms in preterm infants.

CNS and Other Systemic Infections

Both *U. urealyticum* and *M. hominis* cause meningitis in the newborn.[7] Although their overall prevalence as CNS pathogens has not been thoroughly evaluated, evidence suggests that they may be among the most common causes of CSF infections in premature infants within the first few days of life. Congenital infection has been documented in some cases (*Fig. 7.16*).

U. urealyticum in the CSF is significantly associated with severe intraventricular hemorrhage and is often found in the presence of hydrocephalus. Chronic CSF infection of more than one month's duration has been observed with both *M. hominis* and *U. urealyticum*. Changes in the CSF may be similar to those seen in bacterial meningitis, namely low glucose, elevated protein, and mononuclear or polymorphonuclear pleocytosis, or there may be no abnormalities detected whatsoever. The range of infection varies from a mild subclinical course with no sequelae to more severe neurologic damage leading to permanent handicaps.

M. hominis is also a cause of pericardial effusion, adenitis, and subcutaneous abscesses, associated with breaks in the skin due to fetal-monitoring electrodes or forceps wounds.

BACTEREMIA AND OTHER EXTRAGENITAL INFECTIONS

There are numerous individual reports of *M. hominis* and *U. urealyticum* gaining access to the bloodstream. In the case of *U. urealyticum*, this has been reported in postabortal and postpartum bacteremia, as well as in newborn infants with respiratory distress and/or pneumonia. Bacteremia due to *M. hominis* has been demonstrated in a variety of conditions following renal transplantation, trauma, and genitourinary manipulations. Wound infections, brain abscesses, and osteomyelitis have also been reported.

The true incidence of extragenital infections caused by *M. hominis* or *U. urealyticum* is unknown as these micro-organisms are not sought routinely. Most reported cases have been discovered by 'accident' due to the occasional growth of *M. hominis* on blood agar or in routine blood cultures, or after specific mycoplasmal cultures have been set up following the exclusion of other possible infectious causes.

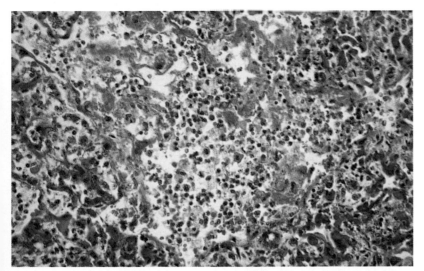

Fig. 7.15 Lung tissue (hematoxylin and eosin × 100) collected at autopsy from a 1-week-old term infant. *U. urealyticum* was isolated in pure culture from blood, tracheal aspirate, and pleural fluid prior to death, and from lung and brain tissue at post mortem. There is a mixed mononuclear and polymorphonuclear cell infiltrate with abundant macrophages, fibrin deposition, and early interstitial fibrosis.

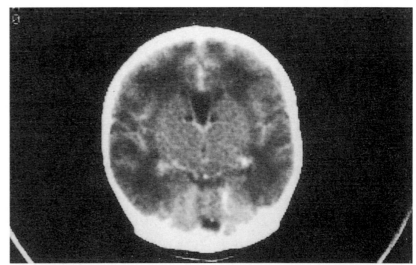

Fig. 7.16 Cranial CT scan of an infant 9 days after birth. *M. hominis* was isolated from the CSF 6 days after birth. There is decreased attenuation, predominantly involving the supratentorial white matter symmetrically, with a few punctate lesions of increased attenuation suggestive of small focal hemorrhage or early calcification. These findings are compatible with diffuse intrauterine infection or a degenerative process.

ARTHRITIS AND OTHER EXTRAGENITAL DISEASE IN IMMUNOCOMPROMISED HOSTS

There is evidence to suggest that mycoplasmas are responsible for a considerable proportion of cases of arthritis in individuals with hypogammaglobulinemia.[8] The organisms have been isolated repeatedly from affected joints in the absence of any other microbial agent.

In some reported cases, the arthritis was persistent, lasting from several months to over a year. Aggressive, erosive arthritis that progresses can occur despite anti-inflammatory therapy and γ-globulin replacement. In some cases involving *U. urealyticum*, the arthritis has been associated with subcutaneous abscesses, persistent urethritis, and chronic urethrocystitis/cystitis. Most cases have required aggressive antibiotic therapy, but some of the strains involved have been, or have become, resistant to multiple antibiotics.

Septic arthritis, surgical wound infections, septicemia, and peritonitis due to *M. hominis* appear to occur rather frequently in patients following organ transplantation and in others undergoing immunosuppressive therapy. Sternal wound infections due to *M. hominis* in heart-lung transplant patients seem to be particularly common. Polyarthritis with recovery of both *U. urealyticum* and *M. hominis* has been seen in a kidney allograft patient on an immunosuppressive regimen. However, further evidence that ureaplasmas cause a problem in immunosuppressed patients or in those with AIDS is lacking.

LABORATORY TESTS

Infections caused by mycoplasmas are sometimes discovered accidentally, either by observing pin-point colonies of *M. hominis* on conventional blood agar, or because treatment directed at common bacterial pathogens has failed, leading to the suspicion that mycoplasmas might be involved. Unfortunately, a mycoplasmal etiology is often considered only as a last resort.

Mycoplasmas should be considered in diseases in which they have been shown to play a role and when common bacteria have neither been revealed by Gram staining nor isolated. For conditions in which there is no strong suggestion of a mycoplasmal etiology, it is difficult to justify either examination for the organisms or anti-mycoplasmal treatment. In particular, isolation of either *M. hominis* or *U. urealyticum* from the female lower genital tract or urine (other than that collected by catheter or suprapubic aspiration) is not meaningful.

Mycoplasmas are very demanding in terms of laboratory culture requirements. The diagnosis of mycoplasmal infections in general bacteriology laboratories is hampered because the organisms are not visible on Gram staining, there has been a paucity of commercially available, reliable culture media specifically designed for mycoplasmal growth, and the organisms grow poorly or not at all in conventional bacteriologic media. *M. hominis* can be recovered occasionally from blood cultures or other clinical material without resort to special media, but this approach is unreliable. Ureaplasmas, *M. genitalium*, *M. fermentans*, and *M. penetrans* are more fastidious than *M. hominis* and cannot be recovered from clinical material unless specific techniques and media are used. If a mycoplasmal infection is suspected, care should be taken to collect a suitable specimen, to ensure that it is transported or stored under conditions known to maintain mycoplasmal viability, and to ensure that its examination is performed by a laboratory experienced in the cultural isolation and identification of mycoplasmas, or their detection by PCR technology.[3–5,9] Reliable information will be obtained only if these conditions are met.

SPECIMENS FOR CULTURE: ANATOMIC SITES

Specimens, including urethral and vaginal discharges, prostatic secretion, urine, tracheal secretion, sputum, pleural fluid, synovial fluid, CSF, or blood, are acceptable for mycoplasmal culture depending on the nature of the clinical condition. Other suitable specimens include placenta or any tissue collected from a biopsy or at autopsy (brain, lung, liver, kidney) if there is reason to suspect the presence of mycoplasmas.

SPECIMEN COLLECTION AND TRANSPORT

Only calcium alginate-, dacron-, or polyester-tipped swabs should be used, and the swab must always be extracted from the specimen. Blood should be collected free of anticoagulants.

Unlike many conventional bacteria, mycoplasmas, due to their lack of a cell wall, are extremely susceptible to adverse environmental conditions, especially drying, osmotic changes, and toxic metabolites. Particular care must be taken to ensure that specimens are not subjected to extreme environmental fluctuations. No specific transport medium is necessary for tissue or fluid specimens if they can be inoculated directly onto mycoplasmal agar medium or into broth medium within a reasonable period of time (i.e., no more than 1 hour after collection). However, if specimens are allowed to remain at room temperature and are not inoculated into appropriate transport medium, this may result in a significant loss of mycoplasmal viability or overgrowth of bacterial contaminants. When possible, specific mycoplasmal medium should be provided for direct inoculation of clinical specimens at the time they are collected. If specimens are collected in a facility that does not have immediate access to mycoplasmal broth for transport, satisfactory alternatives include 2SP medium (0.2 M sucrose in 0.02 M phosphate buffer, pH 7.2), trypticase soy broth with 0.5% bovine serum albumin, and commercially available Stuart's medium. Body fluids should be inoculated in an approximately 1:10 ratio (usually 0.1 ml of fluid per 0.9 ml of broth transport medium). Ideally, some uninoculated material should also be sent to the laboratory. Specimens should be kept refrigerated at 4°C and protected from drying in a sealed container until they can be transported to the laboratory. If transport is not possible within a maximum of 24 hours after collection, the specimen should be stored at −70°C and transported frozen on dry ice. Mycoplasmas are stable for indefinite periods if kept frozen at −70°C in a stable protein-containing broth medium. Storage at −20°C is less reliable as a significant gradual loss of viable organisms may occur.

DETECTION BY CULTIVATION AND POLYMERASE CHAIN REACTION

Although by definition mycoplasmas are free-living (capable of growth on or in cell-free media), they are fastidious and demanding in their requirements for special media. Various media are available. Those sold commercially may be useful but often are not as sensitive as media produced in mycoplasma-experienced laboratories. In using any medium, but in particular one obtained commercially, it is important to exclude mycoplasmal contamination. Fetal calf serum and horse serum used in most media are occasionally contaminated with mycoplasmas of animal origin.

Mycoplasmas are very sensitive to inhibitors present in some batches of horse serum, yeast extract, and even mycoplasmal media bases, and it is common for the standard medium in a laboratory to be temporarily inadequate for cultivation of mycoplasmas. Without proof of adequacy, negative cultures have little meaning. It is essential that rigorous quality-control procedures are followed, using recent clinical isolates and stock strains (including multiple serotypes, especially with ureaplasmas). Consultation with a mycoplasma reference laboratory may be essential or, at least, helpful.

Clinical specimens for mycoplasmal culture should always be diluted serially in broth to at least 10^{-3} and each dilution inoculated onto agar. Dilution is necessary to overcome potential inhibitory substances or metabolites, including antibiotics, which may be present in the body fluid or tissue, and to facilitate quantitative estimation of the number of organisms present. In theory, greater isolation sensitivity may be obtained by centrifuging urine and performing serial dilutions on an aliquot from the sediment. Tissues should preferably be minced rather than ground for cultivation to circumvent potential growth inhibitors that are more likely to be released with grinding.

Mycoplasmas isolated from the genitourinary tract have different metabolic properties and cultivation requirements. Thus, they have different pH ranges for optimal growth, as well as different biochemical substrates from which they derive energy. *U. urealyticum* generates ATP by urea hydrolysis, *M. hominis* metabolizes arginine to ammonia, and *M. genitalium* metabolizes glucose. *M. fermentans* and *M. penetrans* metabolize both arginine and glucose. No single medium formulation will optimally support the growth of all these micro-organisms. Myco-plasmal growth medium ordinarily contains animal serum, peptones, yeast extract, and metabolic substrates such as glucose, arginine, or urea. Shepard's 10 B broth and A8 agar media[10] have been employed success-fully for several years to cultivate both *M. hominis* and *U. urealyticum*

(*Fig. 7.17*). SP-4 broth and agar media will support the growth of *M. hominis, U. urealyticum, M. fermentans, M. penetrans,* and *M. genitalium* and are used with appropriate additives and at an appropriate pH (*Fig. 7.18*). Antibiotics, such as penicillin or nystatin, are incorporated routinely in the media to inhibit bacterial and fungal contamination.

Very little information is available concerning the recovery of *M. genitalium, M. fermentans,* and *M. penetrans* from clinical material. They are thought to grow best in an atmosphere containing 95% nitrogen and 5% CO_2, but extremely slow multiplication, in particular that of *M. genitalium,* requires that incubation be prolonged over a period of weeks.

M. hominis and *U. urealyticum* are much easier to recover from clinical specimens. Their relatively rapid growth rate, particularly that of the latter, makes the identification of most positive cultures possible within 1–5 days. Broth cultures may be incubated at 37°C under atmospheric conditions, and agar plates under 95% nitrogen and 5% CO_2. Urea-plasmas, in particular, are susceptible to a rapid decline in viability in

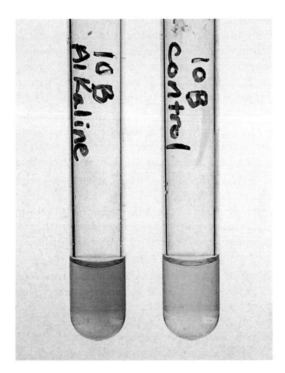

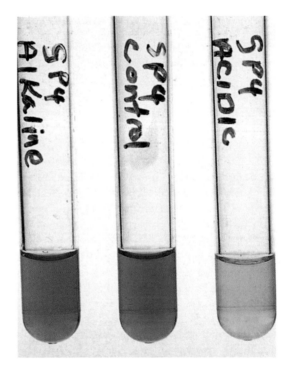

Fig. 7.17 Shepard's 10 B broth. This broth, containing phenol-red pH indicator, is used to detect and cultivate *M. hominis* and *U. urealyticum*. At a pH of 6.0, the broth is yellow. Multiplication of *M. hominis* or *U. urealyticum* with hydrolysis of arginine or urea, respectively, results in an elevation of the pH and a change in color from yellow to pink without a significant increase in turbidity.

Fig. 7.18 SP-4 broth. This broth may be used for the cultivation of *M. hominis, U. urealyticum, M. fermentans, M. penetrans,* or *M. genitalium*. It is normally prepared at a pH of 7.4–7.5. Multiplication of *M. hominis* with arginine hydrolysis elevates the pH, resulting in a color change from red to deep fuschia, while growth of a glucose-metabolizing mycoplasma, such as *M. genitalium,* results in a decrease in pH due to acidic end-products and a change in color from red to yellow.

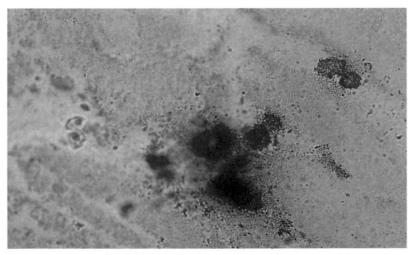

Fig. 7.19 Colonies of *U. urealyticum* growing on A8 agar. The granular brown appearance is due to urease activity and the release of ammonia in the presence of $CaCl_2$ indicator. The colonies are rather amorphous, as is often the case with ureaplasma colonies produced as a result of an initial isolation attempt from clinical material.

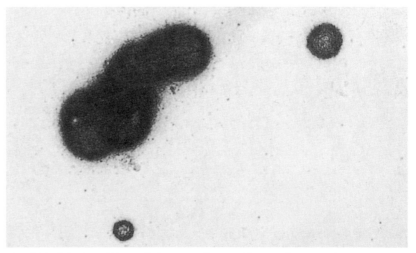

Fig. 7.20 Colonies of *U. urealyticum* growing on A8 agar after several passages on artificial medium. Note the characteristics of these discrete colonies compared to those on the initial isolation plate shown in Fig. 7.19.

culture, which is likely to result from a combination of urea depletion, ammonia production, and elevated pH due to urease activity. The occurrence of growth in 10 B medium is suggested by an alkaline shift due to the urease activity of ureaplasmas or arginine hydrolysis by *M. hominis* causing the phenol-red indicator to turn the color of the medium from yellow to pink (*Fig. 7.17*). Growth in SP-4 broth by glucose-metabolizing mycoplasmas is evident by a red-to-yellow (acidic) change in color, or red to deeper red (alkaline) change by arginine-metabolizing mycoplasmas (*Fig. 7.18*). Aliquots of broth cultures showing color changes should be subcultured to agar. This broth-to-agar technique has been shown to be the most sensitive for recovery of genital mycoplasmas.

Primers specific for each of the genital mycoplasmas have been identified. Detection by the PCR is the method of choice for *M. genitalium*[11] and *M. fermentans*, the former, in particular, being extremely difficult to isolate in primary culture. However, a recent successful approach in the case of *M. genitalium* was to introduce specimens into Vero cell cultures with subculture to mycoplasmal medium when the PCR signified multiplication of organisms.

SPECIES IDENTIFICATION

Colonies of *U. urealyticum* can be identified more easily on A8 agar in which CaCl$_2$ indicator is incorporated, urease activity releasing ammonia with the production of dark brown colonies (*Figs 7.19* and *7.20*). *M. hominis* colonies are urease-negative and have a typical 'fried egg' appearance (*Figs 7.21* and *7.22*). Unlike the colonies of conventional bacteria, small mycoplasmal colonies require a stereomicroscope to determine their presence and characterize their morphology.

Apart from determining the glucose-, arginine-, or urea-metabolizing capacity of an isolated mycoplasma, there are no other biochemical tests that can readily distinguish between the species and, apart from the ureaplasmas, their colonies are likely to be morphologically indistinguishable. Thus, serologic or PCR identification methods must be used.

Serologic tests are of two basic types. The first involves the use of viable organisms, antiserum inhibiting the growth or metabolic functions of the mycoplasmal species or type against which it has been prepared. Examples include the growth-inhibition and metabolism-inhibition (*Fig. 7.23*) methods, and the mycoplasmacidal test. Growth-inhibition undertaken on agar is specific but rather insensitive, making it useful for speciation of mycoplasmas (*Fig. 7.24*) but of limited, if any, value for antibody measurement. Metabolism-inhibition and mycoplasmacidal tests are sufficiently specific to identify organisms and are also sensitive enough for antibody measurement. In the second group of serologic methods, organisms are identified by demonstrating the reaction of specific antibody with whole fixed organisms or their antigens. The most widely used of these procedures is colony immunofluorescence (*Fig. 7.25*).

A problem faced with any of these techniques arises from the serological heterogeneity encountered within a mycoplasmal species. Many serotypes react specifically with antibody, necessitating the use of more than one antiserum if all strains within a species are to be identified correctly.

SEROTYPING

There is some suggestion that certain serotypes of *U. urealyticum* are more likely to be associated with disease than are others, but definitive evidence is lacking. Furthermore, the serological approach to serotyping used in the past was laborious and not practical routinely. However, the development of PCR technologies has facilitated much more rapid biotyping and serotyping.

STAINS

Stains that bind to DNA can often aid in detection of mycoplasmas prior to culture results (*see Fig. 7.12*). Extranuclear fluorescence in fluid specimens treated with DNA fluorochrome stains, such as Hoechst 33258, can be used to identify the presence of micro-organisms. DNA fluorochrome will stain any prokaryotic DNA that is present and Gram staining can be performed to exclude conventional bacteria. Comparison of the specimen with a known positive control will help to establish the presence of a mycoplasma, but confirmation by culture is essential for a definitive diagnosis.

Mycoplasmas in exudates can be stained with Giemsa, but most often such preparations are difficult to interpret due to cellular debris and artifacts. Colonies on agar may be seen more easily after use of the Dienes stain (*see Fig. 7.22*).

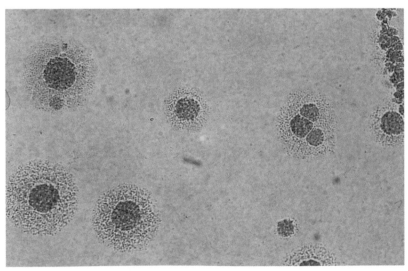

Fig. 7.21 Unstained colonies of *M. hominis* on A8 agar. Such mycoplasmal colonies on agar exhibit a characteristic 'fried egg' appearance due to growth into the agar in the center of the colony. Colonies measure 50–500 µm in diameter. Colonial morphology is dependent to a large extent on local growth conditions and medium components.

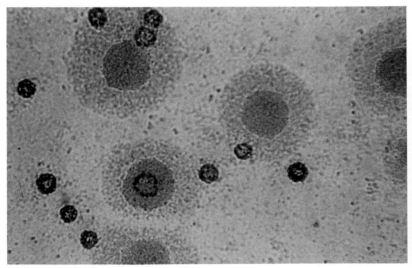

Fig. 7.22 Colonies of *M. hominis* and *U. urealyticum* on A8 agar stained by the Dienes method.

SEROLOGIC DIAGNOSIS

Almost without exception, patients with invasive *M. hominis* infections seroconvert or show a significant rise in the titer of existing antibody. This response can be measured by the metabolism-inhibition assay (*see Figs 7.23* and *7.26*), enzyme-linked immunosorbent assays, or other serologic procedures. Both acute and convalescent sera should be examined, since results based on single specimens are difficult or impossible to interpret.

The assays mentioned are available for detection of antibodies to *U. urealyticum*. However, the determination of ureaplasmal serologic responses is limited to research laboratories. Furthermore, until more information is available about the usefulness of such antibody detection, serodiagnosis cannot be recommended for routine diagnostic purposes.

TREATMENT

Some discussion of appropriate chemotherapy[4,5,12] is necessary as *M. genitalium*, *M. hominis* and *U. urealyticum* are recognized causes of some genital and extragenital disease entities. Patients should be evaluated for mycoplasmas if they are suspected of having a condition for which mycoplasmas may be a cause (for example, urethritis in men, PID in women, meningitis in newborns). Detection of *M. genitalium* by the PCR or a positive culture for either *M. hominis* or *U. urealyticum*, particularly in the absence of other micro-organisms, is sufficient justification for treatment in most instances. Empiric treatment may be necessary in conditions, such as PID, in which obtaining specimens from the affected site may not be feasible, and also because suitable mycoplasmal diagnostic facilities may be lacking in many areas. However, the known antimicrobial resistance among some clinical isolates of both *M. hominis* and *U. urealyticum* means that chemotherapy without validation by in vitro susceptibility testing tends to be risky. In the case of *M genitalium,* an isolate will not be available for testing if, as likely, detection has been by means of PCR technology. The technique used most widely to test the drug susceptibility of the aforementioned mycoplasmas is the broth-dilution method undertaken usually in microtiter plates (*Fig. 7.26*).

A summary of the antimicrobial susceptibilities of *U. urealyticum*, *M. hominis* and *M. genitalium* is given in *Table 7.6*. These mycoplasmas, together with *M. fermentans,* are resistant to sulfonamides, trimethoprim, and all antibiotics that act by inhibiting cell-wall synthesis.

Chloramphenicol and aminoglycosides have poor or no activity against any of these mycoplasmas, apart from streptomycin which is effective against *M. genitalium*. *M. hominis* is susceptible to clindamycin but completely resistant to erythromycin, while the reverse is true for ureaplasmas. This differential susceptibility is sometimes helpful in separating mixed cultures so that the additional drug susceptibilities of each mycoplasmal component can be tested. Tetracyclines of various kinds are the drugs usually used to treat infections by any of the aforementioned mycoplasmas, if there are no contraindications. However, as many as 40% of clinical isolates of *M. hominis* may be tetracycline resistant. Approximately 80–90% of ureaplasmal strains are sensitive to tetracycline, though the incidence of resistant strains may be increasing. If a mycoplasma is resistant to one drug in the tetracycline group, it is usually resistant to others as well. Erythromycin-resistant strains also occur but high-level resistance is thought to be uncommon. There may be a correlation between tetracycline resistance and erythromycin resistance. Doxycycline is better absorbed than tetracycline and has a longer half-life.

Standard doses of tetracyclines usually penetrate the meninges and synovial fluid and achieve levels exceeding the minimal inhibitory concentration (MIC) for susceptible mycoplasmal or ureaplasmal strains. Clindamycin provides an alternative therapy for *M. hominis* infections not involving the CNS, in which there is a contraindication to using a tetracycline, or in cases of tetracycline resistance. In treating conditions known to be sexually transmitted, such as NGU, the index case as well as all sexual contacts should receive antibiotics to prevent reinfection.

The infant with *M. hominis*-induced meningitis presents a difficult therapeutic problem. Normally, tetracycline therapy is contraindicated in children of less than 8 years of age, but no other currently available drug is approved for use or shown to be effective in this condition. However, there are precedents for using intravenous tetracycline or doxycycline to treat infants with mycoplasmal or ureaplasmal meningitis, in which the organisms were eradicated.

Erythromycin is the drug of choice for ureaplasmal infections in neonates. Although erythromycin penetrates poorly into the CNS, *U. urealyticum* has been eradicated from CSF with erythromycin in one instance following treatment failure with doxycycline.

The development of resistance by many strains of *U. urealyticum* and *M. hominis* to the aforementioned 'first-line' antibiotics has prompted investigation of many new antimicrobial compounds as they have become available.

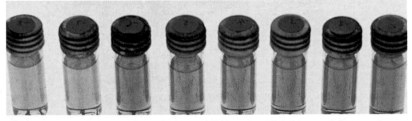

Fig. 7.23 An example of a metabolism-inhibition test. This is essentially growth-inhibition carried out in liquid medium. Organisms that multiply in liquid medium containing a specific substrate metabolize the substrate, and the products alter the pH of the medium as indicated by a change in color of an appropriate pH indicator. Specific antibody inhibits multiplication of the organisms and therefore indirectly prevents the color change from occurring. The test may be used for determining titers of specific antibody by using a constant number of organisms and multiple dilutions of serum. The titer of the serum is recorded as the highest dilution that prevents the change in color of the medium. In addition, the test can be used for the classification and characterization of clinical isolates by using antisera with known antibody titers.

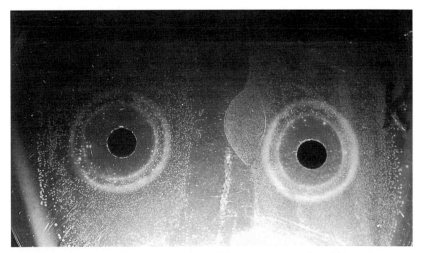

Fig. 7.24 An example of an agar growth-inhibition test. Specific rabbit antiserum placed in wells in the agar medium (filter paper discs impregnated with antisera are more often used) has, after incubation, produced zones in which development of colonies of the homologous mycoplasma has been inhibited. In this case, antibody has also reacted with mycoplasmal antigen to produce rings of precipitation.

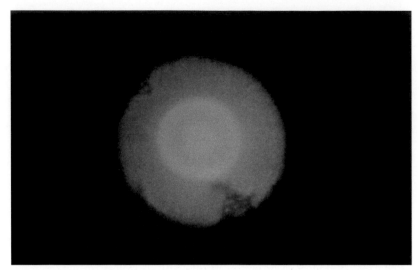

Fig. 7.25 A typical 'fried egg' mycoplasma colony fluorescing after being stained with a fluorescein-conjugated specific rabbit antiserum.

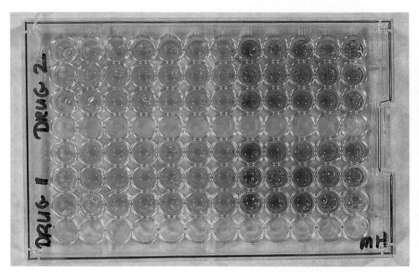

Fig. 7.26 An example of a broth-dilution antibiotic sensitivity test undertaken in a microtiter plate. This test allows large numbers of isolates to be tested simultaneously against several antibiotics and provides reproducible results. The method depends on the inhibition of mycoplasmal growth by specific dilutions of antibiotic. Growth or inhibition of growth is indicated by the presence or absence, respectively, of a color change in the culture medium containing phenol-red pH indicator. Antiserum, instead of antibiotic, may be used to measure antibody quantitatively.

Antimicrobial	U. urealyticum MIC* (µg/ml)	M. hominis MIC* (µg/ml)	M. genitalium MIC* (µg/ml)
Doxycycline	0.05–1	0.1–0.4	≤ 0.01–0.3
Minocycline	0.03	0.4–0.8	ND**
Oxytetracycline	0.4–2	0.5–6.4	ND
Tetracycline	0.05–8	0.2–6.8	ND
Erythromycin	0.1–1.6	> 1000	≤ 0.01
Clarithromycin	≤ 0.004–> 256	16–> 256	≤ 0.01
Azithromycin	0.5–4	4–64	≤ 0.001
Clindamycin	1–50	0.2–1.6	0.2–1
Lincomycin	25–> 500	0.2–1.6	1–10
Rosaramicin	0.008–4	< 0.025–0.4	ND
Spiramycin	32	2–16	≤ 0.01
Chloramphenicol	0.4–3.1	4–25	1–10
Gentamicin	3.1–12.5	1.6–12.5	4–32
Kanamycin	1.6–12.5	1.6–12.5	4–32
Streptomycin	0.4–3.1	4–32	< 1
Spectinomycin	16	< 0.3–10	1–4
Nitrofurantoin	12.5–> 1000	500	ND
Polymixin	12.5–> 1000	1000	ND
Rifampicin	> 1000	> 1000	> 1000
Vancomycin	500–> 1000	500–> 1000	ND
Penicillin	> 4000	> 1000	> 1000
Trimethoprim/ sulfamethoxazole	Inactive	Inactive	Inactive
Ciprofloxacin	0.5–> 64	0.125–4	2
Lomefloxacin	0.5–16	0.5–8	ND
Ofloxacin	0.2–25	0.125–64	1–2

* MIC = minimal inhibitory concentration
** ND = no data

Table 7.6 Susceptibility of *U. urealyticum*, *M. hominis* and *M. genitalium* to various antimicrobials.

Clarithromycin and azithromycin have activity in vitro against *M. genitalium* and *U. urealyticum* but not *M. hominis*. *M. fermentans* is susceptible to azithromycin but not clarithromycin. No published data are available concerning the in vivo clinical efficacy of clarithromycin against *U. urealyticum* infections. However, a single dose of oral azithromycin has been approved for the treatment of NGU due to *C. trachomatis* and it is probably more effective than doxycycline in *M. genitalium*-associated urethritis. Furthermore, it has been shown to

Drug	Adults	Children
Tetracycline	250–500 mg qid	25–50 mg/kg/day, divided into 4 equal doses
Doxycycline	Loading dose of 200 mg; then 100 mg/bid	Loading dose of 4 mg/kg, then 2–4 mg/kg/day divided into 1–2 doses
Clindamycin*	150–450 mg qid	10–25 mg/kg/day, divided into 3 to 4 equal doses
Erythromycin**	250–500 mg qid	20–50 mg/kg/day, divided into 4 equal doses
Azithromycin**	1 g single dose	not recommended
Ofloxacin	200–400 mg bid	not recommended

* Effective only for M. hominis *and* M. genitalium
** Effective only for U. urealyticum *and* M. genitalium

Table 7.7 Oral treatment options for mycoplasmal and ureaplasmal infections.

be as effective clinically as doxycycline in patients with urethritis due to *U. urealyticum*, which reflects its activity in vitro against this micro-organism.

An advantage of fluoroquinolones is that mycoplasmal resistance to them is not documented as frequently as resistance to tetracyclines or macrolides. Ciprofloxacin is marginally less active against *M. hominis*, and *U. urealyticum* in particular, than ofloxacin. A 7-day course of oral ofloxacin appears to be adequate for the treatment of urethritis, but most studies have focused on *C. trachomatis* rather than *U. urealyticum*. Sexual contacts of the index case of urethritis should also receive treatment, just as for any other type of sexually transmitted disease.

Guidelines for the duration and routes of drug administration have not been systematically evaluated for either local genitourinary or systemic extragenital mycoplasmal or ureaplasmal infections. These should be determined individually according to the type and location of infection, as well as the age and clinical condition of the patient and specific recommendations of the manufacturer. *Table 7.7* outlines various oral treatment options. In general, treatment for 10–14 days is recommended. For neonates with meningitis or other systemic infections, parenteral therapy using the same dosage guidelines is advisable, with follow-up cultures to ensure eradication of the organisms. Immuno-compromised persons with systemic mycoplasmal infections, including those of the joints and the genitourinary or respiratory tract, may harbor multiple-resistant strains. Prolonged parenteral therapy, possibly requiring increased dosages, followed by weeks to months of oral therapy may be necessary. This may seem overly aggressive, but there is evidence to indicate that such infections may sometimes be extremely difficult to eradicate. Arthritis due to these organisms can eventually lead to progressive it is irreversible joint damage if, left alone or treated inadequately.

References

1. Razin S, Yogev D, Naot Y. Molecular biology and pathogenicity of mycoplasmas. *Microbiol Mol Biol Rev* 1998; **62**:1094–1156.
2. Lo S-C, Hayes MM, Wang RY-H, Pierce PF, Kotani H, Shih JW-K. Newly discovered mycoplasma isolated from patients infected with HIV. *Lancet* 1991; **338**:1415–1418.
3. Krause DC, Taylor-Robinson D. Mycoplasmas which infect humans. In: Maniloff J, McElhaney RN, Finch LR, Baseman JB (eds): *Mycoplasmas. Molecular Biology and Pathogenesis*. Washington DC, American Society for Microbiology Press, pp 417–444, 1992.
4. Taylor-Robinson D. Infection due to species of *Mycoplasma* and *Ureaplasma*: an update. *Clin Infect Dis* 1996; **23**:671–684.
5. Waites KB, Taylor-Robinson D. *Mycoplasma* and *Ureaplasma*. In: Murray PR, Barron EJ, Pfaller MA, Tenover FC, Yolken RH (eds): *Manual of Clinical Microbiology*, 7th Edition, Washington DC, American Society for Microbiology Press, pp 782–794, 1999.
6. Lo S-C. Mycoplasmas and AIDS. In: Maniloff J, McElhaney RN, Finch LR, Baseman JB (eds): *Mycoplasmas. Molecular Biology and Pathogenesis*. Washington DC, American Society for Microbiology Press, pp 525–545, 1992.
7. Cassell GH, Waites KB, Crouse DT. Genital mycoplasmal infections. In: Remington JS, Klein JO (eds): *Infectious Diseases of the Fetus and Newborn Infant*. Philadelphia, W. B. Saunders, pp 619–670, 1994.
8. Furr PM, Taylor-Robinson D, Webster ADB. Mycoplasmas and ureaplasmas in patients with hypogammaglobulinaemia and their role in arthritis: microbiological observations over 20 years. *Ann Rheum Dis* 1994; **53**:183–187.
9. Tully JG, Razin S (eds). *Molecular and Diagnostic Procedures in Mycoplasmology: Diagnostic Procedures*. New York, Academic Press, Vol 2, 1996.
10. Shepard MC. Culture media for ureaplasmas. In: Razin S, Tully JG (eds): *Methods in Mycoplasmology*. New York, Academic Press, Vol I, pp 137–146, 1983.
11. Taylor-Robinson D, Gilroy CB, Jensen JS. The biology of *Mycoplasma genitalium*. *Venereology* 2000; **13**:119–127.
12. Taylor-Robinson D, Bebear C. Antibiotic susceptibilities of mycoplasmas and treatment of mycoplasmal infections. *J Antimicrob Chemother* 1997; **40**:622–630.

Pelvic Inflammatory Disease

8

J Paavonen and D Schwartz

INTRODUCTION

Pelvic inflammatory disease (PID) refers to infection of the uterus, fallopian tubes, and adjacent pelvic structures not associated with surgery or pregnancy; however, the terminology used is not uniform. In addition to PID, many other terms are commonly used to describe different manifestations of pelvic infection, such as endometritis, salpingitis, salpingo-oophoritis, adnexitis, parametritis, pyosalpinx, tubo-ovarian abscess, tubo-ovarian complex, pelvic peritonitis, perihepatitis, and periappendicitis.[1]

PID carries high morbidity. Long-term sequelae of PID, specifically tubal factor infertility (TFI) and ectopic pregnancy are common and cause major problems in later life. Repeated episodes of PID are associated with a steep increase in the risk of permanent tubal damage. The risks of permanent tubal damage relate to the severity of PID before the start of treatment, and clinical improvement may not directly translate into prevention of tubal damage. However, it should be emphasized that PID and its sequelae are largely preventable.

The CDC definition of PID reads as follows: PID comprises a spectrum of inflammatory disorders of the upper female genital tract, including any combination of endometritis, salpingitis, tubo-ovarian abscess, and pelvic peritonitis. Sexually transmitted organisms, especially *Neisseria gonorrhoeae* and *Chlamydia trachomatis* are implicated in most cases, however, microorganisms that can be part of the vaginal flora (e.g., anaerobes, *Gardnerella vaginalis*, *Haemophilus influenzae*, enteric Gram-negative rods, and *Streptococcus agalactiae*) can also cause PID. In addition, mycoplasmas might play a role in PID.[2]

The International-Infectious Disease Society for Obstetrics and Gynecology-USA (I-IDSOG-USA) recommends the use of the term 'upper genital tract infection' (UGTI), followed by the designation of the etiologic agent, instead of the currently employed term, 'pelvic inflammatory disease'. In addition, they believe that there should be greater emphasis on signs and symptoms related to subclinical or occult UGTI. Therapeutic recommendation for the treatment of UGTI should be given to various stages of this diverse disease entity.[3]

EPIDEMIOLOGY

The exact incidence of PID is unknown because the disease can not be diagnosed reliably from clinical symptoms and signs. Most cases of PID may be asymptomatic or subclinical. Therefore, hospital discharge registries are poor surrogate markers for the true prevalence of PID. Factors associated with PID mirror those for uncomplicated sexually transmitted infections. Risk factors and risk markers for PID include young age, multiple sexual partners, intrauterine device (IUD) insertion, vaginal douching, tobacco smoking, chlamydial and gonococcal cervicitis, and bacterial vaginosis (BV). Barrier contraceptive use protects against PID. Oral contraceptive (OC) use modifies the manifestations of PID towards less symptomatic disease, and OC use may in fact protect against manifest PID.

One important current trend is the shift from inpatient PID towards outpatient PID. Hospitalizations of women with PID have rapidly decreased in the past two decades (*Fig. 8.1*). However, this does not necessarily mean that the overall incidence of PID has decreased, and may only reflect the change in clinical manifestations or management of PID. Recently, a new clinical PID entity, so called 'silent' or 'subclinical' PID, has been described. For example, hospitalizations for acute PID in Finland have decreased by 50% between 1990 and 1999 although the rate of sexual transmitted chlamydial infections has steadily increased.

Another recent trend in developed countries is the shift in the microbial etiology of PID. The relative role of *C. trachomatis* as a cause of PID has increased, whereas the role of *N. gonorrhoeae* has decreased.

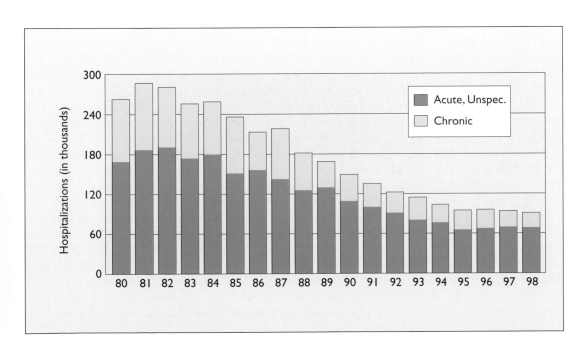

Fig. 8.1 Pelvic inflammatory disease (PID) hospitalizations of women 15–44 years of age in the United States, 1980–1998 from National Hospital Discharge Survey, National Center for Health Statistics, CDC. 1999.

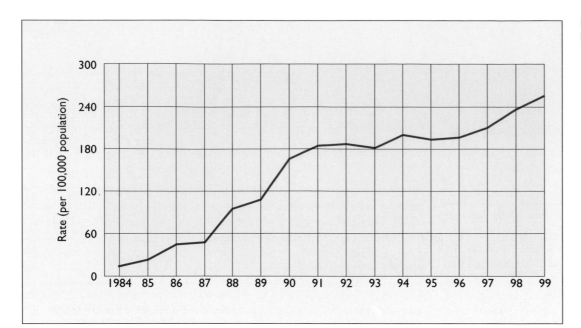

Fig. 8.2 *Chlamydia trachomatis* — reported rates in the United States, 1984–1999 from STD Surveillance, CDC, 1999.

Population	Rate (95% CI)	No. of studies
• STD clinic	40% (25–55)	1
• Gynecologic inpatients	32% (21–43)	9
• Gynecologic outpatients	31% (18–46)	3
• Emergency clinic	43% (26–61)	3
• Primary care clinic	25% (13–40)	1

Modified from Simms and Stephenson: Sex Transm Inf 2000; 76:80–87.[15]

Table 8.1 Prevalence of genital *C. trachomatis* in women with laparoscopically proved PID

In many developed countries, gonorrhea is now a rare disease,[4] whereas rates of chlamydial infection remain high or are increasing (*Fig. 8.2*). Recent screening studies have shown strikingly high rates of *C. trachomatis* among asymptomatic populations. In industrialized countries *C. trachomatis* is now the predominant sexually transmitted organism causing PID (*Table 8.1*).

The topic of intrauterine device (IUD) and upper genital tract infection has recently been systematically reviewed.[5] Concern about upper genital tract infection related to intrauterine devices limits their wider use. Methodological flaws in early observational studies exaggerated the risk of PID associated with IUD use. This misunderstanding has inadvertently affected women's health around the world by limiting access to a highly effective contraceptive device and thus indirectly adding to the burden of unintended pregnancy. Choice of an inappropriate comparison group, overdiagnosis of PID in IUD users, and inability to control for the confounding effects of risk-taking sexual behavior have exaggerated the apparent risk. Women with asymptomatic gonorrhea or chlamydial infection having an IUD inserted have a higher risk of salpingitis than do uninfected women having an IUD inserted. However, the risk is similar to that of infected women not having an IUD inserted. A cohort study of HIV-positive women using a copper IUD suggests that there is no significant increase in the risk of complications or HIV shedding. Furthermore, there appears to be no important effect of IUD use on tubal infertility. Clinical issues and available evidence of IUD and upper genital tract infection are summarized in *Table 8.2*.[5]

MICROBIOLOGY

The most important causative microorganisms of PID are *C. trachomatis*, *N. gonorrhoeae*, and bacteria associated with vaginal infections. The proportion of PID caused by *C. trachomatis* or *N. gonorrhoeae* reflects the background prevalence of these organisms in the target population. If left untreated, it has been estimated that 10% to 30% of women with untreated gonococcal or chlamydial cervicitis develop PID.[6] However, this is probably an overestimation for *C. trachomatis* infection as the models have used probabilities and assumptions for the consequences of untreated infection, which have been derived from a group of women who were culture positive. The assumption is that being culture positive for *C. trachomatis* is the same as being positive in a nucleic acid amplification test (NAAT), which is unlikely in relation to bacterial load alone. None of the models have used cohorts of women who have been screened for *C. trachomatis* using a sensitive NAAT and then followed over time.

Bacterial vaginosis (BV) is the most common cause of abnormal vaginal discharge. BV is characterized by a complex change in vaginal ecology. The concentration of hydrogen peroxide-producing lactobacilli has decreased with a concomitant increase in the concentrations of *Gardnerella vaginalis*, *Mobiluncus* species, other anaerobic Gram-negative rods and genital mycoplasmas. On the other hand, aerobic vaginitis (AV) is characterized by an overgrowth of virulent aerobic or facultative bacteria, most notably *Escherichia coli*, group B streptococci, and enterococci (see Chapter 9). Both types of vaginal infection lead to a massive increase in the concentration of microbial by-products, which are thought to destroy cervical host defense barriers, leading to the ascent of microorganisms and their by-products to the upper genital tract. Non-chlamydial, non-gonococcal microorganisms detected in the upper genital tract of women with laparoscopically proven PID are most commonly microorganisms known to be associated with BV or AV.[7] Other less commonly associated microorganisms include *Actinomyces* spp., which have been typically linked to IUD usage. In less developed countries or populations with a high prevalence of tuberculosis, PID may be associated with *Mycobacterium tuberculosis*, due to dissemination of the microorganism via the bloodstream rather than via ascending spread from the lower genital tract. In some areas of the world, granulomatous salpingitis may be caused by helminths such as *Schistosoma* spp.

Issue	Highest level of evidence	Strength of conclusion	Conclusion
IUD as cause of PID	II-2	A	Risk related to insertion process
Tailstring as cause of PID	I	A	Monofilament tailstring not a vector for infection
IUD insertion in presence of gonorrhea or chlamydial infection	II-2	C	Limited data, but no evidence of increased risk compared with gonorrhea or chlamydial infection without an IUD insertion
IUD use by women with HIV infection	II-2	B	No significant effect on overall complications or viral shedding
Aquisition of C. trachomatis by IUD user	II-2	B	No increase in risk
Acquisition of N. gonorrhoeae by IUD user	II-2	C	Limited data
Levonorgestrel-releasing IUD and upper genital tract infection	II-2	C	Conflicting data on protection against PID
Treatment of PID with IUD in situ	I	B	No impaired response to antibiotic therapy
Infertility after discontinuation	II-2	B	No substantial increase in risk

Table 8.2 Clinical issues and available evidence on the association between IUD and PID.[4]

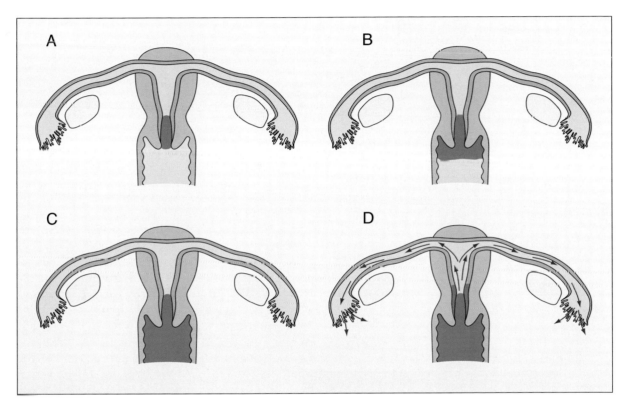

Fig. 8.3 Pathogenesis of pelvic inflammatory disease (PID). PID begins with chlamydial and/or gonococcal cervicitis (A). This is followed by an alteration in the cervicovaginal microenvironment (B), leading to bacterial vaginosis (C). Finally, the original cervical pathogens, the flora causing bacterial vaginosis, or both ascend into the upper genital tract (D). The cross-hatched areas indicate the affected portions of the genital tract.[1]

PATHOGENESIS

PID is an ascending infection in which pathogenic microorganisms ascend from the lower genital tract to the upper genital tract (*Fig. 8.3*). Anatomically, the female genital tract is composed of the external and internal genitalia (*Fig. 8.4*). Internal genitalia include the vagina, uterus, fallopian tubes, and ovaries. Hormonal changes over the stages of a woman's life influence the mucosal components and cyclical environment of this system and also influence the risk for acquiring certain infections. The cervix is probably the most important structural and possibly functional barrier to infectious agents that may ascend from the lower genital tract and vagina into the uterus. The external mucosal surface of the cervix (ectocervix), extends into the vagina, and consists of stratified, non-keratinized, and squamous epithelial cells, which undergo cyclical modifications during the normal menstrual cycle in women of reproductive age. The endocervix has a mucosal surface consisting of a single stratum of mucus-secreting columnar epithelial cells. It has been hypothesized that this cervical mucus may be a natural barrier to the ascending spread of microorganisms, such as *N. gonorrhoeae*,

C. trachomatis, and vaginal bacteria into the uterus. The normal fallopian tubal mucosa also consists of ciliated and nonciliated epithelial cells (*Fig. 8.5*).

The mechanisms by which infecting microorganisms ascend into the upper female genital tract may vary according to the organism and remain a complex issue. In the setting of gonococcal PID and salpingitis, it is thought that infection probably extends via a direct canalicular route from the endocervix into the endometrium and subsequently into the fallopian tubes. This causes edema and incites an intense polymorphonuclear leukocyte response. In studies of gonococcal PID, the organism is more frequently recovered during and immediately after the menstrual period. Using an in vitro organ system model and scanning electron microscopy (*Fig. 8.6*), it has been shown that the gonococcus readily attaches to the microvilli of nonciliated mucosal epithelial cells, and then enters cells, resulting in cell damage and sloughing of the ciliated cells (*Fig. 8.7*). Much of the cell damage may be attributed to the acute inflammatory response. Animal models have also been developed to study the pathogenesis of chlamydial PID.

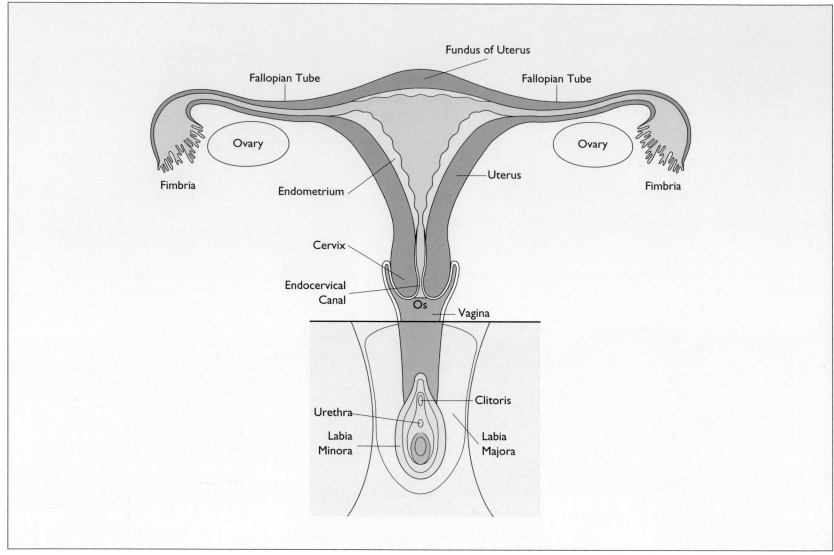

Fig. 8.4 Anatomic depiction of normal internal and external female genitalia.

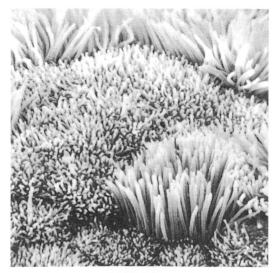

Fig. 8.5 Scanning electron micrograph of cultured human fallopian tube tissue showing both nonciliated cells with microvilli and ciliated cells. (Courtesy of MD Cooper, Southern Illonois University School of Medicine.)

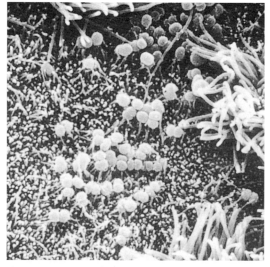

Fig. 8.6 Scanning electron micrograph of gonococci attaching to the microvilli of cultured human fallopian tube tissue. Note that gonococci are only attached to the nonciliated cells. (Courtesy of MD Cooper, Southern Illonois University School of Medicine.)

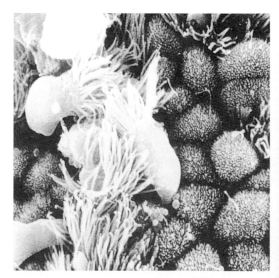

Fig. 8.7 Scanning electron micrograph showing ciliated epithelial cells sloughing from the cultured human fallopian tube mucosa. Some gonococci are still attached to the nonciliated cells, which show some damage as evidenced by their exaggerated borders and abnormal appearance. (Courtesy of MD Cooper, Southern Illonois University School of Medicine.)

Experimental chlamydial infection induced in nonhuman primates results in a complex process of immune-mediated responses leading to overt tubal damage. Previous research using scanning electron microscopy has documented the process of chlamydial attachment to nonciliated epithelial cells (*Fig. 8.8*). Intracellular replication of *C. trachomatis* results in the release of elementary bodies by rupture of the infected cells (*Fig. 8.9*). Comparable data are not available on the pathogenesis of non-gonococcal, non-chlamydial PID.

Several studies have suggested that the risk for developing PID may increase at menses, and that hormonal factors may play a role in the pathogenesis of PID by affecting the structural and functional barriers preventing infection of the upper female genital tract. It has been postulated that initial infection with *C. trachomatis*, *N. gonorrhoeae*, or both, increases the risk for developing endometritis and PID by the ascending spread of these microorganisms, and the concomitant or subsequent ascending infection with vaginal facultative and anerobic bacteria, including organisms associated with BV or AV.

Since age is an important risk factor for PID, specific age-related hormonal or other host immune response-related factors in the cervix or cervical mucus may determine whether or not a cervicovaginal infection ascends to the upper genital tract causing manifest PID. Endometritis is an early manifestation of PID, and most but not all women with PID have plasma cell endometritis (*Fig. 8.10*). Next, salpingitis develops, which can lead to pyosalpinx (*Fig. 8.11*) or tubo-ovarian abscess formation. Perihepatitis is associated with PID in 10–20% of the cases (*Fig. 8.12*).

PATHOLOGY

The spectrum of gross and microscopic pathologic changes occurring in the upper genital tract organs as a result of PID are seen in *Figs 8.13–8.20*. *Figs 8.13–8.16* illustrate the spectrum of acute salpingitis and pyosalpinx. Acute salpingitis is one of the most severe manifestations of PID and often results in pyosalpinx. With resolution of acute salpingitis, there may be a series of structural alterations to the tube, termed chronic salpingitis, which are associated with the well known major complications of PID (*Fig. 8.17*). The mucosal plicae form fibrinous adhesions to one another which progress to bridging between folds (*Fig. 8.18*). Tubo-ovarian adhesions may also form, with occlusion of the tubal ostium, and there may be associated peritoneal inflammation. Eventually, a hydrosalpinx may result (*Figs 8.19–8.23*). Ovarian involvement in PID is almost always a complication of salpingitis, and typically presents as a unilateral or bilateral tubo-ovarian abscess (*Figs 8.22–8.25*). Although less common than a tubo-ovarian abscess, an abscess confined to the ovary may also occur.

A major complication of PID is tubal pregnancy. The unruptured fallopian tube is dilated and has a blue discoloration due to hematosalpinx. Almost two-thirds of tubal pregnancies contain an identifiable embryo (*Fig. 8.26*). Continued growth of the conceptus often results in tubal rupture around the eighth week of gestation, resulting in potentially life-threatening hemorrhage. A few tubal pregnancies may proceed to longer gestations (*Fig. 8.27*).

M. tuberculosis is the most common etiologic agent of granulomatous salpingitis, and for reasons which are not completely understood, the

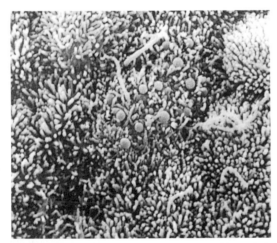

Fig. 8.8 Scanning electron micrograph of chlamydial elementary bodies attaching to the microvilli of nonciliated epithelial cells of the human fallopian tube mucosa. (Courtesy of MD Cooper, Southern Illonois University School of Medicine.)

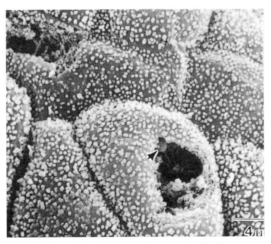

Fig. 8.9 Scanning electron micrograph of a human fallopian tube organ culture infected with *Chlamydia trachomatis*. Note the large hole where the cell has ruptured. The arrow points to an elementary body that remains within the interior of the cell. (Courtesy of MD Cooper, Southern Illonois University School of Medicine.)

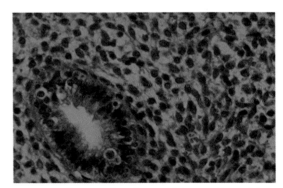

Fig. 8.10 Plasma cell endometritis in a patient with chlamydial infection. Hematoxylin-eosin; original magnification × 132.

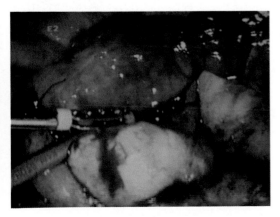

Fig. 8.11 Laparoscopic view of pyosalpinx. Note enlarged fallopian tube proximal from the fimbriated end. (Courtesy of Pontus Molander, MD.)

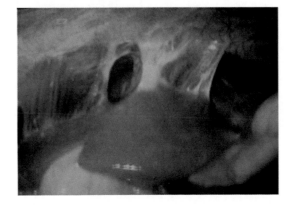

Fig. 8.12 Laparoscopic view of perihepatitis. Note violin string adhesions. (Courtesy of Pontus Molander, MD.)

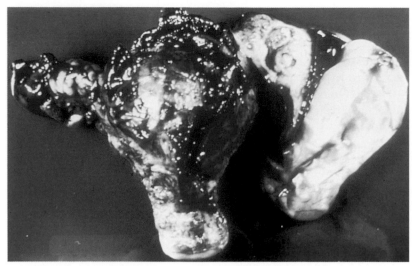

Fig. 8.13 A gross surgical specimen of uterus and infected fallopian tube removed from a patient with salpingitis and ruptured pyosalpinx abscess.

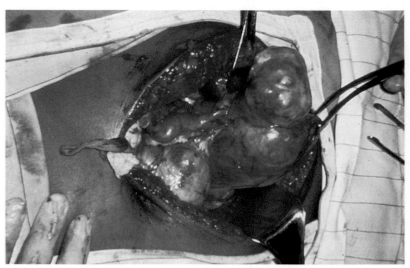

Fig. 8.14 Total abdominal hysterectomy bilateral salpingo-oophorectomy specimen showing unilateral pyosalpinx.

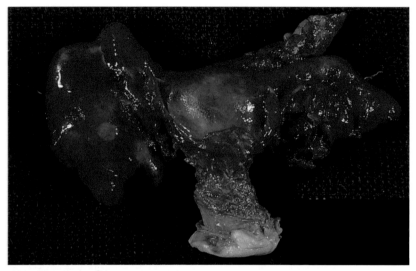

Fig. 8.15 Total abdominal hysterectomy bilateral salpingo-oophorectomy specimen showing unilateral pyosalpinx.

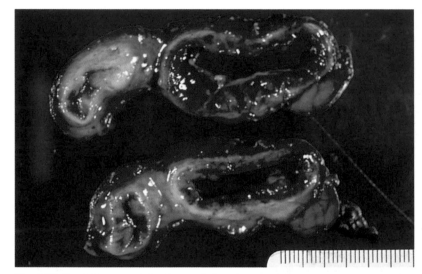

Fig. 8.16 Exudative pyosalpinx from salpingectomy.

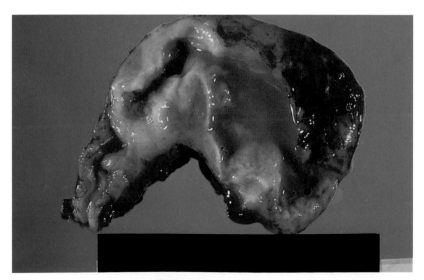

Fig. 8.17 Cross-section of a fallopian tube with chronic salpingitis, showing a thickened wall lined with fibrinohemorrhagic exudate. Salpingitis is the most common STD-associated syndrome associated with infertility.

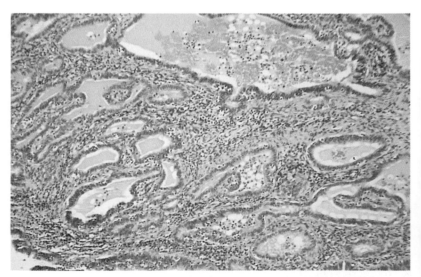

Fig. 8.18 The characteristic microscopic findings of chronic salpingitis are seen here, including thickening and fusion of the plical folds, and plasma cell infiltration of the lamina propria (hematoxylin and eosin × 100).

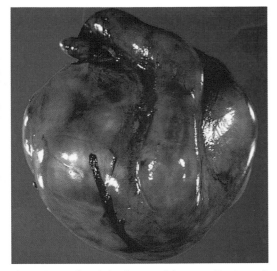

Fig. 8.19 Hydrosalpinx is one of the complications of salpingitis. This case is a typical example of hydrosalpinx, showing a tube, especially the ampullatory portion, with dilation and obliteration of the ostium.

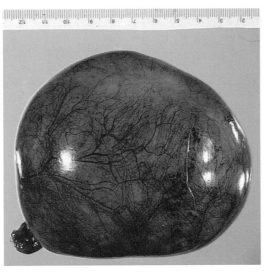

Fig. 8.20 Severe hydrosalpinx. There is marked luminal dilation, and the wall is thin and translucent.

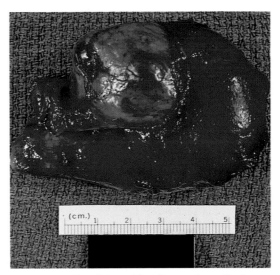

Fig. 8.21 Hydrosalpinx with tubo-ovarian adhesions.

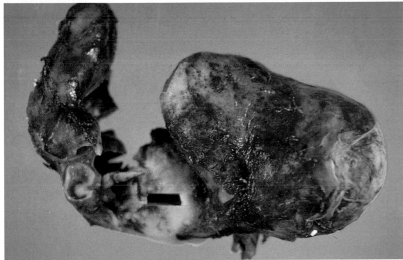

Fig. 8.22

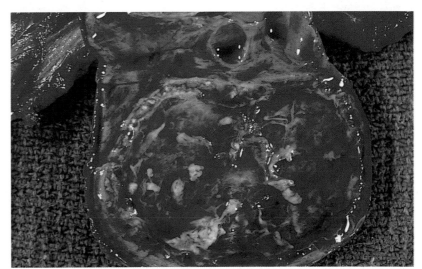

Fig. 8.23

Figs 8.22 and 8.23 Salpingo-oophorectomy specimen with chronic ovarian abscess and hydrosalpinx, before (**Fig. 8.22**) and after (**Fig. 8.23**) opening the specimen. The 'retort' shape of the specimen is typical for this process. The chronicity of the ovarian abscesses is evident from the presence of residual smooth walled cystic cavities lined by fibrin.

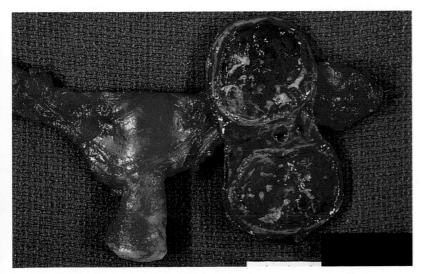

Fig. 8.24 Unilateral tubo-ovarian abscess. The majority of acute and chronic inflammatory lesions of the ovary are infectious, and are a manifestation of PID.

Fig. 8.25 Close-up of abscess in Fig. 8.24 showing hemorrhage, fibrin, and suppurative material.

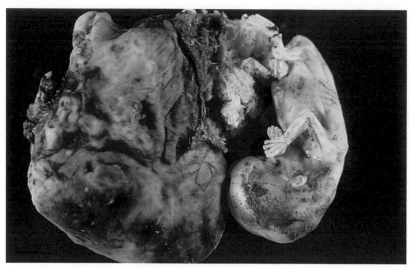

Fig. 8.26 Ectopic pregnancy is a potentially life-threatening complication of PID and salpingitis. In this tubal pregnancy, the placental implantation site into the tube is evident. Among 15–24-year-olds, one in 24 will develop an ectopic pregnancy after her first episode of PID.

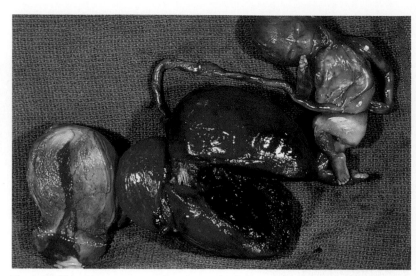

Fig. 8.27 This shows an unusually advanced tubal pregnancy, which ruptured into the abdominal cavity, associated with hematosalpinx. Damage to the fallopian tube from PID is estimated to confer a 7–10-fold greater risk of ectopic pregnancy.

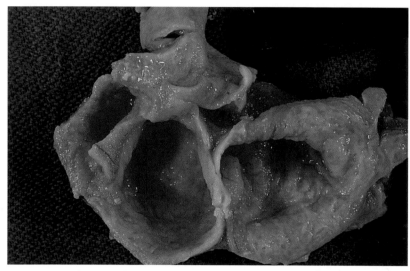

Fig. 8.28 The most common cause of granulomatous salpingitis is *Mycobacterium tuberculosis*. In this case of mycobacterial salpingitis, the tubal lumen is dilated, the mucosal surface is roughened, and the wall is thickened and fibrous. About 10–20% of women who die from tuberculosis have tubal involvement.

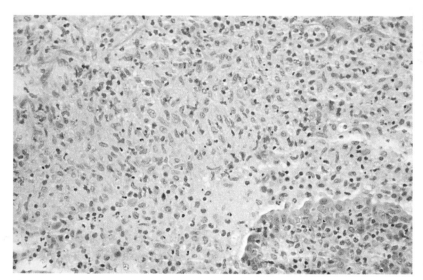

Fig. 8.29 Granulomatous salpingitis from a patient with *M. tuberculosis* infection, showing the replacement of normal tubal architecture by an inflammatory lesion containing mainly histiocytes and lymphocytes (hematoxylin and eosin × 200).

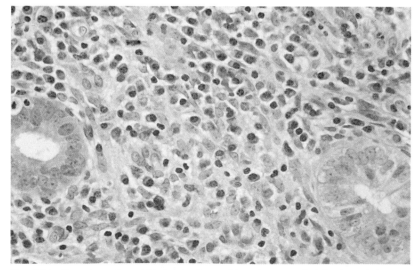

Fig. 8.30 Chronic endometritis in a patient with actinomycotic infection of the endometrium and fallopian tube, associated with an intrauterine device (IUD). Numerous plasma cells infiltrate the stroma (hematoxylin and eosin × 400).

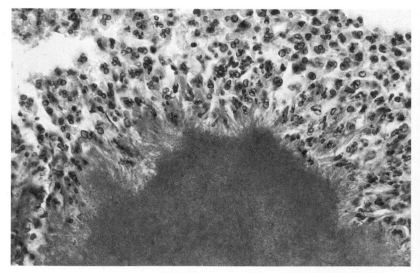

Fig. 8.31 Actinomycotic grain and surrounding acute inflammation from fallopian tube infection. The edge of the grain has radiating eosinophilic material, termed the Splendore-Hoeppli phenomenon (hematoxylin and eosin × 400).

mycobacteria preferentially lodge in the fallopian tube rather than in other parts of the female genital tract. The tube becomes enlarged and nodular, and dense adhesions may form between the tube and ovary (*Fig. 8.28*). The tubal mucosa may appear roughened and micronodular, and microscopically there is granulomatous inflammation, often with multinucleated giant cells (*Fig. 8.29*). Another cause of granulomatous

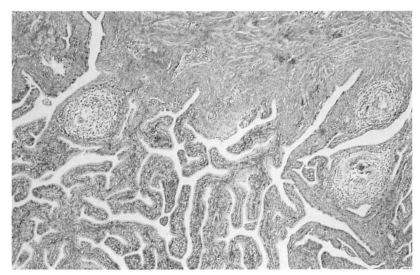

Fig. 8.32 Salpingitis due to *Schistosoma haematobium*. Well-circumscribed granulomas, containing parasite ova, are present within the stroma of several plical folds (hematoxylin and eosin × 40).

- History of low abdominal pain
- Cervical motion tenderness
- Uterine tenderness
- Bilateral adnexal tenderness
- Negative pregnancy test

Table 8.3 Criteria for syndromic diagnosis of PID

Minimum criteria
   Lower abdominal tenderness
   Adnexal tenderness
   Cervical motion tenderness

Additional criteria*
   Oral temperature >38.3°C (101°F)
   Abnormal cervical or vaginal discharge
   Elevated erythrocyte sedimentation rate
   Elevated C-reactive protein
   Laboratory documentation of cervical infection with *Neisseria gonorrhoeae* or *Chlamydia trachomatis*

Definitive criteria**
   Histopathologic evidence of endometritis on endometrial biopsy
   Tubo-ovarian abscess on sonography or other radiologic tests
   Laparoscopic abnormalities consistent with PID

*More elaborate diagnostic evaluation is often needed because incorrect diagnosis and management might cause unnecessary morbidity. These additional criteria may be used to increase the specificity of the diagnosis of the minimum criteria listed previously.
**The definitive criteria for diagnosing PID are warranted in selected cases.

Table 8.4 Centers for Disease Control and Prevention criteria for the diagnosis of pelvic inflammatory disease

---

salpingitis is actinomycotic infection. Actinomycotic infections of the fallopian tube are usually associated with the use of an IUD and actinomycosis of the endometrium (*Figs 8.30 and 8.31*). As in other infections that result in PID, chronic endometritis may also be present. Grossly, an enlarged fibrous mass involving either the tube and/or the ovary is usually present. The inflammatory mass may contain pus-filled sinus cavities, and have adhesions to other structures in the pelvic cavity. The microscopic finding of actinomycotic grains within the inflamed tube or ovary is diagnostic, but microbiologic culture is necessary. Other infectious causes of salpingitis include schistosomiasis, which is rare in North America and Europe but is still a common cause of granulomatous salpingitis worldwide (*Fig. 8.32*).

CLINICAL MANIFESTATIONS

The clinical spectrum of PID ranges from asymptomatic or sub-clinical endometritis to symptomatic salpingitis, pyosalpinx, tubo-ovarian abscess, pelvic peritonitis, and sometimes perihepatitis. Bilateral lower abdominal pain is the most common presenting symptom. Perihepatitis causes right quadrant upper abdominal pain mimicking acute cholecystitis. Other common symptoms are abnormal vaginal discharge, metrorrhagia, postcoital bleeding, dysuria, fever, and nausea. However, symptomatic PID only represents the tip of the iceberg. Increasing attention has recently been focused on so-called 'atypical' or 'silent' PID. For instance, only a fraction of women with tubal factor infertility (TFI) have history of PID suggesting that silent PID may also lead to the development of permanent tubal damage. It has been shown that up two thirds of women with chlamydial cervicitis and no symptoms or signs of PID had plasma cell endometritis on endometrial biopsy, which is consistent with sub-clinical PID. Furthermore, minimally symptomatic patients usually seek medical care late, which increases the risk for tubal damage and long-term sequelae. Studies have shown that not only frank PID but also sub-clinical PID is associated with permanent tubal damage.

DIAGNOSIS

The major clinical criteria for the syndromic diagnosis of PID are history of low abdominal pain, cervical motion tenderness, uterine tenderness, and bilateral adnexal tenderness, and negative pregnancy test (*Table 8.3*).[8] CDC criteria for the diagnosis of PID are listed in *Table 8.4*. The clinical diagnosis of PID has severe limitations since the clinical criteria have low diagnostic accuracy. Thus, false-positive and false-negative diagnoses are common. Multiple studies have shown that the sensitivity of the clinical diagnosis based on history and pelvic examination is low or very low when laparoscopy is used as the gold standard for diagnosis (*Table 8.5*). Therefore, clinicians should have a high index of suspicion of PID while evaluating women with pelvic pain.

Increasing concern about the silent PID has changed the recommendations for PID diagnosis from laboratory- and laparoscopy-based diagnosis towards so-called syndromic diagnosis (*Table 8.3*). Syndromic diagnosis may increase diagnostic sensitivity and lead to earlier therapy, although, on the other hand, it may also lead to unnecessary treatment with antibiotics. However, the syndromic diagnosis of PID is clearly broad and imprecise.

Laparoscopy, endometrial biopsy, and transvaginal sonography (TVS), TVS with power Doppler, and magnetic resonance imaging (MRI) can be used to obtain a more accurate diagnosis of PID. However, these facilities are not readily available in the vast majority of clinical settings or may not be justifiable in clinically mild disease. For instance, although laparoscopy was introduced in the 1960s as the gold standard for PID diagnosis, direct visual diagnosis by laparoscopy is not always feasible, requires general anesthesia, and is costly.

Author and reference	Year	Setting	Country	Laparoscopically confirmed/Total (%)
Jacobson	1969	Gyn	Sweden	532/814 (65%)
Chaparro	1978	Gyn	USA	103/223 (46%)
Sweet	1979	Emergency room	USA	26/29 (90%)
Murphy	1981	Gyn	Australia	8/22 (36%)
Allen	1983	Gyn	S. Africa	63/103 (61%)
Wasserheit	1986	STD/Emergency room/Gyn	USA	22/36 (61%)
Brihmer	1987	Gyn	Sweden	187/359 (52%)
Paavonen	1987	Gyn	Finland	36/45 (67%)
Brunham	1988	Gyn	Canada	44/69 (64%)
Heinonen	1989	Gyn	Finland	33/40 (83%)
Sellors	1991	General practice	Canada	28/95 (30%)
Rousseau	1991	Gyn	Canada	41/54 (76%)
Livengood	1992	Emergency room/Gyn	USA	23/33 (70%)
Weström	1992	Gyn	Sweden	1186/1679 (71%)
Morcos	1993	Gyn	USA	134/176 (76%)
Stacey	1994	STD	UK	7/32 (22%)
Soper	1994	Emergency room/Gyn	USA	84/102 (82%)
Bevan	1995	STD/Emergency room/Gyn	UK	104/147 (71%)
Tukeva	1999	Gyn	Finland	21/30 (70%)

Modified from Munday PE. J Infect 2000; 40: 31–41.[9]

Table 8.5 Correlation between clinical and laparoscopic findings in women suspected of having pelvic inflammatory disease (PID)

Surgical evidence for the diagnosis of PID*
Tubal edema
Tubal exudate
Tubal hyperemia

*By laparoscopy or laparotomy.

Table 8.6 Surgical evidence for the diagnosis of PID*

MINIMUM CRITERIA:
Erythema of fallopian tubes
Edema and swelling of fallopian tubes
Seropurulent exudate from fimbriae and/or on serosal surface of fallopian tubes

SCORING:
Mild: minimum criteria; tubes freely movable and patent
Moderate: minimum criteria more marked; tubes not freely movable; patency uncertain
Severe: inflammatory mass

Table 8.7 Laparoscopic criteria of acute PID

Author	Year	Country	Sensitivity	Specificity
Wölner-Hanssen	1982	Sweden	50%	UNK
Wasserheit	1986	USA	70%	92%
Paavonen	1987	Finland	87%	66%
Heinonen	1989	Finland	58%	57%

Modified from Munday PE. J Infect 2000; 40: 31–41.[9]

Table 8.8 Correlation between laparoscopy and endometrial histopathology in women suspected of having pelvic inflammatory disease

Laparoscopy is considered the 'gold standard' for confirming a diagnosis of PID because it not only allows direct inspection of the fallopian tubes and surrounding pelvic anatomy (*Fig. 8.33*), but also enables microbiologic sampling from the upper genital tract (e.g. fallopian tube, ovary, and peritoneal fluid). Laparoscopy may be used to help characterize fallopian-tube inflammation and the severity of salpingitis (*Tables 8.6 and 8.7*). However, the routine use of laparoscopy to confirm a diagnosis of PID is prohibited by both cost and availability, especially in outpatient clinic settings where most PID is diagnosed. On the other hand, the accuracy of laparoscopy may not be 100% because of expectation bias or because laparoscopy may not detect subtle endosalpingitis.

Endometrial biopsy obtained with an aspiration catheter is a simple outpatient procedure for histopathologic diagnosis of PID (plasma cell endometritis) (*Fig. 8.34*), although the results are not readily available. Endometrial biopsy can provide confirmatory histopathologic diagnosis of endometritis. In contrast to laparoscopy, endometrial biopsy can be performed on an outpatient basis and is considerably less invasive. Studies have found a reasonable correlation between the results of endometrial biopsy and laparoscopic findings (*Table 8.8*).

Clinically, PID must be differentiated from other abdominal and pelvic conditions, including life-threatening conditions, such as acute appendicitis. Thus, laparoscopy should be performed if there is any doubt in the diagnosis. In addition, operative procedures can be performed during laparoscopy, such as liberation of adhesions, peritoneal lavation, drainage and lavation of abscesses, which shorten the need for hospitalization, and may improve outcome. On the other hand, operative laparoscopy facilitates management of other conditions that cause differential diagnostic problems. For instance, endometrioma,

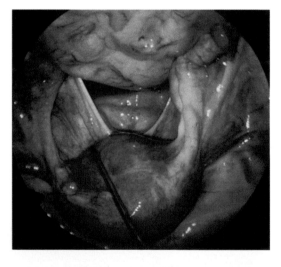

Fig. 8.33 A view through the laparoscope of the female internal pelvic organs and supporting structures (uterus, fallopian tubes, pelvic peritoneum, broad ligament).

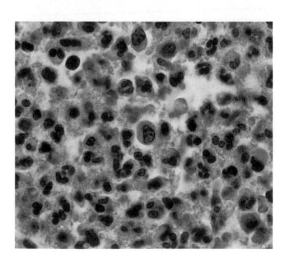

Fig. 8.34 Acute gonococcal endometritis, showing numerous and abundant neutrophils and few plasma cells from endometrial biopsy section (hematoxylin and eosin).

ruptured ovarian cyst, adnexal torsion, and appendicitis can all be managed laparoscopically. Thus, laparoscopy also augments the management of non-PID cases, which are difficult to discriminate from acute PID by clinical examination alone.

It should be emphasized that although laparoscopy is generally accepted as the gold standard for the diagnosis of PID, it has never been properly validated. Therefore the inter- and intra-observer reproducibility of laparoscopic diagnosis is not known. Such observer reproducibility studies of laparoscopic diagnosis of PID are needed.

Transvaginal sonography (TVS), and magnetic resonance imaging (MRI) are other techniques introduced to augment the clinical diagnosis of PID. TVS with Power Doppler is a powerful tool in the diagnosis of PID but it requires special skills and is therefore highly observer dependent. MRI seems to be as accurate as TVS in the diagnosis of inpatient PID when laparoscopy is used as the gold standard.[10] However, MRI is seldom available in settings where PID cases are seen. Tubal enlargement can be easily seen on MR images and is characterized by tortuous folding of fluid-filled structures on T2-weighted images.[11] In one recent study the sensitivity of MRI in the diagnosis of PID was 95%, the specificity was 89%, and the overall accuracy was 93%.[10] The MRI findings

in cases of PID were as follows: fluid-filled tube (*Fig. 8.35*), pyosalpinx, tubo-ovarian abscess (*Fig. 8.36*), or polycystic-like ovaries with free pelvic fluid.

TVS is a noninvasive bedside procedure that is routinely performed in patients with pelvic pain. Earlier studies have shown that TVS performs well in the diagnosis of PID when the criteria include thickened fluid-filled tubes. TVS is superior to trans-abdominal sonography in the diagnosis of pelvic abnormalities. Recent innovation of the sonographic Doppler technique, namely power Doppler, improves the detection of blood flow, particularly low-velocity flow. The detection of inflammation-induced hyperemia by the power Doppler technique has not been well-studied even though early results are encouraging. Power Doppler already has a variety of applications in obstetrics and gynecology.

Specific TVS findings, including wall thickness >5 mm, cog-wheel sign, incomplete septa, and the presence of cul-de-sac fluid, discriminate women with acute PID from women with no PID. Power Doppler TVS reveals hyperemia in women with acute PID (*Fig. 8.37*), since it is rarely present in women without acute PID. Pulsatility indices are significantly lower in the acute PID group than in controls (*Table 8.9*). The combined

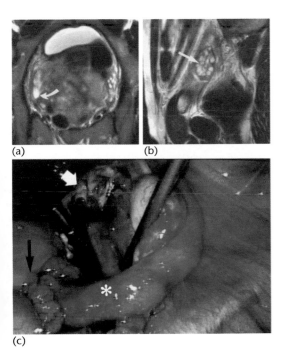

Fig. 8.35 Images in a 15-year-old girl with salpingitis.
(a) T2-weighted axial oblique MR image shows a fluid-filled tube. A small amount of liquid in the tube (arrow) lying on the right ovary has high signal intensity. (b) Sagittal T2-weighted MR image shows a polycystic-like ovary (arrow).
(c) laparoscopic verification shows salpingitis and enlarged ovaries. The fallopian tube (*) is edematous, especially the fimbriae (black arrow). The tube has been lifted up from the ovary (white arrow).
(Reproduced from Ref. 10.)

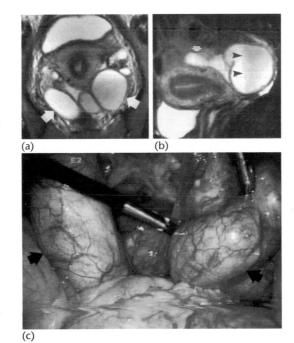

Fig. 8.36 Images in a 35-year-old woman with a bilateral pyosalpinx.
(a) T2-weighted axial oblique MR shows a bilateral pyosalpinx (arrows). The dilated tubes have high signal intensity. The walls are slightly thicker than those in salpingitis but are not irregular. (b) Sagittal STIR MR image shows a small amount of free pelvic fluid (arrow) and layering (arrowheads) in the high-signal-intensity pyosalpinx.
(c) Laparoscopic verification shows both pus-filled, dilated fallopian tubes (arrows).
(Reproduced from Ref. 10.)

| Laparoscopic diagnosis | TVS findings | | | | | | Power Doppler TVS findings | |
| | Wall thickness | | Wall structure | | | Cul-de-sac fluid | Breakdown of adnexal anatomy | PI* (mean ± SE) | Hyperemia |
	<5 mm	>5 mm	Cog-wheel sign	Beads-on-a-string	Incomplete septa				
Salpingitis (*n* = 6)	0	0	0	0	0	3 (50%)	0	0.85 ± 0.06	6 (100%)
Pyosalpinx (*n* = 9)	0	9 (100%)	7 (78%)	0	8 (89%)	5 (56%)	0	0.82 ± 0.09	9 (100%)
TOA** (*n* = 5)	0	5 (100%)	4 (80%)	0	4 (80%)	4 (80%)	5 (100%)	0.83 ± 0.05	5 (100%)
Cases with acute PID (*n* = 20)	0	14 (70%)	11 (55%)	0	12 (60%)	12 (60%)	5 (20%)	0.84 ± 0.04	20 (100%)
Controls (*n* = 20)***	18 (90%)	2 (10%)	1 (5%)	16 (80%)	17 (85%)	3 (15%)	0	1.50 ± 0.10*	2 (10%)
P value	< 0.01	< 0.01	< 0.01	< 0.01	< 0.08	< 0.01	< 0.02	< 0.01	< 0.01

*PI = pulsatility index; **TOA = tubo-ovarian abscess; ***Controls had sactosalpinx.
Modified from Molander et al Ultrasound Obstat Gyaecol 2001; 17:233–238.[12]

Table 8.9 Conventional TVS and power Doppler TVS findings in patients with acute PID and in patients with hydrosalpinx

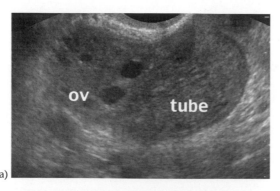

(a)

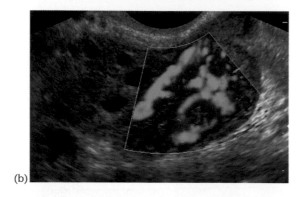

(b)

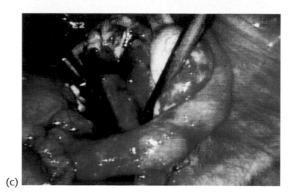

(c)

Fig. 8.37 Acute salpingitis (a) A small echogenic mass in close proximity to ovarian (ov) is seen. Fluid content is not detected. (b) Power Doppler shows increased vascularity highly suggestive of hyperemia and acute inflammation. (c) Laparoscopy confirms the diagnosis of acute salpingitis. (Reproduced from Ref. 12.)

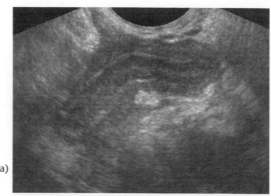

(a)

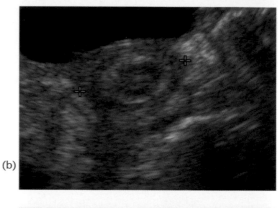

(b)

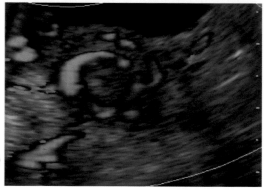

(c)

Fig. 8.38 (a) Transverse vaginal sonographic image showing a typical submucosal ring of an inflamed appendix. Transverse diameter is 18 mm. (b) Transverse vaginal Power Doppler image shows hyperemia. (c) Laparoscopy shows inflamed appendix, proximal end partly released. (Courtesy of Pontus Molander, MD.)

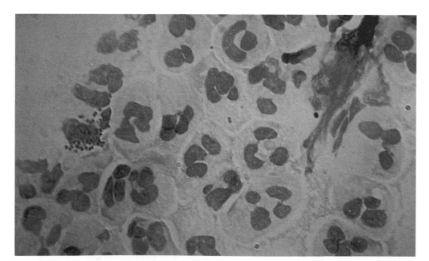

Fig. 8.39 Gram-stained smear of endocervical secretions. Note the polymorphonuclear leukocytes with numerous Gram-negative 'intracellular diplococci'.

use of TVS and power Doppler augments the diagnosis of PID among women referred for low abdominal pain.[12]

Power Doppler TVS can also distinguish between acute appendicitis and PID while avoiding the limitations of trans-abdominal ultrasound. In a preliminary study of six patients with laparoscopically proven acute appendicitis, power Doppler TVS showed either a typical submucosal ring with thick walls (*Fig. 8.38*) or a heterogeneous complex with surrounding hyper-echogenic soft tissue. In this study, hyperemia was present in all cases and normal adnexal structures could be visualized next to the inflamed appendix.[13]

LABORATORY STUDIES

The detection of *C. trachomatis* or *N. gonorrhoeae* in patients with lower abdominal pain, vaginal discharge, and pelvic tenderness is highly suggestive of PID. The endocervical Gram-stained smear (*Fig. 8.39*), if positive for typical Gram-negative, intracellular diplococci, may assist in the diagnosis of PID. Several non-culture tests, including DNA probes, NAATs, and enzyme immunoassays (EIAs) have been developed for the detection of *N. gonorrhoeae* in clinical specimens (see Chapter 6). However, in most routine clinical practices, the laboratory diagnosis of *N. gonorrhoeae* is still based on culture and Gram stain.

Author	Year	ESR* Sensitivity/ specificity (significance)	WBC** Sensitivity/ specificity (significance)	CRP*** Sensitivity/ specificity (significance)
Jacobson	1969	76%/46% ($P < 0.001$)		
Haji	1979			100%/98%
Svensson	1980		72%	
Wölner-Hanssen	1983	76%/31% ($P \leq 0.005$)	44%/32% (P = ns)	
Lehtinen	1986	81%/57% (P = 0.025)		74%/67% ($P < 0.0001$)
Hemila	1987			93%/83%
Schmidt-Rhode	1990	88%/58%	57%/83%	98%
Rousseau	1991		61%/53%	
Sellors	1991	P = 0.006	P = ns	$P < 0.0001$
Livengood	1992	83%/50% (P = ns)	61%/40% (P = ns)	
Wasserheit	1992	45%/83% (P = 0.011)		85%/90% (P = 0.001)
Soper	1992		70%	
Miettinen	1993	51%[#]		46%
Bevan	1995	40%/86% ($P \leq 0.01$)	54%/56% (P = ns)	
Korn	1995	52%/62%	30%/89%	
Peipert	1996	70%/52%	57%/88%	71%/55%

ns = non-significant.
*Erythrocyte sedimentation rate ≥ 15 mm/hour; **White blood cell count > 10,000;
***C-reactive protein; various values used; #ESR > 40 mm/hour.
Modified from Munday PE. J Infect 2000; 40: 31–41.[9]

Table 8.10 Evaluation of laboratory markers in the diagnosis of pelvic inflammatory disease (PID)

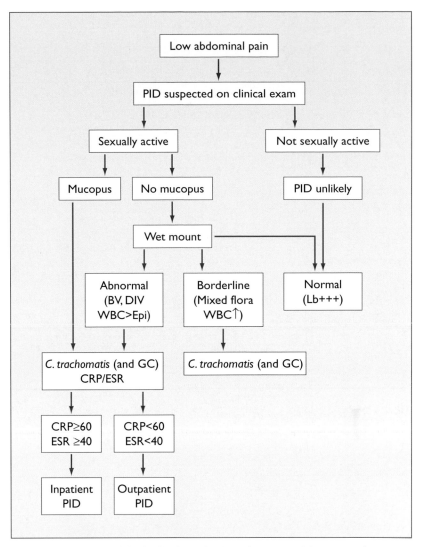

Fig. 8.40 Flow chart of the bed-side evaluation of patients with suspected PID based on findings on speculum examination and wet mount examination. BV = bacterial vaginosis; DIV = desquamative inflammatory vaginitis (aerobic vaginitis); WBC>EPI = the number of white blood cells exceeds the number of epithelial cells per field; Lb+++=high amoung of normal lactobacilli; GC = Neisseria gonorrhoeae; CRP = C-reactive protein; ESR = erthrocyte sedimentation rate; Mucopus = mucopurulentlent endocervical discharge.

Cell culture has long been the 'gold standard' for the confirmatory diagnosis of *C. trachomatis*. However, recently developed NAATs, such as PCR and LCR have largely replaced cell culture and antigen tests in the diagnosis of uncomplicated *C. trachomatis* infection (see Chapter 4 and Appendix 4). NAATs, especially LCR and PCR on first void urine (FVU), are highly effective at detecting both symptomatic and asymptomatic chlamydial infection. Cell culture or antigen tests, which are still used in many clinics miss a large proportion of cases. If screening for chlamydial infection is to be effective, such programs should detect as many cases as possible. Therefore, NAATs using FVU would be the best option. New techniques are constantly being introduced and evaluated. A recent review of the accuracy and efficacy of screening tests for *C. trachomatis* clearly showed that NAATs are excellent diagnostic tests with high accuracy.[14]

Other laboratory tests, which are not specific for PID but are often abnormal or elevated in an acute infection or inflammation and which may help in the diagnosis and monitoring of PID, include the erythrocyte sedimentation rate (ESR), quantitative C-reactive protein (CRP), and the total white blood cell (WBC) count. Combining ESR and CRP increases the ability to discriminate severe PID from moderate to mild PID. Evaluation of laboratory markers in the diagnosis of PID based on multiple studies shows reasonable accuracy for ESR and CRP, but not for WBC (*Table 8.10*).

A simple algorithm developed for primary care bedside diagnosis could augment the management of women with clinical findings consistent with PID. The algorithm is based on the assumption that the presence of lower genital tract infection is a prerequisite for PID (*Fig. 8.40*). Thus, the presence or absence of cervical mucopus on speculum examination and presence or absence of abnormal findings on wet mount examination of vaginal discharge are the key steps of such a flow chart. Systematic use of these simple observations during clinical evaluation are likely to increase the accuracy of the clinical bedside diagnosis of PID.

TREATMENT OF PID

Due to the complex microbiology of PID, a therapeutic approach using broad-spectrum antimicrobial agents is recommended. Problems that often complicate the management of PID include a difficult clinical diagnosis, inaccessibility of clinical sites for microbiologic tests, patient compliance in taking prescribed medications, and delayed access to health-care providers skilled and trained in the management of PID (*Table 8.11*). Unfortunately, PID patients are often managed badly by physicians with little interest in the condition.[15] The optimum therapy regimen should include agents known to be active against

Difficult clinical diagnosis

Sites of infection inaccessible for routine confirmatory testing

Polymicrobial nature

Optimal antibiotic selection

Poor patient compliance with multiple-day therapy and follow-up

Delayed access to appropriate treatment and prevention services

Lack of partner referral for timely evaluation and treatment

Table 8.11 Problems frequently encountered with PID management

Regimen A
    Ofloxacin 400 mg po bid for 14 days or Levofloxacin 500 mg po once daily for 14 days
                            With or without
    Metronidazole 500 mg po bid for 14 days

Regimen B
    Ceftriaxone 250 im once or Cefoxitin (or equivalent cephalosporin) 2 g im plus Probenecid 1 g po in a single dose concurrently once plus Doxycycline 100 mg po bid for 14 days
                            With or without
    Metronidazole 500 mg po bid for 14 days

Table 8.12 Recommended PID outpatient therapy regimens. From CDC 2002 STD treatment guidelines.

Parenteral Regimen A
    Cefotetan 2 g iv bid or Cefoxitin 2 g iv qid plus Doxycycline 100 mg po or iv bid

Parenteral Regimen B
    Clindamycin 900 mg iv tid plus gentamycin loading dose iv or im (2 mg/kg of body weight) followed by a maintenance dose (1.5 mg/kg) tid. Single daily dosing may be substituted. Parenteral therapy may be discontinued 24 hours after demonstrable clinical improvement, and continuing oral therapy should consist of Doxycycline 100 mg bid or Clindamycin 400 mg qid to complete a total of 14 days of therapy.

Alternative Parenteral Regimens
    Ofloxacin 400 mg iv bid or Levofloxacin 500 mg iv once daily with or without Metronidazole 500 mg iv tid
                            Or
    Ampicillin/Sulbactam 3 g iv qid plus Doxycycline 100 mg po or iv bid

Table 8.13 Recommended PID inpatient therapy regimens. From CDC 2002 STD treatment guidelines.

Uncertain diagnosis
Surgical emergencies
Suspected pelvic abscess
Severe illness
Pregnancy
Adolescence
Patient noncompliance
Outpatient therapy failure
Inability to arrange interim re-evaluation

Table 8.14 Acute PID: indications for hospitalization

C. trachomatis, *N. gonorrhoeae*, and the broad-spectrum of aerobic and anaerobic bacteria commonly detected in the UGT of women with PID. The choice of antimicrobial therapy should therefore be guided by knowledge of underlying or presumed etiologic agents, and data on the incidence and prevalence of antimicrobial resistance in confirmed PID pathogens, such as *N. gonorrhoeae*. Recent in vitro susceptibility studies of *N. gonorrhoeae* obtained from women with PID in the USA have demonstrated that in vitro resistance to penicillin and tetracycline occurs in 20–25% of isolates tested.

The CDC provides recommendations for outpatient and inpatient therapy of PID.[2] For example, recommended outpatient regimens include a single dose of ceftriaxone, 250 mg intramuscularly plus oral doxycycline, 100 mg twice daily for 14 days, with or without oral metronidazole, 500 mg twice daily (*Table 8.12*). Inpatient therapy regimens recommended by the CDC include cefoxitin (or a comparable cephalosporin) plus doxycycline, or clindamycin plus gentamicin, in appropriate doses (*Table 8.13*). Male sex partners should receive prophylactic treatment for gonococcal and chlamydial infection, and should be counseled on the proper use of condoms to reduce further exposure to and transmission of STDs. PID patients and their sexual partners should also receive information and counseling on the prevention of HIV infection as well as STDs, and should be offered HIV testing. The decision to choose outpatient management rather than hospitalization for PID should ideally be based on specific clinical criteria. *Table 8.14* provides a summary of criteria for the hospitalization of women with PID. Regardless of the decision to treat PID on an outpatient or inpatient basis, all women with PID should be re-evaluated within 48–72 hours following the initiation of therapy and again following completion of therapy. All recommended antibiotic therapies are effective in achieving short-term clinical cure, but their success in preventing long-term sequelae is not known.[16] The guidelines have not yet been critically evaluated in large, randomized, clinical trials. Another problem is that the guidelines have not been effectively implemented and are often not followed by clinicians.

Combination treatment with doxycycline plus metronidazole is usually effective both for inpatient and outpatient PID, it is well tolerated, easy to administer (orally or intravenously), rarely causes enterocolitis, and is not very costly. One important disadvantage is that it may not provide adequate coverage against gonococci, particularly in populations with high background rates of gonococcal infection caused by strains of *N. gonorrhoeae* exhibiting high-level resistance to tetracyclines. Then, a single-dose therapy for gonorrhea should be given (e.g., ciprofloxacin 500 mg). Intrauterine devices should be removed once antimicrobial treatment is started. Contraceptive counseling should be provided.

Most patients with PID are managed as outpatients. Hospitalization of PID patients is recommended if the diagnosis is in doubt, pelvic abscess is diagnosed, severe symptoms preclude outpatient treatment, or if there is no response to outpatient treatment. Whether inpatient treatment improves the long-term outcome of PID is currently not known. The PID Evaluation and Clinical Health (PEACH) study is an ongoing multicenter randomized clinical trial designed to compare inpatient versus outpatient antimicrobial therapy for the treatment of PID. It is the largest prospective study of PID ever conducted in North America, and the first trial to evaluate the effectiveness and cost-effectiveness of currently recommended treatment guidelines in relation to long-term reproductive sequelae.

One systematic review has found that several regimens of parenteral followed by oral antibiotic treatment are effective in resolving the acute symptoms and signs associated with PID (*Table 8.15*). There was no good evidence supporting an optimal duration of treatment, or comparing oral versus parenteral treatment. Similarly, there is no evidence to support or refute empirical antibiotic treatment for suspected PID.[16]

Surgical management of PID ranges from laparoscopy to laparotomy that is sometimes used to manage cases of ruptured tubo-ovarian abscess

Drug regimen	No. of studies	No. of women	Clinical/microbiological cure rate (%)
Inpatient treatment (initially parenteral, switching to oral)			
Clindamycin + aminoglycoside	11	470	91/97
Cefoxitin + doxycycline	8	427	91/98
Cefoxitin + doxycycline	31	174	95/100
Ceftizoxine + tetracycline	1	18	88/100
Cefotaxime + doxycycline	1	19	94/100
Ciprofloxacin	4	90	94/96
Ofloxacin	1	36	100/97
Sulbactam/ampicillin + doxycycline	1	37	95/100
Amoxillin/clavulanic acid	1	32	93/–
Metronidazole + doxycycline	2	36	75/71
Outpatient treatment (oral unless indicated otherwise)			
Cefoxitin (intramuscular) + probenecid + doxycycline	3	219	89/93
Ofloxacin	2	165	95/100
Co-amoxiclav	1	35	100/100
Sulbactam/ampicillin	1	36	70/70
Ceftriaxone (intramuscular) + doxycycline	1	64	95/100
Ciprofloxacin + clindamycin	1	67	97/94

*Modified from Ross J. Br Med J 2001; **322**: 658–659.[15]*

Table 8.15 Cure rates for antibiotic treatment of acute pelvic inflammatory disease. Aggregated data from systematic reviews of randomized controlled trials and case series

and severe peritonitis. Conservative laparoscopic modalities include procedures like irrigation and drainage. More extensive surgical management of PID is rarely needed. Possible indications for the surgical management of PID are summarized in *Table 8.16*.

OUTCOME

The worldwide increase in the incidence of PID during the past few decades has led to the secondary epidemics of tubal factor infertility and ectopic pregnancy. The proportion of TFI of all infertility ranges from approximately 37% in developed countries to up to 85% in developing countries. After a single episode of PID, the risk for tubal factor infertility is approximately 7%. Each additional episode of PID doubles or triples the risk.[17] TFI remains the leading indication for in vitro fertilization in developed countries. Ectopic pregnancy is the main cause of maternal mortality in the first trimester of pregnancy in developing countries. Women with a history of PID have approximately six-fold increased risk of tubal pregnancy compared to women with no history of PID. Chronic pelvic pain occurs in a large proportion of women with past PID. Women with a history of PID are approximately 10 times more likely to be admitted for pelvic pain, and hysterectomy rates are eight times higher than in other women.[18] Thus, women with PID suffer substantial long-term gynecological morbidity later in their lives (*Table 8.17*).

PREVENTION STRATEGIES

Because *C. trachomatis* is the major cause of PID, it is logical to focus PID prevention efforts on chlamydial infections. Thus, screening for *C. trachomatis* is of paramount importance in the prevention of PID. Clinicians have an important role in the primary prevention of PID

Failure to improve after adequate therapy
Pelvic abscess refractory to medical therapy
Ruptured abscess and peritonitis
Uncertain diagnosis

Table 8.16 Potential indications for surgery in the management of PID

Health problem	Relative risk increase
• Ectopic pregnancy	6×
• Tubal factor infertility	14×
• Chronic abdominal pain	10×
• Risk for hysterectomy	8×

*Modified from Buchan et al. Br J Obstet Gynecol 1993; **100**: 558–559.[17]*

Table 8.17 Major health problems associated with PID

through lifestyle counseling and health education and by asking questions about risk-taking sexual behavior, encouraging screening tests for those at risk, ensuring that male sex partners are evaluated and treated, and by counseling about safe sex practices. However, primary prevention by health education has not proven to be very effective so far. More emphasis should be directed towards primary prevention. Effective health education programs should be implemented especially among adolescents.

Secondary prevention by screening for *C. trachomatis* is likely to have a critical role in the prevention of PID. Chlamydial infection fills the general prerequisites for disease prevention by screening because they are highly prevalent, are associated with significant morbidity, can be diagnosed, and are treatable. One recent randomized controlled trial showed that intervention with selective screening for *C. trachomatis* effectively reduced the incidence of PID by 64% during one year of follow-up.[19]

Use of FVU specimens (or vulvar or vaginal swabs) and NAATs for diagnosis, and single dose treatment with azithromycin should further enhance efforts to prevent PID. However, it remains to be seen whether such interventions have a significant effect on the incidence of ectopic pregnancy and TFI.[20]

C. trachomatis screening programs in Sweden have resulted in a dramatic decrease in the rates of *C. trachomatis* infection, followed by a rapid decrease in the rate of hospitalizations for PID.[21] More importantly, 5–10 years later this was followed by a significant decrease in the rate of ectopic pregnancy, especially in young age groups[22,23] (*Fig. 8.41*). These examples show that *C. trachomatis* screening is effective in a real-life situation. However, it is not yet known whether *C. trachomatis* screening produces a corresponding fall in the related incidence of TFI. Although *C. trachomatis* screening seems to be a straightforward approach, many research questions need to be addressed before nationwide screening programs can be implemented (*Table 8.18*).

PID IN PATIENTS WITH HIV INFECTION

Increasing rates of HIV transmission among intravenous drug users and heterosexuals have contributed to rise in the incidence of HIV infection in women of childbearing age. From 6% to 22% of women in the United States who are diagnosed with PID are HIV-infected,[24,25] rates which are up to ten times greater than those among sexually active women without PID.[26] In some African countries the rate of HIV

Vaginal Infections

9

S Hillier and J Sobel

INTRODUCTION

Vaginal symptoms occur frequently and are a major reason many women seek health care. Vaginal symptoms such as abnormal discharge may be caused by either vaginal or cervical infections, or alternatively may be due to noninfectious causes. The most common cause of vaginal discharge is bacterial vaginosis followed by yeast vulvovaginitis. Although trichomoniasis is relatively common in comparison to bacterial STDs in STD clinics and some prenatal clinics, it is generally agreed to be the least frequent of the three vaginal infections. Desquamative inflammatory vaginitis, of unknown etiology, is a recently described cause of purulent vaginitis. Causes of noninfectious vaginitis include a lack of estrogen postpartum or after the menopause, or allergic vaginitis (*Table 9.1*).

The vagina is a dynamic ecosystem which is sterile at birth and becomes colonized within a few days with a predominantly Gram-positive flora, consisting of anaerobic bacteria, staphylococci, streptococci, and diphtheroids. The vaginal pH in premenarchal females is near neutral (pH 7.0) until puberty. At puberty, under the influence of estrogen, the vaginal epithelium increases to a thickness of about 25 cell layers and the glycogen levels in the epithelium and vagina increase. With the increase in glycogen the predominant flora change to lactobacilli

(*Fig. 9.1*), and the vaginal pH decreases to less than 4.5. This low pH is maintained until the menopause, when the vaginal epithelium thins, a mixed flora of anaerobic bacteria, staphylococci, and diphtheroids becomes re-established, and the vaginal pH rises above 6.0.

Women with *Lactobacillus*-predominant flora usually contain these bacteria at a concentration of 10 million organisms per gram of vaginal fluid. While staphylococci and diphtheroids are relatively common, they are present at 1,000-fold lower concentrations, namely approximately 10,000 organisms per gram of vaginal fluid. The anaerobic coccus, *Peptostreptococcus*, is also recovered from nearly all women, but at concentrations similar to that of aerobic cocci. Anaerobic Gram-negative rods, such as *Prevotella bivia*, *Bacteroides ureolyticus*, and *Porphyromonas* spp. are found in 30–60% of normal women at concentrations of less than one million per gram. Thus, in the normal woman with adequate levels of estrogen, lactobacilli account for more than 95% of micro-organisms present in the vagina. This is apparent by direct visualization of Gram-stained vaginal fluid (*Fig. 9.1*).

An early hypothesis by Döderlein maintained that the predominant lactic acid-producing lactobacilli in the vagina have a protective function against pathogenic bacteria, and that an abnormal vaginal discharge results from partial replacement of the normal flora by less acidophilic microorganisms. Consistent with this hypothesis, lactobacilli have been shown to have *in vitro* inhibitory effects on other microorganisms. Glycogen is deposited on the vaginal epithelium under the influence of estrogen, and is then metabolized to glucose by the host. The glucose is converted to lactic acid by the lactobacilli, which acidifies the vagina to a level inhospitable to many other species of bacteria.

In addition to lactic acid, lactobacilli produce a number of compounds which inhibit other bacteria, such as hydrogen peroxide (H_2O_2), lactacin, acidolin and others. The H_2O_2 generated may directly inhibit

Type	Etiology
Infectious	
Bacterial vaginosis	Mixed *Gardnerella vaginalis*, anaerobes (*Prevotella, Porphyromonas, Bacteroides, Fusobacterium, Peptostreptococcus, Mobiluncus*), and genital mycoplasmas
Candida vulvovaginitis	90% *Candida albicans*, 10% *non-albicans Candida* species, rarely other fungi
Trichomoniasis	*Trichomonas vaginalis*
Rare bacterial	Group A *Streptococcus*
Non-infectious	
Atrophic vaginitis	Post-menopausal, post-partum, post-anti-estrogen therapy etc.
Contact vulvovaginitis	Contact dermatitis (Hypersensitivity)
Chemical irritant vaginitis	Soaps, detergents, topical antimycotics
Allergic vaginitis	Allergens
Desquamative inflammatory vaginitis (DIV)	Unknown (Bacterial? Immune mechanism?)
Erosive lichen planus	Immune mechanisms
Collagen vascular diseases (SLE)	Vasculitis
Pemphigus and pemphigoid syndromes	Immune mechanisms

Table 9.1 Vaginal syndromes and their etiologies.

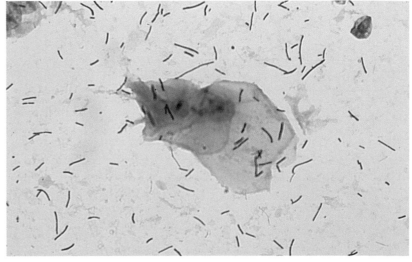

Fig. 9.1 Gram-stained vaginal smear taken from a woman having approximately 10 million (10^7) H_2O_2-producing lactobacilli per gram of vaginal fluid. Note the preponderance of lactobacilli and the lack of other bacterial morphotypes.

other microorganisms.[1] It may also form, in combination with halide (chloride ion) and myeloperoxidase, the potent halide-H_2O_2-myeloperoxidase microbicidal system (*Fig. 9.2*). Women colonized by H_2O_2-generating lactobacilli are less likely to be colonized by *Gardnerella*, genital mycoplasmas, and anaerobes, and are less likely to have bacterial vaginosis. The lactobacilli are autoinhibited by high levels of H_2O_2, so that the levels of H_2O_2-generating lactobacilli are self-regulated in the vagina.

Lactobacilli vary greatly in size but are generally large, straight or curved rods (*Fig. 9.1*). They are Gram-positive, but cells from older cultures may stain Gram-negative or Gram-variable. Lactobacilli are facultative or strictly anaerobic and are usually nonmotile. Although they have complex nutritional requirements, they produce lactic acid as the primary end-product of carbohydrate metabolism. The most common species in the vaginal fluid of women are *Lactobacillus crispatus* and *L. jensenii*, rather than the more commonly cited *L. acidophilus*.[2]

BACTERIAL VAGINOSIS

For many years, *nonspecific vaginitis* was loosely used to refer to vaginal discharges not caused by *Trichomonas vaginalis* or *Candida* spp. In 1955, Gardner and Dukes[3] clinically defined this condition and called it 'Haemophilus vaginalis vaginitis', believing *H. vaginalis* to be the causative organism. This microorganism has since been renamed *Gardnerella vaginalis*. Today, 'Haemophilus vaginalis vaginitis' is referred to as *bacterial vaginosis* (or as *anaerobic vaginosis* in the UK), reflecting the lack of inflammation of the vaginal epithelium in this condition. Others use the term *vaginal bacteriosis*, meaning too many bacteria in the vagina. Bacterial vaginosis is thought to be the result of a complex interaction between many species of bacteria. Gardner and Dukes believed the disease was caused by *G. vaginalis* because they identified the organism in women with bacterial vaginosis but not in women without the disease. In retrospect, they seem to have been unable to recover *G. vaginalis* from the latter group because the medium they used was insensitive and because women with bacterial vaginosis have far greater numbers of the organism than do women without the condition. If sensitive culture techniques[4] are used, as many as 50% of asymptomatic women are found to be colonized with *G. vaginalis*.

The involvement of bacterial species other than *G. vaginalis* in bacterial vaginosis was recognized by Pheifer *et al.*[5] in 1978. They observed that Gram-negative rods (*Prevotella*, *Porphyromonas*, *Bacteroides*, *Fusobacterium*) and *Peptostreptoccus* spp. occurred in increased numbers in the vaginal fluids of women with bacterial vaginosis, and found that metronidazole, which is active against anaerobic bacteria, provides effective therapy. Subsequently, *Mobiluncus* spp. have been found to be highly associated with bacterial vaginosis,[6,7] as has *Mycoplasma hominis*.

The etiologic role of these microorganisms in unclear. However, treatment data suggest that drugs, such as metronidazole or clindamycin which are active against anaerobic bacteria, yield the best clinical response.[4,8–12] Other antimicrobial agents, such as sulfonamides or ampicillin, which are active against *G. vaginalis* but have less activity against anaerobes, are significantly less effective clinically. Although *Mobiluncus* is often resistant to metronidazole, women who have *Mobiluncus* and are treated with this compound have the same rate of cure as women not colonized by *Mobiluncus*.[6] These findings would suggest that anaerobic Gram-negative rods have a more central role in the etiology of bacterial vaginosis than *Gardnerella*, *Mobiluncus*, or the genital mycoplasmas.

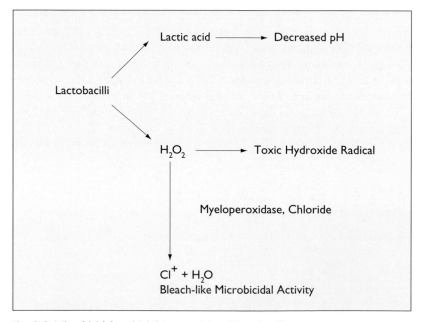

Fig. 9.2 Microbicidal and inhibitory activity of lactobacilli.

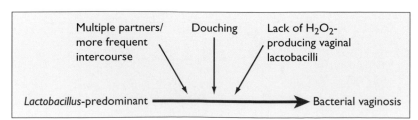

Fig. 9.3 Factors associated with shifts in flora from *Lactobacillus*-predominant to bacterial vaginosis.

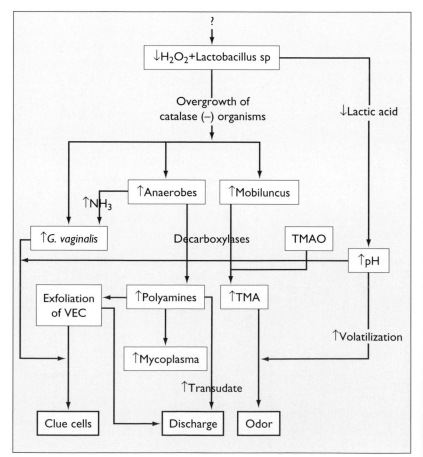

Fig. 9.4 Pathophysiology of bacterial vaginosis.

The development of bacterial vaginosis is the result of a shift in the vaginal ecosystem from one predominated by acid-producing lactobacilli to one characterized by a predominance of *Gardnerella* and anerobic bacteria.[13] The triggers thought to cause this shift in the vaginal ecosystem include multiple sexual partners and/or frequent intercourse, and regular douching (which may kill vaginal lactobacilli) *(Fig. 9.3)*. Women who lack lactobacilli which produce H_2O_2 are also more likely to acquire bacterial vaginosis.[14]

G. vaginalis metabolically produces amino acids, which act as substrates for the production of volatile amines (e.g., putrescine) by anaerobic bacteria; these amines are responsible for the unpleasant odor associated with the disease.[15] The amines, in turn, raise the vaginal pH, so favoring the continued growth of *G. vaginalis* over lactobacilli *(Fig. 9.4)*.

EPIDEMIOLOGY

Bacterial vaginosis is the most common of the vaginitides, yet its epidemiology is not well understood. Although the disease is associated with increased numbers of sexual partners, and detected less frequently among women who are not sexually experienced, it is not considered strictly an STD. The treatment of male sexual partners is not routinely recommended because no study has documented that treatment of the male sexual partner decreases the recurrence of bacterial vaginosis. Recent data suggest that bacterial vaginosis is common among women who have sex with women, especially among those who share sex toys.[16] It is likely, in these cases, that the microbes are transmitted during sexual activity. Although the use of an IUD has been associated with bacterial vaginosis, most affected women have no identifiable risk factors. Without therapy, cases may be self-limited, intermittently recurrent, or chronic.

CLINICAL MANIFESTATIONS

In 1983, the International Working Group on Bacterial Vaginosis formulated clinical criteria for the diagnosis of bacterial vaginosis *(Table 9.2)*. Many cases are so mild that they are not recognized by patients, and are found only on routine examination. Some of these women are only apparently asymptomatic, however, and following treatment will notice the disappearance of a previously inapparent vaginal discharge or odor. This finding may be attributable to the fact that many women consider vaginal malodor to be a hygiene problem rather than a symptom resulting from infection.

Women with bacterial vaginosis may complain of increased vaginal discharge or abnormal vaginal odor. In symptomatic women having bacterial vaginosis and without other genital infections, 90% of women will complain of vaginal discharge, over 70% will complain of odor and 45% will complain of vaginal irritation. The discharge, which typically is milky, clings to the vaginal walls *(Fig. 9.5)*.[17] The vaginal epithelium and vulva appear normal; this lack of inflammation has led to the use of the term *vaginosis* instead of *vaginitis*. The term *vaginosis* does not denote a lack of polymorphonuclear leukocytes in the vaginal wet mount. More than 30 polymorphonuclear leukocytes per high-powered field will be noted in one-third of women with this syndrome.

THREE OF THE FOUR FOLLOWING CRITERIA:

- Clue cells (at least 1 in 5 vaginal epithelial cells with edges obscured by bacteria)
- Vaginal pH > 4.5
- Amine odor spontaneously or after addition of 10% KOH to vaginal fluid
- Thin, homogenous discharge

Table 9.2 Clinical diagnostic criteria for bacterial vaginosis.

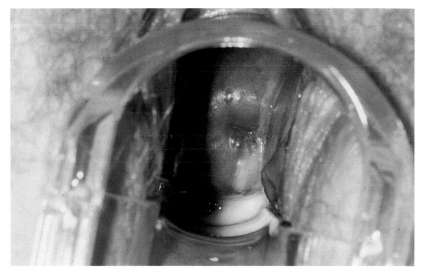

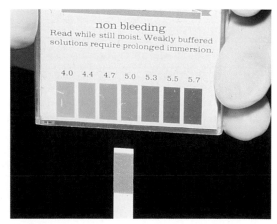

Fig. 9.5 Vaginal examination from a woman with mild bacterial vaginosis. Notice the milky discharge pooling beneath the cervix and the lack of cervical inflammation or vaginal erythema.

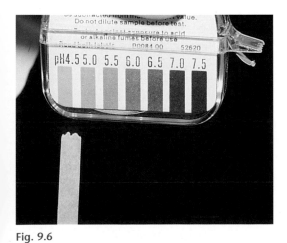

Fig. 9.6

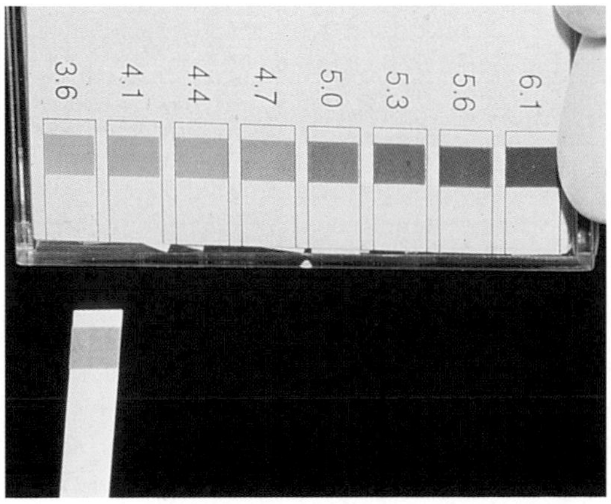

Fig. 9.7

Fig. 9.8

Figs 9.6–9.8 Measurement of vaginal pH is usually performed using commercially available pH strips. A vaginal pH of more than 4.5 is usually considered abnormal, but pH papers with gradations between pH 4.2 and 5.0 (9.7 and 9.8) are usually easier to read than pH paper strips with gradations at each half pH unit (9.6).

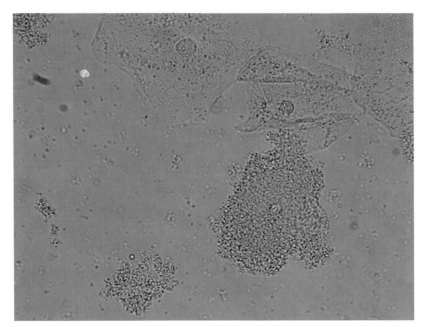

Fig. 9.9 Saline wet mount of vaginal fluid from a woman with bacterial vaginosis. Courtesy of Dr. Elizabeth Lien.

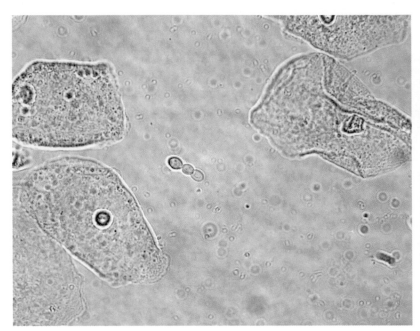

Fig. 9.10 Vaginal wet mount from a woman having clear epithelial cells. Note the presence of building yeasts in the vaginal fluid. Courtesy of Dr. Elizabeth Lien.

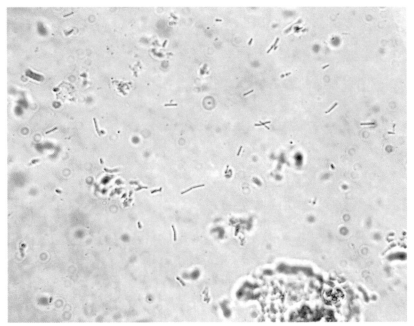

Fig. 9.11 Vaginal fluid wet mount showing presence of large rods. This would be a typical vaginal fluid wet mount from a woman having a *Lactobacillus*-predominant vaginal flora. Courtesy of Dr. Elizabeth Lien.

Bacterial morphotype	Points* scored per morphotype**				
	None	1⁺	2⁺	3⁺	4⁺
Large Gram-positive rod	4	3	2	1	0
Small Gram-negative/variable rod	0	1	2	3	4
Curved Gram-negative/variable rod	0	1	1	2	2

*Score of 0–3 points, normal; 4–6 points, intermediate; 7–10 points, bacterial vaginosis.
**1⁺ < 1/1000× oil immersion field; 2⁺ 1–5; 3⁺ 6–30, 4⁺ >30.

Table 9.3 Standardized scoring method for evaluation of Gram-stained smears for diagnosis of bacterial vaginosis. Nugent RP, Krohn MA, Hillier SL: Reliability of diagnosing bacterial vaginosis is improved by a standardized method of Gram stain interpretation. *J Clin Microbiol* 1991; **29**: 297–301; by permission of the American Society for Microbiology.

Examination of a woman with a complaint of a vaginal discharge or odor should include an evaluation for the clinical criteria of bacterial vaginosis (*Table 9.2*).[17] The odor of the vaginal secretions should be tested by smelling the withdrawn speculum (the 'whiff test'); normal vaginal fluid does not have an unpleasant odor. If this test is negative, a more sensitive procedure for detecting the amines produced is performed by adding a few drops of 10% potassium hydroxide (KOH) to a few drops of vaginal secretions. The mixture should be smelled immediately ('whiffed') for the transient, 'dead fish' odor characteristic of bacterial vaginosis. Potassium hydroxide increases the pH to the point at which the volatilization to trimethylamine occurs. Many women first notice vaginal malodor immediately following intercourse, because semen, which has a pH of 8.0, alkalinizes vaginal fluid so releasing the volatile amines. Women may experience odor during menses as well, due to the increased vaginal pH due to the presence of blood.

The pH of vaginal fluid should be determined by using a strip of narrow-range pH paper (about pH 4.0–5.5), which may be applied to the withdrawn speculum or directly pressed against the vaginal wall with a swab (*Figs 9.6–9.8*). Lastly, a wet mount of vaginal fluid should be done to look for 'clue' cells. These are epithelial cells covered with *G. vaginalis* that Gardner and Dukes called 'clues' to the diagnosis of bacterial vaginosis (*Fig. 9.9*). By comparison, vaginal epithelial cells from women without bacterial vaginosis have clear borders (*Fig. 9.10*). Women having a predominant *Lactobacillus* flora usually have large rods visible in the fluid (*Fig. 9.11*).

When examining a woman for bacterial vaginosis, various potential diagnostic pitfalls should be avoided. The clinical or laboratory assessment may be affected by examination during menses, within a day of sexual intercourse, recent douching, or the use of intravaginal products or systemic antimicrobials. Menses, semen, or douching may affect the pH, and a weakly positive whiff test may be produced by menstrual blood or semen. Care should be taken to ensure that the pH paper does not sample either water used to moisten the speculum or cervical secretions, which are relatively alkaline. It is important to exclude trichomoniasis, which may also have an elevated pH and a positive whiff test because of an accompanying overgrowth of anerobes. Lastly, lactobacilli can cling to epithelial cells, so attention should be given to the morphology of organisms seen on clue cells.

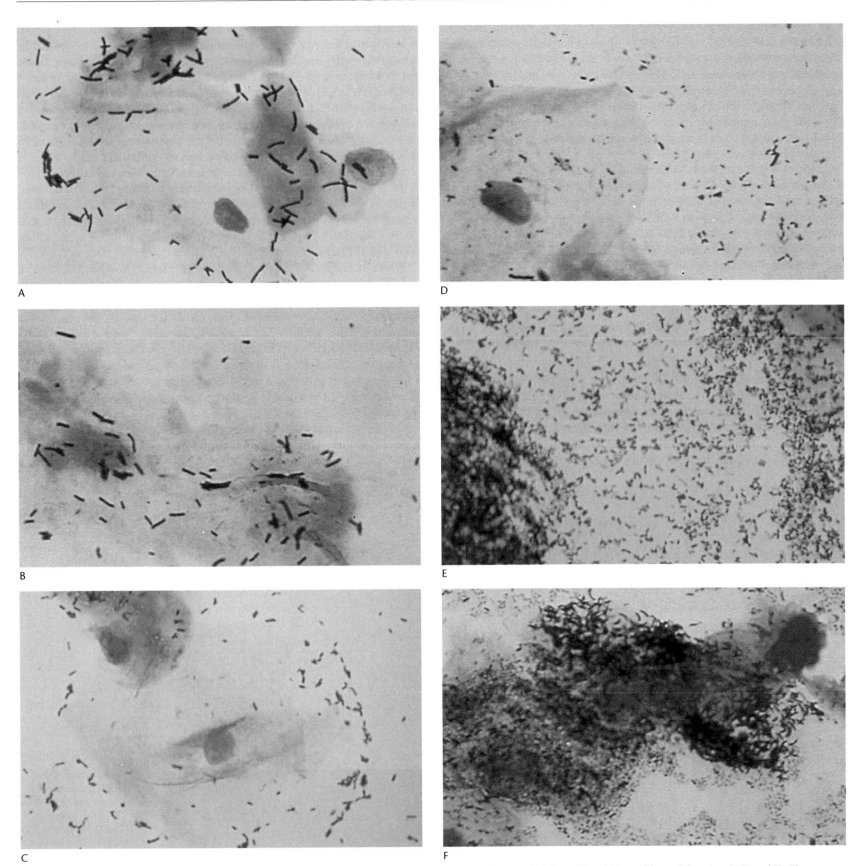

Fig. 9.12 Gram-stained vaginal smears from women with normal vaginal flora (A and B), intermediate vaginal flora (C and D), and bacterial vaginosis (E and F). The scores given to these smears according to the Nugent method are: A = 0; B = 2; C = 4; D = 6; E = 8; and F = 10.

LABORATORY TESTS

The Gram stain is the single best laboratory test for diagnosis of bacterial vaginosis. This method is preferable to culture because it has greater specificity and should be available in any laboratory which is licensed to perform moderately complex tasks. To prepare a vaginal smear for a Gram stain, a swab should be used to obtain vaginal fluid and cells from the vaginal wall (not the cervix). This swab should then be rolled across a slide and the material allowed to air-dry. There is no need to heat-fix the smear prior to shipment to the laboratory. Air-dried vaginal smears are stable at room temperature for months.

In the laboratory, the smear should be heat-fixed and Gram-stained. There are two primary methods for diagnosis of bacterial vaginosis from Gram-stained smears. For the Nugent method (*Table 9.3*), a score of

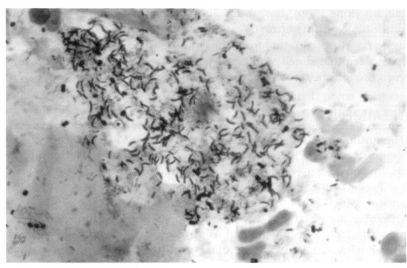

Fig. 9.17 Gram-stained clue cell from a woman with bacterial vaginosis, showing *Mobiluncus curtisii* on the surface.

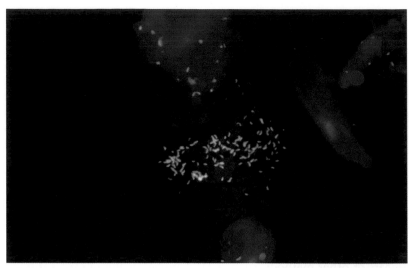

Fig. 9.18 Clue cell from a woman with bacterial vaginosis stained with a fluorescent antibody to *Mobiluncus curtisii*.

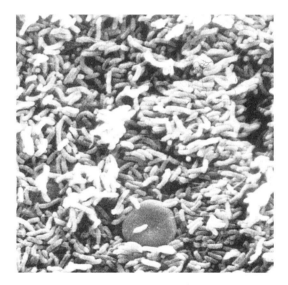

Fig. 9.19 Scanning electron micrograph of *Mobiluncus curtisii*. Notice the red blood cell in the center of the field, with *M. curtisii* on the surface.

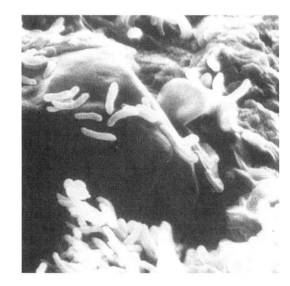

Fig. 9.20 Scanning electron micrograph of *Mobiluncus mulieris*, the longer of the two species of *Mobiluncus*.

Agent and regimen	Efficacy one month post treatment
Metronidazole oral	
500 mg bid for 7 days	78–82%
2 g single dose	72–73%
Intravaginal metronidazole gel	
5 g bid for 5 days	71–73%
Clindamycin oral	
300 mg bid for 7 days	94%
Intravaginal clindamycin cream	
5 g once daily for 7 days	61–85%
Ampicillin	66%
Ofloxacin (300 mg bid for 7 days)	29%
Erythromycin	20%
Tetracycline	20%
Lactate gel	20%
Acetic acid gel	18%
Yogurt	7%
Lactobacilli (10^8 bid for 6 days)	20%
Povidone iodine tablets (200 mg bid for 14 days)	25%

Table 9.4 Effectiveness of different regimens for treatment of bacterial vaginosis.

carefully controlled trials. It is possible that vaginal recolonization with suitable, human-derived strains of lactobacilli may be a useful adjunct to antimicrobial therapy, but so far no commercially available strain has been proven to be beneficial. A number of published studies have linked bacterial vaginosis to complications of pregnancy, including preterm labor, preterm delivery, and amniotic fluid infection, treatment trials using oral netronidazole for prevention of preterm delivery have yielded inconsistant result.[25] While concern about the potential teratogenicity and carcinogenicity of metronidazole has limited its use during pregnancy, this drug is generally regarded as safe for use from the second trimester of pregnancy.

TRICHOMONIASIS

INTRODUCTION

Trichomonas vaginalis is a protozoan that infects the genital tract specifically. Although two other species of trichomonads colonize man (*Trichomonas tenax* in the mouth and *Pentatrichomonas hominis* in the large intestine), these organisms do not occur in the vagina. *T. vaginalis* is ovoid, and approximately 10–20 μm wide (about the size of a white blood cell) (*Fig. 9.21*). The organism has four, free, anterior flagella and

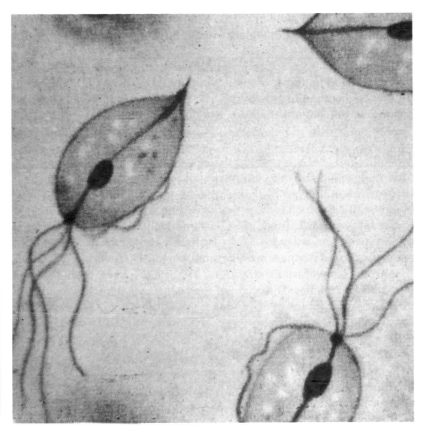

Fig. 9.21 *Trichomonas vaginalis.*

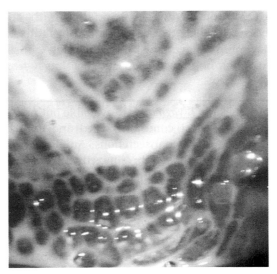

Fig. 9.22 Vaginal erythema and discharge from a patient with trichomoniasis. Note frothiness of discharge.

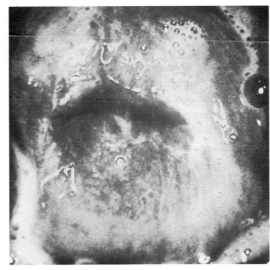

Fig. 9.23 'Strawberry cervix,' seen in about 10% of patients with trichomoniasis. Note frothiness of discharge.

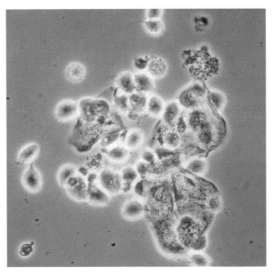

Fig. 9.24 Trichomonads visualized by phase contrast microscopy (× 400).

a fifth flagellum embedded in an undulating membrane that extends around the anterior two-thirds of the cell. The flagella move the protozoan with a jerky movement.

EPIDEMIOLOGY

Women are the main carriers of disease. About one-third of men who are sexual partners of women with *T. vaginalis* have urethral colonization, but men, unlike women, rapidly clear the organism. One study found that 70% of men who had sex with an infected woman 2 days previously were infected, with this percentage dropping to 47% by 14 days or longer. Thus, transmission of the disease depends upon relatively frequent intercourse of men with different partners, and/or occasional long-term infections in some men.[26]

In a study of trichomoniasis in over 13,000 women in the second trimester of pregnancy, the prevalence by culture was 13%. Infection by *T. vaginalis* was associated with Black race, being unmarried, a history of gonorrhea, and having multiple sexual partners during pregnancy. The high prevalence of this sexually transmitted pathogen in pregnant women is of concern because of the recent data suggesting that trichomoniasis is linked with an increased risk of low birth weight. However, treatment of symptomatic trichomoniasis has not been shown to reduce preterm birth.[27]

CLINICAL MANIFESTATIONS

As many as one half of women infected with *T. vaginalis* are asymptomatic. This number depends upon how women are selected for study, how closely the women are questioned for symptoms, and the sensitivity of diagnostic techniques. In symptomatic women, a vaginal discharge is the most common complaint. The discharge usually appears purulent or yellow in color. As in bacterial vaginosis, about 50% of women notice a disagreeable odor, due to the overgrowth of anaerobic microorganisms with resultant amine production. Vulvar itching is also reported by 50% of women with trichomoniasis.

The vaginal mucosa is often erythematous, reflecting the inflammatory nature of the disease process (*Fig. 9.22*). In a few cases, the cervix is inflamed and has punctate hemorrhages (*Fig. 9.23*). Rarely, *T. vaginalis* has been found in the upper genital tract, but the significance of this finding is unknown.

Most men infected with *T. vaginalis* are asymptomatic. About 5–10% of men with nongonococcal urethritis are infected with *T. vaginalis*. The

In men, *Candida* spp. may cause balanitis (inflammation of the glans penis) and balanoposthitis (inflammation of the glans penis and prepuce) (*Fig. 9.32*). *Candida* organisms have been recovered from semen and from the urethras of some men with nonspecific urethritis, but the significance of these findings is unclear.

EPIDEMIOLOGY

Although men can be colonized with *Candida* spp., and many male sexual partners of women with candidiasis are transiently colonized, candidiasis is not recognized as an STD. Instead, symptoms occur in women previously colonized with *C. albicans*. Although the reasons why symptomatic yeast infections occur are not completely understood, pregnancy, diabetes, use of birth control pills, steroid use, immunosuppression associated with HIV infection and transplantation and systemic antimicrobial therapy (which eliminates competing vaginal flora) are recognized predisposing factors to symptomatic infection. However, many women who develop yeast vaginitis will have not had any of the recognized risk factors.

LABORATORY TESTS

C. albicans occurs in both yeast and mycelial forms. Yeasts are oval cells about 4–8 mm in diameter (*Fig. 9.33*). In vaginal specimens, yeasts multiply asexually by forming buds (blastoconidia). If the buds keep forming and elongating, and do not detach from one another, they resemble hyphae and are called pseudohyphae (*Fig. 9.34*). The constrictions between buds in the pseudohyphae differentiate them from true hyphae. The vaginal pH remains normal, 4.0–4.5 in most women with vaginal candidiasis, but some women may have an elevated pH.

The diagnosis of candidiasis is most often made by wet-mount microscopy of vaginal fluid; this can be done when the vaginal fluid is examined for clue cells and trichomonads. Estimates of the sensitivity of wet-mount microscopy range from 40–85%; as with trichomoniasis, sensitivity varies with patient selection, observer experience, and sensitivity of the culture media to which wet-mount results are compared. Symptoms appear to be directly correlated to the quantity of yeasts present, and thus if symptomatic women are studied, the wet mount will appear highly sensitive.[34]

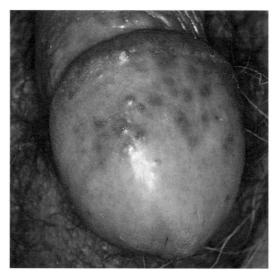

Fig. 9.32 Penile candidal balanitis showing erythematous papules and pustules on the glans penis. Courtesy of Bingham JS: Pocket picture Guide Series. *Sexually transmitted diseases.* London, Gower Medical Publishing Ltd., 1984.

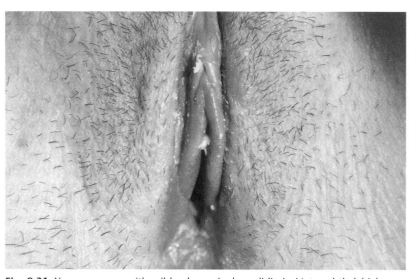

Fig. 9.31 Young woman with mild vulvovaginal candidiasis. Note subtle labial edema extending into clitoral hood.

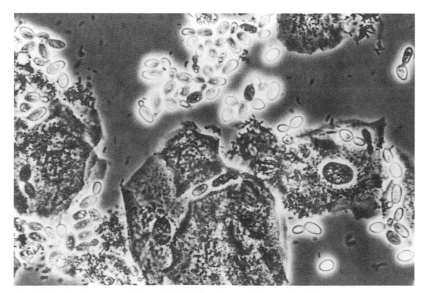

Fig. 9.33 High-power photomicrograph of non-albicans Candida species seen in women with vaginitis (C. glabrata).

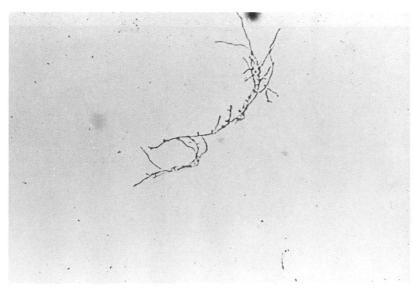

Fig. 9.34 Low-power (× 40) micrograph of C. albicans family hyphae. Seen on saline microscopy.

The wet-mount specimen is examined for yeasts or pseudohyphae under low-power magnification (100×), while subsequent high-power examination (400×) will detect the organisms. Debris from epithelial cells or mucus may be mistaken for or may obscure yeasts, but this potential problem can be eliminated by adding a few drops of 10–15% KOH to the wet-mount specimen. The addition of KOH has been shown to improve both sensitivity and specificity. A Gram stain of vaginal secretions is not as sensitive as wet mount in detecting infection. *Candida* spp. stain intensely Gram-positive (*see Figs 9.35 and 9.36*). *Candida* spp. may be seen on Papanicolaou-stained samples of exfoliated cervical cells. This method is not sensitive, however, and detects only about 50% of cases of symptomatic women.

Culture is the most sensitive diagnostic test, but should be reserved for those instances in which clinical signs or symptoms of yeast infection are present and the wet mount is negative for blastopores or hyphae.[35] Culture is particularly useful in women with refractory and recurrent vaginitis. *Candida* spp. grow on many media, including blood agar. At least two media should be used for greatest yield, one with and one without antimicrobials inhibitory for competing microorganisms. Sabouraud's dextrose, the most widely used medium, supports the growth of all clinically important yeasts. *Candida* spp. will grow at both 25°C and 37°C, so using two temperatures offers no diagnostic advantage. Although *Candida* spp. grow most rapidly at 37°C, more rapidly growing bacteria may obscure fungal colonies at this temperature, and so many authorities prefer to grow *Candida* at 30°C. Pinpoint colonies may be visible at 24 hours but are more apparent at 48–72 hours. Nickerson's agar and its analogs may simplify the identification of *Candida* spp. because the colonies are selectively dark, but this method of identification is not totally reliable. It is important to remember that finding yeast by culture in an asymptomatic woman means only that she may be harboring this organism as part of her normal flora.

TREATMENT

A number of highly effective oral and intravaginal antifungals are available (*Table 9.6*). Nystatin is the least effective with cure rates in the 70–75% range. The remaining antifungals have published efficacies in the 80–88% range. Of the intravaginal imidazoles, clotrimazole, miconazole, butoconazole, tioconazole are available over-the-counter in the USA, while terconazole is available only by prescription. Butoconazole and terconazole have a greater in vitro efficacy against non-*C. albicans* yeasts. However, the clinical significance of this is unclear as the published clinical efficacy for these compounds is similar to that reported for over-the-counter products.

Oral agents which have been used in the USA for treatment of yeast vaginitis include fluconazole, which is supplied as a single 150 mg oral tablet, itraconazole and ketoconazole. Only fluconazole is FDA approved.

Selection of the appropriate antifungal agent and the duration of therapy has been facilitated by the new classification of VVC into complicated and uncomplicated vaginitis (*Table 9.7*). Most women (90%) have uncomplicated VVC being healthy hosts, with mild to moderate, infrequent episodes of vaginitis due to *C. albicans*. Under these circumstances, patients respond to all azoles topical or systemic with a success rate in excess of 90% and regardless of the duration of therapy. Accordingly short course azole therapy, including over-the-counter (OTC) antimycotics are highly useful and effective (*Fig. 9.37*).

Drug	Topical agents and formulation	Dosage regimen
*Butoconazole	2% cream	5 g × 3 d
*Clotrimazole	1% cream	5 g × 7–14 d
	100 mg vag. tab.	1 tab. × 7 d
	100 mg vag. tab	2 tab. × 3 d
	500 mg vag. tab.	1 tab. single dose
*Miconazole	2% cream	5 g × 7 d
	100 mg vag. supp.	1 supp. × 7 d
	200 mg vag. supp.	1 supp. × 3 d
	1200 mg vag. supp.	1 supp. single dose
Econazole	150 mg vag. tab	1 tab. × 3 d
Fenticonazole	2% cream	5 g × 7 d
*Ticonazole	2% cream	5 g × 7 d
	6.5% cream	5 g single dose
Terconazole	0.4% cream	5 g × 7 d
	0.8% cream	5 g × 3 d
	80 mg vag. supp.	80 mg × 3 d
Nystatin	1000,000-U vag. tab.	1 tab. × 14 d

Abbreviations: vag, vaginal; tab, tablets; supp, suppository

	Oral Agents	
Ketoconazole	400 mg bid	× 5 d
Itraconazole	200 mg bid	× 1 d
	200 mg	× 3 d
Fluconazole	150 mg	single dose

*OTC in the United States.

Table 9.6 Therapy for vaginal candidiasis.

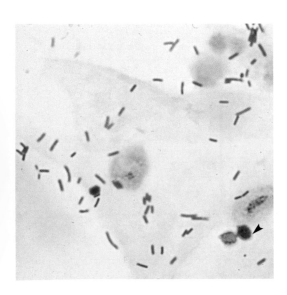

Fig. 9.35 Gram-stained vaginal smear from a woman having a vaginal yeast infection caused by *Candida (Torulopsis) glabrata*, a yeast which does not form hyphae or pseudohyphae. The Gram-positive rods in the background are lactobacilli.

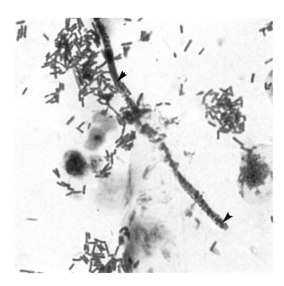

Fig. 9.36 Gram-stained vaginal smear from a woman with vulvovaginal candidiasis. Note large pseudohyphal element and the abundance of Gram-positive rods resembling lactobacilli.

In contrast, women with complicated VVC respond poorly to short-course azole therapy. Accordingly compromised hosts or women with severe vaginitis should receive more prolonged conventional antimycotic treatment.[36]

Treatment of women infected with non-albicans *Candida* species remains highly problematic. In particular vaginitis due to *C. glabrata* is often refractory to azole therapy (50% respond only). Somewhat improved

results are achieved with vaginal boric acid capsules (approximately 70%) although no prospective controlled studies have been undertaken.[37] Anecdotally, the best results appear to follow vaginal therapy with flucytosine cream.

A small subset of women with yeast vulvovaginitis develops recurrent infections, which can cause monthly or even persistent symptoms (*Fig. 9.38*). Longitudinal data suggest that women are usually persistently infected by the same strain or species of yeast.[38] While some of those women have recognized risk factors for yeast infection, most do not.[39] Risk factors should be considered, but a thorough search for subclinical diabetes mellitus is not warranted. The pathogenesis of recurrent vulvovaginal candidiasis is described in *Figure 9.39*.

One approach to the management of recurrent yeast vulvovaginitis is the use of antifungal agents prophylactically prior to, or immediately after menses. In placebo-controlled trials, women who use prophylactic

Uncomplicated	Complicated
Sporadic/infrequent VVC and	Recurrent VVC or
Mild to moderate VVC and	Severe VVC or
Likely to be *C. albicans* and	Non-albicans candidiasis or
Normal, nonpregnant host	Abnormal host e.g., uncontrollable diabetes Debilitation, Immunosuppression

VVC = vulvovaginal candidiasis.

Table 9.7 Classification of vulvovaginal candidiasis.

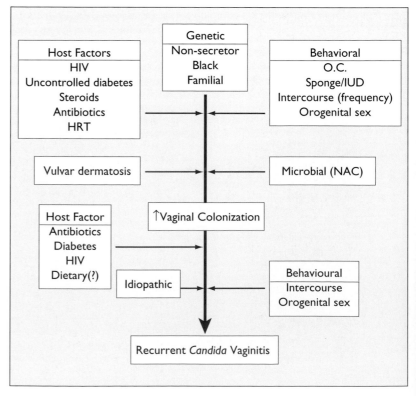

Fig. 9.38 Chronic vulvovaginal candidiasis. Note subtle multiple asymmetrical linear fissures lateral to labia minora.

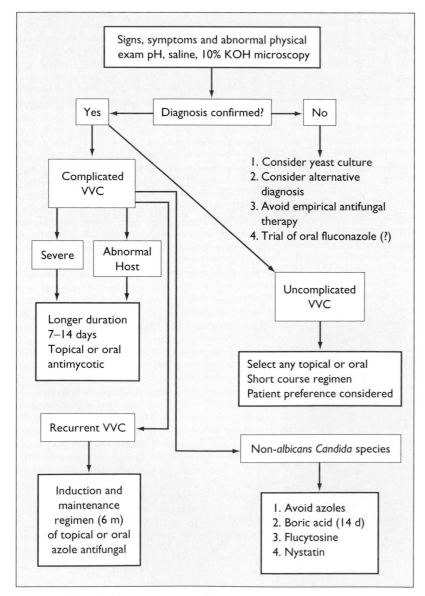

Fig. 9.37 Algorithm for management of acute vulvovaginal candidiasis.

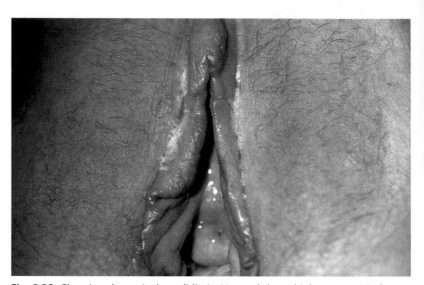

Fig. 9.39 Pathogenesis of recurrent vulvovaginal candidiasis.

antifungals will have fewer episodes of recurrence, but these women will develop increased episodes of yeast vaginitis after stopping prophylactic therapy. Thus, the prophylactic use of antifungals should be viewed as providing suppression rather than cure. Another approach is to prescribe antifungals empirically at the onset of symptoms. Although this approach results in more episodes of yeast vaginitis, the total amount of antifungal used and the total costs for drugs is substantially less.

During pregnancy, yeast vaginitis should be treated with one of the pregnancy category A (nystatin) or B (clotrimazole, miconazole) antifungals. Oral fluconazole should not be used in pregnancy.

Epidemiology
Usually Caucasian
More frequent peri-menopausal, post-partum
Long duration of symptoms
Symptoms
Purulent yellow-green discharge
Dyspareunia
Signs
Variable vestibulitis
Diffuse vaginal erythema and focal erosions
Changes often resemble 'strawberry' rash
Laboratory
Vaginal pH > 4.5 (usually >6)
Amine test negative
↑ 3–4+ vaginal PMN's
↑ parabasal cells + naked nuclei
Lack of lactobacilli
Gram positive cocci
Therapy
2% clindamycin vaginal suppositories (cream) daily × 14 days
or
10% hydrocortisone cream, 5 g nightly × 14 days
Note: No improvement with HRT
Relapse
Maintenance regimen of clindamycin/hydrocortisone

Table 9.8 Desquamative inflammatory vaginitis.

DESQUAMATIVE INFLAMMATORY VAGINITIS

INTRODUCTION

The most recently described cause of infectious vaginitis is desquamative inflammatory vaginitis.[40,41] As this syndrome has been described recently, and occurs rarely in comparison to other types of infectious vaginitis, comparatively little is known about this syndrome.

EPIDEMIOLOGY

Desquamative inflammatory vaginitis occurs more frequently in peri-menopausal or postmenopausal women than in women of reproductive age. This syndrome has been documented much more frequently in Caucasian than in African-American women, even when the study population has a majority of African-American women (*Table 9.8*).[40] Women with desquamative inflammatory vaginitis suffer severe symptoms, with profound effect on daily life.[41] Women with this condition are more likely to report a history of surgery or treatment for blocked fallopian tubes or hysterectomy although the biologic basis for this association is unclear.

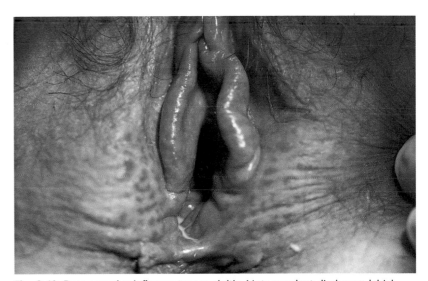

Fig. 9.40 Desquamative inflammatory vaginitis. Note purulent discharge, labial edema and multiple erythematous focal erosive lesions of vulva.

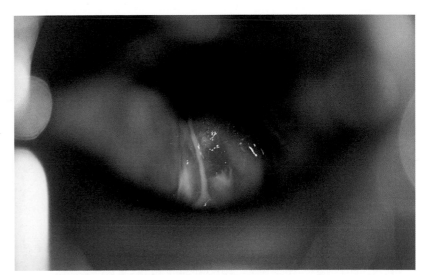

Fig. 9.41 Desquamative inflammatory vaginitis. Multiple erythematous focal vaginal lesions also seen on cervix. Lesions are of variable size and show focal erosion on biopsy.

Fig. 9.42 Clinical picture of desquamative inflammatory vaginitis. Note purulent discharge and erosive lesion of vaginal wall.

CLINICAL FEATURES

Women with desquamative inflammatory vaginitis often present with complaints of vaginal irritation and dyspareunia lasting months or even years. On examination, these women will have profound vaginal erythema (*Figs 9.40-9.42*). While the vaginal pH will usually be greater than 4.5, amine odor is almost universally absent, indicating a lack of anaerobic microorganisms. A purulent yellow-green discharge may be present.

Diagnosis is made on the basis of elevated pH and a lack of amine odor coupled with the microscopic evaluation of vaginal fluid. The wet-mount examination is characterized by the presence of parabasal cells and naked nuclei, suggesting severe desquamation of the vaginal epithelium. A Gram-stained vaginal smear usually shows the presence of many polymorphonuclear leukocytes, the absence of lactobacilli, and the presence of abundant Gram-positive cocci. Although group B streptococci have been reported in 60–70% of women with desquamative inflammatory vaginitis, their causal role remains unproven.

Treatment with 2% clindamycin, as an intravaginal cream or suppository, used once daily for 2 weeks will treat most cases effectively. Unfortunately, a high relapse rate is reported. Patients can be re-treated with clindamycin and some require a maintenance clindamycin regimen. Alternatively, good success is reported with an intensive regimen of intravaginal corticosteroids.

CONCLUSIONS

Vaginal symptoms are common in women, and lead them to seek medical care or to pursue self-diagnosis and treatment. The majority of symptoms are not due to infectious causes and assumption that all symptoms are due to infection is invalid. A careful pelvic examination, measurement of vaginal pH, evaluation of vaginal odor after addition of 10% KOH, and routine microscopy are essential components of office diagnosis. Cultures are not useful at all in the diagnosis of bacterial vaginosis. They are only occasionally indicated for yeast vaginitis, but are vastly superior to wet mount for *Trichomonas*. Several different treatment options are available for these infections, but additional care should be taken when choosing a therapy for use during pregnancy.

References

1. Norrod PE, Morse SA. Presence of hydrogen peroxide in media used for the cultivation of *Neisseria gonorrhoeae*. *J Clin Microbiol* 1982; **15**:103.
2. Antonio MAD, Hawes SE, Hillier SL. The identification of viginal *Lactobacillus* species and the demographic and microbiologi characterics of women colorized by these species. *J Infect Dis* 1999; **180**:1950–1956.
3. Gardner HL, Dukes CD. *Haemophilus vaginalis* vaginitis. *Ann NY Acad Sci* 1959; **83**:280.
4. Totten PA, Amsel R, Hale J, Piot P, Holmes KK. Selective differential human blood bilayer media for isolation of *Gardnerella (Haemophilus) vaginalis*. *J Clin Microbiol* 1982; **15**:141–147.
5. Pfeifer TA, Forsyth PA, Durfee MA *et al*. Nonspecific vaginitis: role of *Haemophilus vaginalis* and treatment with metronidazole. *N Engl J Med* 1978; **198**:1429–1434.
6. Spiegel CA, Eschenbach DA, Amsel R, Holmes KK. Curved anaerobic bacteria in nonspecific vaginosis and their response to antibiotic therapy. *J Infect Dis* 1983; **148**:817–822.
7. Thomason JL, Schreckenberger PC, Spellacy WN, *et al*. Clinical and microbiological characterization of patients with nonspecific vaginosis associated with motile, curved anaerobic rods. *J Infect Dis* 1984; **149**:801–809.
8. Covino JM, Black JR, Cummings M, Zwicki B, McCormack WM. Comparative evaluation of ofloxacin and metronidazole in the treatment of bacterial vaginosis. *Sex Transm Dis* 1993; **20**(3):262–264.
9. Hillier SL, Krohn MA, Watts DH, Wölner-Hanssen P, Eschenbach DA. Microbiological efficacy of intravaginal clindamycin cream for the treatment of bacterial vaginosis. *Obstet Gynecol* 1990; **76**:407–413.
10. Livengood CH, III, Thomason JL, Hill GB. Bacterial vaginosis: treatment with topical intravaginal clindamycin phosphate. *Obstet Gynecol* 1990; **76**:118–123.
11. Schmitt C, Sobel JD, Meriwether C. Bacterial vaginosis: treatment with clindamycin cream versus oral metronidazole. *Obstet Gynecol* 1992; **79**:1020–1023.
12. Hanson JM, McGregor JA, Hillier SL, *et al*. Metronidazola for bacterial vaginosis: A comparison of vaginal geal vs. oral therapy. *J Repro Med* 2000; **45**:889–896.
13. Hillier SL, Krohn MA, Rabe LK, Klebanoff SJ, Eschenbach DA. The normal vaginal flora, H_2O_2-producing lactobacilli, and bacterial vaginosis in pregnant women. *Clin Infect Dis* 1993; **16**(suppl. 4):S273–281.
14. Hawes SE, Hillier SL, Benedetti J, *et al*. Hydrogen peroxide-producing lactobacilli and acquisition of vaginal infections. *J Infect Dis* 1996; **174**:1058–1063.
15. Wolrath H, Forsum U, Larsson PG, Borén H. Analysis of bacterial vaginosis-related arnines in vaginal fluid by gas chromatography and mass spectrometry. *J Clin Microbiol* 2001; **39**:4026–4031.
16. Marrazzo JM, Koutsky LA, Eschenback DA, Agnew K, Stino K, Hillier SL. Characterization of vaginal flora and bacterial vaginosis in women who have sex with women. *J Infect Dis* 2002; **185**:1307–1313.
17. Eschenbach DA, Hillier SL, Critchlow CW, Stevens CE, Koutsky LA, DeRouen T, Holmes KK. Diagnosis and clinical features associated with bacterial vaginosis. *Am J Obstet Gynecol* 1988; **158**:819–828.
18. Nugent RP, Krohn MA, Hillier SL. Reliability of diagnosing bacterial vaginosis is improved by a standardized method of Gram stain interpretation. *J Clin Microbiol* 1991; **29**:297–301.
19. Bump RC, Zuspan FP, Buesching WJ, III, Ayers LW, Stephens T. The prevalence, six-month persistence and predictive values of laboratory indicators of bacterial vaginosis (nonspecific vaginitis) in asymptomatic women. *Am J Obstet Gynecol* 1984; **150**:917–924.
20. Chaltopadhyay B. The role of *Gardnerella vaginalis* in 'non-specific' vaginitis. *J Infect Dis* 1984; **9**:113.
21. Greenwood JR. Current taxonomic status of *Gardnerella vaginalis*. *Scand J Inf Dis* 1983; **40**(suppl.):11.
22. Spiegel CA, Roberts M. *Mobiluncus* gen. nov., *Mobiluncus curtisii* subsp. *curtisii* sp. nov., *Mobiluncus curtisii* subsp. *holmesii* subsp. nov., and *Mobiluncus mulieris* sp. nov., curved rods from the human vagina. *Int J Syst Bacteriol* 1984; **34**:177–184.
23. Roberts MC, Hillier SL, Schoenknecht F, Holmes KK. Comparison of Gram stain, DNA probe and culture for the identification of species of *Mobiluncus* in female genital specimens. *J Infect Dis* 1985; **152**:74–77.
24. Boeke AJP, Dekker JH, van Eijk JTM, Kostense PJ, Bezemer PD. Effect of lactic acid suppositories compared with oral metronidazole and placebo in bacterial vaginosis: a randomised clinical trial. *Genitourin Med* 1993; **69**:388–392.
25. Carey JC, Klebanoff MA, Hauth JC *et al*. Metroridazole to prevent preterm delivery in pregnant women with asymptomatic bacterial vaginosis. *N Engl J Med* 2000; **342**:534–540.
26. Weston TET, Nicol CS. Natural history of trichomonal infection in males. *Br J Vener Dis* 1963; **39**:251–257.
27. Klebanoff MA, Carey JC, Hauth JC. Failure of metronidazole to prevent precterm delivery among pregnant women with asymptotmatic Trichomones vaginalis infection. *N. Engl J Med* 2001; **345**:487–493.
28. Krieger JN, Tam MR, Stevens CE, *et al*. Diagnosis of trichomoniasis. Comparison of conventional wet-mount examination with cytologic studies, cultures, and monoclonal antibody staining of direct specimens. *JAMA* 1988; **259**:1223–1227.
29. Patel Sr, Wiese W, Patel SC, Ohl C, Byrd JC, Estrada CA. Systematic review of diagnostic tests for vaginal trichomoniasis. *Infect Dis Obstet Gynecol* 2000; **8**:248–257.
30. Nyirjesy P, Sobel JD, Weitz V, Leaman DJ, Gelone SP. Difficult-to-treat trichomoniasis: results with paromomycin cream. *Clin Infect Dis* 1998; **26**:986–988.
31. Sobel JD. Vulvovaginal candidiasis — what we do and do not know. *Ann Intern Med* 1984; **101**:390.
32. Sobel JD. Vulvovaginitis due to *Candida glabrata*: an emerging problem. *Mycoses* 1998; **41** (Suppl 2):18–22.
33. Sobel JD. Non-trichomonal purulent vaginitis: clinical approach. *Curr Rep Infect Dis* 2000; **2**:501–505.
34. Lebherz TB, Ford LC. *Candida albicans* vaginitis: The problem is diagnosis, the enigma is treatment. *Chemotherapy* 1982; **28**(suppl. 1):73.
35. Sobel JD, Faro S, Force RW, Foxman B, Ledger WJ, Nyirjesy PR, Reed BD, Summers PR. Vulvovaginal candidiasis: epidemiologic, diagnostic and therapeutic considerations. *Am J Obstet Gynecol* 1998; **178**:203–211.
36. Sobel JD, Kapernick PS, Zervos MJ *et al*. Treatment of complicated *Candida* vaginitis; comparison of single and sequential doses of fluconazole. *Am J Obstet Gynecol* 2001; **185**:363–369.

37. Sobel JD, Chaim W. Therapy of *T. glabrata* vaginitis: retrospective review of boric acid therapy. *Clin Infect Dis* 1997; **24**:649–652.

38. O'Connor MI, Sobel JD. Epidemiology of recurrent vulvovaginal candidiasis: identification and strain differentiation of *Candida albicans*. *J Infect Dis* 1986; **154**:358–362.

39. Foxman B, Somsel P, Tallman P, Gillespie B, Raz R, Colodner R, Kandula D, Sobel JD. Urinary tract infection among women aged 40-65: behavioral and sexual risk factors. *J Clin Epidem* 2001; **54**:710–718.

40. Sobel JD. Desquamative inflammatory vaginitis: a new subgroup of purulent vaginitis responsive to topical 2% clindamycin therapy. *Am J Obstet Gynecol* 1994; **171**:1215.

41. Newbern EC, Foxman B, Leaman D, Sobel JD. Desquamative inflammatory vaginitis: an exploratory case-control study. *Ann Epidemiol* 2002; **12**:346–352.

Human Immunodeficiency Virus Infection and the Acquired Immunodeficiency Syndrome: Viral Pathogenesis, Laboratory Diagnosis and Monitoring

10

R Coombs

INTRODUCTION TO HUMAN RETROVIRUSES

The family *Retroviridae* comprise a large group of ubiquitous single-stranded RNA viruses that infect all classes of vertebrates. A defining feature of retroviruses is the integration of the reverse-transcribed viral cDNA into the host cell's genome to establish a persistent, life-long infection. The integrated viral cDNA, termed the *provirus*, serves as the template for viral replication. The genetic relatedness of retroviruses can be ascertained from the amino acid sequence similarities in the reverse transcriptase enzyme of these retroviruses (*Fig. 10.1*). Human immuno-deficiency viruses (HIV) type-1 and -2 are two of the six recognized exogenous retroviruses that infect humans. Only three retroviruses from two of the seven retrovirus genera produce well-defined clinical disease: namely, the deltaretrovirus, primate T-lymphotropic virus (PTLV, formerly HTLV) type-I and the lentiviruses, HIV-1 and -2. Neither PTLV-II nor the spumavirus, human foamy virus (HFV, which is likely acquired accidentally as a zoonotic infection following severe primate bites), have been associated with well-defined human disease.[1,2]

ORIGINS OF HIV

Recent studies have convincingly shown that there have been three separate interspecies transfers of the lentivirus, simian immuno-deficiency virus (SIV$_{cpz}$), from chimpanzees (*Pan troglodytes*) to humans, which occurred within the last century and resulted in the establishment of HIV-1 groups M, N and O.[3,4] Similarly, HIV-2 has its origins with multiple interspecies transfers of SIV$_{sm}$ from the primate sooty mangaby (*Cerocebus atys*) to man and to primates in captivity (e.g., SIV$_{mac}$ in the rhesus monkey, *Macaca mulatta*).

HIV STRUCTURE

HIV particles are approximately 100-nm in diameter and have a lipid envelope comprised of components from the host cell-derived plasma membrane (*Fig. 10.2*). The envelope renders the virus particles very susceptible to inactivation by environmental drying, detergents and various chemical disinfectants. The lipid envelope surrounds a dense core and associated capsid and nucleocapsid that contains two copies of the unique single-stranded RNA genome (*Fig. 10.3*). The HIV genome length is approximately 10 kilo bases (kb) and is complexed with the virus encoded reverse transcriptase, integrase, *vpr* (*vpx* for HIV-2) and a primer tRNA, which is derived from the host-cell. The HIV virion incorporates a cellular protein, cyclophilin A, which is bound to the viral capsid matrix protein p17 and is necessary for successful viral disassembly in the cellular cytoplasm.[5] The tightly packaged virion core (matrix, capsid and nucleocapsid) protects the enclosed RNA genome from degradation by RNAse in plasma and other body fluids. As a durable marker of HIV-1 replication, the measurement of viral particle-associated RNA plays a central role in monitoring HIV disease progression and response to therapy.[6]

The HIV RNA genome and cDNA provirus contains both noncoding and coding sequences (*Fig. 10.4*). The noncoding sequences, which are important recognition signals for DNA or RNA synthesis, integration and polyadenylation, are located at the 5'- and 3'-terminal ends of the genome. All retroviruses are terminally redundant and contain identical sequences called long terminal repeats (LTRs). The coding sequences include *gag* (group-specific structural antigens), *pol* (RNA-dependent DNA polymerase or reverse transcriptase, integrase and protease), and *env* (envelope structural proteins).

The *gag* gene encodes a precursor polypeptide that is cleaved by the viral-encoded protease to form several internal structural proteins, *viz.*, matrix protein (MA), capsid protein (CA) and nucleic acid binding protein (NC). The *pol* gene encodes for a precursor polypeptide that is similarly cleaved by the virus-specific protease to form three enzymes: the protease, reverse transcriptase and integrase. The *env* gene encodes for a 160 kilodalton (kD) precursor protein, which is cleaved post-transcriptionally into two noncovalently associated envelope glyco-proteins. The first *env* protein is a highly charged glycoprotein (gp120), which is external to the viral envelope and binds to the cell-specific viral receptors (e.g., CD4 receptor in the case of HIV) and ancillary co-receptors (e.g., chemokine receptors for HIV-1). A portion of the *env* gene is highly variable (of the five domains, V1–V5, the V3 loop is the most highly variable) and responsible for defining multiple variants or 'quasi-species' that contribute to viral evasion from neutralizing antibodies produced by the host in response to viral infection. The second *env* protein (gp41) is a hydrophobic transmembrane glycoprotein that anchors the oligomeric surface subunit glycoprotein to the viral envelope membrane. The virion surface is studded with

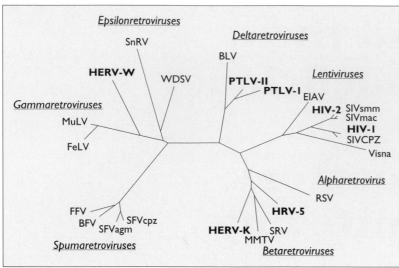

Genus	Examples
Alpharetrovirus	Rous sarcoma virus (RSV)
Betaretroviruses	**Human retrovirus 5 (HRV-5)** Simian retrovirus (SRV) Mouse mammary tumor virus (MMTV) **Human endogenous retrovirus -K (HERV-K)**
Gammaretroviruses	Murine leukemia virus (MuLV) Feline leukemia virus (FeLV) **HERV-W**
Deltaretroviruses	**Primate T-lymphotropic virus (PTLV)-1,-2** Bovine leukemia virus (BLV)
Epsilonretroviruses	Snake retrovirus (SnRV) Walleye dermal sarcoma virus (WDSV)
Lentiviruses	Equine infectious anemia virus (EIAV) **Human immunodeficiency virus (HIV)-1** Simian immunodeficiency virus (SIV) **HIV-2** Visna/maedi virus
Spumaretroviruses	Feline foamy virus (FFV) Bovine foamy virus (BFV) Simian foamy virus (SFV) **Human foamy virus (SFVcpz or HFV)**

* Human retroviruses are indicated in bold

Fig. 10.1 Phylogenetic tree of retroviruses. Humans can be or have been infected with several retroviruses from five of the seven retrovirus genera. The clinically most important retrovirus infections (PTLV, HIV) are acquired by exogenous infection; i.e., by sexual, mother-to-infant, breast-feeding or parenteral routes as are the clinically least important (HRV-5 and HFV). Multiple copies of endogenous DNA proviral sequences are integrated into chromosomal DNA and are transmitted in the germline (HERV-K, HERV-W and several others not shown). Interestingly, these endogenous proviral sequences represent 0.1% or more of human DNA sequences and were acquired sometime in our evolutionary past. Adapted from references 1 and 2.

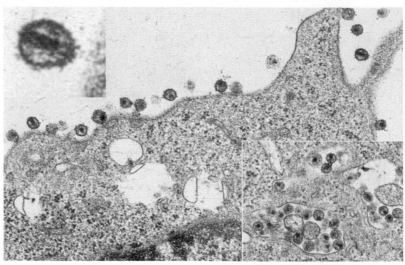

Fig. 10.2 An electron micrograph showing several HIV-1 particles in a culture of infected U931 cells. The enveloped virions contain the conical-shaped nucleocapsid characteristic of lentiviruses. The virions are approximately 100 nm in size.

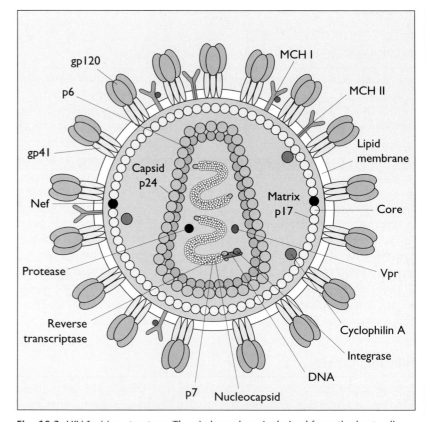

Fig. 10.3 HIV-1 virion structure. The viral envelope is derived from the host cell plasma membrane, contains both viral glycoproteins (gp120 and gp41) and several host cell-derived proteins, most notably, major histocompatibility complex class I and II proteins. After budding from the infected cell, the virion core undergoes extracellular maturation, whereby precursor polyproteins *gag-pol* (gp160) and *gag* (p66/55) are processed by the virion-associated protease to yield several smaller proteins. As a result of this maturation process, the virion undergoes a morphological change to the mature particle, which contains a conical capsid. Within the capsid, the nucleocapsid core contains two copies of the single-stranded viral RNA genome; in addition, virions contain cell-derived tRNA^{lys} primer and short strands of complementary DNA, which are synthesized by the virion-associated reverse transcriptase. Of the accessory proteins encoded by HIV-1 and -2, nef and either vpr and vpx, respectively, are packaged into virions. In addition, a cell-associated protein, cyclophilin A, is associated with the core matrix protein p17. Adapted from references 124 and 125.

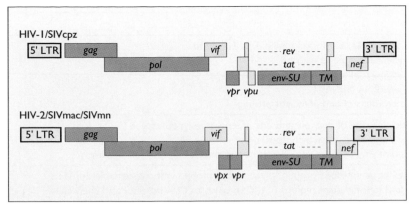

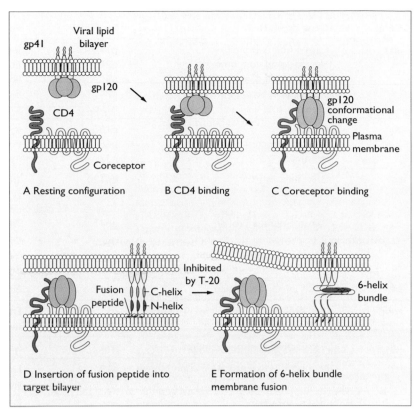

Fig. 10.4 Genome structure of HIV-1 and HIV-2. The linear double-stranded proviral DNA forms of HIV-1 and HIV-2 show similar patterns of genomic organization. The structural genes *gag*, *pol* and *env* give rise to several proteins: matrix (MA), capsid (CA), nucleic-acid-binding (NC), protease (PR), reverse transcriptase (RT), surface subunit glycoprotein (SU) and a smaller transmembrane protein (TM). In addition, HIV *pol* encodes an integrase (IN). Additional regulatory gene products are translated. HIV-1 and -2 have six accessory gene products: *tat*, *rev*, *vif*, *nef*, *vpr* and either *vpu* (in HIV-1) or *vpx* (in HIV-2). Further details about these HIV gene products are given in *Table 10.1*. Adapted from reference 125.

Fig. 10.5 Binding and fusion of HIV-1 with a CD4+ target cell. In unbound virions, the gp41 exists in a stable, nonfusogenic conformation in which the fusion peptides of gp41 are buried within the envelope trimer complex (A). When gp120 binds to the CD4 receptor (B), a conformational change exposes the chemokine receptor binding sites on gp120 (either CCR5 or CXCR4) (C), which in turn triggers a transition of gp41 to the prehairpin intermediate with exposure of the fusion peptide attached to the trimeric coiled-coil N-peptide region. The fusion peptide inserts into the target membrane (D). In this form, the C-peptide has not associated with the N-peptide because of continued association with gp120; at this stage, the intermediate is vulnerable to C-peptide inhibition (e.g., T 20). With the release of the gp120 block, the C-peptide region of gp41 binds to the N peptide region coiled-coil, the complex adopts a helical conformation of the fusion-active hairpin (6-helix bundle), which brings the two membranes into apposition (E). The precise mechanism of membrane fusion is not clear but after fusion is complete, the fusion peptide and transmembrane segment of gp41 lie in the same membrane. A similar mechanism presumably applies to the fusion of an HIV-1 infected cell that expresses viral envelope on the plasma membrane surface with an uninfected CD4+ target cell, which leads to syncytium formation among infected and uninfected cells *in vitro*. Adapted from references 8 and 126.

approximately 72 knobs; each is comprised of three heterodimers of the gp120*env*/gp41*env* complex.[7] Fusion of the retroviral envelope with the target cell plasma membrane is facilitated by the transmembrane glycoprotein through conformational change mediated by a helix coiled-coil mechanism[8] (*Fig. 10.5*).

Several HIV proteins are responsible for regulating viral replication and the host-cell response to infection. Briefly, these retroviral regulatory proteins express the following functions (*Table 10.1*). The *tat* protein augments the expression of virus from the LTR region. The *rev* protein regulates RNA splicing and RNA transport. The *nef* protein down-regulates CD4 protein, which is the cellular receptor for HIV, alters host T-cell activation pathways by decreasing MHC class I antigen expression, and enhances viral infectivity. The *vif* protein is necessary for the proper assembly of the HIV nucleoprotein core and without *vif*, viral cDNA is not efficiently produced. The *vpr* protein (HIV-1) and *vpx* (HIV-2) facilitate transport of the viral cDNA into the nucleus and produce G2 growth arrest and differentiation, which are necessary for optimal viral infection. As such, *vpr* and *vpx* facilitate the infection of nondividing cell by HIV. The *vpu* protein promotes the degradation of CD4 protein in the endoplasmic reticulum and stimulates the release of virions from infected cells.

HIV REPLICATION

HIV has two replication steps (*Fig. 10.6*). The first replication step uses viral-encoded proteins that enter the cell packaged within the virion nucleocapsid and eventually results in formation of the integrated cDNA, which is termed the provirus. The second replication step uses the host-cell enzymatic machinery to replicate the viral RNA genome, transcribe and translate viral proteins from the provirus. The replication of HIV leads to critical cell dysfunction, cell death and immuno-suppression with progression to clinical disease in most instances. Importantly, both steps in viral replication offer specific targets for current antiretroviral therapies (ART).

In the first phase of viral replication, HIV binds to the CD4 cell-surface receptor in conjunction with an associated chemokine co-receptor. Following fusion of the virion envelope with the cell plasma membrane, the HIV core enters the cell cytoplasm and the viral RNA is reverse transcribed to a slightly longer, double-stranded cDNA that enters the nucleus and integrates permanently at a single random site in the cell chromosome. The integration of linear viral cDNA occurs during division of the cell. However, HIV is able to infect resting cells, albeit less efficiently than activated cells in the S-phase of the cell cycle. The inhibition of reverse transcription by nucleotide, nucleoside or non-nucleoside reverse transcriptase inhibitors, when used in combination, is a cornerstone of current anti-HIV-1 therapeutics.

The second replication phase includes the production of viral genomic RNA (vRNA), mRNA and protein synthesis, which almost exclusively uses host-cell enzymatic machinery under the influence of viral gene regulatory products listed in *Table 10.1*. Assembly of virions begins in the endoplasmic reticulum, is followed by migration to the plasma membrane and release from the cell surface by budding. The budding viral envelope, which has a phospholipid composition different from the plasma membrane of the cell, may incorporate some cell-membrane surface proteins (e.g., beta-2 microglobulin, major histocompatability complex class II proteins, etc.), along with the viral specific glyco-proteins. Extracellular HIV undergoes further maturation by continued proteolytic cleavage of the nucleocapsid polypeptides, which results in the mature infectious virion with a distinctive conical-shaped capsid (*Fig. 10.2*). The inhibition of the viral protease by viral-specific protease

These elements are remnants of ancestral retroviral infection and move throughout the host genome as retrotransposons. In addition, most of the HIV cDNA either remains extrachromosomal as linear cDNA fragments or circularized forms. The degree of viral transcription and translation depends on the infected CD4+ cell's stage of differentiation. That stage, in turn, is probably related to exogenous antigen stimulation, cytokines (e.g., IL-2) and viral regulatory proteins (e.g., vpr) that promote cell differentiation and activation of viral promotors; for example, nuclear factor-kappa beta (NF-kβ)-inducible transcription factors. Integration of human retroviruses differs from that of certain other animal retroviruses in that no transforming genes (oncogenes) are associated with the viral genome and the proviral genome is not regularly inserted next to a host-transforming gene. Moreover, clinically important human retroviruses are exogenous and not transmitted in germ cells as are some endogenous vertebrate retroviruses.

CYTOPATHIC EFFECT AND IMMUNE DYSFUNCTION

For HIV, an initial period of intense viral replication is followed by either an acute and rapidly progressive disease in a minority of patients

or a persistent infection with the development of late disease in the majority of patients. However, therapeutic induction of a chronic infection and very slow disease progression appears to be a viable long-term clinical objective if patients are treated with effective antiretroviral therapy that suppresses viral replication to levels that allow for partial, if not complete, preservation or restoration of immune function.

The disease manifestations of HIV are governed by cell and tissue tropism with the clinical signs and symptoms of infection that arise directly or indirectly from viral replication within these cells and tissues. The *sine qua non* of HIV infection is CD4 cell depletion, immune dysfunction and development of opportunistic infections and malignancies. CD4 cell depletion occurs by direct viral replication, cell lysis

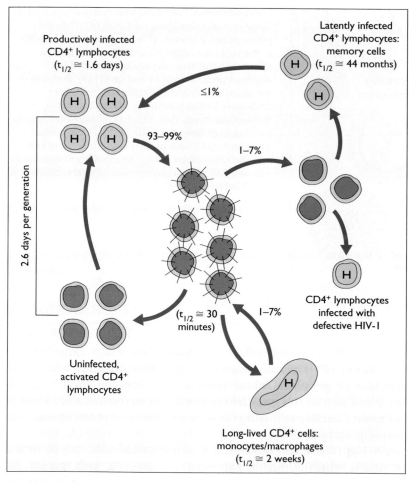

Fig. 10.7 Viral replication dynamics in vivo. Given the extremely stable level of plasma viremia and of infected cells, it appears that large amounts of virus (~10^{10} to 10^{11} virions) are produced and cleared very rapidly from the circulation each day. Most of the circulating cell-free plasma virus originates from recently infected cells, <7% from longer-lived cells such as monocytes/macrophages, and <1% from latently infected cells such as memory T-lymphocytes. The estimated half-life ($t_{1/2}$) of plasma virus is 30 minutes and that of productively infected lymphocytes is 1.6 days. The plasma viral RNA produced from productively infected CD4+ lymphocytes declines to < 500 RNA copies/mL rather quickly after the start of antiretroviral therapy (i.e., in 90% of patients by 6-months).[116] However, because a latently infected reservoir of virus is established soon after primary infection, even with more complete suppression of viral replication (i.e., < 50 RNA copies/mL of plasma), the latently infected pool of infected cells would theoretically take more than 60 years to clear. Thus, eradication of HIV is more a theoretical than practical consideration with current antiretroviral regimens. Adapted from references 9 and 129–131.

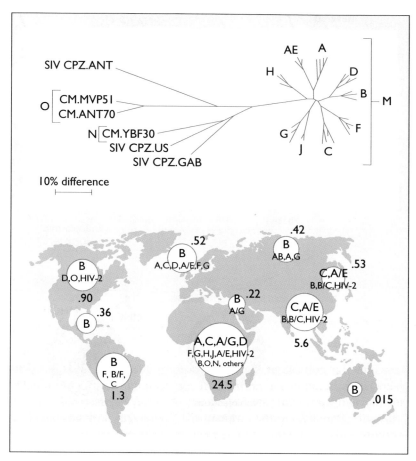

Fig. 10.8 Schematic of HIV-1 groups and clades and their geographic distribution. The phylogenetic relationships among primate lentiviruses is shown with the scale bar indicating an approximate genetic divergence of 10%. There are three groups of HIV-1: group M (major), which is responsible for most of the infection in the Americas and Europe; group O (outlier), a rare form found in Cameroon and Gabon; and group N (novel or non-M-non-O), which was identified in a Cameroonian female. All three HIV-1 groups are closely related to SIV$_{cpz}$ strains that infect chimpanzees and indicate at least three independent introductions of SIV$_{cpz}$ into humans within the past 100 years. The group M viruses comprise 9 subtypes (or clades) and four major circulating recombinant forms (AE, prevalent in Southeast Asia; AG from west and central Africa; AGI from Cyprus and Greece; and AB from Russia).[11] However, the circulating recombinant forms are expanding in number as more full-genome sequences of HIV-1 become available (e.g., FD from Democratic Republic of Congo, formerly Zaire; BC from China and several additional complex recombinants that combine three or more subtypes).[132] The geographic distribution of adults and children living with HIV/AIDS with the estimated number of infected persons × 10^6 (total HIV/AIDS infections 34.3 million as of June 2000).[133] For the distribution of HIV-1 subtypes, the relative abundance is shown by the font size. In Africa, >75% of identified stains have been of subtypes A, C, and D, with C being the most common. There are regional differences within Africa, with subtype C predominately in South Africa and subtypes A and D in East Africa, for example. On a worldwide basis, subtype C accounts for approximately half of all infections. An updated listing of HIV subtypes by country is available from the Los Alamos database <http://hiv-web.lanl.gov/geography/index.html>. Adapted from references 132–134.

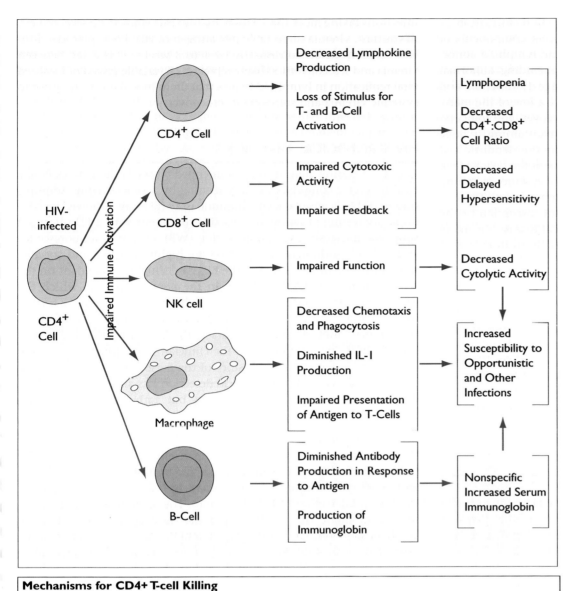

Fig. 10.9 Effect of HIV on immune system: Impaired effector functions of the HIV-infected CD4+ T cell. The CD4+ T-helper cell is the essential immune system conductor. As such, normal CD4+ T cell function includes the secretion of hematopoietic colony-stimulating factors, factors that induce non-lymphoid cell functions, chemotactic factors, induction of cytotoxic T-cell function, secretion of T-cell growth factors such as IL-2 and IL-4, and secretion of differentiation factors for lymphoid cells. The normal effector functions include activation of macrophages, induction of B-cell function and antibody secretion, secretion of cytokines that regulate or suppress immune responses, induction of natural killer (NK) cell function and direct or indirect cytolysis of target cells. The killing of the CD4+ T cells by HIV occurs by both direct and indirect mechanisms.[124]

Mechanisms for CD4+ T-cell Killing

DIRECT

Direct cell killing	• Disruption of cell membrane by massive viral budding • Syncytium formation • Accumulation of unintegrated viral DNA • Interference with cellular RNA processing • Elimination of HIV-infected cells by virus-specific immune responses

INDIRECT

Apoptosis	• Alterations of signaling mechanisms within cells may prime cells for apoptosis • Fas-dependent and Fas-independent pathways may be triggered by HIV • Increased susceptibility of uninfected bystander cells to apoptosis
Immune attack of uninfected cells	• Innocent bystander phenomenon whereby free viral antigens on the surface of infected cells (gp 120 env) may bind to the CD4 receptor og uninfected cells making them targets for both antibody and cell-mediated destruction • Molecular mimicry between HIV-1 envelope constitutents and host proteins may result in autoimmune responses
HIV-inhibited hematopoiesis	• Infection of CD34+ steam cells • Viral proteins and HIV-induced cytokines impair CD34+ survival and clonogenic potential
Thymus damage	• Inhibition of thymopolesis by infection of immature CD4 and CH8 cells (CD3-CD4-CD8- "triple negative" cells and CD3-CD4+-CD8- progenitor cells) • Damage to the thymic epithellial cells and disruption of thymic microenvironment contributes to the failure of CD4+ T-cell regeneration
Lymph node damage	• Destruction of geminal centers and lymph node structure
T-cell anergy	• Block of T-cell proliferation after contact with soluble HIV proteins leads to reduced clonal expansion

Indeterminate immunoblots

With the increased use of HIV-1 antibody screening in low-risk populations, including health-care workers, it is essential for the health care provider to interpret HIV-1 test results accurately. Between 4% and 20% of serum samples that are repeatedly reactive by HIV-1 EI assay are interpreted as indeterminate by Western blot.[38,39] Most of these remain indeterminate after repeat testing and do not indicate HIV-1 infection. However, indeterminate Western blots (IWBs) in HIV-1-infected persons may result from early antibody formation against viral core antigens during primary infection or early detection of HIV-1 antibody by the more sensitive third generation EI assays before there is confirmation by immunoblot, and rarely are due to the loss of core-specific antibody late in infection because of severe immunosuppression.[40,41]

The early, selective use of supplemental tests for HIV-1 proviral cDNA or plasma RNA may help determine the infection status of high-risk individuals before full seroconversion occurs.[34,42,43] Usually, most seroconversion should be identified within 1 to 3 months of primary infection with the use of appropriate supplemental testing.[44] Importantly, negative supplemental tests may also help alleviate the anxiety associated with an indeterminate HIV-1 serology.

Rapid antibody testing

Rapid, reliable and less expensive alternatives to the EI assay with confirmatory immunoblot have been sought for use in acute care settings, emergency rooms, sexually transmitted disease clinics, medical field settings, and developing countries. Consideration should be given to the introduction of rapid screening for HIV-1 antibody into certain clinical settings, such as sexually transmitted disease clinics, as this will greatly enhance testing programs by preventing the need for delayed counseling of seronegative patients and by providing preliminary results to seropositive patients.[45] These preliminary results may encourage patients to return for confirmatory test results and to adopt risk-reducing behavior sooner than occurs using currently accepted testing algorithms.[46] In addition, the rapid HIV-1 screening of source contacts following occupational exposures to blood will minimize or completely prevent the unnecessary use of antiretroviral prophylaxis therapy for the exposed health care worker, drug-related toxicity, cost and anxiety following the exposure if the rapid test is negative.[47,48] Rapid serologic testing will likely become the standard of diagnostic care, and physicians and other health care professionals should become familiar with the indications for rapid testing. However, consideration should also be given to the collection of urine or saliva, which are both acceptable and for some people preferable alternatives to blood, for HIV-1 antibody testing.[49-54]

Detection of HIV-1 subtype antibodies

The envelope protein of HIV-1 isolates from different geographic locations world-wide can differ in more than 35% of amino-acid positions.[55] As a consequence of this diversity, HIV-1 strains are divided into three groups M, O and most recently, group N.[56] Within the 'major' group M, multiple subtypes (or clades) designated A–K have been defined (Fig. 10.8). Group M and its subtypes have been more clearly defined than the other groups; subtype B is the most common subtype in the United States and Europe, while subtypes A, C and E are prominent in Africa and Asia. To date, in the United States, infection with group O is uncommon and no group N infections have been reported.[57] Diagnostic kit reagents have been modified to insure optimal sensitivity and specificity for group M and O virus antibody.

Detection of HIV-2 antibodies

Although HIV-2 infection is less geographically dispersed than HIV-1, and the HIV-2 epidemic is primarily focused in West Africa, HIV-2 is not uncommon in the epidemic in India. HIV-1 and HIV-2 genomes share about 60% homology in conserved genes such as gag and pol, and

35–45% homology in the env genes. The core proteins of HIV-1 and HIV-2 display frequent cross-reactivity whereas the envelope proteins are more type-specific. Despite this cross-reactivity, first and second generation anti-HIV-1 EI assays used for screening of blood donors in the United States are estimated to detect only 55 to 91% of HIV-2 infections. Western blots for HIV-1 antibodies may be positive, negative or indeterminate with HIV-2-positive sera. For the confirmation of HIV-2 EI assay reactivity, p26gag and gp36env correspond to their HIV-1 counterparts p24gag and gp41env, respectively. Several commercially available EI assays now test for both HIV-1 and HIV-2 antibody.

The following procedures are recommended if testing for both HIV-1 and HIV-2 is performed by means of a combination HIV-1/HIV-2 EI assay. A repeatedly reactive specimen by HIV-1/HIV-2 EI assay should be tested by HIV-1 WB or other licensed HIV-1 supplemental test. A positive test by HIV-1 WB test confirms the presence of antibodies to HIV-1 and testing for HIV-2 is recommended only if HIV-2 risk factors are present. If the HIV-1 WB is negative or indeterminate, an HIV-2 EI assay should be performed. If the HIV-2 EI assay is reactive, an HIV-2-specific WB should be performed. In addition, polymerase chain reaction amplification may be helpful to determine infection with HIV-1, HIV-2 or both viruses.

DIRECT DETECTION OF HIV-1

The relative sensitivities of the various direct detection methods for HIV-1 are best illustrated by evaluating the time to virus detection for pediatric infection. Maternal antibody is passed across the placenta to the neonate and thus from birth through the first year of life, diminishing levels of maternal HIV antibody are detected. Thus, pediatric HIV diagnosis relies on the direct detection of HIV by virus culture, antigen or nucleic acid (Table 10.2).

Culture

The detection of HIV-1 by mixed-lymphocyte coculture has extremely high specificity but lower sensitivity in patients with high CD4+ cell counts compared to viral nucleic acid detection methods (see below). The lower sensitivity of HIV-1 coculture compared to currently available nucleic acid detection methods, cost, time constraints, and highly specialized technical nature, leaves HIV-1 culture restricted primarily to research laboratories. However, there may be a rekindled interest in using HIV-1 coculture for assessing viral containment following potent antiretroviral therapy, for obtaining primary clinical HIV-1 isolates for determining viral syncytium-inducing phenotype, drug susceptibility phenotype and viral fitness.[58]

HIV-1 p24 Antigen

With the advent of nucleic acid amplification methods for monitoring HIV-1, the measurement of HIV-1 p24 antigen has a much more limited

HIV-1 assay	Time to detection		
	1–14 days	1–4 months	6 months
		Mean sensitivity (%)*	
Culture	41	89	91
DNA PCR	40	80	97
p24 antigen	27	40	56
ICD p24 antigen	32	97	87
RNA PCR	32	91	100

PCR, polymerase chain reaction; ICD, immune complex dissociated.
*Data is based on nine published studies. Adapted from reference 144.

Table 10.2 Relative sensitivities of various virological assays for the early diagnosis of HIV-1 infection in infants from birth to 6 months of age.

role than it once did. Now the primary use for p24 antigen detection is to identify subjects in the antibody-negative window period of acute HIV-1 infection. Although antigen detection is a less expensive alternative to viral RNA detection for this purpose, both viral RNA and peripheral blood mononuclear cell culture are significantly more sensitive than detection of p24 antigenemia,[59] even with the added sensitivity of p24 antigen acid-dissociation.[60] However, a tyramide signal-amplification boosted EI Assay for quantification of p24 antigen reportedly has equivalent sensitivity to viral RNA reverse transcriptase polymerase chain reaction (RT-PCR) amplification at 200–400 RNA copies/mL.[61] Currently, the greatest use of p24 antigen testing is for screening the United States blood supply. This screening program was introduced in 1996 and is now augmented by a plasma HIV-1 RNA screening assay to further lower the residual risk of HIV-1 infection, which was estimated to be < 1 in 500,000 units (95% confidence interval 200,000 to 2,800,000),[62] before the addition of viral RNA testing.

HIV-1 nucleic acid

The detection of HIV nucleic acid (proviral cDNA or viral RNA) by commercially available amplification technologies provides a specific and sensitive direct detection method to identify persons who are infected but who have not seroconverted,[59,63] to identify infected infants[64] and to resolve indeterminate HIV-1 antibody serology.[38] In addition, the quantification of plasma viral RNA has assumed a critically

important clinical role for assessing disease prognosis and response to antiretroviral therapy.[65–69]

Viral DNA in peripheral blood mononuclear cells

Qualitative HIV-1 DNA polymerase chain reaction (PCR) amplification is the most commonly used assay method for the diagnosis of HIV-1 infection in neonates and infants.[70,71] The Roche Amplicor™ HIV-1 test (Roche Diagnostic Systems, Inc., Branchburg, NJ.) is the only FDA-licensed commercial kit for clinical use.

The major advantages of HIV-1 DNA PCR over culture are its increased sensitivity and more rapid reporting time; that is, one day for DNA PCR compared to two–four weeks for culture. There is always a possible risk of false-positive reactivity due to contamination of the specimen with amplicons (so-called carry-over product contamination) or specimen handling errors,[72] although this is decreased somewhat by the use of the uracyl N-glycosylase enzyme in the commercial assay. False negatives can also occur because of inhibition of the PCR reaction by either hemoglobin or heparin or because of fewer target cells in the assay than expected. To control for the latter, and improve the precision of the assay, testing for HIV-1 DNA should also include concurrent amplification of a cell-associated host gene such as HLA-DQ or the beta-globin locus. Diagnostic laboratories should participate in a quality assurance program to insure that problems with sensitivity and specificity are quickly identified.

Procedure step	Target amplification		Signal amplification
	RT-PCR or US-RT-PCR[a]	NASBA[b]	bDNA[c]
Sample preparation	• Sample plus internal quantitative standard (IQS) is lysed to release virion RNA • Sample centrifugation before addition of standard and lysis buffer is used to increase sensitivity	• Sample and 3 calibrators are absorbed onto silicon dioxde gel and eluated before lysis of virions to release virion RNA	• Sample is concentrated by centrifugation before detergent disruption of virions to release virion RNA
Amplification	• Probes 142 bases in *gag* • HIV-1 genome is reverse transcribed to cDNA and amplified by PCR many times to exponentially produce short-length amplicons • IQS adjusts for recovery and allows for quantification	• Probes approximately 1200 bases in *gag* and *pol* • A series of 3 enzymes is used to make an RNA-DNA HIV-1 target. The reaction is isothermic and continuous • The sample and the 3 calibrators are amplified simultaneously, thus adjusting for recovery	• Probes multiple regions of *pol* • HIV-1 RNA is captured on 48-well microtiter plate • Target and preamplifier probes bind the viral RNA • Branched DNA amplifiers bind the preamplifier probes • No adjustment is made for recovery
Detection	• The amplicon products are attached to a 48-well microtiter plate and biotinylated • An optical density is determined for the sample and the standard, from which a copy number is calculated	• The amplicons are captured on beads and detected by means of electrochemiluminescence • Calculation of copy number is based on the relative amount of the sample compared with the 3 internal calibrators	• Multiple alkaline phosphatase probes amplify the signal, which is detected by measuring light emission from a chemiluminescent substrate • An external standard curve is used for calculating the RNA copy number
Detection level	• 200 copies/mL • 50 copies/ml[e]	• 80 copies/mL	• 50 copies/mL
Quantification level[d]	• 500 copies/mL • 200 copies/mL[e]	• 500 copies/mL	• 100 copies/mL

[a]RT-PCR, reverse transcription polymerase chain reaction, Roche Amplicor HIV-1 Monitor Test; US, UltraSensitive specimen preparation protocol.[137,145]
[b]NASBA, nucleic acid sequence-based amplification, Organon Teknika NucliSens HIV-1 RNA assay.[146]
[c]bDNA, branched DNA, Bayer VERSANT™ HIV-1 RNA 3.0 assay.[141]
[d]The limit of quantification represents the level at which the intra assay variation is less than 0.15 $\log_{10}$ RNA copies/mL such that the 95% confidence limits for the difference between two estimates is equivalent to ±0.5 $\log_{10}$ RNA copies/mL or approximately a 3-fold difference in viral RNA that can be reliably measured.[137,141] This interpretation differs from the kit manufacturers who claim a lower level of quantification based on less strict criteria.
[e]The values are for the Roche HIV-1 Monitor UltraSensitive specimen preparation protocol.[145,147]
Adapted from reference.[148]

Table 10.3 Descriptive differences between plasma HIV-1 RNA quantification assays

13. Huang Y, Paxton WA, Wolinsky SM, *et al*. The role of a mutant CCR5 allele in HIV-1 transmission and disease progression. *Nat Med* 1996; **2**:1240–1243.

14. Samson M, Libert F, Doranz BJ, *et al*. Resistance to HIV-1 infection in caucasian individuals bearing mutant alleles of the CCR-5 chemokine receptor gene. *Nature* 1996; **382**:722–725.

15. Dean M, Carrington M, Winkler C, *et al*. Genetic restriction of HIV-1 infection and progression to AIDS by a deletion allele of the CCR5 structural gene. Hemophilia Growth and Development Study, Multicenter AIDS Cohort Study, Multicenter Hemophilia Cohort Study, San Francisco City Cohort, ALIVE Study. *Science* 1996; **273**:1856–1862.

16. Michael NL, Louie LG, Rohrbaugh AL, *et al*. The role of CCR5 and CCR2 polymorphisms in HIV-1 transmission and disease progression. *Nat Med* 1997; **3**:1160–1162.

17. Michael NL, Chang G, Louie LG, *et al*. The role of viral phenotype and CCR-5 gene defects in HIV-1 transmission and disease progression. *Nat Med* 1997; **3**:338–340.

18. Geijtenbeek TB, Kwon DS, Torensma R, *et al*. DC-SIGN, a dendritic cell-specific HIV-1-binding protein that enhances trans-infection of T cells. *Cell* 2000; **100**:587–597.

19. Geijtenbeek TB, Torensma R, van Vliet SJ, *et al*. Identification of DC-SIGN, a novel dendritic cell-specific ICAM-3 receptor that supports primary immune responses. *Cell* 2000; **100**:575–585.

20. Koenig S, Fauci AS. Immunology of human immunodeficiency virus. In: Holmes KK, Sparling PF, Mardh P-A, *et al*., eds. *Sexually transmitted diseases*. New York, N. Y.: McGraw-Hill, 1999:231–249.

21. Quinn TC, Wawer MJ, Sewankambo N, *et al*. Viral load and heterosexual transmission of human immunodeficiency virus type 1. Rakai Project Study Group. *N Engl J Med* 2000; **342**:921–929.

22. Coombs RW, Speck CE, Hughes JP, *et al*. Association between culturable human immunodeficiency virus type 1 (HIV- 1) in semen and HIV-1 RNA levels in semen and blood: evidence for compartmentalization of HIV-1 between semen and blood. *J Infect Dis* 1998; 177:320–330.

23. Tajima K, Cartier L. Epidemiological features of HTLV-I and adult T cell leukemia. *Intervirology* 1995; **38**:238–246.

24. Nduati R, John G, Mbori-Ngacha D, *et al*. Effect of breastfeeding and formula feeding on transmission of HIV-1: a randomized clinical trial. *JAMA* 2000; **283**:1167–1174.

25. Shepard RN, Schock J, Robertson K, *et al*. Quantitation of human immunodeficiency virus type 1 RNA in different biological compartments. *J Clin Microbiol* 2000; **38**:1414–1418.

26. Pillay K, Coutsoudis A, York D, Kuhn L, Coovadia HM. Cell-free virus in breast milk of HIV-1-seropositive women. *J Acquir Immune Defic Syndr* 2000; **24**:330–336.

27. Cohen MS, Hoffman IF, Royce RA, *et al*. Reduction of concentration of HIV-1 in semen after treatment of urethritis: implications for prevention of sexual transmission of HIV- 1. AIDSCAP Malawi Research Group. *Lancet* 1997; **349**:1868–1873.

28. McClelland RS, Wang CC, Mandaliya K, *et al*. Treatment of cervicitis is associated with decreased cervical shedding of HIV-1. *Aids* 2001; **15**:105–110.

29. Wang CC, McClelland RS, Reilly M, *et al*. The effect of treatment of vaginal infections on shedding of human immunodeficiency virus type 1. *J Infect Dis* 2001; **183**:1017–1022.

30. Speck CE, Coombs RW, Koutsky LA, *et al*. Risk factors for HIV-1 shedding in semen. *Am J Epidemiol* 1999; **150**:622–631.

31. Busch MP, Satten GA. Time course of viremia and antibody seroconversion following human immunodeficiency virus exposure. *Am J Med* 1997; **102**:117–124; discussion 125–126.

32. Atkins D. Screening for human immunodeficiency virus infection. In: DiGuiseppi C, Atkins D, Woolf SH, eds. *US Preventive Services Task Force: Guide to Clinical Preventive Services*. Alexandria, Virginia: International Medical Publishing, 1996:303–323.

33. Ascher DP, Roberts C. Determination of the etiology of seroreversals in HIV testing by antibody fingerprinting. *J Acquir Immune Defic Syndr* 1993; **6**:241–244.

34. Celum CL, Coombs RW, Jones M, *et al*. Risk factors for repeatedly reactive HIV-1 EIA and indeterminate Western blots. A population-based case-control study. *Arch Intern Med* 1994; **154**:1129–1137.

35. Janssen RS, Satten GA, Stramer SL, *et al*. New testing strategy to detect early HIV-1 infection for use in incidence estimates and for clinical and prevention purposes. *JAMA* 1998; **280**:42–48.

36. Centers for Disease Control and Prevention (CDC). Interpretive criteria used to report Western blot results for HIV-1-antibody testing–United States. *MMWR Morbidity and Mortality Weekly Report* 1991; **40**:692–695.

37. Burke DS, Brundage JF, Redfield RR, *et al*. Measurement of the false positive rate in a screening program for human immunodeficiency virus infections. *N Engl J Med* 1988; **319**:961–964.

38. Celum CL, Coombs RW, Lafferty W, *et al*. Indeterminate human immunodeficiency virus type 1 Western blots: seroconversion risk, specificity of supplemental tests, and an algorithm for evaluation. *J Infect Dis* 1991; **164**:656–664.

39. MacDonald KL, Jackson JB, Bowman RJ, *et al*. Performance characteristics of serologic tests of human immunodeficiency virus type-1 (HIV-1) antibody among Minnesota blood donors. *Ann Intern Med* 1989; **110**:617–621.

40. Montagnier L, Brenner C, Chamaret S, *et al*. Human immunodeficiency virus infection and AIDS in a person with negative serology. *J Infect Dis* 1997; **175**:955–959.

41. Zaaijer HL, Bloemer MH, Lelie PN. Temporary seronegativity in a human immunodeficiency virus type 1-infected man. *J Med Virol* 1997; **51**:80–82.

42. Brown AE, Jackson B, Fuller SA, Sheffield J, Cannon MA, Lane JR. Viral RNA in the resolution of human immunodeficiency virus type 1 diagnostic serology. *Transfusion* 1997; **37**:926–929.

43. Eble BE, Busch MP, Khayam-Bashi H, Nason MA, Samson S, Vyas GN. Resolution of infection status of human immunodeficiency virus (HIV)-seroindeterminate donors and high-risk seronegative individuals with polymerase chain reaction and virus culture: absence of persistent silent HIV type 1 infection in a high-prevalence area. *Transfusion* 1992; **32**:503–508.

44. Coutlée F, Olivier C, Cassol S, *et al*. Absence of prolonged immunosilent infection with human immunodeficiency virus in individuals with high-risk behaviors. *Am J Med* 1994; **96**:42–48.

45. Kassler WJ, Dillon BA, Haley C, Jones WK, Goldman A. On-site, rapid HIV testing with same-day results and counseling. *Aids* 1997; **11**:1045–1051.

46. Irwin K, Olivo N, Schable CA, Weber JT, Janssen R, Ernst J. Performance characteristics of a rapid HIV antibody assay in a hospital with a high prevalence of HIV infection. CDC-Bronx-Lebanon HIV Serosurvey Team. *Ann Intern Med* 1996; **125**:471–475.

47. Beltrami EM, Williams IT, Shapiro CN, Chamberland ME. Risk and management of blood-borne infections in health care workers. *Clin Microbiol Rev* 2000; **13**:385–407.

48. Centers for Disease Control and Prevention (CDC). Public Health Service guidelines for the management of health-care worker exposures to HIV and recommendations for postexposure prophylaxis. Centers for Disease Control and Prevention. *MMWR* 1998; **47**:1–33.

49. Constantine NT, Zhang X, Li L, Bansal J, Hyams KC, Smialek JE. Application of a rapid assay for detection of antibodies to human immunodeficiency virus in urine. *Am J Clin Pathol* 1994; **101**:157–161.

50. Martinez PM, Torres AR, Ortiz de Lejarazu R, Montoya A, Martin JF, Eiros JM. Human immunodeficiency virus antibody testing by enzyme-linked fluorescent and western blot assays using serum, gingival-cervicular transudate, and urine samples. *J Clin Microbiol* 1999; **37**:1100–1106.

51. Peralta L, Constantine N, Griffin Deeds B, Martin L, Ghalib K. Evaluation of youth preferences for rapid and innovative human immunodeficiency virus antibody tests. *Arch Pediatr Adolesc Med* 2001; **155**:838–843.

52. Granade TC, Phillips SK, Parekh B, *et al*. Detection of antibodies to human immunodeficiency virus type 1 in oral fluids: a large-scale evaluation of immunoassay performance. *Clin Diagn Lab Immunol* 1998; **5**:171–175.

53. Sy FS, Rhodes SD, Choi ST, *et al*. The acceptability of oral fluid testing for HIV antibodies. A pilot study in gay bars in a predominantly rural state. *Sex Transm Dis* 1998; **25**:211–215.

54. King SD, Wynter SH, Bain BC, Brown WA, Johnston JN, Delk AS. Comparison of testing saliva and serum for detection of antibody to human immunodeficiency virus in Jamaica, West Indies. *J Clin Virol* 2000; **19**:157–161.

55. Korber B, Hoelsher M. *HIV-1 subtypes: implications for epidemiology, pathogenicity, vaccines and diagnostics* – Workshop report from the European Commission (DG XII, INCO-DC) and the joint United Nations programme on HIV/AIDS. AIDS 1997; 11:UNAIDS17–UNAIDS36.

56. Simon F, Mauclere P, Roques P, *et al*. Identification of a new human immunodeficiency virus type 1 distinct from group M and group O. *Nat Med* 1998; **4**:1032–1037.

57. Sullivan PS, Do AN, Ellenberger D, *et al*. Human immunodeficiency virus (HIV) subtype surveillance of African-born persons at risk for group O and group N HIV infections in the United States. *J Infect Dis* 2000; **181**:463–469.

58. Martinez-Picado J, Savara AV, Sutton L, D'Aquila RT. Replicative fitness of protease inhibitor-resistant mutants of human immunodeficiency virus type 1. *J Virol* 1999; **73**:3744–3752.

59. Schacker T, Collier AC, Hughes J, Shea T, Corey L. Clinical and epidemiologic features of primary HIV infection. *Ann Intern Med* 1996; **125**:257–264.

60. Schupbach J, Tomasik Z, Nadal D, et al. Use of HIV-1 p24 as a sensitive, precise and inexpensive marker for infection, disease progression and treatment failure. Int J Antimicrob Agents 2000; **16**:441–445.

61. Ledergerber B, Flepp M, Boni J, et al. Human immunodeficiency virus type 1 p24 concentration measured by boosted ELISA of heat-denatured plasma correlates with decline in CD4 cells, progression to AIDS, and survival: comparison with viral RNA measurement. J Infect Dis 2000; **181**:1280–1288.

62. Schreiber GB, Busch MP, Kleinman SH, Korelitz JJ. The risk of transfusion-transmitted viral infections. The Retrovirus Epidemiology Donor Study. N Engl J Med 1996; **334**:1685–1690.

63. Phair JP, Margolick JB, Jacobson LP, et al. Detection of infection with human immunodeficiency virus type 1 before seroconversion: correlation with clinical symptoms and outcome. J Infect Dis 1997; **175**:959–962.

64. Shearer WT, Quinn TC, LaRussa P, et al. Viral load and disease progression in infants infected with human immunodeficiency virus type 1. Women and Infants Transmission Study Group. N Engl J Med 1997; **336**:1337–1342.

65. Coombs RW, Welles SL, Hooper C, et al. Association of plasma human immunodeficiency virus type 1 RNA level with risk of clinical progression in patients with advanced infection. AIDS Clinical Trials Group (ACTG) 116B/117 Study Team. J Infect Dis 1996; **174**:704–712.

66. Hammer SM, Squires KE, Hughes MD, et al. A controlled trial of two nucleoside analogues plus indinavir in persons with human immunodeficiency virus infection and CD4 cell counts of 200 per cubic millimeter or less. AIDS Clinical Trials Group 320 Study Team. N Engl J Med 1997; **337**:725–733.

67. Katzenstein DA, Hammer SM, Hughes MD, et al. The relation of virologic and immunologic markers to clinical outcomes after nucleoside therapy in HIV-infected adults with 200 to 500 CD4 cells per cubic millimeter. AIDS Clinical Trials Group Study 175 Virology Study Team. N Engl J Med 1996; **335**:1091–1098.

68. Mellors JW, Rinaldo CR, Gupta P, White RM, Todd JA, Kingsley LA. Prognosis in HIV-1 infection predicted by the quantity of virus in plasma. Science 1996; **272**:1167–1170.

69. O'Brien WA, Hartigan PM, Martin D, et al. Changes in plasma HIV-1 RNA and CD4+ lymphocyte counts and the risk of progression to AIDS. Veterans Affairs Cooperative Study Group on AIDS. N Engl J Med 1996; **334**:426–431.

70. Bremer JW, Lew JF, Cooper E, et al. Diagnosis of infection with human immunodeficiency virus type 1 by a DNA polymerase chain reaction assay among infants enrolled in the Women and Infants' Transmission Study. J Pediatr 1996; **129**:198–207.

71. Owens DK, Holodniy M, McDonald TW, Scott J, Sonnad S. A meta-analytic evaluation of the polymerase chain reaction for the diagnosis of HIV infection in infants. JAMA 1996; **275**:1342–1348.

72. Frenkel LM, Mullins JI, Learn GH, et al. Genetic evaluation of suspected cases of transient HIV-1 infection of infants. Science 1998; **280**:1073–1077.

73. Allain JP. Will genome detection replace serology in blood screening for microbial agents? Baillières Best Pract Res Clin Haematol 2000; **13**:615–629.

74. Steketee RW, Abrams EJ, Thea DM, et al. Early detection of perinatal human immunodeficiency virus (HIV) type 1 infection using HIV RNA amplification and detection. New York City Perinatal HIV Transmission Collaborative Study. J Infect Dis 1997; **175**:707–711.

75. Owens DK, Holodniy M, Garber AM, et al. Polymerase chain reaction for the diagnosis of HIV infection in adults. A meta-analysis with recommendations for clinical practice and study design. Ann Intern Med 1996; **124**:803–815.

76. Rich JD, Merriman NA, Mylonakis E, et al. Misdiagnosis of HIV infection by HIV-1 plasma viral load testing: a case series. Ann Intern Med 1999; **130**:37–39.

77. Schwartz DH, Laeyendecker OB, Arango-Jaramillo S, Castillo RC, Reynolds MJ. Extensive evaluation of a seronegative participant in an HIV-1 vaccine trial as a result of false-positive PCR. Lancet 1997; **350**:256–259.

78. Weber B, Fall EH, Berger A, Doerr HW. Reduction of diagnostic window by new fourth-generation human immunodeficiency virus screening assays. J Clin Microbiol 1998; **36**:2235–2239.

79. Michael NL, Herman SA, Kwok S, et al. Development of calibrated viral load standards for group M subtypes of human immunodeficiency virus type 1 and performance of an improved AMPLICOR HIV-1 MONITOR test with isolates of diverse subtypes. J Clin Microbiol 1999; **37**:2557–2563.

80. Coste J, Montes B, Reynes J, et al. Comparative evaluation of three assays for the quantitation of human immunodeficiency virus type 1 RNA in plasma. J Med Virol 1996; **50**:293–302.

81. Gomes P, Taveira NC, Pereira JM, Antunes F, Ferreira MO, Lourenco MH. Quantitation of human immunodeficiency virus type 2 DNA in peripheral blood mononuclear cells by using a quantitative-competitive PCR assay. J Clin Microbiol 1999; **37**:453–456.

82. Loussert-Ajaka I, Simon F, Farfara I, Descamps D, Collin G, Brun-Vezinet F. Detection of circulating human immunodeficiency virus type 2 in plasma by reverse transcription polymerase chain reaction. Res Virol 1995; **146**:409–414.

83. Schutten M, van den Hoogen B, van der Ende ME, Gruters RA, Osterhaus AD, Niesters HG. Development of a real-time quantitative RT-PCR for the detection of HIV-2 RNA in plasma. J Virol Methods 2000; **88**:81–87.

84. Takehisa J, Osei-Kwasi M, Ayisi NK, et al. Phylogenetic analysis of HIV type 2 in Ghana and intrasubtype recombination in HIV type 2. AIDS Res Hum Retroviruses 1997; **13**:621–623.

85. Kartsonis NA, D'Aquila RT. Clinical monitoring of HIV-1 infection in the ERA of antiretroviral resistance testing. Infect Dis Clin North Am 2000; **14**:879–899.

86. Brown AJ, Richman DD. HIV-1: gambling on the evolution of drug resistance? Nat Med 1997; **3**:268–271.

87. Durant J, Clevenbergh P, Halfon P, et al. Drug-resistance genotyping in HIV-1 therapy: the VIRADAPT randomised controlled trial. Lancet 1999; **353**:2195–2199.

88. Baxter JD, Mayers DL, Wentworth DN, et al. A randomized study of antiretroviral management based on plasma genotypic antiretroviral resistance testing in patients failing therapy. CPCRA 046 Study Team for the Terry Beirn Community Programs for Clinical Research on AIDS. Aids 2000; **14**:F83–93.

89. Para MF, Glidden DV, Coombs RW, et al. Baseline human immunodeficiency virus type 1 phenotype, genotype, and RNA response after switching from long-term hard-capsule saquinavir to indinavir or soft-gel-capsule saquinavir in AIDS clinical trials group protocol 333. J Infect Dis 2000; **182**:733–743.

90. Hirsch MS, Brun-Vezinet F, D'Aquila RT, et al. Antiretroviral drug resistance testing in adult HIV-1 infection: recommendations of an International AIDS Society-USA Panel. JAMA 2000; **283**:2417–2426.

91. Nijhuis M, Schuurman R, Boucher CAB. Homologous recombination for rapid phenotyping of HIV. Current Opinion in Infectious Diseases 1997; **10**:474–479.

92. Hertogs K, de Bethune MP, Miller V, et al. A rapid method for simultaneous detection of phenotypic resistance to inhibitors of protease and reverse transcriptase in recombinant human immunodeficiency virus type 1 isolates from patients treated with antiretroviral drugs. Antimicrob Agents Chemother 1998; **42**:269–276.

93. Petropoulos CJ, Parkin NT, Limoli KL, et al. A novel phenotypic drug susceptibility assay for human immunodeficiency virus type 1. Antimicrob Agents Chemother 2000; **44**:920–928.

94. Schuurman R. State of the art of gentoypic HIV-1 drug resistance. Current Opinion in Infectious Diseases 1997; **10**:480–484.

95. Larder BA, Kemp SD, Harrigan PR. Potential mechanism for sustained antiretroviral efficacy of AZT-3TC combination therapy. Science 1995; **269**:696–699.

96. Henrard DR, Phillips JF, Muenz LR, et al. Natural history of HIV-1 cell-free viremia. JAMA 1995; **274**:554–558.

97. Hogervorst E, Jurriaans S, de Wolf F, et al. Predictors for non- and slow progression in human immunodeficiency virus (HIV) type 1 infection: low viral RNA copy numbers in serum and maintenance of high HIV-1 p24-specific but not V3-specific antibody levels. J Infect Dis 1995; **171**:811–821.

98. Chun TW, Stuyver L, Mizell SB, et al. Presence of an inducible HIV-1 latent reservoir during highly active antiretroviral therapy. Proc Natl Acad Sci USA 1997; **94**:13193–13197.

99. Finzi D, Hermankova M, Pierson T, et al. Identification of a reservoir for HIV-1 in patients on highly active antiretroviral therapy. Science 1997; **278**:1295–1300.

100. Wong JK, Hezareh M, Gunthard HF, et al. Recovery of replication-competent HIV despite prolonged suppression of plasma viremia. Science 1997; **278**:1291–1295.

101. Stellbrink HJ, van Lunzen J, Hufert FT, et al. Asymptomatic HIV infection is characterized by rapid turnover of HIV RNA in plasma and lymph nodes but not of latently infected lymph-node CD4+ T cells. Aids 1997; **11**:1103–1110.

102. Peeters MF, Colebunders RL, Van den Abbeele K, et al. Comparison of human immunodeficiency virus biological phenotypes isolated from cerebrospinal fluid and peripheral blood. J Med Virol 1995; **47**:92–96.

103. Jurriaans S, Van Gemen B, Weverling GJ, et al. The natural history of HIV-1 infection: virus load and virus phenotype independent determinants of clinical course? Virology 1994; **204**:223–233.

104. Tillmann HL, Heiken H, Knapik-Botor A, et al. Infection with GB virus C and reduced mortality among HIV-infected patients. N Engl J Med 2001; **345**:715–724.

105. Xiang J, Wunschmann S, Diekema DJ, *et al*. Effect of coinfection with GB virus C on survival among patients with HIV infection. *N Engl J Med* 2001; **345**:707–714.

106. Rosenberg PS, Goedert JJ, Biggar RJ. Effect of age at seroconversion on the natural AIDS incubation distribution. Multicenter Hemophilia Cohort Study and the International Registry of Seroconverters. *Aids* 1994; **8**:803–810.

107. Gao X, Nelson GW, Karacki P, *et al*. Effect of a single amino acid change in MHC class I molecules on the rate of progression to AIDS. *N Engl J Med* 2001; **344**:1668–1675.

108. Kroner BL, Goedert JJ, Blattner WA, Wilson SE, Carrington MN, Mann DL. Concordance of human leukocyte antigen haplotype-sharing, CD4 decline and AIDS in hemophilic siblings. Multicenter Hemophilia Cohort and Hemophilia Growth and Development Studies. *Aids* 1995; **9**:275–280.

109. Ioannidis JP, Cappelleri JC, Lau J, Sacks HS, Skolnik PR. Predictive value of viral load measurements in asymptomatic untreated HIV-1 infection: a mathematical model. *Aids* 1996; **10**:255–262.

110. Fessel WJ. Human immunodeficiency virus (HIV) RNA in plasma as the preferred target for therapy in patients with HIV infection: a critique. *Clin Infect Dis* 1997; **24**:116–122.

111. Ho DD, Neumann AU, Perelson AS, Chen W, Leonard JM, Markowitz M. Rapid turnover of plasma virions and CD4 lymphocytes in HIV-1 infection. *Nature* 1995; **373**:123–126.

112. Wei X, Ghosh SK, Taylor ME, *et al*. Viral dynamics in human immunodeficiency virus type 1 infection. *Nature* 1995; **373**:117–122.

113. Musey L, Hughes J, Schacker T, Shea T, Corey L, McElrath MJ. Cytotoxic-T-cell responses, viral load, and disease progression in early human immunodeficiency virus type 1 infection. *N Engl J Med* 1997; **337**:1267–1274.

114. Rosenberg ES, Billingsley JM, Caliendo AM, *et al*. Vigorous HIV-1-specific CD4+ T cell responses associated with control of viremia. *Science* 1997; **278**:1447–1450.

115. Schacker TW, Hughes JP, Shea T, Coombs RW, Corey L. Biological and virologic characteristics of primary HIV infection. *Ann Intern Med* 1998; **128**:613–620.

116. Gulick RM, Mellors JW, Havlir D, *et al*. Treatment with indinavir, zidovudine, and lamivudine in adults with human immunodeficiency virus infection and prior antiretroviral therapy. *N Engl J Med* 1997; **337**:734–739.

117. Marschner IC, Collier AC, Coombs RW, *et al*. Use of changes in plasma levels of human immunodeficiency virus type 1 RNA to assess the clinical benefit of antiretroviral therapy. *J Infect Dis* 1998; **177**:40–47.

118. Department of Health and Human Services (DHHS) and the Henry J. Kaiser Family Foundation. *Guidelines for the use of antiretroviral agents in HIV-infected adults and adolescents (www.hivatis.org)*. Washington, D.C.: U.S. Public Health Service, 2001.

119. Mellors JW, Munoz A, Giorgi JV, *et al*. Plasma viral load and CD4+ lymphocytes as prognostic markers of HIV-1 infection. *Ann Intern Med* 1997; **126**:946–954.

120. Bangsberg DR, Hecht FM, Charlebois ED, *et al*. Adherence to protease inhibitors, HIV-1 viral load, and development of drug resistance in an indigent population. *Aids* 2000; **14**:357–366.

121. Reichelderfer PS, Coombs RW. Cartesian coordinate analysis of viral burden and CD4+ T-cell count in human immunodeficiency virus type-1 infection. *Antiviral Res* 1998; **38**:181–194.

122. Deeks SG, Wrin T, Liegler T, *et al*. Virologic and immunologic consequences of discontinuing combination antiretroviral-drug therapy in HIV-infected patients with detectable viremia. *N Engl J Med* 2001; **344**:472–480.

123. Ledergerber B, Egger M, Opravil M, *et al*. Clinical progression and virological failure on highly active antiretroviral therapy in HIV-1 patients: a prospective cohort study. Swiss HIV Cohort Study. *Lancet* 1999; **353**:863–868.

124. Cohen OJ, Fauci AS. Pathogenesis and medical aspects of HIV-1 infection. In: Knipe DM, Howley MD, eds. *Fields Virology*. Vol. 2. Philadelphia: Lippincott Williams and Wilkins, 2001:2043–2094.

125. Streicher HZ, Reitz MSJ, Gallo RC. Human immunodeficiency viruses. In: Mandel GL, Bennett JE, Donlin R, eds. *Mandell, Douglas, and Bennett's Principles and practice of infectious diseases*. Vol. 2. New York, N. Y.: Churchill Livingstone, 2000:1874–1887.

126. Freed EO, Martin MA. HIVs and their replication. In: Knipe DM, Howley MD, eds. *Fields Virology*. Vol. 2. Philadelphia: Lippincott Williams and Wilkins, 2001:1971–2041.

127. Dimitrov DS, Willey RL, Sato H, Chang LJ, Blumenthal R, Martin MA. Quantitation of human immunodeficiency virus type 1 infection kinetics. *J Virol* 1993; **67**:2182–2190.

128. Furtado MR, Callaway DS, Phair JP, *et al*. Persistence of HIV-1 transcription in peripheral-blood mononuclear cells in patients receiving potent antiretroviral therapy. *N Engl J Med* 1999; **340**:1614–1622.

129. Perelson AS, Essunger P, Cao Y, *et al*. Decay characteristics of HIV-1-infected compartments during combination therapy. *Nature* 1997; **387**:188–191.

130. Ramratnam B, Bonhoeffer S, Binley J, *et al*. Rapid production and clearance of HIV-1 and hepatitis C virus assessed by large volume plasma apheresis. *Lancet* 1999; **354**:1782–1785.

131. Pierson T, McArthur J, Siliciano RF. Reservoirs for HIV-1: mechanisms for viral persistence in the presence of antiviral immune responses and antiretroviral therapy. *Annu Rev Immunol* 2000; **18**:665–708.

132. McCutchan FE. Understanding the genetic diversity of HIV-1. *Aids* 2000; **14**:S31–44.

133. UNAIDS. *Report on the global HIV/AIDS epidemic June 2000*. Geneva: http:/www.unaids.org, 2000:1–135.

134. Fauci AS, Lane HC. Human immunodeficiency virus (HIV) disease: AIDS and realted disorders. In: Braunwald E, Fauci AS, Kasper DL, Hauser SL, Longo DL, Jameson JL, eds. *Harrison's principles of internal medicine*. New York: McGraw-Hill, 2001:1852–1913.

135. Mellors JW, Kingsley LA, Rinaldo CR, *et al*. Quantitation of HIV-1 RNA in plasma predicts outcome after seroconversion. *Ann Intern Med* 1995; **122**:573–579.

136. Tang Y-W, Persing DH. Molecular detection and identification of microoganisms. In: Murray PR, Baron EJ, Pfaller MA, Tenover FC, Yolken RH, eds. *Manual of Clinical Microbiology*. Washington, D.C.: American Society for Microbiology, 1999:215–244.

137. Yen-Lieberman B, Brambilla D, Jackson B, *et al*. Evaluation of a quality assurance program for quantitation of human immunodeficiency virus type 1 RNA in plasma by the AIDS Clinical Trials Group virology laboratories. *J Clin Microbiol* 1996; **34**:2695–2701.

138. Erali M, Hillyard DR. Evaluation of the ultrasensitive Roche Amplicor HIV-1 monitor assay for quantitation of human immunodeficiency virus type 1 RNA. *J Clin Microbiol* 1999; **37**:792–795.

139. Sun R, Ku J, Jayakar H, *et al*. Ultrasensitive reverse transcription-PCR assay for quantitation of human immunodeficiency virus type 1 RNA in plasma. J Clin Microbiol 1998; **36**:2964–2969.

140. Natarajan V, Watters D, L. DR. *Quantitation of viremia in human immunodeficiency virus infection by viral RNA estimation*. Manual of Clinical Laboratory Immunology. Washington, D.C.: ASM Press, 1997:773–780.

141. Erice A, Brambilla D, Bremer J, *et al*. Performance characteristics of the QUANTIPLEX HIV-1 RNA 3.0 assay for detection and quantitation of human immunodeficiency virus type 1 RNA in plasma. *J Clin Microbiol* 2000; **38**:2837–2845.

142. Collins ML, Irvine B, Tyner D, *et al*. A branched DNA signal amplification assay for quantification of nucleic acid targets below 100 molecules/ml. *Nucleic Acids Res* 1997; **25**:2979–2984.

143. Vergis EN, Mellors JW. Natural history of HIV-1 infection. *Infect Dis Clin North Am* 2000; **14**:809–825.

144. Henrard D, Reichelderfer P. Assays for the diagnosis of HIV infection. In: Merigan TCJ, Bartlett JG, Bolognesi D, eds. *Textbook of AIDS medicine*. Philadelphia: Williams and Wilkins, 1999:661–671.

145. Brambilla DJ, Granger S, Jennings C, Bremer JW. Multisite comparison of reproducibility and recovery from the standard and ultrasensitive Roche AMPLICOR HIV-1 MONITOR assays. *J Clin Microbiol* 2001; **39**:1121–1123.

146. Bremer J, Nowicki M, Beckner S, *et al*. Comparison of two amplification technologies for detection and quantitation of human immunodeficiency virus type 1 RNA in the female genital tract. Division of AIDS Treatment Research Initiative 009 Study Team. *J Clin Microbiol* 2000; **38**:2665–2669.

147. Mulder J, Resnick R, Saget B, *et al*. A rapid and simple method for extracting human immunodeficiency virus type 1 RNA from plasma: enhanced sensitivity. *J Clin Microbiol* 1997; **35**:1278–1280.

148. Coombs RW, Reichelderfer P. Use of plasma HIV-1 RNA to assess prognosis and monitor therapy in HIV-1 infection. In: Merigan Jr TC, Bartlett JG, Bolognesi D, eds. *Textbook of AIDS Medicine*. Philadelphia: Williams and Wilkins, 1999:673–685.

149. Greene, WC and Peterlin, BM. Charting HIV's remarkable voyage through the cell: basic science as a passport to future therapy. *Nature Medicine* 2002; **8**:673–680.

Human Immunodeficiency Virus Infection and the Acquired Immunodeficiency Syndrome: Epidemiology

11

P Fleming

INTRODUCTION

June 5, 2001 marked 20 years since the first report in the Centers for Disease Control and Prevention's (CDC) *Morbidity and Mortality Weekly Report* of an unusual cluster of cases of *Pneumocystis carinii* pneumonia in young homosexual men in Los Angeles.[1] In the weeks and months that followed, other such reports of unusual opportunistic infections, previously known to occur among severely immunocompromised patients, were reported from several U.S. cities.[2] Upon investigation of the clinical, biological and behavioral characteristics of the affected men, health officials theorized that a previously unrecognized disease agent, probably transmitted sexually, was suppressing immune function and increasing susceptibility to infection with other agents.

The syndrome became known as the Acquired Immunodeficiency Syndrome (AIDS). Surveillance for AIDS cases was established and reports from physicians and local health departments to the CDC were investigated. Within two years, the epidemiology of cases made clear that the putative agent was transmitted through: sexual contact between men, and between men and women; needle sharing among injecting drug users; receipt of blood transfusions or blood products; and from mother to child perinatally.[3,4] Equally important, the epidemiology made clear that it was not transmitted through insect vectors, casual contact, or through air, food, or water. Early prevention measures were established by public health authorities and affected communities mobilized to alert their members to the need to reduce sex and drug risks. The causative agent (a retrovirus named the human immunodeficiency virus [HIV]) was discovered, an antibody test was developed, universal screening of the blood supply was implemented in March of 1985, and in that same year, the surveillance case definition for AIDS was revised to include laboratory evidence of HIV.[5] Nevertheless, approximately half a million persons had already been infected in the U.S. by the mid-1980s and annual HIV incidence was at its peak.[6] It would take the next decade and a half to understand more completely how this infectious disease could emerge, diffuse so rapidly into a global epidemic, and so profoundly challenge the ability of society, medicine and governments to respond.

The 1990s witnessed the development of numerous effective antiretroviral treatments that improved survival and quality of life.[7–9] At the same time, targeted programs were developed to bring a portfolio of effective prevention interventions to at-risk communities.[10,11] While infected and at-risk populations in western Europe and North America benefited from prevention and treatment advances won as a result of the investment of substantial public and private resources, the epidemic spread unchecked through Africa, and now poses a significant threat in parts of Asia, India, Latin America, eastern Europe and China.[12] HIV is pandemic. It has already claimed over 20 million lives worldwide. The global search is on for biomedical interventions to prevent transmission, pharmacologic agents to treat disease, a safe, effective vaccine, and rapid methods to diagnose infection. In many geographic areas, efforts to prevent and control HIV are hampered by inadequate resources, competition instead of cooperation, lack of political commitment, and ignorance. Ideally, HIV is totally preventable through behavior change. In the U.S., prevention programs promote behavioral risk reduction, substance abuse prevention and treatment, increased HIV testing, and sustained access to prevention and treatment programs. Health care providers remain key to fighting the HIV epidemic through assessing patient risk, counseling and voluntary testing, and referring patients for prevention and treatment as appropriate. Worldwide, investment in vaccine research and affordable treatment for the large number already infected is urgently needed to stop the spread of HIV and reduce mortality.

HIV prevention and control are public health challenges that can be achieved. At the start of the third decade of the HIV pandemic, much is understood about HIV in terms of the epidemiology, virology, pathogenesis, immune response, and clinical course. In this chapter, we review the epidemiology of HIV in the U.S., as well as highlight the global threat of HIV.

CASE DEFINITION AND CLASSIFICATION

CASE DEFINITION (Table 11.1)

Investigations of the earliest AIDS cases yielded a working case definition that largely included severe life-threatening opportunistic infections (OIs) such as *Pneumocystis carinii* pneumonia, disseminated herpes simplex virus infection, cerebral toxoplasmosis. Early cases were diagnosed based on definitive laboratory or clinical tests indicative of one of the AIDS-defining OIs.[13] In 1985, the AIDS surveillance case definition was revised to include laboratory evidence of infection with HIV.[5] By 1987, the definition was revised again to include presumptive diagnoses of some of the most common OIs in the presence of laboratory tests diagnostic of HIV infection. Other conditions were added, including HIV encephalopathy and wasting, bringing the total number of AIDS-defining conditions to 23 for adults and adolescents ≥13 years of age, and 24 for children <13 years of age.[14] By the early 1990s, federal funds for treatment and care were tied to the number of AIDS cases and many community groups called for an expanded AIDS case definition in order to include a much larger number of HIV-associated conditions. At the same time, clinical management of HIV was increasingly reliant on monitoring T-lymphocyte subsets to track the course of immune-suppression and the risk of OIs. In 1993, the definition was expanded to include HIV-infected persons with evidence

This revised definition of HIV infection, which applies to any HIV (e.g., HIV-1 or HIV-2), is intended for public health surveillance only. It incorporates the reporting criteria for HIV infection and AIDS into a single case definition. This definition is not presented as a guide to clinical diagnosis or for other uses.

I. In adults, adolescents, or children aged greater than or equal to 18 months*, a reportable case of HIV infection must meet at least one of the following criteria:

Laboratory Criteria

- Positive result on a screening test for HIV antibody (e.g., repeatedly reactive enzyme immunoassay), followed by a positive result on a confirmatory (sensitive and more specific) test for HIV antibody (e.g., Western blot or immunofluorescence antibody test)
  or
- Positive result or report of a detectable quantity on any of the following HIV virologic (nonantibody) tests: HIV nucleic acid (DNA or RNA) detection (e.g., DNA polymerase chain reaction [PCR] or plasma HIV-1 RNA)**; HIV p24 antigen test, including neutralization assay; HIV isolation (viral culture)

OR

Clinical or Other Criteria (if the above laboratory criteria are not met)

- Diagnosis of HIV infection, based on the laboratory criteria above, that is documented in a medical record by a physician
  or
- Conditions that meet criteria included in the case definition for AIDS***

II. In a child aged less than 18 months, a reportable case of HIV infection must meet at least one of the following criteria:

Laboratory Criteria

Definitive

- Positive results on two separate specimens (excluding cord blood) using one or more of the following HIV virologic (nonantibody) tests: HIV nucleic acid (DNA or RNA) detection; HIV p24 antigen test, including neutralization assay, in a child greater than or equal to 1 month of age; HIV isolation (viral culture)
  or

Presumptive

A child who does not meet the criteria for definitive HIV infection but who has:

- Positive results on only one specimen (excluding cord blood) using the above HIV virologic tests and no subsequent negative HIV virologic or negative HIV antibody tests

OR

Clinical or Other Criteria (if the above definitive or presumptive laboratory criteria are not met)

- Diagnosis of HIV infection, based on the laboratory criteria above, that is documented in a medical record by a physician
  or
- Conditions that meet criteria included in the 1987 pediatric surveillance case definition for AIDS ****

III. A child aged less than 18 months born to an HIV-infected mother will be categorized for surveillance purposes as "not infected with HIV" if the child does not meet the criteria for HIV infection but meets the following criteria:

Laboratory Criteria

Definitive

- At least two negative HIV antibody tests from separate specimens obtained at greater than or equal to 6 months of age
  or
- At least two negative HIV virologic tests***** from separate specimens, both of which were performed at greater than or equal to 1 month of age and one of which was performed at greater than or equal to 4 months of age
  AND
  NO other laboratory or clinical evidence of HIV infection (i.e., has not had any positive virologic tests, if performed, and has not had an AIDS-defining condition)
  or

Presumptive

A child who does not meet the above criteria for definitive 'not infected' status but who has:

- One negative EIA HIV antibody test performed at greater than or equal to 6 months of age and NO positive HIV virologic tests, if performed
  or
- One negative HIV virologic test***** performed at greater than or equal to 4 months of age and NO positive HIV virologic tests, if performed
  or
- One positive HIV virologic test with at least two subsequent negative virologic tests*****, at least one of which is at greater than or equal to 4 months of age; or negative HIV antibody test results, at least one of which is at greater than or equal to 6 months of age
  AND
  NO other laboratory or clinical evidence of HIV infection (i.e., has not had any positive virologic tests, if performed, and has not had an AIDS-defining condition)
  OR

Clinical or Other Criteria (if the above definitive or presumptive laboratory criteria are not met)

- Determined by a physician to be 'not infected', and a physician has noted the results of the preceding HIV diagnostic tests in the medical record
  AND
  NO other laboratory or clinical evidence of HIV infection (i.e., has not had any positive virologic tests, if performed, and has not had an AIDS-defining condition)

IV. A child aged less than 18 months born to an HIV-infected mother will be categorized as having perinatal exposure to HIV infection if the child does not meet the criteria for HIV infection (II) or the criteria for 'not infected with HIV' (III).

---

*Children aged greater than or equal to 18 months but less than 13 years are categorized as "not infected with HIV" if they meet the criteria in **III**.

** In adults, adolescents, and children infected by other than perinatal exposure, plasma viral RNA nucleic acid tests should **NOT** be used in lieu of licensed HIV screening tests (e.g., repeatedly reactive enzyme immunoassay). In addition, a negative (i.e., undetectable) plasma HIV-1 RNA test result does not rule out the diagnosis of HIV infection.

***AIDS-defining conditions for adults and adolescents 13 years and older include: Candidiasis of bronchi, trachea, or lungs; Candidiasis, esophageal; Carcinoma, invasive cervical; Coccidioidomycosis, disseminated or extrapulmonary; Cryptococcosis, extrapulmonary; Cryptosporidiosis, chronic intestinal; Cytomegalovirus disease (other than in liver, spleen or nodes); Cytomegalovirus retinitis; HIV encephalopathy; Herpes simplex: chronic or bronchitis, esophagitis or pneumonitis; Histoplasmosis, disseminated or extrapulmonary; Isosporiasis, chronic intestinal; Kaposi's sarcoma; Lymphoma, Burkitt's; Lymphoma, immunoblastic; Lymphoma, primary in brain; Mycobacterium avium complex or M. kansasii, disseminated or extrapulmonary; M. tuberculosis, pulmonary; M. tuberculosis, disseminated or extrapulmonary; Mycobacterium of other species, disseminated or extrapulmonary; Pneumocystis carinii pneumonia; Pneumonia, recurrent; Progressive multifocal leukoencephalopathy; Salmonella septicemia, recurrent; Toxoplasmosis of brain; Wasting syndrome due to HIV.

****AIDS-defining conditions for children less than 13 years old include the conditions listed above and: Bacterial infections, multiple or recurrent (including Salmonella septicemia) and Lymphoid interstitial pneumonia or pulmonary lymphoid hyperplasia; but they **exclude** the conditions above that were added to the adult/adolescent case definition in 1993: invasive cervical carcinoma, extrapulmonary M. tuberculosis, and recurrent pneumonia.

***** HIV nucleic acid (DNA or RNA) detection tests are the virologic methods of choice to exclude infection in children aged less than 18 months. Although HIV culture can be used for this purpose, it is more complex and expensive to perform and is less well standardized than nucleic acid detection tests. The use of p24 antigen testing to exclude infection in children aged less than 18 months is not recommended because of its lack of sensitivity.

An original paper copy of the document containing this definition can be obtained from the Superintendent of Documents, U.S. Government Printing Office (GPO), Washington, DC 20402–9371; telephone: (202)512–1800. Contact GPO for current prices.

Table 11.1 2000 Revised Surveillance Case Definition for HIV Infection

of severe immunosuppression based on a count of <200 CD4 T-lymphocytes per microliter of blood.[15] Effectively, this meant that a diagnosis of AIDS could occur approximately 18–24 months earlier in the course of disease than under the 1987 case definition. In addition, pulmonary *Mycobacterium tuberculosis*, invasive cervical cancer, and recurrent pneumonia in HIV-infected persons were included as AIDS-defining conditions. The 1993 expansion of the AIDS case definition was associated with the peak of AIDS diagnoses in the U.S. However, the AIDS case definition for children was not changed in 1993.

Following the advent of the era of highly active antiretroviral therapy (HAART) in the mid-1990s, AIDS incidence trends were no longer indicative of underlying trends in HIV incidence.[16–20] AIDS data also underestimated the need for treatment and other services.[21] Proposals to expand the AIDS case definition to include all persons diagnosed with HIV infection were first made in 1985, when the HIV antibody test was developed; again in 1992, prior to the implementation of the revised 1993 AIDS case definition; and again in 1997, when CDC published the first reports of substantial treatment-associated declines in AIDS incidence and deaths.[19–20] In 1999, CDC published guidelines for national HIV case surveillance, including best standards and practices for HIV case reporting as well as a revised integrated HIV/AIDS surveillance case definition for children and adults (*Table 11.1*).[22] The HIV/AIDS case definition includes current laboratory tests for monitoring HIV infection in children and adults.

CLASSIFICATION SYSTEM

Clinical classification systems for children and adults have likewise reflected advances in clinical management. For adults and adolescents, the 1993 classification system includes a 9-cell grid with 3 immunologic stages (CD4 <200/microliter, 200–499, ≥500) and 3 clinical stages (asymptomatic or acute HIV infection, symptomatic, AIDS-defining).[15]

The classification system for children was last revised in 1994 to a 12-cell grid in which the immunologic categories include age-specific CD4 thresholds categorized as none, moderate and severe immunosuppression.[23,24] The clinical categories include no symptoms, mild, moderate and severe.

EPIDEMIOLOGY

THE GLOBAL EPIDEMIC

The Joint United Nations Program on AIDS (UNAIDS) estimates that 36 million HIV-infected persons were alive throughout the world in 2000[12] (*Fig. 11.1*). Most (96%) live outside the rich countries of North America, Western Europe, and Australia. Africa is the most severely affected continent accounting for approximately 70% of the estimated number of prevalent infections worldwide. The spread of the epidemic in Africa occurred earlier than in other parts of the developing world; thus, Africa has already experienced high rates of AIDS and deaths. This has resulted in decreased life expectancies, increased infant mortality rates, and a growing number of orphaned children. Because most infections are acquired through sexual transmission among the adolescent and young adult segments of the population, most severe illnesses and deaths occur among young and middle-age adults. Many countries with high or rising HIV seroprevalence rates have not yet experienced the full impact of the epidemic because they have recent or emerging epidemics (*Fig. 11.2*). The majority of infected persons are asymptomatic and risk furthering the spread of HIV, in addition to the certainty of increased AIDS cases and deaths in the future. In addition to the threat of sexual

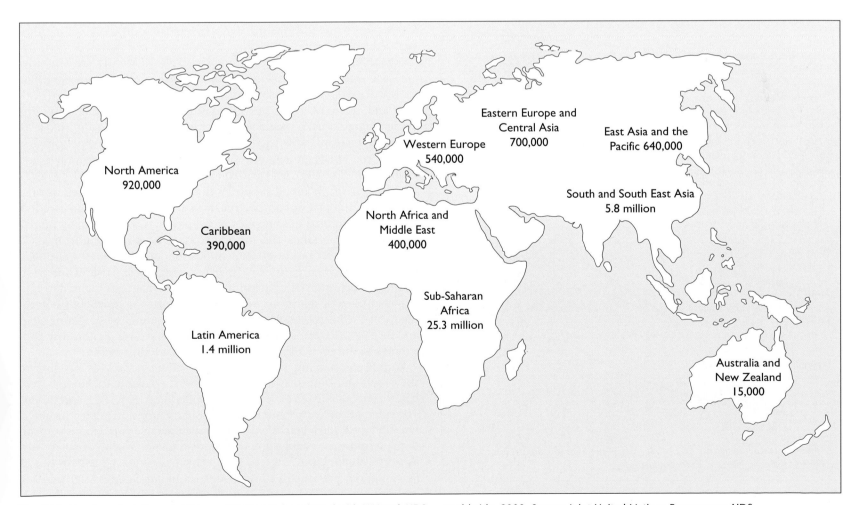

Fig. 11.1 Number of adults and children estimated to be infected with HIV and AIDS — worldwide, 2000. Source: Joint United Nations Program on AIDS.

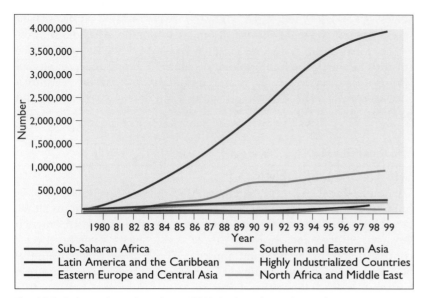

Fig. 11.2 Estimated number of new HIV infections, by region and year — worldwide, 1980–1999. Source: Joint United Nations Program on AIDS.

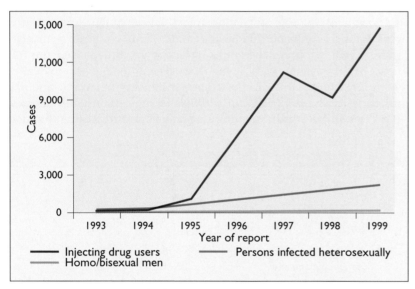

Fig. 11.3 HIV infections newly diagnosed in adults/adolescents by transmission group, 1993–99, eastern Europe. Source: EuroHIV.

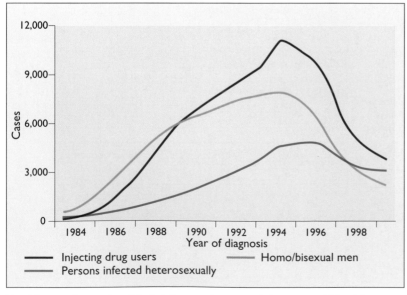

Fig. 11.4 AIDS cases in adults/adolescents by transmission group, 1984–99, western Europe. Source: EuroHIV.

transmission of HIV potentiated by high background rates of sexually transmitted diseases, some countries in Asia and Eastern Europe have substantial injecting drug-using populations and are reporting increasing numbers of HIV and AIDS cases (*Fig. 11.3*). In Latin America and the Caribbean region, a complex epidemiologic pattern includes HIV spread through sex between men, sex between men and women, and needle sharing among injecting drug users. However, some Latin American countries have sufficient resources to provide access to anti-retroviral treatments and declines in death rates have been reported from selected countries. In 1999, the most recent year for which estimates of the number of new HIV infections are available, sub-Saharan Africa accounted for about two-thirds of the approximately 6 million new cases of HIV world-wide. Asia and Eastern Europe represent the other geographic areas with growing rates of HIV infections. In contrast, in most of the highly industrialized countries, estimated rates of new infections have stabilized. However, even in these countries, the epidemic is dynamic as rates may decline in one risk group but increase in another. Migrants from countries with high HIV prevalence may introduce new viral sub-types and transmission patterns, and demographic changes in some sub-groups may predict increasing numbers of cases even in the absence of an increase in rates of transmission.

The rate of AIDS per 100,000 population in the U.S. remains the highest in the industrialized world; 14.7 reported AIDS cases per 100,000 population in 2000.[25] Even in the HAART era, AIDS incidence in the U.S. is markedly higher than in Western Europe, Canada, and Australia. These other countries did not adopt the immunologic criterion that was added to the U.S. AIDS case definition in 1993. Nevertheless, AIDS incidence rates are substantially lower than in the U.S. and there is considerable variation in rates among Western European countries.[26–27] For example, in 1999, the most recent year for which data were available (except for 1998 for France), AIDS incidence rates per 100,000 population were: Portugal, 8.8; Spain, 7.1; Italy, 3.6; France, 3.0; United Kingdom, 1.2. The epidemic in the highly industrialized countries is principally attributed to sex between men and needle sharing among injecting drug-users (*Fig. 11.4*). All these countries are faced with similar challenges to their ability to monitor the epidemic. As HAART delays progression to AIDS among persons diagnosed with HIV and receiving care, additional steps needed to understand the epidemiology of HIV include promoting testing early in the course of disease to increase knowledge of HIV status among infected persons and revising national surveillance systems to monitor the number and characteristics of HIV cases as well as AIDS cases.[22,28]

The safety of the blood supply in the United States has been assured through voluntary donor deferral and universal screening practices since 1985 and heat treatment of blood products, with virtually no risk of HIV infection since the introduction of donor screening by PCR testing has greatly narrowed the window of detection of HIV antibody in recently infected persons.[29] However, a significant risk of infection through transfusion of contaminated blood remains in many developing countries. In addition, even with advances in short-course treatments that reduce perinatal transmission when administered during labor and delivery, HIV transmission through breastfeeding significantly contributes to the epidemic in infants in the developing world.[30]

Worldwide, varying patterns of HIV sub-types provide insights to the origin and transmission of HIV.[31,32] The epidemic in Africa is very heterogeneous with the occurrence of subtypes A, B, C, D, E and others. The epidemic in North America and Western Europe originated in Africa, but sub-type B spread rapidly throughout vulnerable populations early on in these countries, establishing this strain as predominant. More recently, as North America and Western Europe have experienced large waves of in-migration, particularly from countries in Africa and Asia, the U.S. and Europe have experienced local transmission of non-B subtypes. Some studies suggest there are sub-type specific differences in virulence and transmissibility. Targeted vaccine development efforts are taking into account specific regions of the HIV genome that are common across strains with the goal of producing vaccines that are effective broadly in the population.

THE EPIDEMIC IN THE UNITED STATES

The cumulative total of AIDS cases reported in the U.S. was 774,467 as of December 31, 2000.[25] The characteristics of persons with AIDS have changed as the epidemic has evolved from one that initially affected mostly white gay men to a very heterogeneous epidemic with significant local and regional variation. Following the virtual elimination of HIV infections acquired through the receipt of blood or blood products, sex- and drug-associated transmission accounted for nearly all new HIV cases. AIDS cases have been reported from every state and the epidemic increasingly disproportionately affects racial/ethnic minorities, particularly black and Hispanic adolescents and adults. AIDS surveillance is currently the only national measure of the epidemic's effect at the population level. In the past, the time for progression of HIV disease followed a statistical distribution, from an acute phase at acquisition of infection, to asymptomatic infection, to disease symptoms, to severe end-stage disease characterized by immune-suppression and opportunistic illness, to death. Although some persons progressed to AIDS rapidly, the median time to AIDS-defining opportunistic illnesses was estimated to be about 10 years. Statistical models estimated the number of HIV infections that must have occurred annually in order to produce the observed number of AIDS cases; this procedure, known as back-calculation, estimated that approximately one million persons had been infected with HIV by the end of 1992.[6] With the advent of HAART, AIDS cases now represent a biased set of persons with HIV infection.[33] Those persons successfully maintained AIDS-free on HAART are not represented in the national AIDS surveillance data. Instead, the data represent persons not diagnosed with HIV until they have AIDS, those who may lack access to testing and care, and those for whom treatments are failing, likely due to a combination of viral resistance and problems adhering to complex treatment regimens.[34] HAART has also improved survival of patients following an AIDS diagnosis and has contributed to a dramatic decline in deaths of persons with AIDS.[35] In addition to AIDS case reports, anonymous unlinked HIV seroprevalence surveys, reporting of HIV cases in some states, and targeted studies of seroincidence (e.g.,

cohorts, studies of seroconverters, repeat testers at public clinics) provided useful data to monitor emerging trends in the epidemic.[36] The most useful seroprevalence data, from the anonymous Survey of Child-bearing Women, helped to estimate the national prevalence of women with HIV infection, the number of infected children born each year, and the geographic distribution of HIV-infected women who delivered liveborn infants each year; unfortunately, this survey was discontinued in 1996.

HIV/AIDS disproportionately affects young adults. Most persons with AIDS in the U.S. have been diagnosed in their mid-thirties (*Fig. 11.5*). Although the introduction of highly effective treatment regimens during the mid-1990s resulted in an increase in the median age at AIDS diagnosis (from 39 years for those diagnosed in 1994 to 43 years for those diagnosed in 1999), the vast majority of HIV infections were acquired by infected persons during their twenties.[37,38] These represent the ages at which young persons become sexually active, have the highest rates of partner change, and initiate drug-using behaviors. In addition, these ages represent the peak rates of other sexually transmitted diseases (STDs) such as chlamydia and gonorrhea, and some ulcerative STDs, notably genital herpes, which are associated with behavioral risks for HIV and with increased biologic risks for transmission of HIV infection.[39,40] Without timely access to testing, diagnosis and treatment, HIV-related morbidity and mortality take their toll on young adults in their most productive years of life. As recently as 1995, HIV/AIDS was the leading cause of death among adults aged 25–44 years (*Fig. 11.6*), followed by a remarkable decline in the rank of HIV/AIDS as a cause of death after the introduction of HAART.

Of the 41,690 adults and adolescents reported to the CDC with AIDS during 2000, 25% were women, 68% were racial/ethnic minorities (including 47% black non-Hispanic, 20% Hispanic, 0.9% Asian/Pacific Islander, and 0.5% American Indian/Alaska Native). The proportion of AIDS cases that represents persons of racial/ethnic minority groups has steadily increased[25] (*Fig. 11.7*). In addition, the rate per 100,000 population of AIDS cases reported during 2000 highlights the disproportionate impact that the HIV epidemic continues to have on minority communities with rates in blacks (58.1) and Hispanics (22.5) that are 9 and 3.4 times higher, respectively, than whites (6.6). The rates in Asians/Pacific Islanders and American Indians/Alaska Natives were 3.4 and 9.8, respectively. The proportion of female AIDS cases has steadily

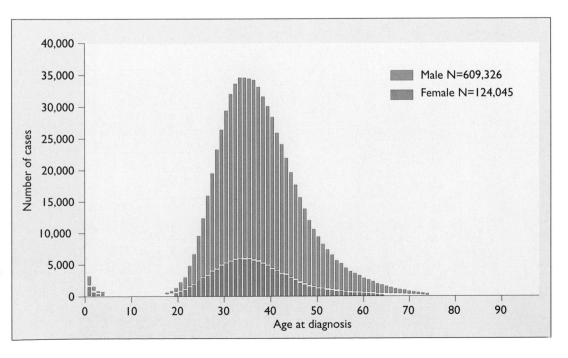

Fig. 11.5 AIDS cases by age and sex, reported 1981–1999, United States. Source: CDC Division of HIV/AIDS Prevention.

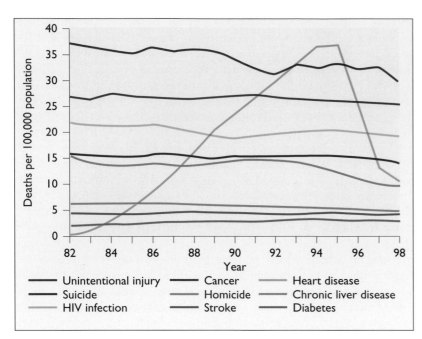

Fig. 11.6 Trends in annual rates of death from leading causes of death among persons 25–44 years old, 1982–1998, United States. Source: CDC National Center for Health Statistics.

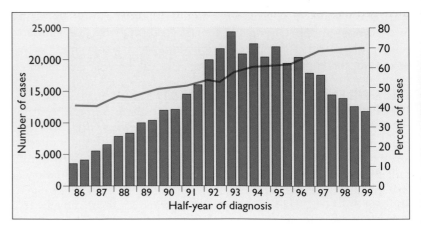

Fig. 11.7 AIDS incidence in racial/ethnic minorities and percentage of AIDS cases, January 1986–June 1999, United States. Source: CDC Division of HIV/AIDS Prevention.

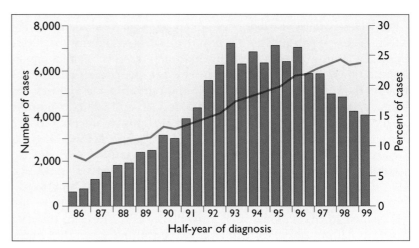

Fig. 11.8 AIDS incidence in women and percentage of AIDS cases, January 1986–June 1999, United States. Source: CDC Division of HIV/AIDS Prevention.

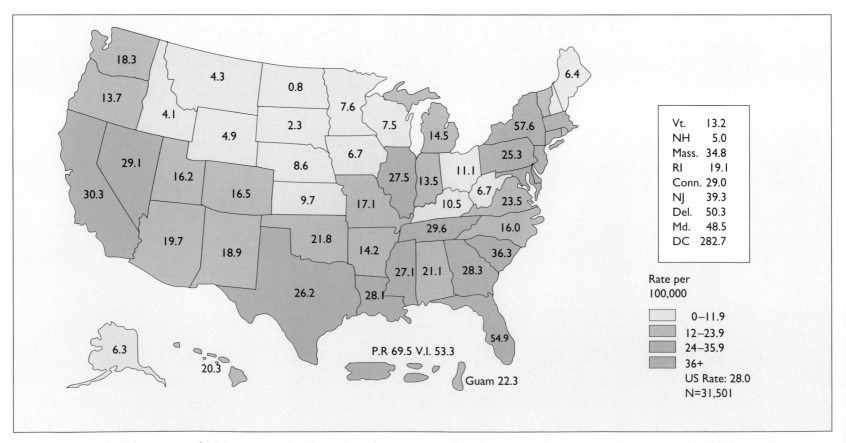

Fig. 11.9 Male adult/adolescent annual AIDS rates per 100,000 population for cases reported in 2000, United States. Source: CDC Division of HIV/AIDS Prevention.

increased (*Fig. 11.8*), reflecting principally the impact of heterosexual HIV transmission. The epidemic differentially affects the high-population coastal states; rates of reported AIDS cases per 100,000 population for 2000 for both men and women were highest in the northeast, southeast and west coast (*Figs 11.9* and *11.10*).

Of adult and adolescent men (*n* = 31,501) and women (*n* = 10,459) reported with AIDS during 2000, 24% and 36% were reported without information on HIV exposure category. Documentation of behavioral risks for HIV in medical records from a complete patient history, including discussion of sex and drug-using risks, remains the most critical step in assuring that national, state and local HIV/AIDS surveillance data accurately reflect the dynamics of the epidemic. After health department staff contact providers and review patient records, risk exposure data can be obtained on nearly all persons with AIDS. However, such efforts are labor-intensive and costly and are not feasible in all jurisdictions. Therefore, at the national level, statistical adjust-

ments to the recently reported data account for delays in reporting of cases and delays in collecting complete risk information in order to estimate the characteristics of incident AIDS cases.[25] Using adjusted data, among men diagnosed with AIDS during 1999 (estimated *n* = 32,389), 53% were men who have sex with men (MSM), 27% were injecting drug users (IDU), 6% were men with the dual risks MSM and IDU, and 13% were heterosexual contacts (HET) of women known to have HIV/AIDS or to be in a recognized risk category. Among women (estimated *n* = 10,309), 62% were HET and 35% were IDU. Very few newly diagnosed persons with HIV/AIDS are identified as having hemophilia, coagulation disorder, transfusion or transplantation as their probable mode of exposure to HIV. Thus, male–male sexual contact remains the most common risk for HIV acquisition and transmission for men, despite increases in recent years in the proportion of men with AIDS who acquired HIV heterosexually (*Fig. 11.11*). AIDS prevalence by risk group for men is shown in *Fig. 11.12*. However, among women, the

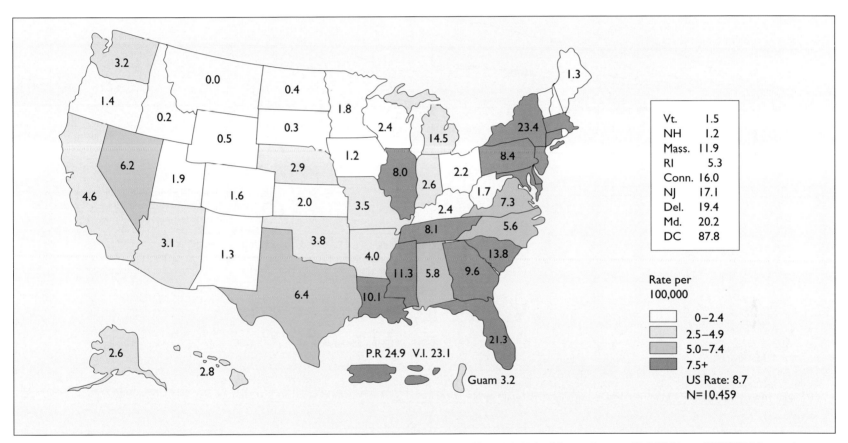

Fig. 11.10 Female adult/adolescent annual AIDS rates per 100,000 population for cases reported in 2000, United States. Source: CDC Division of HIV/AIDS Prevention.

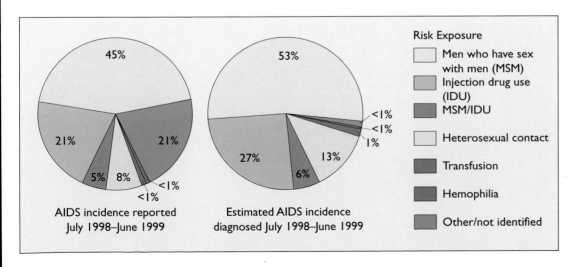

Fig. 11.11 AIDS cases in adult/adolescent men, reported July 1998–June 1999, and estimated AIDS incidence, diagnosed July 1998–June 1999, by risk exposure, United States. Source: CDC Division of HIV/AIDS Prevention.

epidemic primarily reflects heterosexually acquired HIV infections; the majority of these are associated with partners with a history of drug injecting (*Fig. 11.13*). AIDS prevalence by risk group for women is shown in *Fig. 11.14*. For both men and women, preventing and treating substance abuse and reducing high-risk needle-sharing behaviors among drug users remains an important step to combating HIV transmission in some populations and geographic areas, particularly among black and Hispanic communities and those geographically

concentrated along the East coast. The HAART era is associated with declines in AIDS incidence in MSM, IDU and HET risk categories, although declines have been most precipitous for MSM and least for HET (*Fig. 11.15*). Declines in AIDS incidence slowed in 1998 and 1999 and AIDS incidence leveled at approximately 40,000 cases per year during the late 1990s.

Nearly all HIV/AIDS cases in children are perinatally acquired. HIV can be transmitted from mother to infant in utero, intrapartum, or

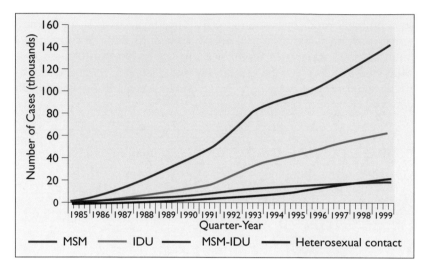

Fig. 11.12 Estimated AIDS prevalence among men, by risk exposure, 1985–1999, United States. Source: CDC Division of HIV/AIDS Prevention.

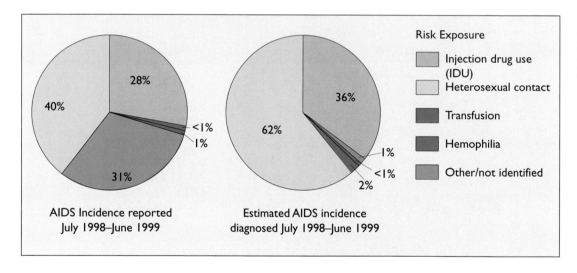

Fig. 11.13 AIDS cases in adult/adolescent women, reported July 1998–June 1999, and estimated AIDS incidence, diagnosed July 1998–June 1999, by risk exposure, United States. Source: CDC Division of HIV/AIDS Prevention.

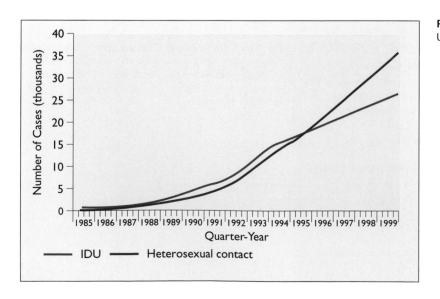

Fig. 11.14 Estimated AIDS prevalence among women, by risk exposure, 1985–1999, United States. Source: CDC Division of HIV/AIDS Prevention.

postpartum through breastfeeding. Since the finding that the treatment of pregnant women and their newborns with zidovudine (ZDV) reduces the risk of HIV transmission to the infant from about 25% to <8%, recommendations for universally offering voluntary HIV testing and ZDV prophylaxis to pregnant women have resulted in remarkable declines of more than 80% from the peak incidence of perinatally acquired AIDS cases in 1992[41–43] (*Fig. 11.16*). In addition, the avoidance of breastfeeding by pregnant women identified as HIV-infected through antenatal screening, revised obstetrical practices such as elective C-sections, and treatment with HAART for maternal health during pregnancy are associated with further reductions in the risk of perinatal HIV transmission. However, to eliminate perinatal HIV transmission will require intensive programmatic efforts to bring substance-using women into prenatal care to offer HIV testing and treatment. Studies have shown that such women are least likely to access prenatal care and therefore are less likely to have been offered testing and treatment prior to labor and delivery.[44] The potential to introduce short-course treatment interventions to the mother during labor and delivery and to the neonate holds the promise of further reducing perinatal HIV transmission.[45]

While adjusted AIDS incidence has declined substantially (*Fig. 11.17*), i.e., a 40% decline from nearly 70,000 AIDS cases in 1995, the year

before the widespread use of HAART, to nearly 42,000 cases in 1999, deaths of persons with AIDS declined even more precipitously during this period. From 1995 to 1999, deaths declined 67%, from nearly 51,000 to nearly 17,000. Persons diagnosed with AIDS are likely to receive medical care and to benefit most from advances in HIV treatment and management. The decline in the number of deaths was substantially greater than would have been expected in the absence of effective treatment of persons with AIDS; the number of observed deaths in 1996 was estimated to be 19% lower than would have been expected based on the number of AIDS cases and the observed distribution of survival times following an AIDS diagnosis in the pre-HAART era.[46] Survival increased substantially following the introduction of HAART. For patients diagnosed with an AIDS-defining opportunistic infection (OI), the probability of surviving at least 24 months increased from 49% for those diagnosed in 1993 to 80% for those diagnosed in 1997.[35] The greatest gains in survival were for those diagnosed with AIDS in 1996 compared to those diagnosed in 1995. Patients on HAART therapy have increased CD4 T-lymphocyte counts, decreased HIV-1 RNA plasma viral loads, and decreased incidence of AIDS-defining OIs. Thus, although both HIV-related morbidity and mortality decreased substantially in 1996 and 1997 due to a combination of factors, including both effective treatment and expected declines following the

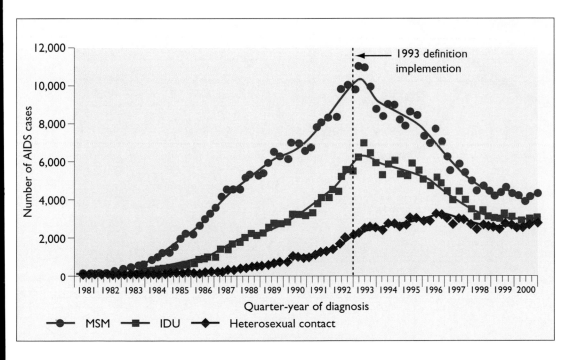

Fig. 11.15 Estimated number of AIDS cases among men who have sex with men (MSM), injecting drug users (IDU) and persons exposed through heterosexual contact, by quarter year of diagnosis, 1981–2000, United States. Source: CDC Division of HIV/AIDS Prevention.

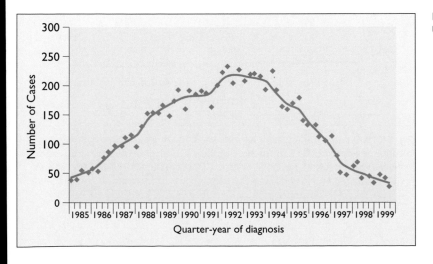

Fig. 11.16 Perinatally-acquired AIDS cases by quarter year of diagnosis, 1985–1999, United States. Source: CDC Division of HIV/AIDS Prevention.

earlier peak of HIV incidence in the U.S., the recent leveling in AIDS incidence and death trends is of concern. The current levels of AIDS incidence and deaths in the U.S. remain the highest in the industrialized world. Systematic efforts to promote risk recognition and assessment, increased access to voluntary testing and behavioral risk reduction for those who test negative and timely access to standard-of-care for those who test positive are essential to achieving further reductions in HIV-related morbidity and mortality. Recently, there have been a number of reports of adverse events associated with selected treatment regimens. For example, reports of treatment-associated deaths of pregnant women, deaths due to mitochondrial dysfunction in infants who were perinatally exposed to combination therapies, and various side effects such as lipodystrophy, metabolic dysfunctions, and hepatotoxicity have raised concerns regarding the potential for serious health risks associated with long-term treatment of HIV disease.[47–49]

The epidemiologic curves representing AIDS incidence and deaths are remarkably similar in Europe (*Fig. 11.18*) and the U.S. (*Fig. 11.17*). As deaths declined more precipitously than AIDS cases, the prevalence of

AIDS increased (*Fig. 11.17*). A fundamental principle of epidemiology is that the prevalence of a disease is equal to the incidence rate times the duration of the illness ($P = I \times D$). With increased survival of persons with AIDS, AIDS prevalence has steadily increased and was estimated to be approximately 330,000 in mid-2000. However, despite increases in AIDS prevalence, persons with AIDS represent only about one-third of the estimated 800,000-900,000 HIV-infected persons now living in the U.S. AIDS prevalence in future years will be affected not only by improved survival following an AIDS diagnosis, but by the underlying rate of new infections, the number of infected persons diagnosed, and the success of treatment to delay or prevent progression to AIDS among such persons. CDC has recommended that all states add HIV-infection to their list of notifiable diseases and that states require providers to report persons who are diagnosed with HIV, not just those with an AIDS diagnosis. Thirty-five states and Territories have implemented confidential HIV case reporting and these states have since reported over 125,000 cases of HIV (without AIDS). Although HIV case reports do not by themselves measure either total incidence or prevalence, trends in

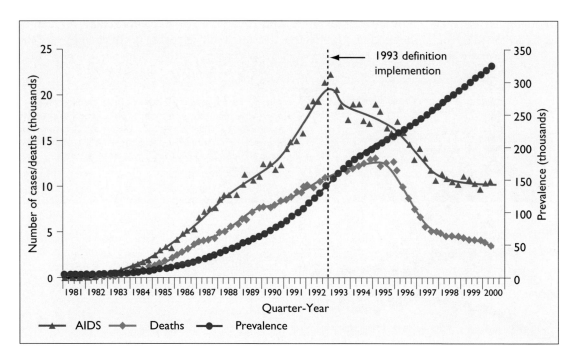

Fig. 11.17 Estimated AIDS incidence, deaths, and prevalence, by quarter year of diagnosis/death, 1981–June 2000, United States. Source: CDC Division of HIV/AIDS Prevention.

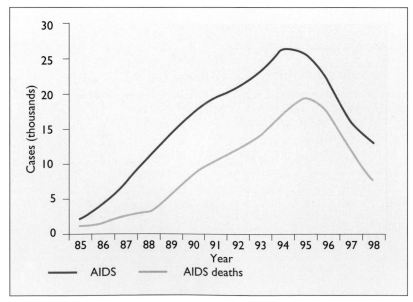

Fig. 11.18 Trends in AIDS incidence and reported AIDS deaths, WHO European Region. Source: EuroHIV

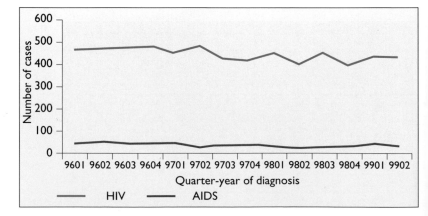

Fig. 11.19 Estimated number of persons aged 13–24 years diagnosed with HIV infection, by disease status at the time of the initial diagnosis of HIV — 25 states, January 1996 through June 1999. Source: CDC Division of HIV/AIDS Prevention.

the diagnosis of HIV infection in young adults less than 25 years of age are useful to identify populations most in need of prevention and care interventions. They also help monitor more recent trends in HIV incidence in these states, because young persons diagnosed with HIV represent recent HIV infections[50] (*Fig. 11.19*).

Other strategies to monitor trends in the epidemic include monitoring HIV prevalence in selected high-risk populations such as young adults entering the Job Corps (*Fig. 11.20*), and young adults applying for military service (*Fig. 11.21*).[36] More recently, a method called the Serologic Testing Algorithm for the detection of Recent HIV Seroconversions (STARHS) was developed to determine whether a positive HIV detection test represents a recently acquired infection (e.g., within the last 4 months) or someone who was infected at some time in the past.[51] This method may enable direct estimation of HIV incidence rates in the population if it can be applied to all new HIV diagnoses nationally. Research studies using STARHS have found high rates of HIV incidence among young MSM, particularly black MSM, in selected settings in some U.S. cities.[52,53] Such data on HIV incidence rates would be extremely valuable in monitoring the epidemic and in planning for prevention and care programs at the local level if the STARHS method can be applied at the population level. Prior to the expansion of the AIDS surveillance case definition in 1993, through back-calculation from AIDS incidence, several investigators estimated that HIV incidence in the early 1990s was at least 40,000 cases.[6,37] Because trends in seroprevalence among high-risk youth and in the number of new HIV diagnoses in young adults (<25 years of age) were nearly stable during most of the 1990s, national trends in HIV incidence are assumed to have been relatively stable since the early 1990s.[54] While local increases or decreases in HIV incidence in selected populations or risk groups are frequently reported, data are not currently available at the population level to predict whether such local trends will become more widespread. Recent reports of increased rates of STDs in MSM in some cities, high HIV incidence rates in black MSM in some cities, and high rates of HIV infection in young women, especially blacks, in selected states, emphasize the importance of renewed attention to primary HIV prevention.[53,55–57] Lacking a curative treatment or a highly effective vaccine, behavioral risk reduction with appropriate counseling, testing, and referral remains the most effective prevention strategy for the immediate future.[58] The role of primary care physicians in achieving reductions in HIV incidence cannot be over-emphasized. The vigilance of specialists and emergency-care physicians in detecting symptomatic HIV cases and providing prompt testing, diagnosis and treatment are likewise critical to lessening the burden of morbidity and mortality and also to facilitating linkages to counseling and risk reduction programs to prevent further HIV transmission.[28]

References

1. CDC. *Pneumocystis* pneumonia — Los Angeles. *MMWR* 1981; **30**:250–252.
2. CDC. Kaposi's sarcoma and *Pneumocystis* pneumonia among homosexual men — New York City and California. *MMWR* 1981; **30**:305–308.
3. CDC. Prevention of acquired immune deficiency syndrome (AIDS): report of inter-agency recommendations. *MMWR* 1983; **32**:101–104.
4. CDC. Acquired immunodeficiency syndrome (AIDS) update – United States. *MMWR* 1983; **32**:309–311.
5. CDC. Revision of the case definition of acquired immunodeficiency syndrome for national reporting — United States. *MMWR* 1985; **34**:373–375.
6. Brookmeyer R. Reconstruction and future trends of the AIDS epidemic in the United States. *Science* 1991; **253**:37–42.
7. CDC. PHS task force recommendations for the use of antiretroviral drugs in pregnant women infected with HIV-1 for maternal health and for reducing perinatal HIV-1 transmission in the United States. *MMWR* 1998; **47**(No. RR-2):1–39.
8. CDC. Guidelines for the use of antiretroviral agents in pediatric HIV infection. *MMWR* 1998; **47**(RR-4):1–43.
9. CDC. Report of the NIH panel to define principles of therapy of HIV infection and Guidelines for the use of antiretroviral agents in HIV-infected adults and adolescents. *MMWR* 1998; **47**(RR-5):1–82.
10. CDC. Public Health Service guidelines for counseling and antibody testing to prevent HIV infection and AIDS. *MMWR* 1987; **36**:509–515.
11. Francis DP, Anderson RE, Gorman ME et al. Targeting AIDS prevention and treatment toward HIV-1-infected persons: the concept of early intervention. *JAMA* 1989; **262**:2572–2576.
12. CDC. The global HIV/AIDS epidemic, 2001. *MMWR* 2001; **50**:434–439.
13. CDC. Update on acquired immune deficiency syndrome (AIDS) — United States. *MMWR* 1982; **31**:507–514.
14. CDC. Revision of the CDC surveillance case definition for acquired immuno-deficiency syndrome. *MMWR* 1987; **36**(suppl 1):1–15.
15. CDC. 1993 Revised classification system for HIV infection and expanded surveillance case definition for AIDS among adolescents and adults. *MMWR* 1992; **41**(No. RR-17):1–19.
16. Hammer SM, Katzenstein DA, Hughes MD et al. A trial comparing nucleoside monotherapy with combination therapy in HIV-infected adults with CD4 cell counts from 200 to 500 per cubic millimeter. *N Engl J Med* 1996; **335**:1081–1090.
17. Carpenter CC, Fischel MA, Hammer SM et al. Antiretroviral therapy for HIV infection in 1997: updated recommendations of the International AIDS Society — USA panel. *JAMA* 1997; **277**:1962–1969.

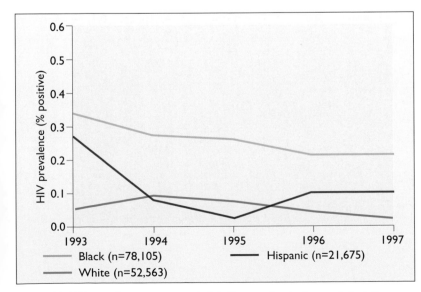

Fig. 11.20 HIV prevalence among male Job Corps entrants, by race/ethnicity, 1993–1997. Source: CDC Division of HIV/AIDS Prevention.

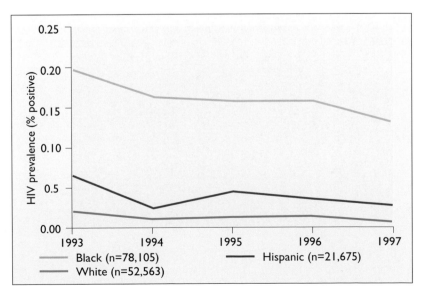

Fig. 11.21 HIV prevalence among male military applicants, by race/ethnicity, 1993–1997. Source: CDC Division of HIV/AIDS Prevention.

18. CDC. 1997 USPHS/IDSA guidelines for the prevention of opportunistic infections in persons infected with human immunodeficiency virus. *MMWR* 1997; **46**(No. RR-12):1–48.
19. CDC. Update: trends in AIDS incidence, deaths, and prevalence — United States, 1996. *MMWR* 1997; **46**:165–173.
20. CDC. Update: trends in AIDS incidence — United States, 1996. *MMWR* 1997; **46**:861–867.
21. Bozzette SA, Berry SH, Duan N *et al.* The care of HIV-infected adults in the United States. *N Engl J Med* 1999; **339**:1897–1904.
22. CDC. Guidelines for national HIV case surveillance, including monitoring for HIV and AIDS. *MMWR* 1999; **48**(RR-13):1–31.
23. CDC. Classification system for human immunodeficiency virus (HIV) infection in children under 13 years of age. *MMWR* 1987; **36**:225–236.
24. CDC. 1994 Revised classification system for human immunodeficiency virus infection in children less than 13 years of age. *MMWR* 1994; **43**(RR-12):1–9.
25. CDC. *HIV/AIDS Surveillance Report*, 2000; **12**(No.1):1–41.
26. Downs AM. Heisterkamp SH, Brunet JB *et al.* Reconstruction and prediction of the HIV/AIDS epidemic among adults in the European Union and in the low prevalence countries of central and eastern Europe. *AIDS* 1997; **11**:649–662.
27. European Centre for the Epidemiological Monitoring of AIDS. HIV/AIDS surveillance in Europe. *End-year report 1999*, 1999; No 62:1–50.
28. Janssen RS, Holtgrave DR, Valdiserri RO et al. The serostatus approach to fighting the HIV epidemic: prevention strategies for infected individuals. *Am J Public Health* 2001; **91**:1019–1024.
29. Lackritz EM, Jacobs TA, Stramer SL *et al.* Results of national testing of US blood donations for HIV-1 p24 antigen. *Conf Retroviruses and Opportunistic Infections* (4th) January 22–26, 1997 (Abstract 751).
30. Hu DJ, Heyward WL, Byers RH *et al.* HIV infection and breast-feeding: policy implications through a decision analysis model. *AIDS* 1992; **6**:1505–1513.
31. Hu DJ, Dondero TJ, Rayfield MA *et al.* The emerging genetic diversity of HIV: the importance of global surveillance for diagnostics, research, and prevention. *JAMA* 1996; **275**:210–216.
32. CDC. Identification of HIV-1 Group O infection — Los Angeles County, California, 1996. *MMWR* 1996; **45**:561–565.
33. Kaplan JE, Hanson D, Dworkin MS *et al.* Epidemiology of human immunodeficiency virus-associated opportunistic infections in the United States in the era of highly active antiretrovival therapy. *Clinical Inf Dis* 2000; **30**:S5–S14.
34. Fleming PL, Wortley PM, Karon JM, DeCock KM, Janssen RS. Tracking the HIV epidemic: current issues, future challenges. *Am J Public Health* 2000; **90**:1037–1041.
35. Lee LM, Karon JM, Selik R, Neal JJ, Fleming PL. Survival after AIDS diagnosis in adolescents and adults during the treatment era, United States, 1984–1997. *JAMA* 2001; **285**:1308–1315.
36. CDC. National HIV prevalence surveys, 1997 summary. Atlanta, GA: CDC; 1998:1–25.
37. Rosenberg PS. Scope of the AIDS epidemic in the United States. *Science* 1995; **270**:1372–1375.
38. Rosenberg PS, Biggar RJ. Trends in HIV incidence among young adults in the United States. *JAMA* 1998; **279**:1894–1899.
39. CDC. 1998 Guidelines for treatment of sexually transmitted diseases. *MMWR* 1998; **47**(No. RR-1):1–16.
40. CDC. *Tracking the hidden epidemics: trends in STDs in the United States, 2000.* 2000; 1–31.
41. CDC. Recommendations of the Public Health Service Task Force on use of zidovudine to reduce perinatal transmission of human immunodeficiency virus. *MMWR* 1994; **43**(No. RR-11):1–21.
42. CDC. U.S. Public Health Service recommendations for human immunodeficiency virus counseling and voluntary testing for pregnant women. *MMWR* 1995; **44**(No. RR-7):1–14.
43. Lindegren ML, Byers RH, Thomas P *et al.* Trends in perinatal transmission of HIV/AIDS in the United States. *JAMA* 1999; **282**:531–538.
44. CDC. Success in implementing Public Health Service guidelines to reduce perinatal transmission of HIV – Louisiana, Michigan, New Jersey and South Carolina, 1993, 1995, and 1996. *MMWR* 1998; **47**:688–691. Errata. *MMWR* 1998; **47**:718.
45. Shaffer N, Chuachoowong R, Mock PA *et al.* Short-course zidovudine for perinatal HIV-1 transmission in Bangkok, Thailand: a randomized controlled trial. *Lancet* 1999; **353**:773–780.
46. Fleming PL, Ward JW, Karon JM, Hanson DL, DeCock KM. Declines in AIDS incidence and deaths in the USA: a signal change in the epidemic. *AIDS* 1998; **12**(suppl A): S55–S61.
47. Mandelbrot L, Landreau-Mascaro A, Rekacewicz C *et al.* Lamivudine-zidovudine combination for prevention of maternal–infant transmission of HIV-1. *JAMA* 2001; **285**:2083–2093.
48. Lichtenstein K, Ward D, Delaney K *et al.* Clinical factors related to the severity of fat distribution in the HIV outpatient study (HOPS). *Conf Retroviruses and Opportunistic Infections* (7th) January 30–February 2, 2000 (Abstract 23).
49. Mulligan K. Abnormalities of body composition and lipids associated with HAART: pathogenesis, clinical manifestations, and case definitions. *Conf Retroviruses and Opportunistic Infections* (7th) January 30–February 2, 2000 (Abstract S20).
50. CDC. Diagnosis and reporting of HIV and AIDS in states with integrated HIV and AIDS surveillance — U.S. *MMWR* 1998; **47**:309–314.
51. Janssen RS, Satten GA, Stramer SL *et al.* New testing strategy to detect early HIV-1 infection for use in incidence estimates and for clinical and prevention purposes. *JAMA* 1998:**280**:42–48. Erratum: *JAMA* 1999; **281**:1893.
52. Valleroy LA, MacKellar DA, Karon JM *et al.* HIV infection in disadvantaged out-of-school youth: prevalence for U.S. Job Corps entrants, 1990 through 1996. *J Acquir Immune Defic Syndr Hum Retrovirol* 1998; **19**:67–73.
53. CDC. HIV incidence among young men who have sex with men – seven U.S. cities, 1994–2000. *MMWR* 2001; **50**:440–444.
54. Karon JM, Fleming PL, Steketee RW, DeCock KM. HIV in the United States at the turn of the century: an epidemic in transition. *Am J Public Health* 2001; **91**:1060–1068.
55. CDC. Increases in unsafe sex and rectal gonorrhea among men who have sex with men – San Francisco, California, 1994–1997. *MMWR* 1999; **48**:45–48.
56. CDC. Resurgent bacterial sexually transmitted disease among men who have sex with men — King County, Washington, 1997–1999. *MMWR* 1999; **48**:773–777.
57. Lee LM, Fleming PL. Trends in human immunodeficiency virus diagnoses among women in the United States, 1994–1998. *JAMA* 2001; **56**:94–99.
58. CDC. Revised guidelines for HIV counseling, testing, and referral and revised recommendations for HIV screening of pregnant women. *MMWR* 2001; **50**(RR-19):1–57.

Human Immunodeficiency Virus Infection and the Acquired Immunodeficiency Syndrome: Diagnosis and Management

12

D Spach and R Harrington

INTRODUCTION

The human immunodeficiency virus (HIV)/acquired immunodeficiency syndrome (AIDS) epidemic has now been well established for more than 20 years and the global toll of this disease has been devastating. Unfortunately, the impact of HIV and AIDS continues to grow every year, especially in developing countries. Although effective antiretroviral therapy is available to most persons in developed countries, a cure remains elusive and an effective vaccine to prevent HIV infection is not yet available. Medical providers will thus continue to need to stay informed on how to appropriately recognize and diagnose HIV, as well as how to provide effective long-term management. In the past 5 years, the field of HIV and AIDS has changed more rapidly than any other in medicine. The major goals of this chapter are to provide the clinician with up-to-date information on how to better diagnose and manage HIV-related complications, as well as to better understand current concepts on how to effectively use antiretroviral therapy.

PRIMARY (ACUTE) HIV INFECTION

Available data suggest that approximately 50% of persons who acquire HIV develop an acute retroviral illness.[1] The acute retroviral syndrome typically occurs 7–14 days following HIV acquisition, manifesting as a mononucleosis-like (or influenza-like) illness, with the most common symptoms consisting of fever (80–90%), fatigue (70–90%), rash (40–80%) (*Fig. 12.1*), headache (32–70%), lymphadenopathy (40–70%), pharyngitis (50–70%), and myalgias or arthralgias (50–70%).[1] Unfortunately, more than 50% of persons with the acute retroviral syndrome who seek medical care do not receive a correct diagnosis,[2] probably because of the non-specific nature of the acute illness and the lack of awareness of this syndrome. The acute HIV illness typically persists for about 7–10 days, but in unusual circumstances, has persisted for 4 to 8 weeks. Several studies suggest that individuals with a more severe and more prolonged acute HIV illness more often have accelerated HIV disease progression. A recent study of 17 persons with acute HIV infection found that by the time patients are commonly diagnosed with primary HIV infection, peak level HIV replication is already established in blood, oropharyngeal tissues, and genital tract; thus HIV-infected persons are likely highly infectious to others during this acute illness.[3] In addition, this same study found very high levels of HIV in semen among those who had concomitant infection with another sexually transmitted pathogen.

The antibody screening test used for persons with established HIV — the recombinant enzyme-linked immunoassay (ELISA) test — usually is negative in persons with the acute HIV infection syndrome and typically does not turn positive until at least 3 weeks after acquiring HIV.[4] The HIV RNA test, however, is uniformly positive in persons presenting with acute HIV infection, with most having a value greater than 100,000 copies/ml. The diagnosis of acute HIV infection in this so-called 'window period' can be established by the combination of a negative serology test and detection of virus (either a positive HIV RNA test or a positive p24 antigen test).[5] Although the HIV RNA assay has an extremely high sensitivity, occasional false-positive tests occur.[5] These false-positive results, however, generally are low-level positive tests, with HIV RNA levels typically less than 10,000 copies/ml. In contrast, those with true acute HIV infection almost always have an HIV RNA level greater than 50,000 copies/ml. The p24 antigen test has excellent specificity and is less expensive, but is limited by a lower sensitivity (89%) and it becomes positive 3 to 4 days later than the HIV RNA test. When an HIV RNA or p24 antigen test can not be obtained, acute HIV infection can be confirmed by a negative HIV serology test, followed at least 4 weeks later with a positive HIV serology test.

Establishing a diagnosis of acute HIV infection can have major consequences. First, given the finding of peak HIV levels throughout the body during acute HIV infection, this period poses a major risk for transmission, especially considering most persons in this setting are unaware they have acquired HIV. Thus, if the diagnosis of acute HIV infection is established, prompt counseling for safe sex and safe needle practices can be given to the patient. Second, if the acute HIV infection illness is not recognized, subsequent AIDS-related manifestations often do not develop for at least 5 years, and thus the HIV infection may go undiagnosed for years. Last, aggressive combination antiretroviral therapy of HIV starting at the time of the acute HIV illness (and within 6 months of seroconversion) is now recommended in the current Department of Health and Human Services (DHHS) Guidelines.[6]

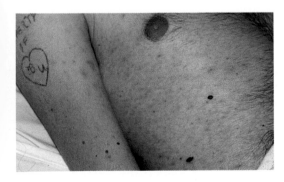

Fig. 12.1 Cutaneous maculopapular eruption associated with acute HIV infection.

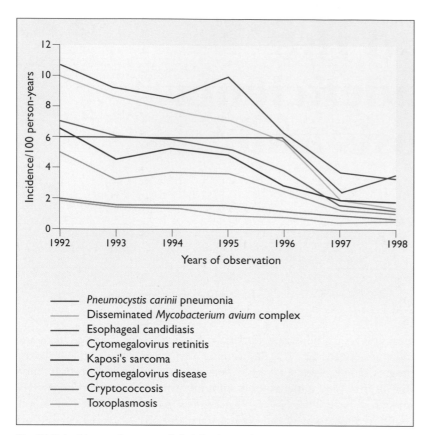

Fig. 12.2 Incidence of opportunistic infections, 1992–1998. Graph shows the incidence per 100 person years.

OPPORTUNISTIC INFECTIONS AND OTHER HIV-RELATED COMPLICATIONS

For 10 years following the 1981 reports of *Pneumocystis carinii* pneumonia (PCP) and Kaposi's sarcoma in gay men and injection drug users living in Los Angeles, San Francisco, and New York City,[7] the incidence of AIDS-associated opportunistic infections (OI) and cancers rose sharply as the HIV epidemic evolved. Antiretroviral and prophylactic therapies slowly stabilized the incidence of opportunistic infections in the early 1990s, but not until after the release of HIV protease inhibitors in 1995 and their widespread use as part of highly active antiretroviral therapy (HAART) did the incidence of OIs drop dramatically (*Fig. 12.2*).[8] Several large United States and European studies have clearly shown that following the widespread use of HAART, steep reductions in AIDS-defining OIs and Kaposi's sarcoma occurred, but with little decline or even an increase in the incidence of other AIDS-associated malignancies. The United States Adult Spectrum of Disease project performed a retrospective analysis of almost 50,000 HIV-infected persons in 11 United States cities and found declining incidence for almost all AIDS-defining infections from 1992 to 1998, with a sharp reduction in these complications occurring from 1995 to 1998.[8] In addition, two multicenter, prospective, observational studies conducted in Europe — the Swiss Cohort Study[9] and the EuroSIDA study[10] — yielded similar results. The Swiss study followed more than 2,400 HIV-infected patients starting HAART in seven centers throughout Switzerland between 1995 and 1997. The investigators tracked OIs in the 6 months before and 15 months after HAART and found the overall incidence of AIDS-defining infections decreased from 15.1 per 100 person-years before HAART to 3.6 per 100 person-years in the 15 months after HAART. Risks factors independently associated with protection against opportunistic infections consisted of a higher baseline CD4+ count, an increase in CD4+ cell count of > 50 cells/mm^3, and control of HIV replication (HIV RNA less than 400 copies/ml) after 6 months of HAART. The other large European study, EuroSIDA, included more than 7,300 patients in 52

centers throughout Europe and also demonstrated a reduced incidence of AIDS-defining infections following the widespread use of HAART, from 30.7 per 100 patient-years in 1994 to 2.5 per 100 patient-years in 1998. In both studies, the reduced incidence was greater for some AIDS-defining illnesses than for others. The most significant declines were seen in Kaposi's sarcoma, *Pneumocystis carinii* pneumonia, *Mycobacterium avium* complex (MAC), esophageal candidiasis, and cytomegalovirus disease, whereas the incidence of non-Hodgkin's lymphoma declined little[9] or actually increased.[10] Both studies also demonstrated protection against the development of AIDS-defining infections by HAART that was independent of increasing CD4+ counts, suggesting that tight control of HIV replication per se provides significant clinical benefit.

Prophylaxis for certain OIs has remained a critical component of care of HIV-infected individuals and recommendations for prophylaxis are listed in *Table 12.1*. Despite the benefits provided by OI prophylaxis and HAART, OIs and AIDS-associated cancers continue to occur disproportionately in certain patient populations. The Adult Spectrum of Disease project found that 32% of patients who developed *Pneumocystis carinii* pneumonia in 1996–1998 had been prescribed prophylaxis appropriately.[8] In these cases, lack of adherence to therapy, borderline CD4+ counts, other immunosuppressive conditions, and drug resistance may have played a role. Of note, however, rates of *Pneumocystis carinii* pneumonia were markedly higher among individuals who were either not in care, or were in care and met criteria for prophylaxis, but were not prescribed appropriate prophylaxis.[8] These data demonstrate that simple, inexpensive measures such as establishing medical care and receiving appropriate OI prophylaxis would likely eliminate many serious AIDS-defining infections. In developing nations, only few patients have access to medical care, let alone HAART, and the spectrum and incidence of AIDS-defining infections has steadily increased during the last 20 years.

With the decreasing incidence of OIs in industrialized countries during the HAART era, the need for primary and secondary prophylaxis for many of the major AIDS-defining infections has significantly decreased.[11–18] In addition, in some instances, HAART has led to improvements and cure of AIDS-defining illnesses without the need for specific disease-directed therapy.[19,20] Moreover, HAART-induced immune system recovery can precipitate 'immune reconstitution syndromes' that are characterized by intense inflammatory reactions associated with known and occult infections.[21] These reactions can be localized, as in cases of suppurative adenitis or cytomegalovirus vitritis, or generalized, as in cases of unrecognized, disseminated mycobacterial disease. These syndromes carry significant morbidity and usually require anti-inflammatory therapy (corticosteroids and/or non-steroidal anti-inflammatory drugs) and in some instances temporary interruption of HAART. Finally, HAART has been associated with a paradoxical increase in the incidence of herpes zoster[22] and oral warts.[23] Individuals developing zoster after HAART were reported to have higher baseline or greater increases in CD8+ cell counts, but a clear explanation for this increased number of infections after antiretroviral therapy is lacking.

DERMATOLOGIC MANIFESTATIONS

Despite advances in antiretroviral therapy, a wide range of dermatologic disorders continue to occur in HIV-infected individuals, including non-infectious and infectious causes. Frequently occurring non-infectious disorders include eosinophilic folliculitis, xerosis, and medication-related cutaneous side effects. Eosinophilic folliculitis typically presents as intensely pruritic papules located on the face, scalp, trunk, and upper extremities; often the lesions are excoriated because of the severe pruritus. The diagnosis is confirmed with a skin biopsy that shows the characteristic perifollicular eosinophilic infiltrate, often with some follicular degeneration. Patients with xerosis develop dry, rough skin with a predilection for the anterior tibial areas, dorsal hands, and

Pathogen	Indication	First choice	Alternatives
*Pneumocystis carinii**	CD4+ count <200/mm³ or Oropharyngeal candidiasis	Trimethoprim-sulfamethoxazole (TMP-SMZ) 1 DS qd TMP-SMZ 1 SS qd	Dapsone 50 mg bid or 100 mg qd Dapsone 50 mg qd + Pyrimethamine 50 mg qw + Leucovorin 25 mg qw Dapsone 200 mg + Pyrimethamine 75 mg + Leucovorin 25 mg qw Aerosolized pentamidine, 300 mg q month via Respirgard II, nebulizer Atovaquone 1,500 mg qd TMP-SMZ, 1 DS tiw
Mycobacterium tuberculosis Isoniazid-sensitive †	TST reaction ≥ 5 mm or prior positive TST result without treatment or contact with case of active tuberculosis	Isoniazid 300 mg + Pyridoxine 50 mg qd × 9 mo Isoniazid 900 mg + Pyridoxine 100 mg biw × 9 mo Rifampin, 600 mg + Pyrazinamide 20 mg/kg qd × 2 mo	Rifabutin 300 mg qd + Pyrazinamide 20 mg/kg qd × 2 mo Rifampin 600 mg qd × 4 mo
Mycobacterium tuberculosis Isoniazid-resistant	Same: high probability of exposure to isoniazid-resistant tuberculosis	Rifampin 600 mg + Pyrazinamide 20 mg/kg qd × 2 mo	Rifabutin 300 mg qd + Pyrazinamide 200 mg/kg qd × 2 mo Rifampin, 600 mg qd × 4 mo Rifabutin, 300 mg qd × 4 mo
Mycobacterium tuberculosis Multidrug-(isoniazid rifampin) resistant	Same; high probability of exposure to multidrug-resistant tuberculosis	Choice of drugs requires consultation with public health authorities	None
Toxoplasma gondii§	IgG antibody to *Toxoplasma* and CD4+ count <100/mm³	TMP-SMZ 1 DS qd	TMP-SMZ 1 SS qd Dapsone 50 mg qd + Pyrimethamine 50 mg qw + Leucovorin 25 mg qw Atovaquone 1500 mg qd ± Pyrimethamine 25 mg qd + Leucovorin 10 mg qd
Mycobacterium avium complex	CD4+ count <50/mm³	Azithromycin 1,200 mg qw Clarithromycin, 500 mg bid	Rifabutin 300 mg qd Azithromycin 1,200 mg qw + Rifabutin 300 mg qd
Varicella zoster virus (vzv)	Significant exposure to chickenpox or shingles for patients who have no history of either condition or, if available, negative antibody to VZV	Varicella zoster immune globulin (VZIG), 5 vials (1.25 mL each) im, administered ≤96 h after exposure, ideally within 48 h	

All regimens are oral unless listed otherwise.

ABBREVIATIONS: po = by mouth; im = intramuscular; iv = intravenous; sc = subcutaneous; qd = daily; qw = weekly; biw. = twice a week; tiw. = three times a week; mo = month; DS = double-strength tablet; SS = single-strength tablet; TMP-SMZ = trimethoprim-sulfamethoxazole; TST = tuberculin skin test.

#Prophylaxis should also be considered for persons with a CD4+ percentage of <14% for persons with a history of an AIDS-defining illness, and possibly for those with CD4+ counts >200 but <250 cells/mL. Patients receiving dapsone should be tested for glucose-6 phosphate dehydrogenase deficiency. A dosage of 50 mg qd is probably less effective than that of 100 mg qd Patients who are being administered therapy for toxoplasmosis with sulfadiazine-pyrimethamine are protected against Pneumocystis carinii pneumonia and do not need additional prophylaxis against PCP.

†Directly observed therapy is recommended for isoniazid, 900 mg biw.; isoniazid regimens should include pyridoxine to prevent peripheral neuropathy. Rifampin should not be administered concurrently with protease inhibitors or nonnucleoside reverse transcriptase inhibitors. Rifabutin should not be given with hard-gel saquinavir or delavirdine; caution is also advised when the drug is coadministered with soft-gel saquinavir. Rifabutin may be administered at a reduced dose (150 mg qd) with indinavir, nelfinavir, or amprenavir; at a reduced dose of 150 mg qod. (or 150 mg three times weekly) with ritonavir; or at an increased dose (450 mg qd) with efavirenz; information is lacking regarding coadministration of rifabutin with nevirapine. Exposure to multidrug-resistant tuberculosis might require prophylaxis with two drugs; consult public health authorities. Possible regimens include pyrazinamide plus either ethambutol or a fluoroquinolone.

Table 12.1 Prophylaxis to prevent first episode of opportunistic disease in adults and adolescents infected with HIV. Strongly recommended as standard of care. Adapted from the 1999 USPHS/IDSA Guidelines for the Prevention of Opportunistic Infections.[89]

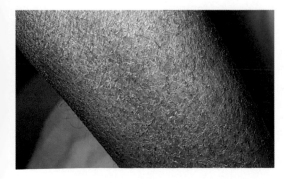

Fig. 12.3 Dry scaling skin showing the typical appearance of xerosis.

forearms (*Fig. 12.3*). Multiple reports have noted dry and itchy skin among a substantial proportion of persons taking indinavir[24] and this association has become one of the most frequent causes of dry skin among HIV-infected persons. In addition, indinavir-associated paronychia have been reported, typically manifesting as pyogranuloma-like lesions on the great toe.[25,26] The pathogenesis of indinavir-associated paronychia may be related to the shared homology between indinavir and the cytoplasmic retinoic acid-binding protein 1 and the function of retinoic acid as a regulator of epithelial cell growth. Many antiretroviral medications have been associated with drug rashes, including nevirapine, efavirenz, and abacavir (*Fig. 12.4*). The most serious complications have involved the Stevens-Johnson-like rashes associated with nevirapine and the rash associated with the abacavir hypersensitivity reaction.[27]

Infectious cutaneous complications associated with HIV include bacterial, fungal, or viral etiologies. Staphylococcal folliculitis is the most common cutaneous bacterial infection that occurs among HIV-infected individuals and typically manifests as pruritic follicular lesions in hair-bearing areas, particularly on the trunk and face. This condition clinically resembles eosinophilic folliculitis, but staphylococcal folliculitis often shows abundant Gram-positive cocci on Gram's stain and the lesions usually respond well to anti-staphylococcal antimicrobial therapy. Another

less common cutaneous disorder, cutaneous bacillary angiomatosis, can be caused by either *Bartonella quintana* or *B. henselae* and may manifest as papular, nodular, pedunculated, or verrucous lesions (*Fig. 12.5*).[28] Although some investigators have isolated the causative organism from skin lesions, the diagnosis is most often made by performing a Warthin-Starry silver stain on a biopsy sample (*Fig. 12.6*). The incidence of bacillary angiomatosis has markedly decreased following the wide-spread use of trimethoprim-sulfamethoxazole for *Pneumocystis carinii* prophylaxis.

Seborrheic dermatitis, a common and early manifestation of HIV infection, is believed to result from a combination of infection with the fungus *Malassezia* spp. plus the host response to this organism (*Fig. 12.7*). The pathogenicity of *Malassezia* probably corresponds more with the subtype of *Malassezia* spp. rather than the density of the organism.[29] The diagnosis is based on the characteristic erythematous, scaly lesion in the distribution of scalp, eyebrows, beard, and facial folds. Other fungal infections, such as cryptococcosis (*Fig. 12.8*) and histoplasmosis, may cause multiple cutaneous lesions when they disseminate. In addition, disseminated infection with *Penicillium marneffei* manifesting as multiple cutaneous lesions, is one of the most common opportunistic infections in certain areas of Asia,[30] particularly in northern Thailand (*Fig. 12.9a, b*).

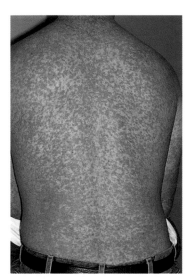

Fig. 12.4 Diffuse erythematous macular drug eruption caused by nevirapine.

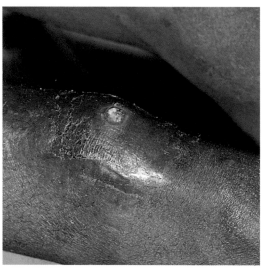

Fig. 12.5 Subcutaneous bacillary angiomatosis lesion that has eroded the skin surface. Reproduced with permission from *International Journal of Dermatology*.

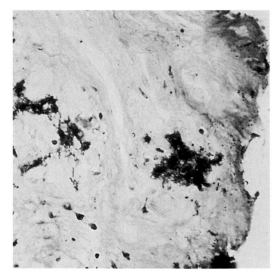

Fig. 12.6 Warthin-Starry stain of a skin biopsy taken from a patient with bacillary angiomatosis showing multiple clumps of organisms. Reproduced with permission from *International Journal of Dermatology*.

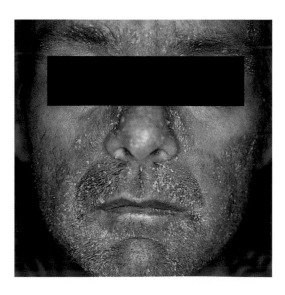

Fig. 12.7 Typical appearance of seborrheic dermatitis manifested by erythema and scaling of the nasolabial folds, facial creases, and eyebrows.

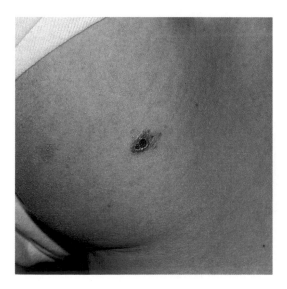

Fig. 12.8 Skin lesion of a patient with disseminated cryptococcal infection.

Molluscum contagiosum, caused by a pox virus, typically presents as umbilicated papular lesions, most commonly on the face, neck, (*Fig. 12.10*) and genital tract. In contrast with immunocompetent individuals who generally have spontaneous resolution of these lesions, patients with HIV infection usually have progressively enlarging and spreading lesions that do not spontaneously resolve (*Fig. 12.11*). Often confused with molluscum contagiosum, human papilloma virus (HPV)-related warts develop as thick, hyperkeratotic papular growths most often seen on the hands (*Fig. 12.12*), feet, vulva, penis, or perianal region. The diagnosis of molluscum and warts is almost always based on the clinical appearance of the lesions. Herpes zoster virus infection can develop at any stage of a patient's HIV disease, and, in some instances, it may be their first HIV-related manifestation. Several reports have shown a significant increase in herpes zoster within 6 months after starting aggressive antiretroviral therapy.[22] Patients with herpes zoster typically develop painful grouped vesicles along a dermatomal distribution that

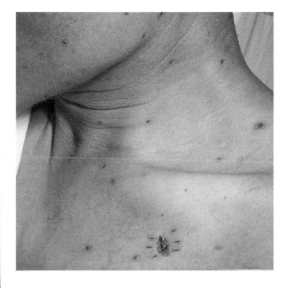

Fig. 12.9A Multiple cutaneous lesions caused by disseminated *Penicillium marneffei* in an HIV-infected patient from Thailand (courtesy of Pornchai Chirachanakul, MD, Bamrasnaradura Infectious Disease Hospital, Thailand).

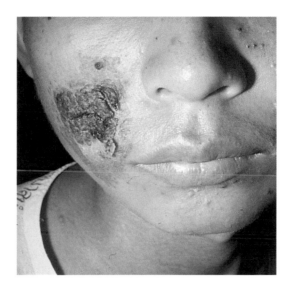

Fig. 12.9B Facial lesions caused by disseminated *Penicillium marneffei* in an HIV-infected patient from Thailand (courtesy of Pornchai Chirachanakul, MD, Bamrasnaradura Infectious Disease Hospital, Thailand).

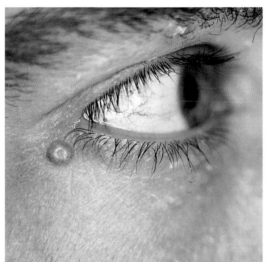

Fig. 12.10 Typical papular, umbilicated molluscum contagiosum lesion.

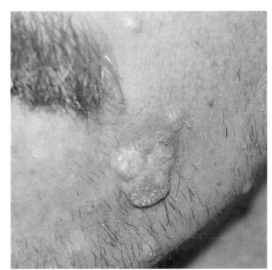

Fig. 12.11 Giant molluscum contagiosum lesion in patient with advanced AIDS.

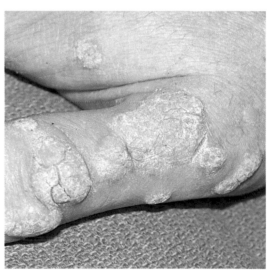

Fig. 12.12 Extensive hyperkeratotic warts located on a patient's hands.

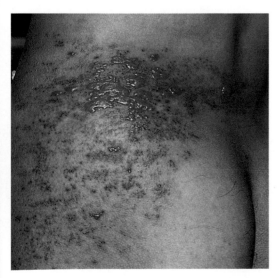

Fig. 12.13A Herpes zoster lesions that show typical grouped vesicular lesions with erythematous base in a dermatomal distribution.

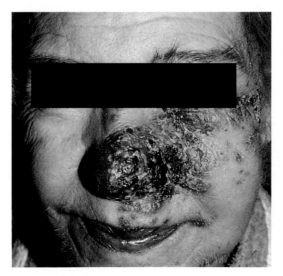

Fig. 12.13B Facial herpes zoster lesions that show crusting as they begin to heal.

will crust as they began to heal (*Fig. 12.13a, b*). Although the clinical presentation is often similar to that of herpes zoster in the immuno-competent patient, HIV-infected persons may have an illness with longer duration, as well as a higher risk of central nervous system involvement and dissemination. The diagnosis is usually made clinically, but can be confirmed using direct fluorescent antibody stains and culture tests, with the highest yield from scraping the base of the lesion to obtain cells. Patients with early-stage HIV disease who develop cutaneous herpes simplex virus infection typically present with symptoms similar to those seen in immunocompetent individuals, but those with advanced immunosuppression more often present with painful and ulcerative lesions (*Fig. 12.14*), rather than vesicular or pustular lesions. These ulcerative lesions can become chronic and are most often located on the face, penis, vulva, or perianal region. The diagnosis is often made clinically, but can be confirmed by culture, antigen detection, direct immunofluorescence, or by PCR testing. Kaposi's sarcoma, now known to be caused by human herpes virus 8,[31] frequently presents as an asymptomatic, indurated, reddish-purple papule or nodule anywhere on the skin, with a particular tendency to appear on the face, genitals, and feet (*Fig. 12.15a–f*). In addition, Kaposi's

sarcoma can develop in other organ systems, such as the lungs or gastrointestinal tract. The clinical diagnosis of Kaposi's sarcoma can be confirmed by biopsy of a lesion showing characteristic histopathology (*Fig. 12.16a–c*).

Most HIV-infected patients who become infested with scabies typically present with multiple pruritic papules often located on the hands (particularly on the wrist and between fingers), the belt line, and, in males, the glans penis (*Fig. 12.17*). An unusual variant of scabies, crusted (Norwegian) scabies, can develop in late-stage AIDS patients and is characterized by non-pruritic hyperkeratotic plaques and an extra-ordinarily large number of mites (*Fig. 12.18*). With any type of scabies, the diagnosis is made by scraping a skin lesion and identifying mites under the microscope (*Fig. 12.19*). A summary of the common derma-tologic disorders and their treatment is shown in *Table 12.2*.

ORAL MANIFESTATIONS

Following the widespread use of aggressive antiretroviral therapy, some oral disorders, namely oral hairy leukoplakia and necrotizing periodontal disease, have decreased in frequency, but others, such as candidiasis and oral aphthae, have not undergone major changes in frequency.[32] Accordingly, diagnosing and treating HIV-associated oral lesions remains an important aspect of HIV clinical care. Oral candidiasis, caused by *Candida albicans*, still occurs very commonly among HIV-infected individuals, especially those with CD4+ counts less than 300 cells/mm^3. Oral candidiasis can appear in one of three different forms: pseudo-membranous (thrush), atrophic (erythematous), and angular cheilitis (*Fig. 12.20a–c*). Symptoms often depend on the severity of candidiasis and may include pain or alterations in taste. Although most experienced clinicians diagnose oral candidiasis on the basis of the clinical appearance of this disorder, a potassium hydroxide (KOH) wet mount or Gram's stain of a scraping showing pseudohyphae can confirm the diagnosis. Oral hairy leukoplakia, another common oral disorder, occurs as a result of Epstein–Barr virus-induced epithelial thickening of the tongue. Often confused with candidiasis, oral hairy leukoplakia generally develops on the side of the tongue and is not removed by scraping (*Fig. 12.21*). The diagnosis is made on the clinical appearance of the lesion. This disorder rarely causes symptoms and rarely requires treatment.

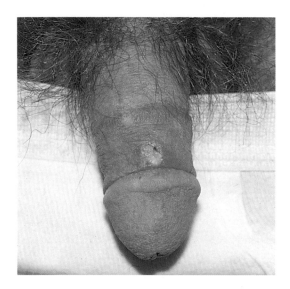

Fig. 12.14 Chronic ulcerative painful herpes simplex lesion on the dorsal shaft of the penis.

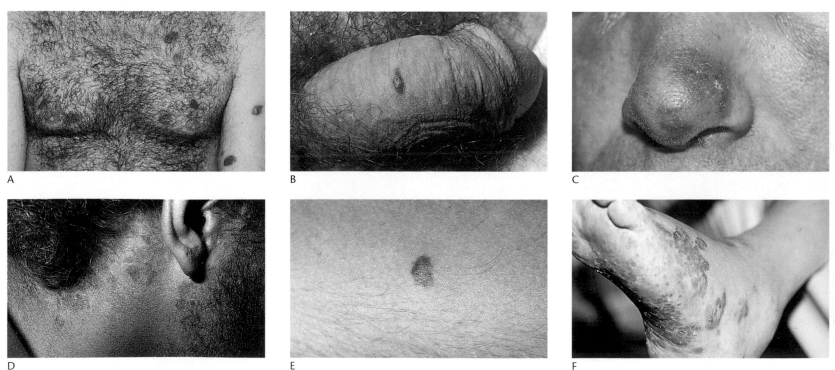

A

B

C

D

E

F

Fig. 12.15A–F Multiple locations and variable appearance of Kaposi's sarcoma lesions.

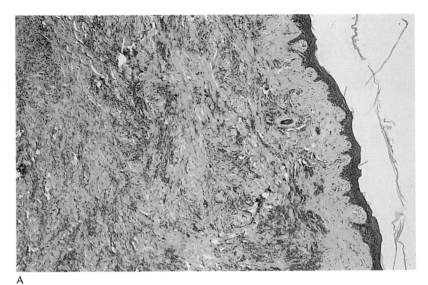

A

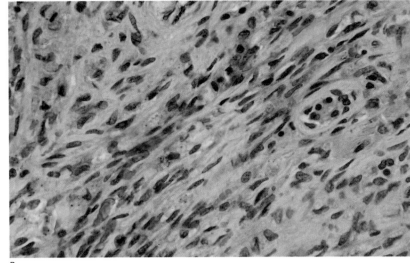

B

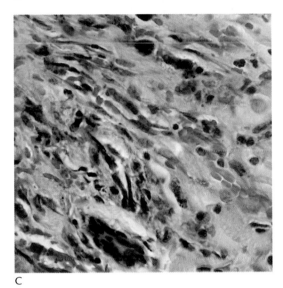

C

Fig. 12.16A, B, C. Histology of Kaposi's sarcoma. (A) Low-power photomicrograph (hematoxylin and eosin × 40) shows poorly circumscribed lesion that diffusely involves reticular dermis and has readily apparent vascular and spindle-cell features. (B) Higher power magnification (hematoxylin and eosin × 400) shows spindle-cell neoplastic component and occasional extravasated erythrocytes. (C) Higher power magnification (hematoxylin and eosin × 400) showing neoplastic vessels, multiple abnormal slit-like vascular spaces, marked cytologic atypia, and extravasated erythrocytes.

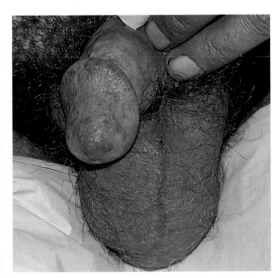

Fig. 12.17 Scabies lesions on the glans penis.

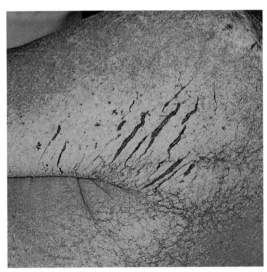

Fig. 12.18 Thick hyperkeratotic lesions of Norwegian scabies. Reproduced with permission from the *New England Journal of Medicine.*

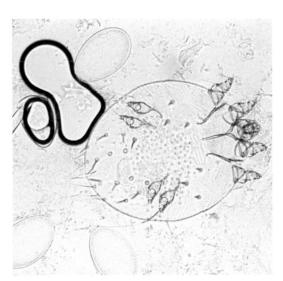

Fig. 12.19 Typical appearance of scabies mite (200×). Reproduced with permission from the *New England Journal of Medicine.*

Condition	Treatment
Xerosis	Mild: emollients (e.g. eucerin) Severe: add mild topical steroid
Kaposi's sarcoma	HAART Systemic chemotherapy (liposomal anthracyclin, paclitaxel, ABV) Local irradiation Liquid nitrogen
Eosinophilic pustular folliculitis	Antihistamines Topical steroids Ultraviolet light therapy 3–5×/week Metronidazole
Bacterial folliculitis	Antibiotics (dicloxacillin, cephalexin, amoxicillin-clavulanic acid); prolonged therapy often needed
Bacilliary angiomatosis	Erythromycin 500 mg po qid × 2–3 months Azithromycin 250–500 po qd × 2–3 months Clarithromycin 500 mg po bid × 2–3 months Doxycycline 100 mg po bid × 2–3 months
Seborrheic dermatitis	Mild; 2% ketoconazole cream bid Moderate-severe; 2% ketoconazole cream bid plus 1% hydrocortisone bid Refractory; ketoconazole 200 mg po qd
Molluscuscum contagiosum	Liquid nitrogen Retin-A 0.025% applied qhs
Warts	Liquid nitrogen Podophyllin Podophylox Imiquimod cream Surgery for severe non-responsive cases
Herpes zoster	Acyclovir 800 mg po 5×/day × 7–10d Famciclovir 500 mg po tid × 7–10d Valacyclovir 1000 mg po tid × 7–10d
Herpes simplex	Acyclovir 400 mg po tid × 7–10d Famciclovir 500 mg po bid × 7–10d Valacyclovir 500 mg po bid × 7–10d
Scabies	Pemethrin (5% cream); apply from neck down and leave on for 8–12 hours, repeat in 1 week Lindane (1% lotion): apply from neck down and leave on for 8–12 hours, repeat in 1 week Ivemectin (Crusted scabies) 200 µg/kg single dose (may need repeat treatment)

Table 12.2 Treatment of common dermatologic disorders.

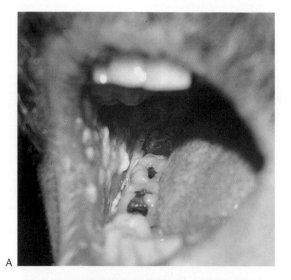

A

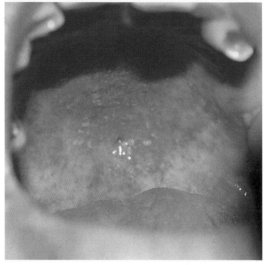

B

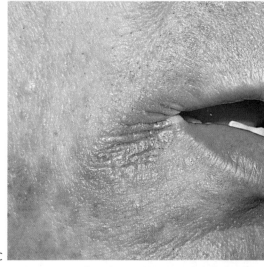

C

Fig. 12.20 A, B, C Three major clinical presentations of oral candidiasis.
(A) Pseudomembranous type with thick plaque-like lesions on the buccal mucosa.
(B) Erythematous (atrophic) type showing diffuse erythema of upper palate.
(C) Angular chelitis type that shows marked fissuring of the corners of the mouth.

Patients with early-stage HIV disease who develop oral herpes simplex infection typically present with symptoms similar to those seen in an immunocompetent individual, namely recurrent vesicular lesions on the lips or pharynx that resolve in 5 to 7 days. Individuals with advanced HIV disease, however, generally develop non-healing ulcerative lesions that may involve the tongue, gums, pharynx, or palate (*Fig. 12.22*). The diagnosis is usually made by either fluorescent antibody testing or by viral culture on a sample obtained from scraping the base of the lesion. Oral herpes simplex virus lesions and non-herpetic oral aphthae may be extremely difficult to distinguish from each other. Non-herpetic oral aphthae typically appear as painful, well-circumscribed, ulcerations, most often present on the labial mucosa, tongue, or soft palate (*Fig. 12.23*). The cause of these oral aphthae remains unknown. Less frequently, patients may develop other oral disorders, such as gingivitis or Kaposi's sarcoma (*Fig. 12.24*). A summary of the common oral disorders and their treatment is shown in *Table 12.3*.

PULMONARY DISORDERS

Streptococcus pneumoniae is the most common bacterial cause of severe pneumonia among HIV-infected individuals, occurring approximately 10 times more frequenty than among persons not infected with HIV. Black HIV-infected patients have the highest rate of invasive pneumococcal disease, with a rate approximately 5-fold greater than whites.[33] Patients often develop pneumococcal pneumonia before they develop other manifestations of immunosuppression, and most have clinical signs and symptoms similar to those in HIV-negative individuals. Chest radiographs show either segmental, lobar, or multilobar consolidation in approximately 75% of patients (*Fig. 12.25*). The major distinctive feature of pneumococcal pneumonia in HIV-infected individuals is the approximate 20-fold higher incidence of pneumococcal bacteremia. Although HIV-infected individuals usually respond well to typical treatment regimens and do not have higher mortality rates than HIV-negative persons,[34] they do have a higher relapse rate. Recent studies suggested no benefit of pneumococcal vaccine in sub-Saharan African patients[35] and in black patients in the United States,[36] but these findings may have predominantly resulted from inadequate vaccine responses in individuals with low CD4+ counts. In contrast, another study showed that HIV-infected individuals who received pneumococcal vaccine and had CD4+ counts greater than 500 cells/mm³ had a 50% decrease in the risk of pneumococcal disease.[37] Taken together, the available data suggest

Condition	Treatment

Candidiasis	Mild: clotrimazole troches: 10 mg 5×/d × 7–10 d
	Moderate-Severe:
	   Fluconazole: 100 mg po qd × 7–10 d
	   Ketoconazole: 200 mg po qd × 7–10 d
	   Itraconazole solution 100 mg bid × 7–10 d

Oral hairy leukoplakia	None
Herpes simplex	Acyclovir 400 mg po tid × 7–10 d (or until lesions heal) Famciclovir 500 gm bid × 7–10 d (or until lesions heal) Valacyclovir 500 to 100 mg bid × 7 to 10 d (or until lesions heal)

Aphthae	Symptomatic: 2% viscous lidocaine pm
	Mild: triamcinolone 0.1% with dental paste applied to lesions 3–4×/d
	Severe or recurrent:
	   Prednisone 40 mg po qd to taper over a month
	   Thalidomide

Gingivitis	Oral hygiene: brushing, flossing Mouth Rinses: 0.12% chlorhexidine tid Severe cases: antimicrobials (metronidazole, penicillin, or clindamycin)
Kaposi's sarcoma	Options include HAART, excision, local radiation, or chemotherapy

Table 12.3 Treatment of common oral disorders.

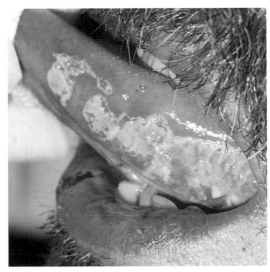

Fig. 12.21 Oral hairy leukoplakia on the side of tongue showing characteristic raised white lesions that generally are not removed by scraping.

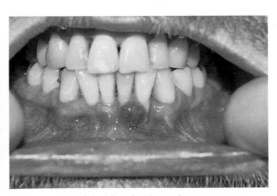

Fig. 12.24 Nodular, firm lesion on lower gums caused by Kaposi's sarcoma.

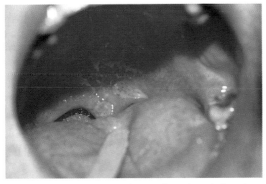

Fig. 12.22 Patient with advanced AIDS and chronic ulcerative oral lesions caused by herpes simplex virus.

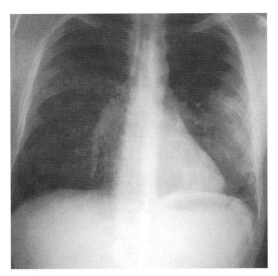

Fig. 12.25 Lobar pneumonia in a patient with pneumococcal pneumonia.

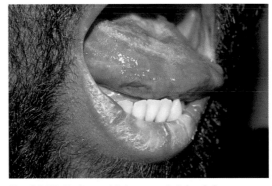

Fig. 12.23 Patient with large, painful aphthae on lateral aspect of tongue

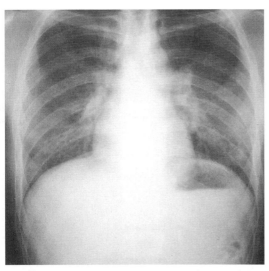

Fig. 12.26 Chest radiograph that shows characteristic diffuse interstitial perihilar infiltrates in a patient with *Pneumocystis carinii* pneumonia.

pneumococcal vaccine should be targeted to those individuals who have a CD4+ count greater than 200 cells/mm³ and ideally should be given as early as possible in the course of HIV disease, preferably when the CD4+ cell count is greater than 500 cells/mm³. Although other bacteria, such as *Haemophilus influenzae*, can cause pneumonia, they occur much less frequently than pneumococcal pneumonia. In contrast to immune-competent persons, those with AIDS have a significant proportion of cases of community-acquired pneumonia caused by *Pseudomonas aeruginosa*.

Pneumocystis carinii pneumonia has remained one of the most common AIDS-defining OIs, despite its marked decrease as a result of effective prophylaxis and antiretroviral therapy. Early in the course of *Pneumocystis carinii* pneumonia, patients usually have nonspecific systemic symptoms, such as fever, night sweats, malaise, and weight loss. Typically, patients then develop a non-productive cough followed by dyspnea. The physical examination is generally non-specific, but on occasion may reveal rales on chest auscultation. Patients with *Pneumocystis carinii* pneumonia usually have CD4+ cell counts less than 200 cells/mm³. The chest radiograph most often shows diffuse or perihilar interstitial infiltrates (*Fig. 12.26*). Less characteristic findings may include upper lobe infiltrates and cystic changes (*Fig 12.27*). In addition, up to 20% of patients with *Pneumocystis carinii* pneumonia present with a normal chest radiograph.

The approach to the evaluation of the patient with suspected *Pneumocystis carinii* pneumonia depends on the index of suspicion for this infection and the clinical stability of the patient. A definitive diagnosis can be made using Papanicolaou smears, silver stains, or monoclonal antibody tests on material obtained from an induced sputum, bronchoalveolar lavage, or rarely, transbronchial biopsy (*Fig 12.28A–D*). Although the diagnostic yield of induced sputum (approximately 60%) is significantly less than with bronchoalveolar lavage (approximately 90%), it is often first performed because it is a non-invasive test. Those patients with negative induced sputum should proceed to bronchoscopy. Because bronchoalveolar lavage has such a high yield, transbronchial biopsy is rarely necessary. Although effective treatment for *Pneumocystis carinii* pneumonia has significantly improved the survival of HIV-infected patients, fatalities still occur (*Fig. 12.29*). Patients with CD4+ counts less than 200 cells/mm³ or a history of *Pneumocystis carinii* pneumonia should receive prophylaxis for this infection. Multiple studies have now shown that persons on highly active antiretroviral therapy who have sustained CD4+ cell count increases to above 200 and sustained suppression of HIV can safely discontinue *Pneumocystis carinii* pneumonia prophylaxis.[15,16]

Although the incidence of tuberculosis has declined recently in the United States, an estimated 6,000 to 9,000 new cases still occur annually[38,39] and tuberculosis remains the most important infection in HIV-infected patients worldwide (*Fig. 12.30*). Tuberculosis can occur at any stage of HIV disease. In general, the presentation of tuberculosis in patients with early-stage HIV differs from that in patients with AIDS. Patients with early-stage HIV disease present similarly to HIV-negative individuals, namely they usually have a positive purified protein derivative (PPD) skin test, chest radiographs show upper lobe involvement (frequently with cavitation) (*Fig. 12.31*), and extrapulmonary disease infrequently occurs. In contrast, patients with CD4+ counts less than 200 cells/mm³ often have an atypical presentation characterized by a negative PPD, middle, lower lobe, or diffuse infiltrates, mediastinal adenopathy, and by extrapulmonary disease. Regardless of the stage of HIV disease, the diagnosis of tuberculosis pneumonia is based on the isolation of *M. tuberculosis* from material obtained from the respiratory tract (usually sputum). Acid-fast smear-positive specimens from individuals clinically suspected to have tuberculosis bolster the diagnosis (*Fig. 12.32*). Smear-positive specimens from patients at intermediate or low risk for tuberculosis who could also be colonized or infected with atypical mycobacteria can present a diagnostic dilemma. In these cases, rapid tests that detect *M. tuberculosis* ribosomal RNA or DNA are of value when they yield a positive result. Patients at all stages of HIV disease generally respond to standard anti-tuberculosis therapy, assuming the infecting strains are not drug resistant. Multidrug-resistant tuberculosis was responsible for outbreaks of disease in New York and Florida in the early 1990s, due primarily to poor adherence to anti-tuberculosis therapy and lax infection control measures. Although the rates of multidrug-resistant tuberculosis have decreased substantially in industrialized countries, non-adherence to therapy remains the greatest risk for a resurgence of this difficult to treat infection. In developing countries, multi-drug-resistant tuberculosis is being seen with increased frequency in a number of hospitals. All HIV-infected patients should undergo PPD testing and those at continued risk for tuberculosis should be tested annually.

Other less common processes may involve the lung. For example, although HIV-infected patients with *Mycobacterium avium* complex (MAC) infection generally present with disseminated disease, focal pulmonary disease can occur, albeit infrequently. In addition, isolation of MAC from the respiratory tract has a good predictive value for the development of MAC bacteremia, even among patients without pulmonary symptoms. Obtaining respiratory cultures for screening purposes, however, is not recommended, mainly because of their low sensitivity. Most patients who develop disease caused by MAC have CD4+ counts less than 50 cells/mm³.

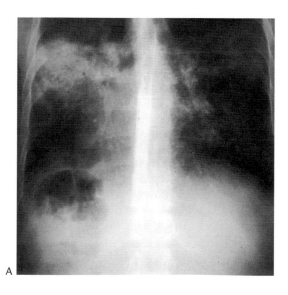

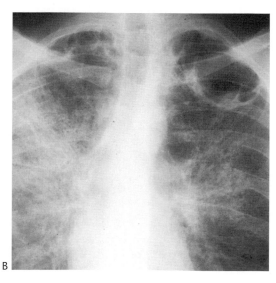

Fig. 12.27 A, B Chest radiograph that shows diffuse interstitial perihilar infiltrates and cystic changes in left upper lobe (courtesy of Douglas Paauw, M.D., Department of Medicine, University of Washington Medical Center, Seattle, WA).

A

B

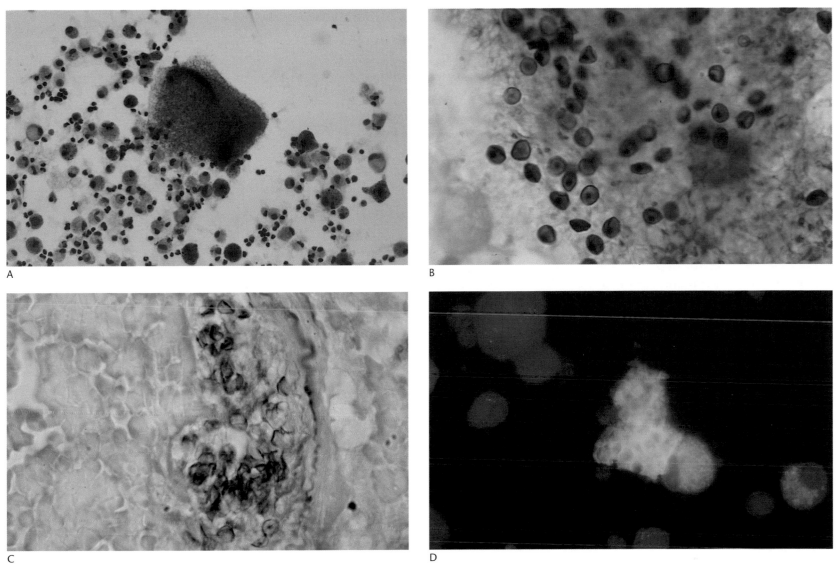

Fig. 12.28 A–D (A) Bronchoalveolar lavage cytospin preparation that shows mass of *Pneumocystis carinii* organisms appearing as green-brown abnormalities; the individual cysts are not apparent. Larger pigmented alveolar macrophages are evident (Papanicolaou stain (× 250). (B) Bronchoalveolar lavage cytospin preparation with the Gomori Methanamine silver stain (× 1000) that shows individual *Pneumocystis carinii* cysts; the cyst walls are stained using this stain and several cells show the characteristic central dot. (C) Transbronchial lung biopsy that identifies cysts, but the morphology often appears more distorted than in smear preparations (Gomori Methanamine silver stain ×1000). (D) Indirect immunofluorescent stain (× 400) using monoclonal antibody specific for *Pneumocystis carinii*; the organisms stain green and are in clusters; the alveolar macrophages stain red (courtesy of Thomas Fritsche, M.D., Ph.D, Department of Microbiology, University of Washington, Seattle, WA).

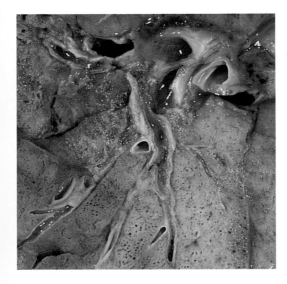

Fig. 12.29 Autopsy lung tissue from patient with AIDS and diffuse *Pneumocystis carinii* pneumonia. The lung tissue shows diffuse consolidation and patchy areas of induration and mucous plugging of bronchioles.

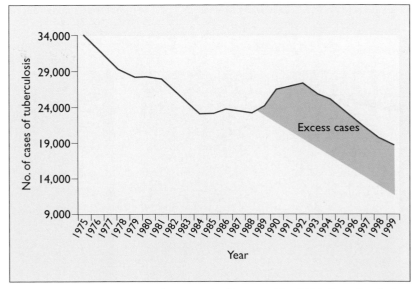

Fig. 12.30 Incidence of tuberculosis in United States, 1975–1999. From Small PM, Fujiwara PI. Management of tuberculosis in the United States. *N Engl J Med* 2001; **345**:189–200.

Cytomegalovirus rarely causes clinically significant pulmonary disease, despite its frequent isolation from the respiratory tract. Moreover, isolation of cytomegalovirus from the respiratory tract has not been shown to be a good predictor for the development of cytomegalovirus disease of the retina or gastrointestinal tract. HIV-infected individuals who develop cytomegalovirus pneumonia nearly always have advanced HIV disease and often have other immunosuppressing conditions such as malignancies, steroid therapy, or chemotherapy. It is not uncommon for these patients to have co-infecting pulmonary pathogens, such as *Aspergillus* spp., in addition to cytomegalovirus. Since culture of respiratory specimens lack specificity for cytomegalovirus-induced pneumonia, the diagnosis rests on histologic evidence of infection demonstrating characteristic cytomegalic inclusions.

Among HIV-infected individuals, infection with *Cryptococcus neoformans* most commonly involves the central nervous system, but because the lungs serve as the portal of entry for this organism, patients may develop pulmonary cryptococcosis. When pulmonary cryptococcosis does occur, approximately 70% of patients have evidence of disseminated infection, with positive cultures from either blood or the cerebrospinal fluid. Patients who develop pulmonary cryptococcosis usually present with non-specific symptoms, such as fever, cough, dyspnea, headache, and weight loss. Chest radiography most often shows either focal or diffuse interstitial infiltrates, but less commonly, nodular patterns, pleural effusions, or lymphadenopathy are apparent (*Fig. 12.33*). The diagnosis depends on identifying cryptococcal organisms from fluid or tissue specimens. In addition, tests for serum cryptococcal antigen are usually positive. *Histoplasma capsulatum* is a rare cause of pulmonary disease, except among those patients from highly endemic areas in the midwestern United States. Almost all HIV-infected patients who develop histoplasmosis present with disseminated disease and approximately 85% have a CD4+ cell count less than 100 cells/mm^3.[40] Approximately 5% of patients, however, will develop focal pulmonary disease. The diagnosis can be made by stain and culture of respiratory specimens, although identification by culture can take up to 6 weeks. In the case of disseminated disease, the histoplasma antigen detection test provides a rapid, reliable method of diagnosis with a sensitivity of 70% in bronchoalveolar lavage fluid, 85% in serum, and 95% in urine.[41]

Kaposi's sarcoma is a serious non-infectious pulmonary disorder that can occur among HIV-infected patients. Pulmonary Kaposi's sarcoma causes symptoms that include dyspnea, cough, and on occasion, hemoptysis. Although most patients have concomitant cutaneous involvement, some may have isolated pulmonary disease. Chest radiographic appearances include diffuse reticular-nodular lesions that have irregular borders, mediastinal enlargement, and less frequently, pleural

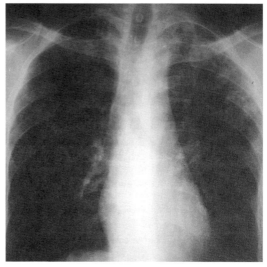

Fig. 12.31 Chest radiograph that shows left upper lobe infiltrate due to *Mycobacterium tuberculosis*.

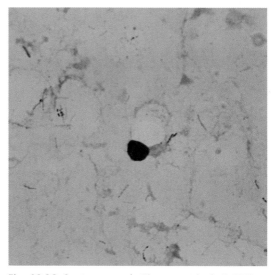

Fig. 12.32 Sputum sample Kinyoun stain (× 1,000) that shows numerous red-purple acid-fast bacilli.

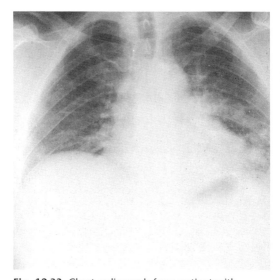

Fig. 12.33 Chest radiograph from patient with pulmonary cryptococcosis that shows nodular pulmonary infiltrates.

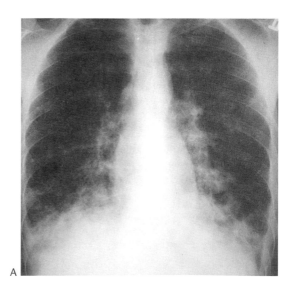

A

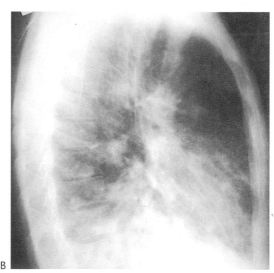

B

Fig. 12.34A (PA view), B (lateral view) Chest radiographs from patient with pulmonary Kaposi's sarcoma that show bilateral interstitial and nodular infiltrates.

effusion (*Fig. 12.34A, B*). The diagnosis is made by viewing endobronchial lesions during bronchoscopy, or by histologic examination of a transbronchial or open lung biopsy specimen. Many patients with Kaposi's sarcoma, including those with visceral disease, respond to treatment with antiretroviral therapy alone, although those with extensive disease may require chemotherapy. Response rates are higher in those with less extensive disease and higher CD4+ counts.[42] A summary of the common pulmonary disorders and their treatment is shown in *Table 12.4*.

GASTROINTESTINAL DISORDERS

Two major types of gastrointestinal manifestation predominate in HIV-infected patients: 1) esophagitis; and 2) diarrhea. The major causes of esophagitis include candida (*Fig. 12.35*), cytomegalovirus (*Fig. 12.36*), herpes simplex virus (*Fig. 12.37*), aphthous lesions, and acid reflux. These disorders, except for acid reflux, most commonly occur in patients with CD4+ counts less than 100 cells/mm^3. On occasion, esophageal Kaposi's sarcoma may mimic these disorders. In general, regardless of the cause of the esophagitis, patients present with odynophagia and retrosternal chest pain. Because candida esophagitis is the most common of these disorders, most recommend empirically treating esophagitis as presumptive candida esophagitis, and if not improved in 3 to 5 days, then proceeding to upper endoscopy with biopsy (*Fig. 12.38*). The treatment of common esophageal disorders is shown in *Table 12.5*.

Among HIV-infected patients, diarrhea is a frequent cause of morbidity. The differential diagnosis is extensive and the more common causes of diarrhea are listed in *Table 12.6*. The diagnosis of the offending pathogen generally requires a stepwise approach (*Table 12.7*). The most common HIV-associated bacterial enteric pathogens, *Salmonella* spp., *Shigella* spp., and *Campylobacter* spp., occur more

frequently among HIV-infected patients than among persons who do not have HIV. These infections usually cause diarrhea and fever and patients often have cultures that are positive from blood as well as from stool. Because HIV-infected patients frequently receive antimicrobials, *Clostridium difficile* also may cause diarrhea.

The parasite *Cryptosporidium parvum*, a coccidian protozoan, can causes severe, watery, cholera-like diarrhea with cramps, and, in some instances, nausea and vomiting. Its life cycle is shown in *Fig. 12.39*. Among HIV-infected patients with CD4+ counts greater than 200 cells/mm^3, cryptosporidiosis usually causes a self-limited diarrheal illness, similar to the illness in normal hosts. In contrast, patients with CD4+ counts less than 200 cells/mm^3 typically develop unremitting diarrhea associated with weight loss and generalized wasting. In one study, cryptosporidia were found in 21% of patients with AIDS and diarrhea. Oocysts can be found in the stool using a modified acid-fast stain (*Fig. 12.40*). Although the diagnosis can also be made by small bowel biopsy (*Fig. 12.41*), this is usually not required. In addition to causing intestinal disease, cryptosporidia are the most common cause of HIV cholangiopathy, an ascending, acalculous (often sclerosing) cholangitis with papillary stenosis causing both extra- and intra-hepatic biliary obstruction and dilatation.

Microsporidia, most commonly *Encephalitozoon bieneusi*, *Encephalitozoon intestinalis* or *Encephalitozoon hellum*, can cause infections in HIV-infected persons, including enteritis, hepatitis, cholangiopathy, peritonitis and disseminated disease. Patients usually have advanced HIV disease with CD4+ counts less than 100 cells/mm^3. The diagnosis can be difficult and is best made using a modified trichrome stain (Weber stain) or calcofluor stain (*Fig. 12.42A, B*). Electron microscopy permits species identification.[43] Another coccidian protozoan, *Isospora belli*, can cause a diarrheal illness similar to cryptosporidiosis. Isosporiasis is most frequently seen in the tropics, particularly in Haiti. Iodine-stained wet mounts and modified acid-fast stool smears may reveal oocysts that are significantly larger than the cryptosporidial oocysts (*Fig. 12.43*).

Giardia lamblia, a common pathogen among HIV-infected patients, causes problems ranging from asymptomatic infection to profuse watery diarrhea, abdominal cramps, bloating, nausea, and severe malabsorption. Direct stool examination may reveal trophozoites or cysts (*Fig. 12.44*). Other tests used to diagnose giardia include stool antigen detection and upper endoscopy with duodenal biopsy. Amebiasis, caused by *Entamoeba histolytica*, may cause proctocolitis with diarrhea, tenesmus, cramps, abdominal pain, and rectal discharge. Amebic colitis may resemble ulcerative colitis (*Fig. 12.45A, B*). For HIV-infected patients, this disorder is found more frequently among men who have sex with other men. When the diagnosis is suspected, multiple stool samples for ova and

Condition	Treatment
Pneumococcal pneumonia	Ceftriaxone 1–2 g IV qd
PCP (Treatment)*	TMP/SMZ: 15–20 mg/kg (TMP)/d po or IV in 3–4 divided doses × 21 d or TMP/Dapsone: TMP 15–20 mg/kg/d in 3–4 divided doses plus Dapsone 100 mg po qd or Pentamidine: 3–4 mg/kg IV qd × 21 d or Clindamycin/Primaquine: clindamycin 600 mg po tid plus primaquine 15 mg base po qd × 21 d or Atovaquone: 750 mg po bid × 21 d
Tuberculosis	Isoniazid: 300 mg po qd × 9–12 months plus Rifampin: 600 mg po qd × 9–12 months plus Pyrazinamide: 20 mg/kg po qd × 2 months plus Ethambutol: 20 mg/kg po qd (discontinue if isolate not drug-resistant)
Kaposi's sarcoma	HAART first Systemic chemotherapy

Patients with marked hypoxia (pO$_2$ less than 70) should receive adjunctive corticosteroid therapy.

Table 12.4 Treatment of common pulmonary disorders.

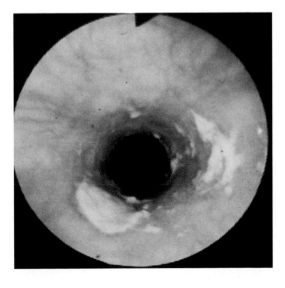

Fig. 12.35 Endoscopic appearance of candida esophagitis. Reproduced with permission from Silverstein, Endoscopy Atlas.

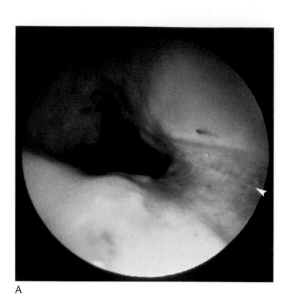

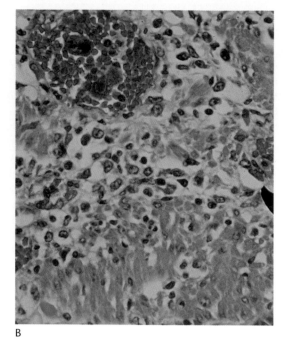

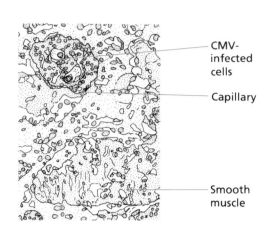

CMV-infected cells

Capillary

Smooth muscle

Fig. 12.36A, B (A) Endoscopic view showing large ulcerated esophageal lesion caused by cytomegalovirus. (B) Typical intranuclear and intracytoplasmic inclusions are seen within two cytomegalovirus-infected endothelial cells. Reproduced with permission from Silverstein, Endoscopy Atlas.

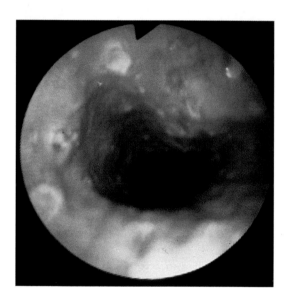

Fig. 12.37 Endoscopic view showing multiple ulcerated esophageal lesions caused by herpes simplex infection. Reproduced with permission from Silverstein, Endoscopy Atlas.

Condition	Treatment
Candida esophagitis	Fluconazole: 200 mg po qd × 3d then 100 mg po qd × 18 d Intraconazole solution 100 mg po bid × 14–21d Amphotericin 0.3 to 0.5 mg/kg/day (IV)
Cytomegalovirus esophagitis	Ganciclovir: 5 mg/kg IV bid × 2–4 weeks then 6 mg/kg IV qd Foscarnet: 60 mg/kg IV tid × 2–4 weeks then 100 mg/kg IV qd Valganciclovir 900 mg PO bid × 2–4 weeks, then 900 mg PO qd
Herpes esophagitis	Acyclovir: 400 mg po tid (may require larger doses or IV dosing) × 14–21 d Famciclovir 500 mg tid × 14–21 d Valacyclovir 1000 mg bid × 14–21 d
Kaposi's sarcoma	HAART first Systemic chemotherapy

Table 12.5 Treatment of common esophageal disorders.

Bacterial	Viral	Parasitic	Neoplastic
Salmonella spp. Shigella spp. Campylobacter spp. Mycobacterium avium-complex Clostridium difficille	Cytomegalovirus HIV	Cryptosporidium parvum Entamoeba histolytica Giardia lamblia Isospora belli	Kaposi's sarcoma Lymphoma

Table 12.6 Common causes of diarrhea in HIV-infected patients.

Initial studies	If initial studies are nondiagnostic consider the following
Stool culture (for Salmonella, Shigella, and Campylobacter	Weber Stain (for microsporidia)
Modified acid-fast stain (for Cryptosporidium and Isospora)	Sigmoidoscopy with biopsy
Microscopic evaluation of stool for ova and parasites × 3	Upper endoscopy with duodenal or small bowel biopsy
Evaluation of stool for Clostridium difficile toxin (if patient has been taking antibiotics recently)	

Table 12.7 Evaluation of diarrhea in HIV-infected patients.

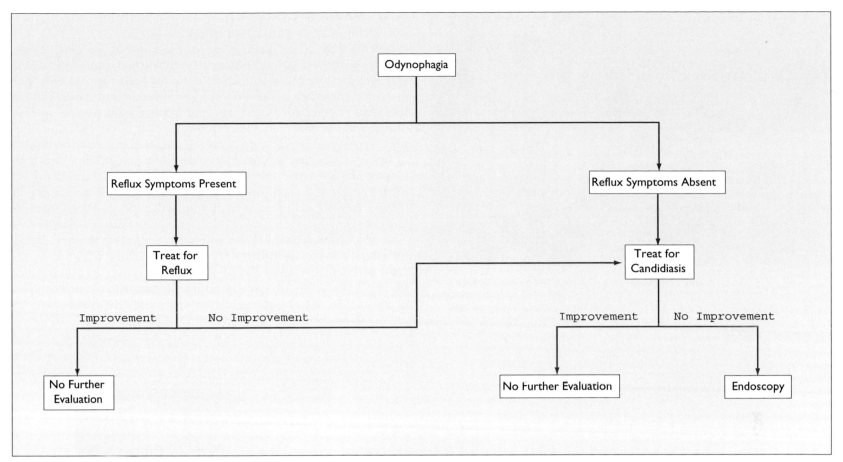

Fig. 12.38 Evaluation of odynophagia.

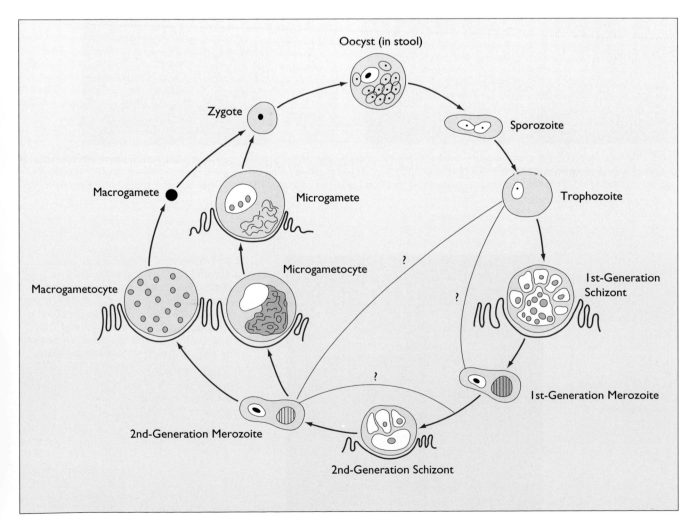

Fig. 12.39 Life cycle of *Cryptosporidium parvum*.

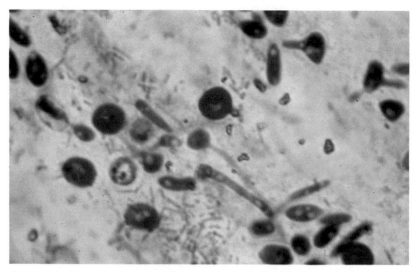

Fig. 12.40 Although cryptosporidia are occasionally identified in unstained and iodine-stained concentrated wet mounts, they are best identified by performing a modifed acid-fast stain on smears. Oocysts appear as circular red organisms 4 to 6 μm in diameter. Sporozoites can occasionally be seen within oocysts. (Modified acid-fast stain, × 1000).

parasites should be collected (*Fig. 12.46*) and, if negative, the diagnosis can usually be made with bowel biopsy.

Patients with lower gastrointestinal tract cytomegalovirus disease almost always have advanced-stage HIV disease and commonly present with diarrhea, weight loss, nausea, vomiting, and pain. As with pulmonary cytomegalovirus disease, stool or lower intestinal swab cultures that yield cytomegalovirus are non-specific since many patients without disease will intermittently shed cytomegalovirus in the gastrointestinal tract. Appearance at endoscopy is variable, showing either normal mucosa or discrete ulcerated lesions. As compared to proctocolitis caused by herpes simplex virus, the ulcerative lesions of cytomegalovirus are usually single or few and deeply penetrating. The diagnosis is made by biopsy showing cytoplasmic inclusion bodies on histologic samples (*Fig. 12.47*).

Mycobacterium avium complex is another important cause of gastrointestinal disease. Identifying *Mycobacterium avium* complex as the cause of enteritis or colitis usually occurs in the context of disseminated *Mycobacterium avium* complex infection. *Mycobacterium avium* complex is also on the list of pathogens that can cause HIV cholangiopathy.

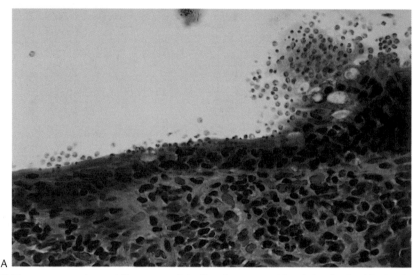
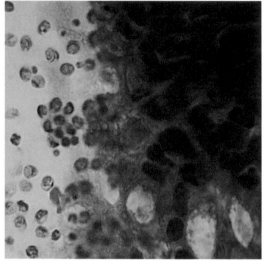

Fig. 12.41 (A) Numerous cryptosporidia are seen infecting the mucosal brush border in this duodenal biopsy. The organisms appear as small, 4 to 6 μm in diameter, round, basophilic bodies (hematoxylin and eosin × 40). (B) Higher magnification (hematoxylin and eosin × 400) showing numerous cryptosporidia adherent to brush border of duodenal mucosal. The organisms do not exhibit acid-fastness in histologic sections, because the stage of the organism infecting small bowel mucosal is different than stage of organism passed in stool.

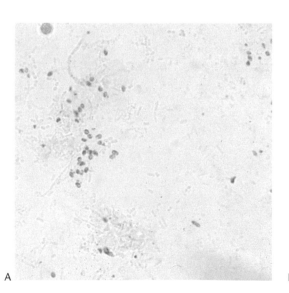
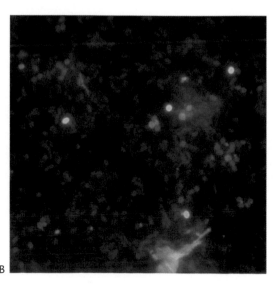

Fig. 12.42 (A) Modified trichrome stain (Weber stain) of stool sample showing red-stained microsporidia. (B) Calcifluor stain showing brightly staining scattered microsporidia organisms that are few in number; abundant, but less intense staining bacteria are present as background material. (Courtesy of Thomas Fritsche, MD, PhD, Department of Microbiology, University of Washington, Seattle, WA.)

Gastrointestinal symptoms usually include nausea, abdominal pain, diarrhea, anemia, and weight loss. Abdominal computed tomographic scans may show associated enlarged retroperitoneal lymph nodes and a thickened bowel wall. A stool culture positive for *Mycobacterium avium* complex suggests the diagnosis of intestinal *Mycobacterium avium* complex, but this should be confirmed by bowel biopsy (*Fig. 12.48*). Rapid diagnosis of disseminated disease can be made by acid-fast stain of bone marrow, liver, or lymph node biopsies. More commonly the diagnosis of disseminated *Mycobacterium avium* complex is made by culturing *Mycobacterium avium* complex from blood, a process that typically takes 12 to 14 days.

Among the tumors of the gastrointestinal tract described in patients with AIDS, Kaposi's sarcoma is the most common. Kaposi's sarcoma lesions can develop in the stomach, small bowel, large bowel, and the anorectal area. These tumors are usually asymptomatic, but in some instances, can bleed, obstruct the bowel lumen, or cause perforation. Because superficial biopsy may not detect submucosal lesions, biopsies are sometimes falsely negative. As with pulmonary Kaposi's sarcoma, many patients with gastrointestinal Kaposi's sarcoma often respond to

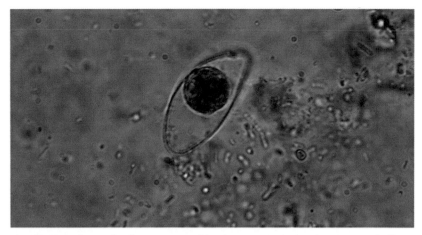

Fig. 12.43 Iodine-stained wet mount of fecal concentrate showing *Isospora belli*. The photomicrograph shows an immature oocyst 25–30 μm in diameter with a single central granular zygote. Similar to cryptospordia, isospora are best identified with a modified acid-fast stain.

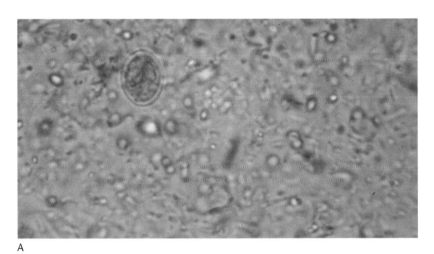

A

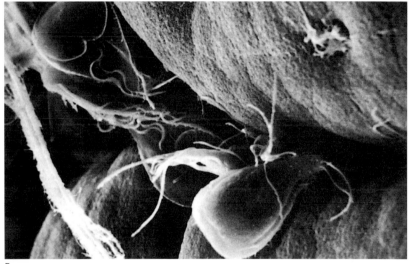

B

Fig. 12.44 (A) Cyst of *Giardia lamblia* showing ovoid shape, prominent cyst wall, granular cytoplasm, and at least two nuclei. (B) Scanning electron micrograph (× 1,550) of Giardia trophozoites in a crevice of a jejunal villus.

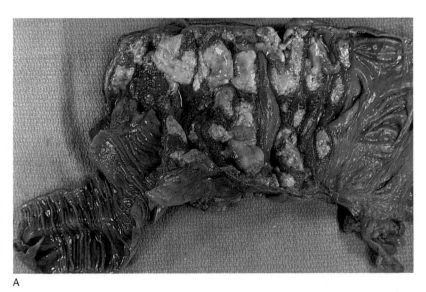

A

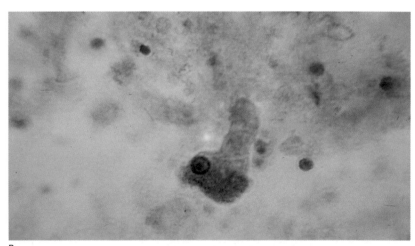

B

Fig. 12.45 (A) Markedly dilated segment of proximal large bowel showing numerous ulcers (whitish-green mucosal defects) caused by *Entamoeba histolytica*; (B) *Entamoeba histolytica* trophozoite. Note the single nucleus (Trichrome stain × 1,000).

antiretroviral therapy alone. The treatment of common intestinal disorders is shown in *Table 12.8*. In addition to developing esophagitis and diarrhea, HIV-infected individuals who have male-to-male sex frequently have abnormalities of the perianal region. These most common conditions include perianal warts (*Fig. 12.49*), herpes simplex virus infection (*Fig. 12.50*), Kaposi's sarcoma, and human papillomavirus-related anal dysplasia and carcinoma.

NEUROLOGIC DISORDERS

HIV-infected patients frequently develop neurologic problems, especially with advanced HIV disease. Any patient with AIDS who presents with new neurologic complaints or a new abnormal neurologic finding should have a clinical evaluation that includes a complete neurological examination, and, if either meningitis, encephalopathy, or a brain mass lesion is suspected, they should have further evaluation that may include brain imaging and lumbar puncture.

Cryptococcal meningitis is the most common central nervous system infection in patients with AIDS. This infection, caused by the fungus *Cryptococcus neoformans*, usually involves patients who have CD4+ counts less than 100 cells/mm³ and typically manifests as a subacute to chronic illness characterized by fever, headache, malaise, altered mental status, and less frequently, photophobia or neck stiffness. Patients with altered mental status, a non-inflammatory cerebrospinal fluid, and a high cerebrospinal fluid cryptococcal antigen titer have a poor prognosis. The diagnosis of cryptococcal meningitis can be confirmed on a cerebrospinal fluid sample using one or more of three available tests: India ink, cryptococcal antigen, or culture. The India ink assay (*Fig. 12.51*) is the most rapid, but has significantly lower sensitivity than the cryptococcal antigen test, and operators inexperienced with the India ink test can confuse white blood cells with yeasts. The cryptococcal antigen test is the standard rapid diagnostic for cryptococcal meningitis and has a sensitivity in cerebrospinal fluid greater than 95%.[44] Individuals with extremely high antigen titers can have a paradoxically negative antigen test due to the prozone phenomenon. In these cases dilution of the cerebrospinal fluid will yield a positive result. For the initial diagnosis, any detectable cryptococcal antigen titer on a cerebro-

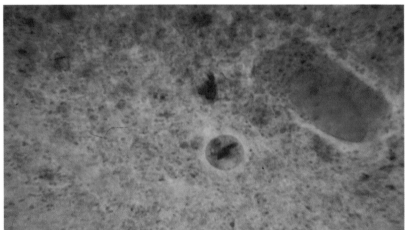

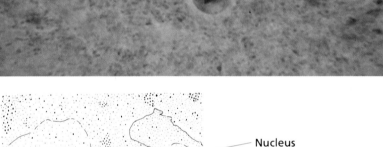

Fig. **12.46** Iodine wet mount (× 400) that shows *Entamoeba histolytica* cyst with one rounded nucleus in left upper portion of organism and several cytoplasmic chromatoidal bodies in middle of organism.

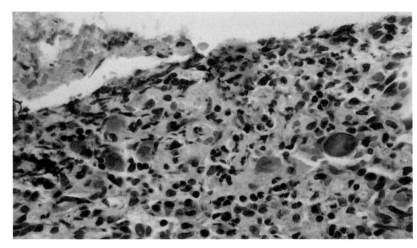

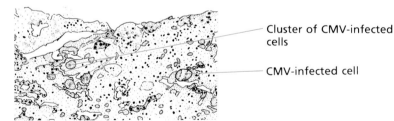

Fig. **12.47** Numerous cytomegalovirus-infected cells present within the lamina propria of colon (hematoxylin and eosin × 400).

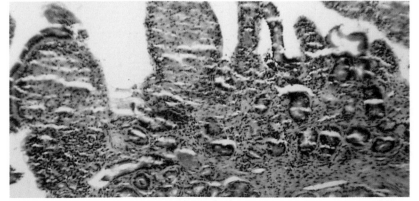

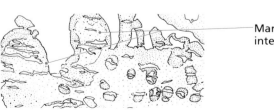

Fig. **12.48** Numerous acid-fast bacilli filling the cytoplasm of histocytes in small bowel; the intestinal infection was caused by *Mycobacterium avium* complex (Ziehl–Nelson stain × 1000).

spinal fluid specimen is reliable evidence of cryptococcal meningitis; patients with cryptococcal meningitis, however, frequently maintain a positive cerebrospinal fluid titer during treatment without evidence of persistent central nervous system infection. Cultures for *C. neoformans*, which generally take at least several days before turning positive, are predominantly used to confirm the initial diagnosis and to follow treatment responses. Serum cryptococcal antigen titers are positive in greater than 95% of patients with cryptococcal meningitis, but are not useful for following patients with known disease.

Toxoplasma encephalitis, caused by the protozoan parasite *Toxoplasma gondii*, is the most common cause of focal central nervous system mass lesions in patients with AIDS. In almost all cases, Toxoplasma encephalitis results from reactivation of latent infection in patients who have CD4+ counts less than 100 cells/mm³. The clinical presentation is characterized by fever, headache, mental status changes, and less often, seizures. Since the definitive diagnosis of toxoplasma encephalitis requires brain biopsy, most cases are diagnosed presumptively based on clinical presentation, radiographic appearance, and response to therapy. Patients

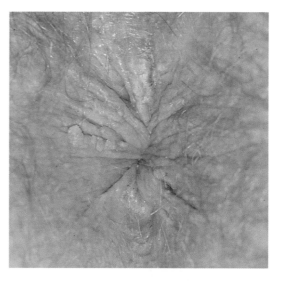

Fig. 12.49 Raised, irregular perianal warts.

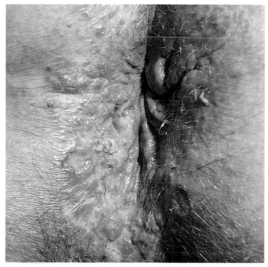

Fig. 12.50 Perianal vesicular and ulcerative lesions caused by herpes simplex virus infection.

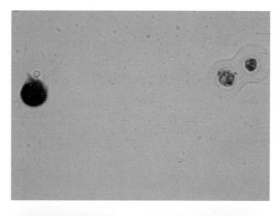

Fig. 12.51 Irregular violet-staining budding yeast with visible capsule, typical of *Cryptococcus neoformans*, present in cerebrospinal fluid specimen. A darkly staining small lymphocyte is present on left side of smear.

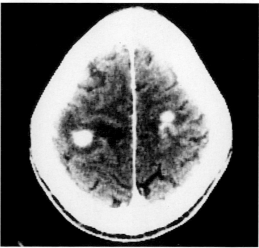

Fig. 12.52 Contrast brain CT scan showing two enhancing lesions compatible with CNS toxoplasmosis.

Condition	Treatment	Response
Salmonellosis	Ciprofloxacin: 500 mg po bid × 21d	Good
Campylobacter	Ciprofloxacin: 500 mg po bid × 14d	Good
Shigellosis	Ciprofloxacin: 500 mg po bid × 14d	Good
Clostridium difficile	Metronidazole: 500 mg po tid × 10d	Good
	or	
	Vancomycin: 125 mg po qid × 10d	Good
Cryptosporidiosis	HAART first	
	Paromomycin: 500 mg po tid × 30d, then	Fair
	500 mg po bid	
	plus	
	Azithromycin: 500 mg po bid × 30d, then	Fair
	500 mg po qd	
Microsporidiosis	HAART first	Unknown
	Albendazole: 400 mg po bid × 4 weeks	
Amebiasis	Metronidazole: 750mg po tid × 10d,	Good
	followed by	
	Paromomycin: 500 mg po tid × 7d	
	or	
	Iodoquinol: 650 mg po tid × 20d	
Isosporiasis	TMP/SMZ: 1 DS po qid × 10d, then	Good
	1 DS po bid × 20d	
Giardiasis	Metronidazole: 500 mg po tid × 10d	Good
Cytomegalovirus	Ganciclovir: 5 mg/kg IV bid × 2–4 weeks	Fair
	or	
(enteritis, colitis)	Foscarnet: 90 mg/kg IV bid × 2–4 weeks	
	or	
	Valcyclovir 900 mg bid × 2–4 weeks	
MAC enteritis	Clarithromycin: 500 mg po bid	
	(or Azithromycin 600 mg po qd)	
	plus	
	Ethambutol: 1,200 mg po qd	Good
	Plus/minus	
	Ciprofloxacin: 500 mg po bid or rifabutin	
	300 mg po qd	
Kaposi's sarcoma	HAART first	Fair
	Systemic chemotherapy	

Table 12.8 Treatment of common intestinal disorders.

with serologic evidence of previous infection with *T. gondii* and CT scans showing multiple ring-enhancing lesions (*Fig. 12.52*) are started on empiric therapy. If the patient does not respond to therapy within 14 days, or if they deteriorate despite therapy, a brain biopsy is generally indicated (*Fig. 12.53A, B*). In addition, brain biopsy may be indicated for patients who have negative serology for *T. gondii*, and a solitary brain lesion on magnetic resonance imaging (MRI). Some authors have suggested that a positive single photon emission computed tomography (SPECT) and positron emission tomography (PET) supports the diagnosis of alternative conditions, such as primary central nervous system lymphoma. Cerebrospinal fluid examination is nonspecific and may be normal. Use of toxoplasma PCR amplification assays and serology for toxoplasma performed on cerebrospinal fluid has not been reliable. Similarly, serum serological testing to determine acute rises in IgM toxoplasma titers is not reliable.

Patients who develop central nervous system lymphoma present with symptoms and signs that resemble those seen in patients with toxoplasma encephalitis. This tumor is usually induced by Epstein–Barr virus and occurs in patients with advanced HIV disease. The diagnosis is first suggested if a patient has only one or two lesions present on CT (or MRI) scanning and a negative toxoplasma serology. In addition, if a patient fails to respond to anti-toxoplasma therapy, the likelihood that the lesion is a lymphoma markedly increases (*Fig. 12.54A, B*). Since more than 90% of primary central nervous system lymphomas are associated with Epstein–Barr virus, PCR for Epstein–Barr virus in cerebrospinal fluid is a useful test and carries a sensitivity and specificity of more than 95%.[45] Definitive diagnosis requires brain biopsy but many experts will treat patients without a biopsy in the presence of a characteristic clinical presentation and a positive Epstein–Barr virus PCR on cerebrospinal fluid.

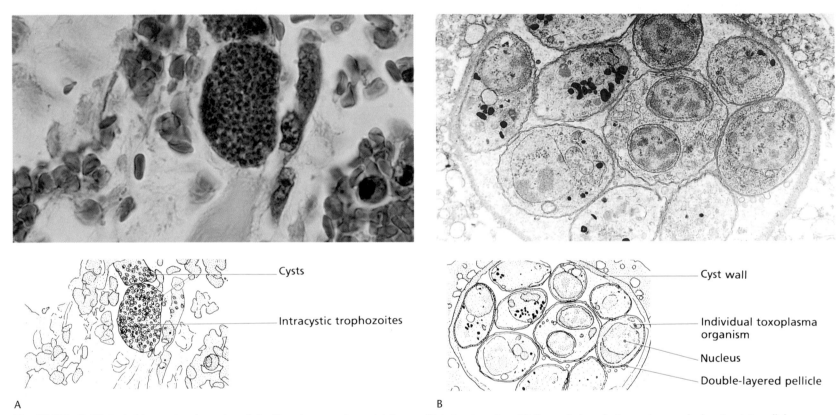

Cysts

Intracystic trophozoites

Cyst wall

Individual toxoplasma organism

Nucleus

Double-layered pellicle

A   B

Fig. 12.53A, B (A) Brain biopsy showing extracellular *Toxoplasma* cysts containing multiple trophozoites. (B) Transmission electron micrograph showing intracellular *Toxoplasma* cyst that contained 10 intracystic organisms.

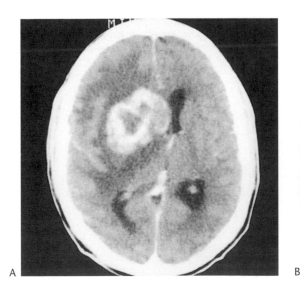
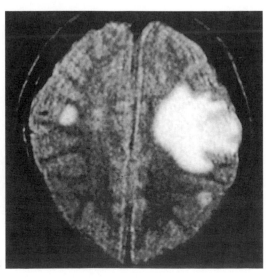

Fig. 12.54 (A) Contrast CT scan showing a large lesion impinging on the ventricles with shift of midline structures. Biopsy of the lesion revealed lymphoma. (B) MRI scan showing a large lesion that was determined to be lymphoma on biopsy.

A   B

Progressive multifocal leukoencephalopathy (PML), a rare, progressive, demyelinating disease, results from reactivation of a papovavirus known as JC virus. This disorder typically only occurs when a patient's CD4+ count decreases to less than 100 cells/mm³. Signs and symptoms are often non-specific and include headache, behavioral changes, mental impairment, dementia, visual field deficits, ataxia, limb weakness, and dysarthria. The diagnosis can strongly be suggested by the characteristic appearance of white matter lesions on CT (*Fig. 12.55*) or MRI scan (*Fig. 12.56*). The MRI scan generally shows more numerous and extensive lesions than CT scan, and, in some instances, the MRI scan is strongly positive when the CT scan does not show any evidence of PML. PCR performed on cerebrospinal fluid for JC virus is highly specific and has a sensitivity greater than 70%.[45] Brain biopsy is needed for definitive diagnosis but this rarely is done because the disease is seldom confused with other conditions.

Patients with early neurosyphilis (meningeal or meningovascular) present with headaches, photophobia, cranial nerve involvement, or stroke, typically within 10 years after the patient developed secondary syphilis. The diagnosis is suspected in patients with positive serologic tests and confirmed with cerebrospinal fluid studies. Late neurosyphilis (paresis and tabes dorsalis) rarely occurs among HIV-infected patients, or in any other patient in the present-day antibiotic era.

HIV itself may cause significant neurologic disease, including aseptic meningitis, peripheral neuropathy, and AIDS-associated dementia. The most common of these, AIDS-associated dementia, usually presents with mental slowing, impaired memory, decreased concentration, and loss of fine motor skills. In most circumstances, the diagnosis is made clinically. Brain CT scan may show atrophy and dilated ventricles. Most cerebrospinal fluid studies are non-specific, although β-2 microglobulin levels are usually elevated. Some studies have demonstrated a correlation between cerebrospinal fluid HIV RNA levels and HIV dementia, although others have not shown a clear-cut correlation. Brain biopsy, when performed, may show evidence of direct HIV invasion of the brain. Treatment of common neurologic disorders is shown in *Table 12.9*.

OPHTHALMIC DISORDERS

An array of ocular manifestations can develop in HIV-infected patients. Cotton wool spots, believed to result from direct retinal microvascular HIV infection, often occur in HIV-infected patients (*Fig. 12.57*). Although these lesions usually do not cause symptoms, they can be confused with cytomegalovirus retinitis, the most common serious ocular finding among HIV-infected patients. This infection results from reactivation of cytomegalovirus in patients who almost always have CD4+ counts less than 50 cells/mm³. Most patients complain of seeing floaters or flashing lights and some notice a visual field deficit. The diagnosis is made with fundoscopic evaluation (*Fig. 12.58*) and biopsy is not required. Other retinal lesions, such as those caused by *T. gondii* (*Fig. 12.59*) or *Pneumocystis carinii*, can occur, but much less often than cytomegalovirus retinitis or cotton wool spots. The treatment of common ocular disorders is summarized in *Table 12.10*.

HEMATOLOGIC/ONCOLOGIC DISORDERS

Among HIV-infected persons, lymphohematologic disorders often occur. Lymphadenopathy frequently develops in HIV-infected patients and may result from one of three major causes: direct HIV invasion of the lymph nodes, non-Hodgkins (or Hodgkin's) lymphoma, and opportunistic infections, such as human herpes virus-8 associated Castleman's disease, tuberculosis, or infection with *Mycobacterium avium* complex.

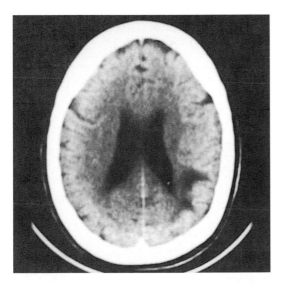

Fig. 12.55 CT scan that shows markedly dilated ventricles. A brain biopsy revealed progressive multifocal leukoencephalopathy.

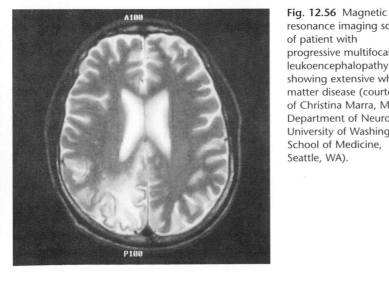

Fig. 12.56 Magnetic resonance imaging scan of patient with progressive multifocal leukoencephalopathy showing extensive white matter disease (courtesy of Christina Marra, MD, Department of Neurology, University of Washington School of Medicine, Seattle, WA).

Condition	Treatment
Cryptococcal meningitis	(Initial) Amphotericin B (0.7–1.0 mg/kg/d IV) ± Flucytosine (100 mg/kg/d po) × 14d followed by Fluconazole (400 mg/d) for a minimum of 10 weeks (Maintenance) Fluconazole: 200 mg po qd
Toxoplasma encephalitis	(Initial) Pyrimethamine: 200 mg po × 1 then 75 mg po qd plus Sulfadiazine: 1.5 gm po qid (or Clindamycin: 600 mg po qid) plus Leucovorin: 10–25 mg qd (Maintenance) Pyrimethamine: 100 mg po × 1 then 25–50 mg po qd plus Sulfadiazine: 1.0 gm po tid (or Clindamycin: 450 mg po tid) plus Leucovorin: 10–25 mg qd
CNS lymphoma	Radiation therapy
PML	HAART
Neurosyphilis	Penicillin: 4 million units IV q4 h × 10–14d or Ceftriaxone: 2g IV qd × 10–14d
AIDS-associated dementia	HAART

Table 12.9 Treatment of common neurologic disorders.

Early in the course of HIV infection, patients may develop significant HIV-related lymphadenopathy, with node histopathology showing hyperplasia and in-situ PCR assays showing HIV-infected lymphocytes and virus-coated dendritic cells. With progressive immunosuppression, the node architecture deteriorates and there is loss of follicle structure and loss of HIV containment. Lymphoma, most often large, immunoblastic B-cell lymphoma, but also Hodgkin's disease and Burkitt's lymphoma, usually present at an advanced stage and often with 'B symptoms' (fever, weight loss, diaphoresis) in addition to enlarged lymph nodes (*Fig. 12.60*). The diagnosis requires a node biopsy (*Fig. 12.61A–C*). Castleman's disease, a lymphoproliferative disorder associated with HHV-8 infection, presents with waxing and waning, often massive, lymphadenopathy.[46,47] HIV-infected patients usually have the multicentric form of Castleman's disease and it is characterized by hepatosplenomegaly, generalized lymphadenopathy, and B symptoms. Lymph node histopathology shows either plasma cell infiltration (most common in multicentric Castleman's disease) or a hyaline-vascular appearance in which circumferential layers of lymphocytes and hyaline are present in a classic onion skin appearance. Enlarged lymph nodes may also result from infection with opportunistic pathogens, such as *M. avium* complex (*Fig. 12.62A–C*), *M. tuberculosis*, and disseminated histoplasmosis (*Fig. 12.63*).

Hematologic abnormalities (anemia, neutropenia, and thrombocytopenia, thrombotic thrombocytopenic purpura (TTP)) can result from either HIV-related effects, OIs, or from medications used to treat HIV-related opportunistic infections. Because patients may have multiple possible causes for their hematologic disorder, the exact cause may be difficult to identify. In some instances, bone marrow examination with aspirate, biopsy, and culture may be a valuable diagnostic tool. *Figure 64* shows bone marrow invaded by *Histoplasma capsulatum*. In some instances, examination of a peripheral blood smear has revealed a diagnosis of disseminated histoplasmosis (*Fig. 12.65*).

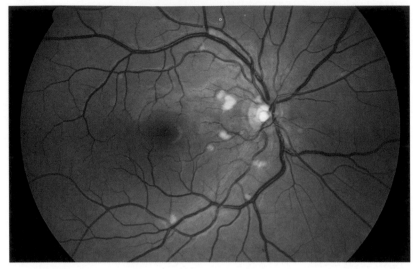

Fig. 12.57 Fundoscopic photograph showing multiple cotton wool spots in an HIV-infected patient.

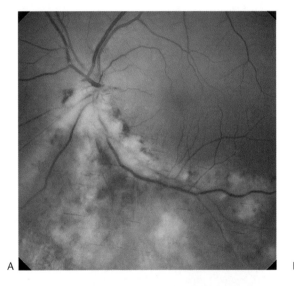

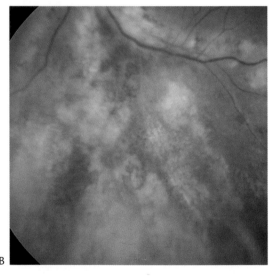

A   B

Fig. 12.58 A, B Fundoscopic photograph showing cytomegalovirus retinitis with typical retinal swelling, hemorrhage, and necrosis.

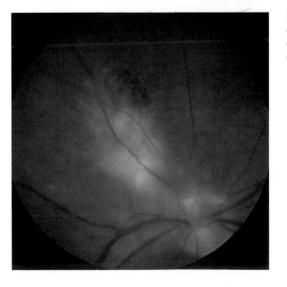

Fig. 12.59 Reactivation of ocular *Toxoplasma* chorioretinitis in an area of previous scarring.

Condition	Treatment
Cytomegalovirus retinitis	Ganciclovir: 5 mg/kg IV bid × 2–3 weeks then 6 mg/kg IV qd or Foscarnet: 60 mg/kg IV tid × 2–3 weeks then 100 mg/kg IV qd or Valganciclovir: 900 mg po bid × 3 weeks, then 900 mg qd or Ganciclovir implants
HIV retinopathy	None required

Table 12.10 Treatment of common ocular disorders.

WOMEN AND HIV

Available data suggest that HIV-infected women and men who have equal access to medical care have similar survival rates and disease progression rates.[48] In addition, women and men have similar rates of HIV-associated illnesses, except for fewer cases of Kaposi's sarcoma among women. Several studies have shown that early in the course of HIV disease, women have relatively lower HIV RNA levels than men when matched for similar CD4+ cell counts.[48] This difference typically equalizes as the disease progresses. HIV infection may produce multiple reproductive health concerns in women, with specific issues developing at different stages of the HIV illness. Frequency, severity, and treatment response of many gynecological problems may be linked to degrees of immunosuppression. Regardless of the stage of HIV infection, early detection, intervention, and aggressive treatment of gynecological problems are warranted in HIV-infected women.

Increased rates of human papillomavirus infection and human papillomavirus-associated cervical dysplasia occur among HIV-infected women when compared with HIV-seronegative women (*Fig. 12.66*). Moreover, invasive cervical carcinoma clearly occurs at an increased frequency and is an AIDS-defining condition. In order to detect early cervical abnormalities, Papanicolaou smears are recommended twice in the first year after diagnosis and, if normal, every year thereafter. The approach to abnormal Papanicolaou smears depends on whether the abnormality is atypical squamous cells of undetermined significance (ASCUS), ASCUS associated with severe inflammation, or low-grade squamous intraepithelial lesion. Ideally, HIV-infected women with such

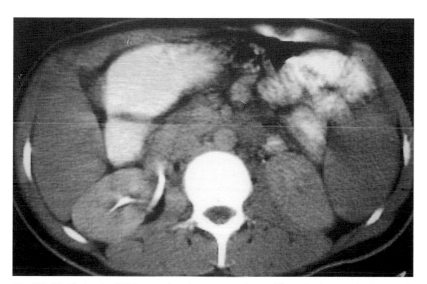

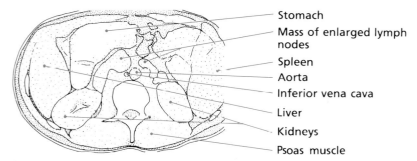

Stomach

Mass of enlarged lymph nodes

Spleen

Aorta

Inferior vena cava

Liver

Kidneys

Psoas muscle

Fig. 12.60 Abdominal CT scan showing retroperitoneal lymphadenopathy in a patient with AIDS.

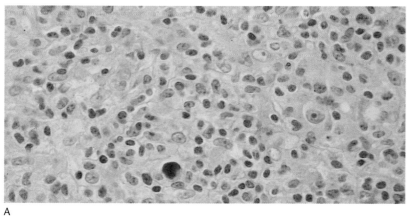

A

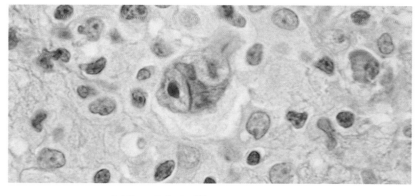

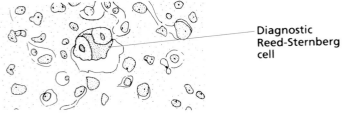

Diagnostic Reed-Sternberg cell

B

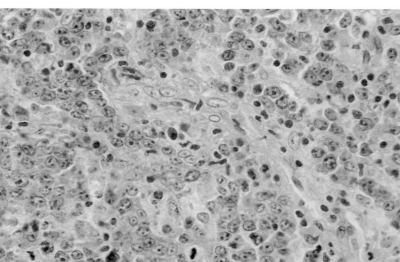

C

Fig. 12.61 (A) Hodgkin's lymphoma, mixed cellularity type from retroperitoneal lymph node (hematoxylin and eosin × 1,000). (B) Hodgkin's lymphoma, mixed cellularity type with evident Reed-Sternberg cell (hematoxylin and eosin × 1,000). (C) Malignant non-Hodgkin's lymphoma, diffuse large-cell type from retroperitoneal lymph node (hematoxylin and eosin × 400).

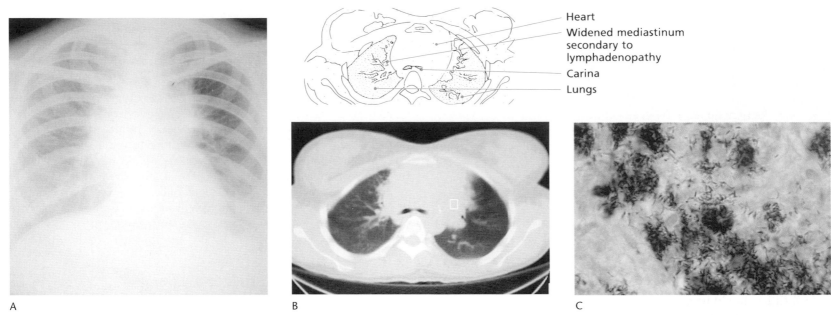

A   B   C

Fig. 12.62 (A) Chest radiograph showing mediastinal lymphadenopathy caused by *Mycobacterium avium* complex. (B) CT scan showing mediastinal lymphadenopathy caused by *Mycobacterium avium* complex. (C) Abundant acid-fast bacilli present in histiocytes of lymph node, with most present intracellularly (Ziehl–Neelson × 1,000).

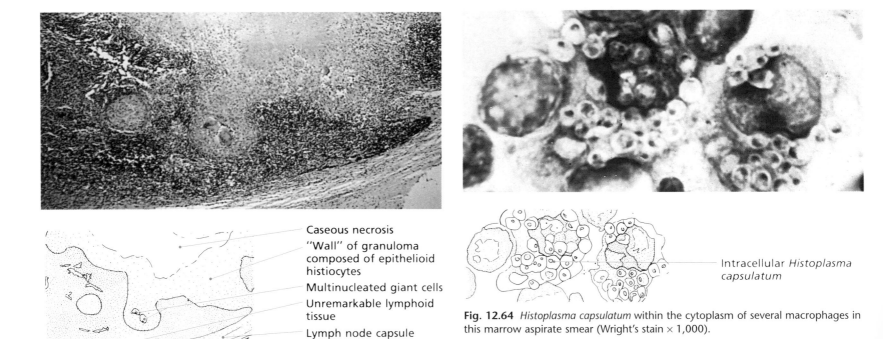

Fig. 12.63 Lymph node showing caseating granulomatous inflammation in AIDS patient with disseminated histoplasmosis (hematoxylin and eosin × 100).

Fig. 12.64 *Histoplasma capsulatum* within the cytoplasm of several macrophages in this marrow aspirate smear (Wright's stain × 1,000).

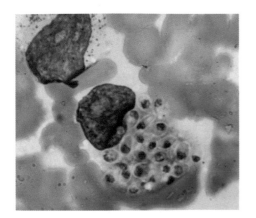

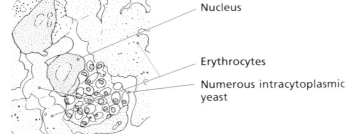

Fig. 12.65 Numerous intracellular *Histoplasma capsulatum* organisms can be seen within the cytoplasm of several macrophages in this peripheral blood smear; the yeasts cells are 2–5 μm in size (Wright's stain × 1,000).

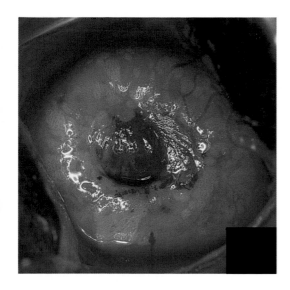

Fig. 12.66 Cervicitis with cervical condylomata acuminata. Viewed through the colposcope.

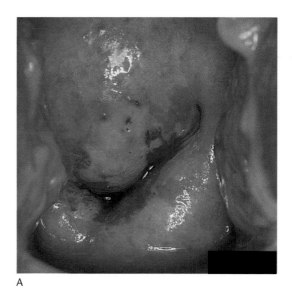

A

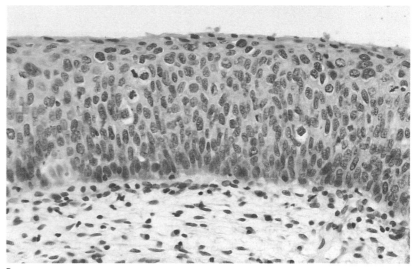

B

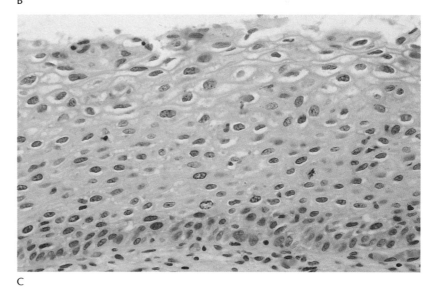

C

Fig. 12.67 (A) Cervicitis in an HIV-infected woman later found to have a high-grade squamous intraepithelial lesion (SIL) on cervical biopsy. (B) Cervical histopathology consistent with high-grade SIL. (C) Cervical histopathology consistent with low-grade SIL.

abnormalities should be evaluated and followed by an individual with significant expertise with abnormal Papanicolaou smears. (*Fig. 12.67A–C*). All HIV-infected women with ASCUS should be referred for colposcopy. Genital warts, or condylomata acuminata, are also caused by human papillomavirus and may develop into extensive refractory lesions in HIV-infected women. Warts on the cervix are usually asymptomatic and may require colposcopy to visualize. Earlier concerns regarding higher prevalence and severity of genital tract infections and menstrual irregularities have not been supported in follow-up studies.

MISCELLANEOUS CLINICAL MANIFESTATIONS

In addition to the major clinical disorders already discussed, HIV can less frequently affect other organ systems, such as renal, endocrine, or cardiac. A variety of renal lesions in patients with HIV infection have been described, but glomerular lesions have been the most common.[49] HIV-associated nephropathy, which consists of nephrotic range proteinuria and focal and segmental glomerulosclerosis, often leads to end-stage renal disease. Other HIV-related renal abnormalities include other glomerular morphologic changes, as well as nonspecific lesions, such as acute tubular necrosis, nephrocalcinosis, interstitial nephritis, and indinavir-associated nephrolithiasis and nephropathy.

Earlier reports have described adrenal insufficiency occurring in HIV-infected patients, predominantly among those with advanced AIDS. The most frequent cause of adrenal insufficiency has been cytomegalovirus infection of the adrenal gland, but other microorganisms including *M. tuberculosis* and *H. capsulatum* can also cause adrenal insufficiency.

The clinical spectrum of cardiac disorders in HIV-related disease includes HIV-induced myocarditis, congestive cardiomyopathy (presumed to be of viral origin), nonbacterial thrombotic endocarditis, Kaposi's sarcoma of the myocardium, and non-Hodgkin's lymphoma of the pericardium. Pulmonary hypertension is an uncommon but devastating diagnosis with a median survival of less than 2 years.[50] Patients present with dyspnea, hypoxia and signs of right-sided heart failure. The pathogenesis is thought to be due to HIV-induced production of lymphokines and growth factors that lead to endothelial cell proliferation.

IMMUNE RECONSTITUTION SYNDROMES

HAART-induced immune system recovery has led to the development of inflammatory reactions associated with a variety of opportunistic infections.[51] These reactions coincide with increasing CD4+ cell counts and often occur within weeks of initiating antiretroviral therapy. They can be associated with known infections or be the first manifestation of an occult infection. Individuals with very low CD4+ counts who present with these syndromes are often very ill and can have high fever, extensive adenopathy, effusions, and significant visceral involvement, indicative of a systemic inflammatory response, usually to a disseminated infection. Patients with higher CD4+ counts usually present with more localized disease, such as mycobacterial adenitis or cytomegalovirus vitreitis, representing an inflammatory response to a confined infection.

The first report of an immune reconstitution syndrome in patients on HAART involved five patients diagnosed with a cytomegalovirus retinitis within 6 months of starting HAART, two of whom developed an inflammatory vitreitis early in the course of their cytomegalovirus disease.[52] Subsequently, other investigators have reported the occurrence of cytomegalovirus immune reconstitution vitreitis (with papillitis, macular edema and epiretinal membrane formation) in up to 63% of patients with a history of cytomegalovirus retinitis who had started HAART.[53] This complication carries significant morbidity since most patients experience decreased visual acuity that only occasionally improves over time.[54]

Patients with mycobacterial infections, including *M. tuberculosis* and atypical mycobacterial disease, can also develop immune reconstitution syndromes. Patients with *Mycobacterium avium* complex usually have occult infections and, with immune reconstitution, develop fever, diaphoresis and adenitis (cervical, axillary, thoracic, and abdominal). If CD4+ counts are low (< 50 cells/mm^3) individuals often have more severe symptoms and *Mycobacterium avium* complex can be cultivated from the blood.[55] Patients with higher CD4+ counts (100 to 150 cells/mm^3) usually have more localized, suppurative disease.[56] Individuals with tuberculosis can also present with local adenitis that usually represents unmasked occult infection. However, the largest study of immune reconstitution syndromes in patients with *M. tuberculosis* involved individuals with known tuberculosis who were already on anti-tuberculous therapy and were subsequently started on antiretroviral therapy. In this study 12 (36%) of 33 patients who started HAART developed an immune reconstitution syndrome (recurrent fever and enlargement of existing lesions or appearance of new lesions) a mean of 15 days after HAART compared with 2 (7%) of 28 historical controls who did not receive HAART.[57] Other infections associated with immune reconstitution syndromes in HIV-infected patients initiating antiretroviral therapy include progressive multifocal leukoencephalopathy,[58] cryptococcal meningitis,[59] hepatitis B virus,[60] histoplasmosis, and Castleman's disease.[61] In most cases, patients with immune reconstitution syndromes can be managed without interruption of HAART (or other necessary anti-infective therapy). Severely symptomatic patients may benefit from anti-inflammatory treatments including non-steroidal anti-inflammatory drugs and corticosteroids.

Although HAART has dramatically reduced the incidence of HIV-associated opportunistic infections, the recovery of protective immunity against individual pathogens varies. Furthermore, certain individuals remain susceptible to particular opportunistic infections despite recovering CD4+ cell counts, either because they have lost the ability to respond to particular antigens[54,62–64] or because they have other generalized immunosuppressing conditions.[65,636] Identifying these individuals, investigating the reasons for their impaired immunity, and developing therapies that correct these deficiencies are some of the challenges for the future.

ANTI-HIV THERAPY

In the mid 1980s, testing began on potential anti-HIV therapy and in 1987 the United States Food and Drug Administration approved zidovudine (AZT), a nucleoside reverse transcriptase inhibitor, for treatment of HIV. Although initial results with zidovudine in patients

with advanced AIDS generated tremendous enthusiasm, it soon became clear that zidovudine, by itself, would be grossly inadequate for long-term management of AIDS. In the early 1990s, two additional nucleoside reverse transcriptase inhibitors, didanosine (ddI) and zalcitabine (ddC), were subsequently approved. Interest then arose for combination therapy, but once again, it became clear that the combination of two reverse transcriptase inhibitors would not be sufficient. A breakthrough occurred in the mid-1990s with the introduction of protease inhibitors and the widespread use of aggressive three-drug combination therapy. Soon thereafter, the non-nucleoside reverse transcriptase inhibitors were added as the third class of antiretroviral therapy medications. Following the widespread use of potent antiretroviral therapies in developed countries, a dramatic decline in AIDS-related deaths has occurred[67,68] (*Fig. 12.68A, B*). Despite these tremendous advances in antiretroviral therapy, several limitations remain, including failure to eradicate HIV, development of resistance, and long-term toxicities such as fat maldistribution.

ANTIRETROVIRAL MEDICATIONS

The currently approved antiretroviral drugs include six nucleoside reverse transcriptase inhibitors, one nucleotide reverse transcriptase

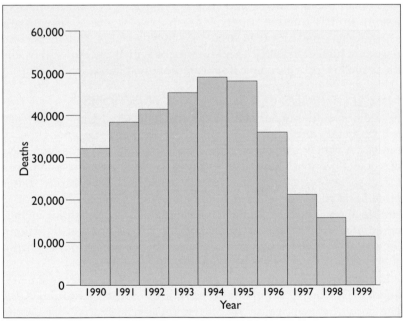

Fig. 12.68A AIDS-related deaths in the United States, 1990–1999.

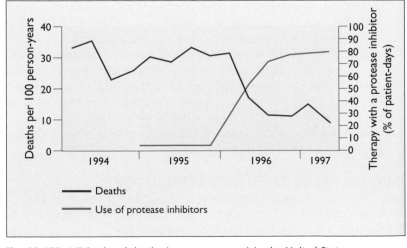

Fig. 12.68B AIDS-related deaths (per person years) in the United States, 1994–1997 and the relationship with use of protease inhibitors.

inhibitor, three non-nucleoside reverse transcriptase inhibitors, and six protease inhibitors (*Table 12.11*). The nucleoside and nucleotide reverse transcriptase inhibitors are commonly referred to as nucleoside (nucleotide) analogs and they structurally resemble the human nucleosides that HIV uses when converting its RNA into DNA. These compounds undergo intracellular phosphorylation and the triphosphorylated form of the compound is the active form of the drug. If HIV incorporates the triphosphorylated nucleoside or nucleotide analog, chain termination results (*Fig. 12.69*). The non-nucleoside reverse transcriptase inhibitors have a mechanism of action distinct from nucleoside reverse transcriptase inhibitors; drugs in this class directly inhibit proper functioning of the reverse transcriptase enzyme. The HIV protease normally plays an important role late in the viral life cycle by post-translational editing and processing. HIV protease inhibitors block this process, leading to synthesis of defective viral particles. During the first several years of use of aggressive antiretroviral therapy, dosing schedules were often very complicated and pill burden typically very high. In more recent years, dosing schedules have become simplified and pill burden decreased. Moreover, with more options available, regimens can more easily be chosen that have better side effect profiles.

GUIDELINES FOR ANTIRETROVIRAL THERAPY

Two prominent sets of antiretroviral therapy guidelines exist: (1) the United States Department of Health and Human Services (DHHS) guidelines and (2) the International AIDS Society (IAS) guidelines. These two guidelines offer very similar overall recommendations, but some minor differences exist. The DHHS antiretroviral therapy guidelines, found at the website address http://www.hivatis.org, were last updated in February 2002 and are updated on a regular basis (*Table 12.12A, B*).[6] These 2002 guidelines recommend starting antiretroviral therapy in patients with any of the following scenarios (a) acute HIV syndrome, (b) HIV diagnosed within 6 months of seroconversion, (c) severe HIV-related symptoms or AIDS, and (d) a CD4 count less than 200 cells/mm[3]. For individuals who have a CD4 count greater than 200 cells/mm[3], but less than 350 cells/mm[3], therapy is generally offered. The IAS antiretroviral therapy guidelines, most recently revised in July 2002, recommend starting antiretroviral therapy for (a) HIV-related symptoms, or (b) CD4+ count less than 200 cells/mm[3].[69] Both sets of guidelines recommend using a minimum of three drugs when starting

therapy, generally two nucleoside reverse transcriptase inhibitors plus either a protease inhibitor, a non-nucleoside reverse transcriptase inhibitor, or two protease inhibitors.

Generic name	Trade name	Dose
Nucleoside RTI		
Abacavir (ABC)	*Ziagen*	300 mg PO bid
Didanosine (ddI)	*Videx*	400 mg PO qd (250 mg qd if < 60 kg)
Lamivudine (3TC)	*Epivir*	150 mg PO bid
Stavudine (d4T)	*Zenit*	40 mg PO bid (30 mg PO bid if < 60 kg)
Zalcitabine (ddC)	*Hivid*	0.75 mg PO tid
Zidovudine (AZT)	*Retrovir*	300 mg PO bid; or 200 mg tid
*Zidovudine + Lamivudine	*Combivir*	One PO bid
*Zidovudine + Lamivudine + Abacavir	*Trizivir*	One PO bid
Nucleotide RTI		
Tenfovir	*Viread*	300 mg PO qd
Non-Nucleoside RTI		
Delavirdine	*Rescriptor*	400 mg PO tid
Efavirenz	*Sustiva*	600 mg PO qd (dose can be split and given 200 mg in am and 400 mg in pm)
Nevirapine	*Viramune*	200 mg PO qd × 14d, then 200 mg PO bid
Protease Inhibitors		
Amprenavir	*Agenerase*	1,200 mg PO bid
Indinavir	*Crixivan*	800 mg PO q8h
Lopinavir + Ritonavir	*Kaletra*	3 PO bid (400 mg lopinavir bid + 100 mg ritonavir bid)
Nelfinavir	*Viracept*	1,250 mg PO bid or 750 mg PO tid
Ritonavir	*Norvir*	600 mg PO bid (dose escalated#)
Saquinavir	*Fortivase*	1,200 mg PO tid

*Standard doses of zidovudine, lamivudine, and abacavir are used in these fixed combinations.
#Ritonavir dose escalation: 300 mg PO bid × 2d, 400 mg PO bid × 3d, 500 mg PO bid × 8d, then 600 mg PO bid.

Table 12.11 Antiretroviral medications reference.[6]

Clinical category	CD4 T cell count	Plasma HIV RNA	Recommendation
Symptomatic (AIDS, severe symptoms)	Any value	Any value	Treat
Asymptomatic	CD4+ T cells <200/mm[3]	Any value	Treat
Asymptomatic	CD4+ T cells >200/mm[3] but <350/mm[3]	Any value	Treatment should generally be offered, though controversy exists*
Asymptomatic	CD4+ T cells >350/mm[3]	(bDNA) or >55,000 (RT PCR) >55,000 (by bDNA or RT PCR)	Some experts would recommend initiating therapy, recognizing that the 3-year risk of developing AIDS in untreated patients is >30%. and some would defer therapy and monitor CD4+ T cell counts more frequently.
Asymptomatic	CD4+ T cells >350/mm[3]	(bDNA) or <55,000 (by bDNA or RT-PCR) <55,000 (RT PCR)	Many experts would defer therapy and observe, recognizing that the 3-year risk of developing AIDS in untreated patients is <15%.

*Clinical benefit has been demonstrated in controlled trials only for patients with CD4+ T cells <200/mm[3]. However, most experts would offer therapy at a CD4+ T cell threshold <350/mm[3]. A recent evaluation of data from the MACS cohort of 231 individuals with CD4+ T cell counts >200 and <350 cells/mm[3] demonstrated that of 40 (17%) individuals with plasma HIV RNA <10,000 copies/ml, none progressed to AIDS by 3 years (Alvaro Munoz, personal communication). Of 28 individuals (29%) with plasma viremia of 10,000–20,000 copies/ml, 4% and 11% progressed to AIDS at 2 and 3 years, respectively. Plasma HIV RNA was calculated as RT-PCR values from measured bDNA values.

Table 12.12A DHHS 2002 Antiretroviral Therapy Guidelines. Indications for the initiation of antiretroviral therapy in the chronically HIV-infected patient reference.[6]

	Column A	Column B
Strongly Recommended	Efavirenz Indinavir Nelfinavir Ritonavir plus Indinavir Ritonavir plus Lopinavir Ritonavir plus Saquinavir	Didanosine + Lamivudine Stavudine + Didanosine* Stavudine + Lamivudine Zidovudine + Didanosine Zidovudine + Lamivudine
Alternative Regimen	Abacavir Amprenavir Delavirdine Nelfinavir + Saquinavir-SGC Nevirapine Ritonavir Saquinavir-SGC	Zidovudine + Zalcitabine
No Recommendation: Insufficient Data	Hydroxyurea with antiretroviral medications Ritonavir + Amprenavir Ritonavir + Nelfinavir Tenofovir	
Not Recommended:	All monotherapies	
Should Not Be Offered:	Saquinavir-HGC	Stavudine + Zidovudine Zalcitabine + Didanosine Zalcitabine + Lamivudine Zalcitabine + Stavudine

Pregnant women may have increased risk of lactic acidosis and liver damage when taking didanosine plus stavudine.
SGC = soft gel capsule (Fortivase).
HGC = hard gel capsule (Invirase).

Table 12.12B DHHS 2002 recommendations for antiretroviral regimens for the treatment of established HIV in adults and adolescents (regimens listed in alphabetical order, not by order of preference). Use one choice from column A and column B.

Patients on antiretroviral therapy need close monitoring to determine their response to therapy and to follow for any possible drug-related adverse effects. The virologic goal is to suppress the plasma HIV RNA levels to less than 50 copies/ml, with the rationale that tight control of HIV diminishes the number of HIV virions that replicate and thus lessens the chances for emergence of resistant strains. Accordingly, HIV RNA monitoring should consist of a baseline value prior to starting therapy, followed by a level every 4 weeks until the HIV RNA is less than 50 copies/ml. The first post-therapy HIV RNA taken at week 4 should show at least a 10-fold decline and most patients should suppress their HIV RNA to less than 50 copies/ml by 16 to 20 weeks. Once the target goal of less than 50 copies/ml has been reached, the HIV RNA levels should be determined approximately every 3 months. Recent work has shown that although low-level viremia often occurs on protease-inhibitor-based regimens, it does not correlate with long-term virologic suppression.[70] Although optimal HIV suppression does not always result from antiretroviral therapy, recent work has shown substantial immunologic benefit among some individuals who achieve only moderately tight control of their HIV RNA levels.[70] The immunologic goal is to restore and preserve immune function. Monitoring of CD4+ counts provides the best estimate of immunologic response and values should be obtained approximately every 3 months. Standard CD4+ cell count measurements do not, however, provide specific information regarding CD4+ cell function and do not differentiate between naïve and memory cells. The ultimate goal of antiretroviral therapy is to improve quality of life and prolong survival.

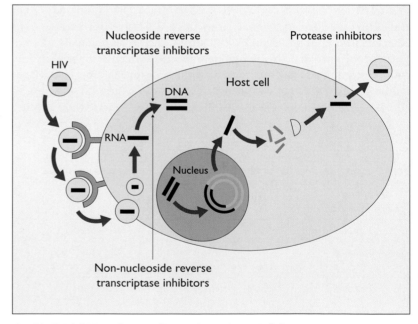

Fig. 12.69 Inhibition of HIV replication by antiretroviral drug.

LIMITATIONS AND COMPLICATIONS OF ANTIRETROVIRAL MEDICATIONS

Despite many tremendous benefits of antiretroviral therapy, current antiretroviral therapy has limitations. Although patients may have plasma HIV RNA suppressed to less than 50 copies/ml for years, there is no evidence that prolonged antiretroviral therapy will eradicate HIV. Indeed, HIV persists in cellular and anatomical reservoirs.[71] Innovative strategies that have attempted to eradicate HIV from reservoirs have not been successful.[72] Since eradication of HIV does not appear realistic, long-term treatment with antiretroviral therapy will be required. Sustained virologic suppression clearly requires long-term strict adherence to antiretroviral therapy,[73] a goal not feasible for many persons infected with HIV. Non-adherence represents the most important factor leading to antiretroviral therapy resistance. Other predictors of HIV suppression include the host immune status, inherent potency of the regimen, antiretroviral cross-resistance from prior therapy, absorption and metabolism of medications, and drug–drug interactions that may affect the concentration of the antiretroviral medications. The first indication of resistance generally comes from a persistent increase in HIV RNA levels (*Fig. 12.70*). Resistance can be determined by one of two assays: phenotypic assays or genotypic assays (see Chapter 11).

The HIV-associated lipodystrophy syndrome has become a troublesome adverse effect of antiretroviral therapy, with prevalence rates ranging between 2 and 83%.[74,75] This syndrome lacks a clear-cut case definition, but includes body fat redistribution and metabolic abnormalities such as hyperlipidemia and insulin resistance. The fat redistribution findings can be grouped as either lipoaccumulation (central adiposity, lipomatosis, breast enlargement and dorsocervical fat pad) or lipoatrophy (loss of fat in the cheeks, extremities and buttocks) and these often occur together (*Fig. 12.71*). Suggested risk factors for lipodystrophy include older age, female sex, longer duration of antiretroviral therapy and reduced HIV viral load. Some investigators have linked the protease inhibitors to the development of diabetes, lipid abnormalities and lipoaccumulation[75] whereas others have suggested the nucleoside reverse transcriptase inhibitors, particularly stavudine, are more often associated with lipoatrophy (possibly due to adipocyte mitochondrial toxicity).[76]

PERINATAL TRANSMISSION

Antiretroviral therapy has had a major impact on the transmission of HIV from mother to child. The Pediatric AIDS Clinical Trials Group 076 study demonstrated HIV transmission rates of 8.3% among HIV-infected pregnant women who received zidovudine compared with 25.5% among those who received placebo.[77] In this trial, the zidovudine regimen consisted of oral zidovudine given after week 14 of gestation, intravenous zidovudine given during labor and delivery, and oral zidovudine given to the newborn until 6 weeks of age. Subsequently, the 'short course zidovudine' study that involved non-breastfeeding HIV-infected women from Thailand found that women who received zidovudine for 4 weeks prior to labor (and during labor) had perinatal transmission of only 9% compared with 19% for women given placebo.[78] A third study from Uganda randomized HIV-infected mothers to either a single 200 mg dose of nevirapine at the onset of labor plus a single 2 mg/kg dose given to the infant 48–72 hours after birth, or to zidovudine given orally during labor and to the infant for 1 week after birth. The HIV transmission rates were 12% in nevirapine group and 21% in the zidovudine group.[79] Follow-up from this study, however, found that among the women who received nevirapine, resistance to the medication developed in 20%, presumably as a result of the very long half-life of nevirapine. In a placebo-controlled trial in Africa that involved HIV-infected women who breastfed, combined regimen of zidovudine and lamivudine was a begun at week 36 of gestation, given orally intrapartum, and for 1 week post-partum to both the infant and the mother.[80] Transmission by age 6 weeks was 17% in the placebo group and 9% in the zidovudine plus lamivudine group. In general, available data would suggest that zidovudine given in utero or

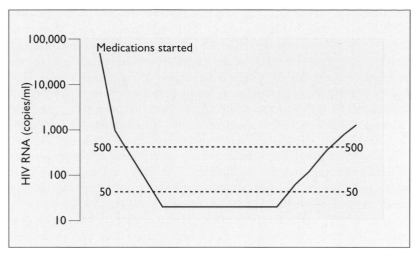

Fig. 12.70 Initial HIV suppression in response to antiretroviral therapy followed by gradual increases in HIV RNA levels that reflect the likely development of resistance.

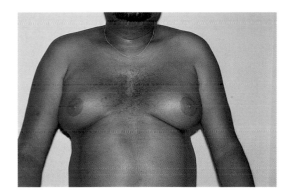

Fig. 12.71 HIV-infected patient with marked lipodystrophy. The patient has marked fat accumulation in abdominal and breast regions.

post-partum only rarely (if at all) affects growth or development of the fetus.[80] Of concern is that French investigators have reported eight cases of mitochondrial dysfunction among infants not infected with HIV who had in utero and/or neonatal exposure to either zidovudine plus lamivudine (four infants) or zidovudine alone (four infants).[81]

Current Public Health Task Force Recommendations for reducing perinatal HIV transmission are based on the specific situation of the HIV-infected pregnant woman.[80] Four specific scenarios have been addressed in these guidelines (*Table 12.13*): (a) HIV-infected pregnant women who have not received prior antiretroviral therapy, (b) HIV-infected women receiving antiretroviral therapy during the current pregnancy, (c) HIV-infected women in labor who have had no prior therapy, and (d) infants born to mothers who have received no antiretroviral therapy during pregnancy or intrapartum. Three cases of fatal lactic acidosis have been observed among pregnant women taking an antepartum combination antiretroviral regimen that included didanosine and stavudine.[80] Accordingly, regimens that contain the combination of didanosine and stavudine should be avoided during pregnancy. The guidelines also recommend that women who have an HIV RNA level greater than 1,000 copies/ml should receive counseling regarding the benefit of scheduled cesarean section in decreasing the risk of transmission of HIV to their child. In contrast, women with HIV RNA less than 1,000 copies/ml should be advised that scheduled cesarean section is unlikely to further substantially decrease their risk of HIV transmission to their child.

OCCUPATIONAL EXPOSURE TO HIV AND POST-EXPOSURE PROPHYLAXIS

Accidental occupational exposure to HIV represents an important issue for all health care workers involved in the care of HIV-infected individuals. The risk of HIV transmission is approximately 0.3% with percutaneous exposure to HIV-infected blood and approximately 0.09% with mucous membrane exposures.[82] In the United States, as of June 2000, 56 health care workers had documented HIV seroconversion as a result of occupational HIV exposure. The recommendation to use antiretroviral therapy for postexposure prophylaxis was driven by data from a retrospective case-control study that found use of zidovudine monotherapy for post-exposure prophylaxis in health care workers reduced the risk of HIV transmission by approximately 81%.[83] Moreover, animal HIV postexposure prophylaxis studies with nucleotide reverse transcriptase inhibitors also support use of these medications for postexposure prophylaxis in humans.[82] To date, no data have been published that test the efficacy of combination antiretroviral therapy for postexposure prophylaxis in health care workers.

In June 2001, revised HIV postexposure prophylaxis guidelines were issued and these guidelines also included recommendations for the management of occupational exposures to hepatitis B virus and hepatitis C virus.[82] Immediately after an exposure, the health care worker should thoroughly clean the site of exposure, followed promptly by the first dose of postexposure antiretroviral therapy. The type of exposure and the status of the host patient are the two major factors that guide the recommendations for postexposure prophylaxis (*Tables 12.14* and *12.15*). The recommended regimens are classified as either basic two drug regimens or expanded three drug regimens. In general, more severe exposures involve either a large-bore hollow needle, deep puncture, visible blood on the device, or a needle used in a source patient's artery or vein. Regardless of which regimen is used, post-exposure antiretroviral prophylaxis should be taken for 28 days. Unfortunately, several studies have shown that health care workers often do not tolerate these regimens and often have difficulty completing the 28 day course.[84] Expert opinion is available at the National Clinicians' Postexposure Prophylaxis Hotline (PEPline), a service run by the University of California–San Francisco/San Francisco General Hospital staff and supported by the Health Resources and Services Administration Ryan White CARE Act, HIV/AIDS Bureau, AIDS Education and Training Centers (Phone: 888-448-4911; internet: http://www.ucsf.edu/hivcntr). Although it is widely believed that combination antiretroviral therapy lowers the risk of HIV transmission with a percutaneous exposure to a rate much lower than 0.3%, eight

Clinical scenario recommendations*	
Scenario	**Recommendation**
Scenario #1: HIV-infected pregnant women who have not received prior antiretroviral therapy.	Pregnant women with HIV infection must receive standard clinical, immunologic, and virologic evaluation. Recommendations for initiation and choice of antiretroviral therapy should be based on the same parameters used for persons who are not pregnant, although the known and unknown risks and benefits of such therapy during pregnancy must be considered and discussed. The three-part AZT chemoprophylaxis regimen, initiated after the first trimester, should be recommended for all pregnant women with HIV infection regardless of antenatal HIV RNA copy number to reduce the risk for perinatal transmission. The combination of AZT chemoprophylaxis with additional antiretroviral drugs for treatment of HIV infection is recommended for infected women whose clinical, immunologic or virologic status requires treatment or who have HIV RNA over 1,000 copies/mL regardless of clinical or immunologic status. Women who are in the first trimester of pregnancy may consider delaying initiation of therapy until after 10–12 weeks' gestation.
Scenario #2: HIV-infected women receiving antiretroviral therapy during the current pregnancy.	HIV infected women receiving antiretroviral therapy in whom pregnancy is identified after the first trimester should continue therapy. AZT should be a component of the antenatal antiretroviral treatment regimen after the first trimester whenever possible, although this may not always be feasible. For women receiving antiretroviral therapy in whom pregnancy is recognized during the first trimester, the woman should be counseled regarding the benefits and potential risks of antiretroviral administration during this period, and continuation of therapy should be considered. If therapy is discontinued during the first trimester, all drugs should be stopped and reintroduced simultaneously to avoid the development of drug resistance. Regardless of the antepartum antiretroviral regimen, AZT administration is recommended during the intrapartum period and for the newborn. Recommendations for resistance testing in HIV-infected pregnant women are the same as for non-pregnant patients: acute HIV infection, virologic failure, or suboptimal viral suppression after initiation of antiretroviral therapy.
Scenerio #3: HIV-infected women in labor who have had no prior therapy.	Several effective regimens are available. These include: 1) single dose nevirapine at the onset of labor followed by a single dose of nevirapine for the newborn at age 48 hours; 2) oral AZT and 3TC during labor, followed by one week of oral AZT/3TC for the newborn; 3) intrapartum intravenous AZT followed by 6 weeks of AZT for the newborn; and 4) the two-dose nevirapine regimen combined with intrapartum intravenous AZT and 6 weeks AZT for the newborn. In the immediate postpartum period, the woman should have appropriate assessments (e.g., CD4+ count and HIV RNA copy number) to determine whether antiretroviral therapy is recommended for her own health.
Scenario #4: Infants born to mothers who have received no antiretroviral therapy during pregnancy or intrapartum.	The 6-week neonatal AZT component of the AZT chemoprophylactic regimen should be discussed with the mother and offered for the newborn. AZT should be initiated as soon as possible after delivery — preferably within 6–12 hours of birth. Some clinicians may choose to use AZT in combination with other antiretroviral drugs, particularly if the mother is known or suspected to have AZT-resistant virus. However, the efficacy of this approach for prevention of transmission is unknown, and appropriate dosing regimens for neonates are incompletely defined. In the immediate postpartum period, the woman should undergo appropriate assessments (e.g., CD4+ count and HIV RNA copy number) to determine if antiretroviral therapy is required for her own health. The infant should undergo early diagnostic testing so that if HIV-infected, treatment can be initiated as soon as possible.

Discussion of treatment options and recommendations should be noncoercive, and the final decision regarding the use of antiretroviral drugs is the responsibility of the woman. A decision to not accept treatment with AZT or other drugs should not result in punitive action or denial of care. Use of AZT should not be denied to a woman who wishes to minimize exposure of the fetus to other antiretroviral drugs and who therefore chooses to receive only AZT during pregnancy to reduce the risk for perinatal transmission.

Table 12.13 Clinical scenarios and recommendations for the use of antiretroviral drugs to reduce perinatal human immunodeficiency virus (HIV) transmission.[80]

Exposure type	Infection status or source				
	HIV-positive Class 1*	HIV-positive Class 2*	Source of unknown HIV status†	Unknown source §	HIV-negative
Less severe¶	Recommend basic 2-drug PEP	Recommend expanded 3-drug PEP	Generally, no PEP warranted; however consider basic 2-drug PEP** for source with HIV risk factors††	Generally, no PEP, warranted; however consider basic 2-drug PEP** in settings where exposure to HIV-infected persons is likely	No PEP warranted
More severe §§	Recommend expanded 3-drug PEP	Recommend expanded 3-drug PEP	Generally, no PEP warranted; however, consider basic 2-drug PEP** for source with HIV risk factors††	Generally, no PEP warranted; however, consider basic 2-drug PEP** in settings where exposure to HIV-infected persons is likely	No PEP warranted

*HIV-positive, Class 1 — asymptomatic HIV infection or known low viral load (e.g., <1,500 RNA copies/mL).

HIV-positive, Class 2 — symtomatic HIV infection, AIDS, acute seroconversion, or known high viral load.

If drug resistance is a concern, obtain expert consultation. Initiation of postexposure prophylaxis (PEP) should not be delayed pending expert consultation, and, because expert consultation alone cannot substitute for face-to-face counseling, resources should be available to provide immediate evaluation and follow-up care for all exposures.

†Source of unknown HIV status (e.g., deceased source person with no samples available for HIV testing).

§Unknown source (e.g., a needle from a sharps disposal container).

¶Less severe (e.g., solid needle and superficial injury).

**The designation 'consider PEP' indicates that PEP is optional and should be based on an individualized decision between the exposed person and the treating clinician.

††If PEP is offered and taken and the source is later determined to be HIV-negative, PEP should be discontinued.

§§More severe (e.g., large-bore hollow needle, deep puncture, visible blood on device, or needle used in patient's artery or vein).

From: Centers for Disease Control and Prevention. Updated U.S. Public Health Service Guidelines for the Management of Occupational Exposures to HBV, HCV, and HIV and Recommendations for Postexposure Prophylaxis. MMWR 2001; 50(No. RR-11):1–52.

Table 12.14 Recommended HIV postexposure prophylaxis (PEP) for percutaneous injuries.

Basic regimens Combination of two medications	Expanded regimen Basic regimen plus one of the following
Zidovudine 300 mg bid (or 200 mg tid) plus Lamivudine: 150 mg bid	Nelfinavir: 1250 mg bid (or 750 mg tid) or Indinavir: 800 mg q8h or #Efavirenz: 600 mg qd or
*Stavudine: 40 mg bid plus Lamivudine: 150 mg bid	#Lopinavir/Ritonavir: 400 mg bid or #Abacavir: 300 mg bid
*Stavudine 40 mg bid plus ^Didanosine: 400 mg qd	

*For persons less than 60 kg, dose should be reduced to 30 mg bid.

^For persons less than 60 kg, dose should be reduced to 250 mg qd.

#The drugs efavirenz, lopinavir/ritonavir, and abacavir should be used with caution and are best used with expert consultation.

Table 12.15 Medications and specific regimens used for postexposure prophylaxis for occupational exposure

failures with combination therapy have been documented to occur in this setting.[82] Health care workers should undergo HIV serologic testing at baseline, 6 weeks, 3 months, and 6 months. Some experts would also recommend testing at 12 months, especially in the setting of concomitant infection with hepatitis C virus infection.

NON-OCCUPATIONAL EXPOSURE TO HIV AND POST-EXPOSURE PROPHYLAXIS

In recent years, the potential use of postexposure prophylaxis for non-occupational exposures has generated considerable controversy. In July 1997, the CDC sponsored meetings of consultants to address use of post-exposure antiretroviral prophylaxis for non-occupational HIV exposures.[85] After extensive discussions and debate, the US Public Health Service could not definitively recommend for or against anti-retroviral agents for non-occupational HIV exposures, mainly because of the lack of data on this intervention. Nevertheless, many clinicians offer HIV antiretroviral prophylaxis following a non-occupational exposure. A recent feasibility study in San Francisco enrolled 401 persons who were prescribed 4 weeks of postexposure antiretroviral prophylaxis for a non-occupational HIV exposure.[86] Ninety-four percent of these exposures involved men having sex with men, all started prophylaxis within 72 hours of the exposure, 97% received dual nucleoside therapy, and 78% completed therapy. When tested 6 months after the exposure, none had seroconverted to HIV. Because seroconversion rates per sexual exposure are low, this study did not prove efficacy of post-exposure prophylaxis, but it did provide useful information on feasibility of this intervention.

VACCINES

The devastating impact of the HIV epidemic on many nations of the world has created a desperate hope for an effective preventive vaccine. Although the first 15 years of the HIV epidemic saw relatively little progress in the HIV vaccine field, significant progress has occurred during the past 5 years. This progress is attributable to an enhanced understanding of HIV pathogenesis, increased private and public sector involvement, a growing cadre of able investigators committed to this research, and a major commitment to develop an effective preventive vaccine. Most early work on HIV vaccines focused on inducing neutralizing antibodies, but recent work has also concentrated on vaccines that generate cellular immunity through cytotoxic T-lymphocyte responses.[87,88] The ideal HIV vaccine should prevent infection in a very high proportion of persons receiving the vaccine. A less desired, but potentially beneficial scenario, would be a vaccine that does not prevent infection, but would slow the progression of the disease, as well as diminish the infectiousness of those who acquire HIV despite vaccination. Several hurdles regarding HIV vaccines still must be overcome, including better understanding of the biological correlates of protective immunity, establishing either humoral or cellular immunity to an array of HIV subtypes, and development of the extensive infra-structure necessary to extensively vaccinate high proportions of susceptible individuals in developing countries.

References

1. Kahn JO, Walker BD. Acute human immunodeficiency virus type 1 infection. *N Engl J Med* 1998; **339**:33–39.

2. Schacker T, Collier AC, Hughes J, Shea T, Corey L. Clinical and epidemiologic features of primary HIV infection. *Ann Intern Med* 1996; **125**:257–264.

3. Pilcher CD, Shugars DC, Fiscus SA *et al*. HIV in body fluids during primary HIV infection: implications for pathogenesis, treatment and public health. *Aids* 2001; **15**:837–845.

4. Niu MT, Jermano JA, Reichelderfer P, Schnittman SM. Summary of the National Institutes of Health workshop on primary human immunodeficiency virus type 1 infection. *AIDS Res Hum Retroviruses* 1993; **9**:913–924.

5. Daar ES, Little S, Pitt J *et al*. Diagnosis of primary HIV-1 infection. Los Angeles County Primary HIV Infection Recruitment Network. *Ann Intern Med* 2001; **134**:25–29.

6. Fauci AS, Bartlett JG, *et al. Guidelines for the Use of Antiretroviral Agents in HIV-Infected Adults and Adolescents*. Report: Department of Health and Human Services and the Henry J. Kaiser Family Foundation; 2001.

7. CDC. A cluster of Kaposi's sarcoma and *Pneumocystis carinii* pneumonia among homosexual male residents of Los Angeles and Orange Counties, California. *MMWR* 1982; **31**:305–307.

8. Kaplan JE, Hanson D, Dworkin MS *et al*. Epidemiology of human immunodeficiency virus-associated opportunistic infections in the United States in the era of highly active antiretroviral therapy. *Clin Infect Dis* 2000; **30**(Suppl 1):S5–14.

9. Ledergerber B, Egger M, Erard V *et al*. AIDS-related opportunistic illnesses occurring after initiation of potent antiretroviral therapy: the Swiss HIV Cohort Study. *JAMA* 1999; **282**:2220–2226.

10. Mocroft A, Katlama C, Johnson AM *et al*. AIDS across Europe, 1994–98: the EuroSIDA study. *Lancet* 2000; **356**:291–296.

11. Currier JS, Williams PL, Koletar SL *et al*. Discontinuation of *Mycobacterium avium* complex prophylaxis in patients with antiretroviral therapy-induced increases in CD4+ cell count. A randomized, double-blind, placebo-controlled trial. AIDS Clinical Trials Group 362 Study Team. *Ann Intern Med* 2000; **133**:493–503.

12. El-Sadr WM, Burman WJ, Grant LB *et al*. Discontinuation of prophylaxis for *Mycobacterium avium* complex disease in HIV-infected patients who have a response to antiretroviral therapy. Terry Beirn Community Programs for Clinical Research on AIDS. *N Engl J Med* 2000; **342**:1085–1092.

13. Furrer H, Egger M, Opravil M *et al*. Discontinuation of primary prophylaxis against *Pneumocystis carinii* pneumonia in HIV-1–infected adults treated with combination antiretroviral therapy. Swiss HIV Cohort Study. *N Engl J Med* 1999; **340**:1301–1306.

14. Furrer H, Opravil M, Bernasconi E, Telenti A, Egger M. Stopping primary prophylaxis in HIV-1-infected patients at high risk of toxoplasma encephalitis. Swiss HIV Cohort Study. *Lancet* 2000; **355**:2217–2218.

15. Ledergerber B, Mocroft A, Reiss P *et al*. Discontinuation of secondary prophylaxis against *Pneumocystis carinii* pneumonia in patients with HIV infection who have a response to antiretroviral therapy. Eight European Study Groups. *N Engl J Med* 2001; **344**:168–174.

16. Lopez Bernaldo de Quiros JC, Miro JM, Pena JM *et al*. A randomized trial of the discontinuation of primary and secondary prophylaxis against *Pneumocystis carinii* pneumonia after highly active antiretroviral therapy in patients with HIV infection. Grupo de Estudio del SIDA 04/98. *N Engl J Med* 2001; **344**:159–167.

17. Schneider MM, Borleffs JC, Stolk RP, Jaspers CA, Hoepelman AI. Discontinuation of prophylaxis for *Pneumocystis carinii* pneumonia in HIV-1-infected patients treated with highly active antiretroviral therapy. *Lancet* 1999; **353**:201–203.

18. Weverling GJ, Mocroft A, Ledergerber B *et al*. Discontinuation of *Pneumocystis carinii* pneumonia prophylaxis after start of highly active antiretroviral therapy in HIV-1 infection. EuroSIDA Study Group. *Lancet* 1999; **353**:1293–1298.

19. Aboulafia DM. Regression of acquired immunodeficiency syndrome-related pulmonary Kaposi's sarcoma after highly active antiretroviral therapy. *Mayo Clin Proc* 1998; **73**:439–443.

20. Hocqueloux L, Agbalika F, Oksenhendler E, Molina JM. Long-term remission of an AIDS-related primary effusion lymphoma with antiviral therapy. *Aids* 2001; **15**:280–282.

21. Behrens GM, Meyer D, Stoll M, Schmidt RE. Immune reconstitution syndromes in human immuno-deficiency virus infection following effective antiretroviral therapy. *Immunobiology* 2000; **202**:186–193.

22. Domingo P, Torres OH, Ris J, Vazquez G. Herpes zoster as an immune reconstitution disease after initiation of combination antiretroviral therapy in patients with human immunodeficiency virus type-1 infection. *Am J Med* 2001; **110**:605–609.

23. Greenspan D, Canchola AJ, MacPhail LA, Cheikh B, Greenspan JS. Effect of highly active antiretroviral therapy on frequency of oral warts. *Lancet* 2001; **357**:1411–1412.

24. Calista D, Boschini A. Cutaneous side effects induced by indinavir. *Eur J Dermatol* 2000; **10**:292–296.

25. Bouscarat F, Bouchard C, Bouhour D. Paronychia and pyogenic granuloma of the great toes in patients treated with indinavir. *N Engl J Med* 1998; **338**:1776–1777.

26. Colson AE, Sax PE, Keller MJ *et al*. Paronychia in association with indinavir treatment. *Clin Infect Dis* 2001; **32**:140–143.

27. Metry DW, Lahart CJ, Farmer KL, Hebert AA. Stevens-Johnson syndrome caused by the antiretroviral drug nevirapine. *J Am Acad Dermatol* 2001; **44**(Suppl 2):354–357.

28. Spach DH, Koehler JE. Bartonella-associated infections. *Infect Dis Clin North Am* 1998; **12**:137–155.

29. Pechere M, Krischer J, Remondat C, Bertrand C, Trellu L, Saurat JH. *Malassezia* spp carriage in patients with seborrheic dermatitis. *J Dermatol* 1999; **26**:558–561.

30. Duong TA. Infection due to *Penicillium marneffei*, an emerging pathogen: review of 155 reported cases. *Clin Infect Dis* 1996; **23**:125–130.

31. Antman K, Chang Y. Kaposi's sarcoma. *N Engl J Med* 2000; **342**:1027–1038.

32. Patton LL, McKaig R, Strauss R, Rogers D, Eron JJ, Jr. Changing prevalence of oral manifestations of human immuno-deficiency virus in the era of protease inhibitor therapy. *Oral Surg Oral Med Oral Pathol Oral Radiol Endod* 2000; **89**:299–304.

33. Nuorti JP, Butler JC, Gelling L, Kool JL, Reingold AL, Vugia DJ. Epidemiologic relation between HIV and invasive pneumococcal disease in San Francisco County, California. *Ann Intern Med* 2000; **132**:182–190.

34. Janoff EN, Breiman RF, Daley CL, Hopewell PC. Pneumococcal disease during HIV infection. Epidemiologic, clinical, and immunologic perspectives. *Ann Intern Med* 1992; **117**:314–324.

35. French N, Nakiyingi J, Carpenter LM *et al*. 23-valent pneumococcal poly-saccharide vaccine in HIV-1-infected Ugandan adults: double-blind, randomised and placebo controlled trial. *Lancet* 2000; **355**:2106–2111.

36. Breiman RF, Keller DW, Phelan MA *et al*. Evaluation of effectiveness of the 23-valent pneumococcal capsular polysaccharide vaccine for HIV-infected patients. *Arch Intern Med* 2000; **160**:2633–2638.

37. Dworkin MS, Ward JW, Hanson DL, Jones JL, Kaplan JE. Pneumococcal disease among human immunodeficiency virus-infected persons: incidence, risk factors, and impact of vaccination. *Clin Infect Dis* 2001; **32**:794–800.

38. Havlir DV, Barnes PF. Tuberculosis in patients with human immuno-deficiency virus infection. *N Engl J Med* 1999; **340**:367–373.

39. Markowitz N, Hansen NI, Hopewell PC *et al*. Incidence of tuberculosis in the United States among HIV-infected persons. The Pulmonary Complications of HIV Infection Study Group. *Ann Intern Med* 1997; **126**:123–132.

40. Hajjeh RA, Pappas PG, Henderson H *et al*. Multicenter case-control study of risk factors for histoplasmosis in human immunodeficiency virus-infected persons. *Clin Infect Dis* 2001; **32**:1215–1220.

41. Wheat LJ, Connolly-Stringfield PA, Baker RL *et al*. Disseminated histo-plasmosis in the acquired immune deficiency syndrome: clinical findings, diagnosis and treatment, and review of the literature. *Medicine (Baltimore)* 1990; **69**:361–374.

42. Dupont C, Vasseur E, Beauchet A *et al*. Long-term efficacy on Kaposi's sarcoma of highly active antiretroviral therapy in a cohort of HIV-positive patients. CISIH 92. Centre d'information et de soins de l'immunodeficience humaine. *Aids* 2000; **14**:987–993.

43. Sheikh RA, Prindiville TP, Yenamandra S, Munn RJ, Ruebner BH. Microsporidial AIDS cholangiopathy due to *Encephalitozoon intestinalis*: case report and review. *Am J Gastroenterol* 2000; **95**:2364–2371.

44. Powderly WG. Cryptococcal meningitis and AIDS. *Clin Infect Dis* 1993; **17**:837–842.

45. Cinque P, Vago L, Dahl H *et al*. Polymerase chain reaction on cerebrospinal fluid for diagnosis of virus-associated opportunistic diseases of the central nervous system in HIV-infected patients. *Aids* 1996; **10**:951–958.

46. Oksenhendler E, Duarte M, Soulier J *et al*. Multicentric Castleman's disease in HIV infection: a clinical and pathological study of 20 patients. *Aids* 1996; **10**:61–67.

47. Shahidi H, Myers JL, Kvale PA. Castleman's disease. *Mayo Clin Proc* 1995; **70**:969–977.

48. Hader SL, Smith DK, Moore JS, Holmberg SD. HIV infection in women in the United States: status at the Millennium. *JAMA* 2001; **285**:1186–1192.

49. Szczech LA. Renal diseases associated with human immunodeficiency virus infection: epidemiology, clinical course, and management. *Clin Infect Dis* 2001; **33**:115–119.

50. Opravil M, Pechere M, Speich R *et al*. HIV-associated primary pulmonary hypertension. A case control study. Swiss HIV Cohort Study. *Am J Respir Crit Care Med* 1997; **155**:990–995.

51. Jacobson MA. Human immunodeficiency virus-associated immune reconstitution disease. *Am J Med* 2001; **110**:662–663.

52. Jacobson MA, Zegans M, Pavan PR *et al*. Cytomegalovirus retinitis after initiation of highly active antiretroviral therapy. *Lancet* 1997; **349**:1443–1445.

53. Karavellas MP, Plummer DJ, Macdonald JC *et al*. Incidence of immune recovery vitritis in cytomegalovirus retinitis patients following institution of successful highly active antiretroviral therapy. *J Infect Dis* 1999; **179**:697–700.

54. Jouan M, Saves M, Tubiana R *et al*. Discontinuation of maintenance therapy for cytomegalovirus retinitis in HIV-infected patients receiving highly active antiretroviral therapy. *Aids* 2001; **15**:23–31.

55. Race EM, Adelson-Mitty J, Kriegel GR *et al*. Focal mycobacterial lymphadenitis following initiation of protease-inhibitor therapy in patients with advanced HIV-1 disease. *Lancet* 1998; **351**:252–255.

56. Phillips P, Kwiatkowski MB, Copland M, Craib K, Montaner J. Mycobacterial lymphadenitis associated with the initiation of combination antiretroviral therapy. *J Acquir Immune Defic Syndr Hum Retrovirol* 1999; **20**:122–128.

57. Narita M, Ashkin D, Hollender ES, Pitchenik AE. Paradoxical worsening of tuberculosis following antiretroviral therapy in patients with AIDS. *Am J Respir Crit Care Med* 1998; **158**:157–161.

58. Miralles P, Berenguer J, Garcia de Viedma D *et al*. Treatment of AIDS-associated progressive multifocal leukoencephalopathy with highly active antiretroviral therapy. *Aids* 1998; **12**:2467–2472.

59. Woods ML, 2nd, MacGinley R, Eisen DP, Allworth AM. HIV combination therapy: partial immune restitution unmasking latent cryptococcal infection. *Aids* 1998; **12**:1491–1494.

60. Mastroianni CM, Trinchieri V, Santopadre P *et al*. Acute clinical hepatitis in an HIV-seropositive hepatitis B carrier receiving protease inhibitor therapy. *Aids* 1998; **12**:1939–1940.

61. Zietz C, Bogner JR, Goebel FD, Lohrs U. An unusual cluster of cases of Castleman's disease during highly active antiretroviral therapy for AIDS. *N Engl J Med* 1999; **340**:1923–1924.

62. Johnson SC, Benson CA, Johnson DW, Weinberg A. Recurrences of cytomegalovirus retinitis in a human immunodeficiency virus-infected patient, despite potent antiretroviral therapy and apparent immune reconstitution. *Clin Infect Dis* 2001; **32**:815–819.

63. Komanduri KV, Feinberg J, Hutchins RK *et al*. Loss of cytomegalovirus-specific CD4+ T cell responses in human immunodeficiency virus type 1-infected patients with high CD4+ T cell counts and recurrent retinitis. *J Infect Dis* 2001; **183**:1285–1289.

64. Torriani FJ, Freeman WR, Macdonald JC *et al*. CMV retinitis recurs after stopping treatment in virological and immunological failures of potent antiretroviral therapy. *Aids* 2000; **14**:173–180.

65. Bender MA, Sax PE. Discontinuing prophylaxis against *Pneumocystis carinii* pneumonia. *N Engl J Med* 2001; **344**:1639; discussion 1640–1641.

66. Le Moal G, Breux JP, Roblot F. Discontinuing prophylaxis against *Pneumocystis carinii* pneumonia. *N Engl J Med* 2001; **344**:1639–1641.

67. CDC. HIV/AIDS Surveillance Report. 2000; **1**:1.

68. Palella FJ, Jr., Delaney KM, Moorman AC *et al*. Declining morbidity and mortality among patients with advanced human immunodeficiency virus infection. HIV Outpatient Study Investigators. *N Engl J Med* 1998; **338**:853–860.

69. Yeni PG, Hammer SM, Carpenter CC, *et al*. Antiretroviral treatment for adult HIV infection in 2002: updated recommendations of the International AIDS Society–USA Panel. *JAMA* 2002; **288**:222–235.

70. Havlir DV, Bassett R, Levitan D *et al*. Prevalence and predictive value of intermittent viremia with combination HIV therapy. *JAMA* 2001; **286**:171–179.

71. Pierson T, McArthur J, Siliciano RF. Reservoirs for HIV-1: mechanisms for viral persistence in the presence of antiviral immune responses and antiretroviral therapy. *Annu Rev Immunol* 2000; **18**:665–708.

72. Davey RT, Jr., Bhat N, Yoder C *et al*. HIV-1 and T cell dynamics after interruption of highly active antiretroviral therapy (HAART) in patients with a history of sustained viral suppression. *Proc Natl Acad Sci USA* 1999; **96**:15109–15114.

73. Paterson DL, Swindells S, Mohr J *et al*. Adherence to protease inhibitor therapy and outcomes in patients with HIV infection. *Ann Intern Med* 2000; **133**:21–30.

74. Carr A, Samaras K, Burton S *et al*. A syndrome of peripheral lipodystrophy, hyperlipidaemia and insulin resistance in patients receiving HIV protease inhibitors. *Aids* 1998; **12**:F51–58.

75. Safrin S, Grunfeld C. Fat distribution and metabolic changes in patients with HIV infection. *Aids* 1999; **13**:2493–2505.

76. Brinkman K, Smeitink JA, Romijn JA, Reiss P. Mitochondrial toxicity induced by nucleoside-analogue reverse-transcriptase inhibitors is a key factor in the pathogenesis of antiretroviral-therapy-related lipodystrophy. *Lancet* 1999; **354**:1112–1115.

77. Connor EM, Sperling RS, Gelber R *et al*. Reduction of maternal–infant transmission of human immunodeficiency virus type 1 with zidovudine treatment. Pediatric AIDS Clinical Trials Group Protocol 076 Study Group. *N Engl J Med* 1994; **331**:1173–1180.

78. Shaffer N, Chuachoowong R, Mock PA *et al*. Short-course zidovudine for perinatal HIV-1 transmission in Bangkok, Thailand: a randomised controlled trial. Bangkok Collaborative Perinatal HIV Transmission Study Group. *Lancet* 1999; **353**:773–780.

79. Guay LA, Musoke P, Fleming T *et al*. Intrapartum and neonatal single-dose nevirapine compared with zidovudine for prevention of mother-to-child transmission of HIV-1 in Kampala, Uganda: HIVNET 012 randomised trial. *Lancet* 1999; **354**:795–802.

80. Recommendations for use of antiretroviral drugs in pregnant HIV-1–infected women for maternal health and interventions to reduce perinatal HIV-1 transmission in the United States. In: *Public Health Service Task Force*; 2001.

81. Blanche S, Tardieu M, Rustin P *et al*. Persistent mitochondrial dysfunction and perinatal exposure to antiretroviral nucleoside analogues. *Lancet* 1999; **354**:1084–1089.

82. CDC. Updated U.S. Public Health Service Guidelines for the Management of Occupational Exposures to HBV, HCV, and HIV and Recommendations for Postexposure Prophylaxis. *MMWR* 2001; **50**(RR-11):1–52.

83. Cardo DM, Culver DH, Ciesielski CA *et al*. A case-control study of HIV seroconversion in health care workers after percutaneous exposure. Centers for Disease Control and Prevention Needlestick Surveillance Group. *N Engl J Med* 1997; **337**:1485–1490.

84. Parkin JM, Murphy M, Anderson J, El-Gadi S, Forster G, Pinching AJ. Tolerability and side-effects of post-exposure prophylaxis for HIV infection. *Lancet* 2000; **355**:722–723.

85. CDC. Management of possible sexual, injecting-drug-use, or other nonoccupational exposure to HIV, including considerations related to antiretroviral therapy. *MMWR* 1998; **47**(RR-17):1–14.

86. Kahn JO, Martin JN, Roland ME *et al*. Feasibility of postexposure prophylaxis (PEP) against human immunodeficiency virus infection after sexual or injection drug use exposure: the San Francisco PEP Study. *J Infect Dis* 2001; **183**:707–714.

87. Kahn J. Building and testing an effective HIV vaccine. *West J Med* 1999; **171**:363–365.

88. Letvin NL. Progress in the development of an HIV-1 vaccine. *Science* 1998; **280**:1875–1880.

89. 1999 USPHS/IDSA guidelines for the prevention of opportunistic infections in persons infected with human immunodeficiency virus. *Clin Infect Dis.* 2000; **30**:S29–65.

Genital Herpes

A Wald, R Ashley, P Pellett and A Moreland

13

INTRODUCTION

Genital herpes is a common, often painful disease that has serious consequences for certain populations. Medical research in the twentieth century significantly expanded our knowledge of the infection and its treatment. Prior to the nineteenth century, the term *herpes* (Greek for 'to creep') was used in medical literature for a variety of skin eruptions. Over time, the meaning of the term narrowed to mean primarily the classic appearance of grouped vesicles on an erythematous base. A viral etiology was eventually suggested by transmission experiments in the early 1900s, and was confirmed and classified in relation to other viral diseases by the 1950s.

Genital herpes infections are caused by the herpes simplex viruses (HSV) that are large (150–200 nm) viruses that consist of approximately 152,000 base pairs of double-stranded DNA encapsulated in a proteinaceous capsid, which is, in turn, surrounded by an electron dense tegument. The core and tegument are encapsulated within a host cell-derived lipid bilayer, studded with virus-specified proteins and glycoproteins (*Figs 13.1* and *13.2*). HSV type 1 (HSV-1) and HSV type 2 (HSV-2), are two of the eight known human herpesviruses (*Table 13.1*). The nucleotide sequences of HSV-1 and HSV-2 are approximately 50% identical and their encoded proteins are closely related. The viruses each encode nearly 80 genes, many of which are not needed for virus growth in cell culture but serve various roles in pathogenesis. No genes are unique to either virus.

HSV-1 is responsible for more than 90% of orolabial herpes and herpes keratitis, while HSV-2 is responsible for approximately 90% of recurrent genital herpes. HSV infection is characterized by viral shedding from affected skin or mucous membranes and by cellular and humoral immune responses. Neutralizing antibodies, which are produced early in the course of infection and persist for variable lengths of time, do not prevent mucocutaneous recurrences, perhaps because extracellular virus is inactivated by these antibodies while intracellular viral replication and direct cell-to-cell transfer of new infectious virus are controlled by

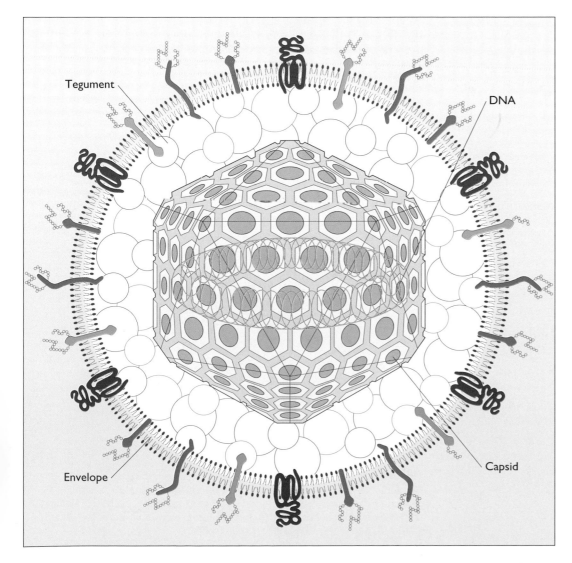

Fig. 13.1 Herpesvirus morphology. Schematic representation.

241

cell-mediated immunity. The exact role of humoral antibodies in reactivation of the infection is not fully understood; however, antibodies appear to attenuate the severity of the disease since recurrences generally are less severe than the primary infection and transplacental passage of antibodies appears to be protective against neonatal herpes. Cell-mediated immune responses undoubtedly play an important role in the manifestation of herpes infections as evidenced by the severe, prolonged, and frequently recurring infections that occur in patients who have impaired cell-mediated immunity.

EPIDEMIOLOGY

Accurate estimates of the prevalence of HSV-2 infection in several populations have only recently become available. A national survey in the USA from 1988 to 1994 found a seroprevalence of 21.9% in individuals of 12 years of age or older, with 17.6% of whites, 45.9% of blacks, and 22.3% of Mexican Americans being HSV-2 seropositive.[1] This reflects an overall 30% increase in HSV-2 seroprevalence since the initial survey that took place from 1976 to 1980. Consistent among the serologic surveys are higher rates of infection among women than men. Of interest are the high rates of infection among people who report

only 2 to 4 lifetime sexual partners, especially among African-American women *(Fig. 13.3)*. This suggests that once HSV-2 prevalence becomes high, individual sexual behavior is a less important determinant of infection. Studies in several Western countries have found a wide range of HSV-2 seroprevalence, from less than 10% in some college students to over 80% in groups of female sex workers.[2] Among HSV-2 seropositive persons, only a small proportion report a history of genital herpes. For example, in the US national survey, only 10% of those with HSV-2 antibodies reported a diagnosis of genital herpes.[1] However, persons without a history of genital herpes are the most common source of new infections both for sexual partners and for neonates,[3,4] and viral shedding studies show that almost all persons with HSV-2 antibodies shed virus in the genital tract.[5] In parallel to the rising seroprevalence of HSV-2 infection, there has been an increase in the number of initial office visits for genital herpes to physicians throughout the 1980s and 1990s[6] *(Figure. 13.4)*.

While issues surrounding genital herpes clinical disease have been most publicized in developed countries and among the affluent, seroprevalence of HSV-2 is even higher among the economically disadvantaged and in the developing world. Recent studies from many areas of Africa show prevalence in the general population that exceeds 50%.[7,8] In addition, molecular techniques have shown that HSV accounts for a large proportion of genital ulcers worldwide, even in regions with endemic syphilis and chancroid. In a 10-city study of genital ulcers in STD clinics around the US, genital herpes was the predominant cause, accounting for greater than 50% of ulcerations in all cities but one.[9] HSV has also been shown to be the predominant agent of genital ulcer disease in STD clinics in Lesotho, India and Thailand.

Importantly, serologic surveys for HSV-2 are likely to underestimate the true prevalence of genital herpes, since HSV-1 can account for 30–50% of primary genital herpes in some Western countries. Especially

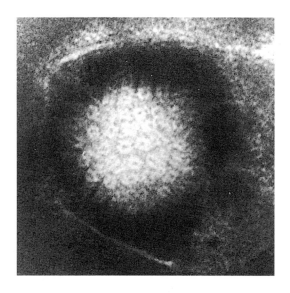

Fig. 13.2 Herpesvirus morphology. Electron micrograph. Courtesy of McKendrick GDW, Sutherland S: An Introduction to Herpes Infections. London, Gower Medical Publishing Ltd, 1983.

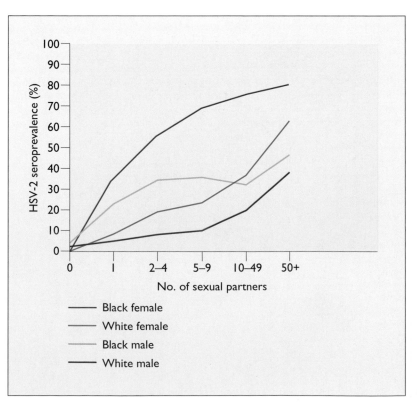

Fig. 13.3 Prevalence of HSV-2 antibody in the USA in 1988–1994, according to gender, race, and number of reported lifetime sex partners. Courtesy of Fleming DT, McQuillan GM, Johnson RE, *et al.* Herpes simplex virus type 2 in the United States, 1976 to 1994. *NEJM* 1997; **337**:1105–1111.

Virus	Principal diseases
Herpes simplex virus type 1 (HSV-1)	Skin and mucosal vesicles and ulcers, especially oral
Herpes simplex virus type 2 (HSV-2)	Skin and mucosal vesicles and ulcers, especially genital
Varicella-zoster virus (VZV)	Chickenpox, shingles
Epstein–Barr virus (EBV)	Infectious mononucleosis, Burkitt's lymphoma
Cytomegalovirus (CMV)	Serious disease in immunosuppressed patients and congenital infection
Human herpesvirus 6 (HHV-6)	Roseola infantum, non-rash febrile illness in young children, and possibly pneumonia in immunosuppressed patients
Human herpesvirus 7 (HHV-7)	Some cases of roseola infantum
Human herpesvirus 8 (HHV-8)	Associated with Kaposi's sarcoma and some lymphomas

Table 13.1 Human herpesviruses.

high frequency of genital HSV-1 has been noted among women and among men who have sex with men.[10] Among newly acquired HSV-1 infections in adults, one-third present with genital herpes, one third present with oral infection, and one third seroconvert to HSV-1 without localized symptoms.[11]

Transmission of HSV infection occurs when viral particles enter the skin or mucous membranes through traumatic microscopic openings or fissures. Friction to genital mucosal surfaces often occurs during intercourse, resulting in a favorable environment for passage of virus into keratinocytes. Once inside a keratinocyte, the virus replicates inside the

cell's nucleus, and then spreads to surrounding cells (*Figs 13.5* and *13.6*). Damage to the involved skin involves epidermal and, on occasion, dermal layers. The virus then enters the peripheral sensory or autonomic nerve endings, and ascends to sensory or autonomic root ganglia, where it establishes a latent infection.[12] Reactivation from latency is common with the virus descending along the involved nerve root back to the genital mucosa or skin. If the reactivation results in clinical lesions, the event is called a 'recurrence'. Alternatively, the virus may reactivate without causing appreciable lesions. Transmission of the infection can occur readily by contact with lesions, but viral replication appears to

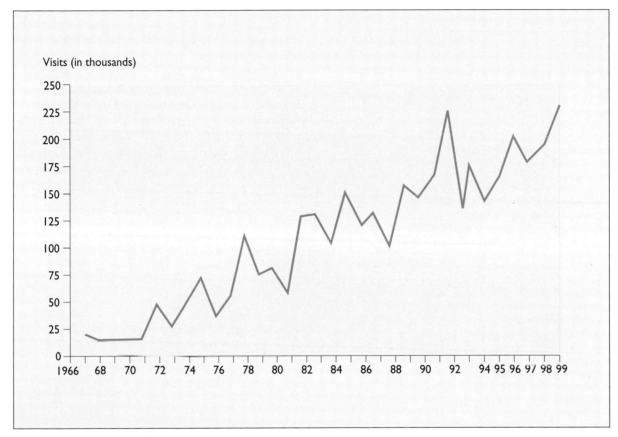

Fig. 13.4 Genital HSV infections: initial visits to physicians' offices, USA, 1966–1999. Source: http://www.cdc.gov/nchstp/dstd/Stats_Trends/1999Surveillance/99PDF/99Section5.pdf (HSV segment) http://www.cdc.gov/nchstp/dstd/Stats_Trends/1999SurvRpt.htm (for whole report). Division of STD Prevention. Sexually Transmitted Disease Surveillance, 1999. Department of Health and Human Services, Atlanta: Centers for Disease Control and Prevention, September 2000.

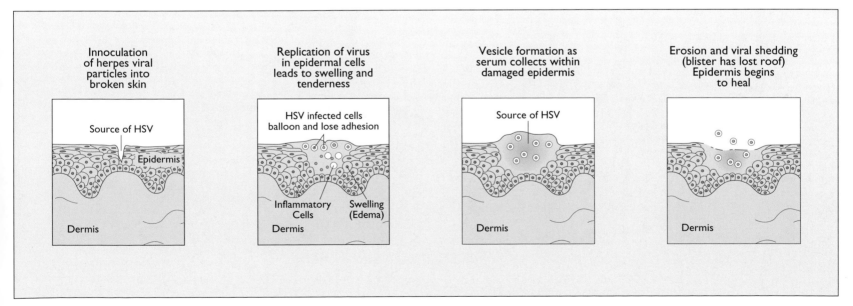

Fig. 13.5 Infection with HSV. Courtesy of Milton Tam, PhD.

achieve sufficient titers to result in transmission even in the absence of symptoms. In fact, transmission occurs most commonly from partners who have a history of genital herpes but did not notice a lesion at the time of transmission, or from partners who are infected but do not recognize that they have genital herpes.[3,13,14] The prominence of asymptomatic viral shedding in the transmission of genital herpes underscores the need for identification of infected persons by antibody tests and for consistent adherence to safer sexual practices.

CLINICAL MANIFESTATIONS

CLASSIFICATION OF GENITAL HERPES

The classification of genital herpes encompasses the clinical presentation of the patient and the virologic and serologic findings. However, the laboratory results are usually not available at the time that the patient is evaluated (*Table 13.2*):

First-episode infection

- Primary HSV-1 or HSV-2
- Non-primary initial HSV-2
- First recognized recurrence of HSV-1 or HSV-2.

Recurrent infection with HSV-1 or HSV-2

First episode infections are those in which the patient does not have a previous history of genital herpes. *Primary genital herpes* can be caused by either HSV-1 or HSV-2; the affected person is seronegative for HSV antibodies. In general, this type of genital herpes is the most severe clinically. *Non-primary initial genital herpes* refers to new acquisition of HSV-2 in a person with prior HSV-1 infection. While the reverse order of acquisition is also possible, acquisition of HSV-1 in a HSV-2-seropositive person is unusual. The presence of antibodies to the heterologous virus attenuates the clinical presentation of the disease so that in general, first-episode nonprimary genital herpes is less severe than first-episode primary genital herpes, but more severe than recurrent disease. The protection is seen both in the spectrum of clinical disease and in the frequency of subclinical shedding in the first months after the infections.[15] However, the distinction between primary and nonprimary genital herpes cannot be made with certainty by clinical observation. About 25% of patients who present with a clinical first episode of genital herpes already have antibodies to the virus which is isolated from the genital area and thus present with *first recognized recurrence*. As the immune response takes some time to develop after initial infection, the presence of antibodies indicates that the

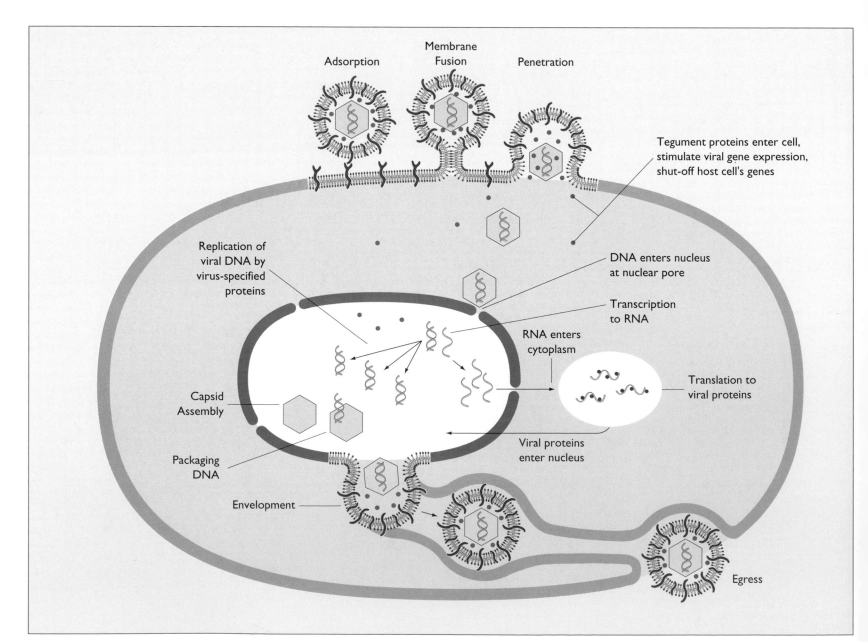

Fig. 13.6 HSV replication cycle.

person has had the infection for some time but has not recognized recurrences.

Recurrent genital herpes refers to repeated episodes of genital herpes in the same person. The recurrence rate for genital infections is higher with HSV-2 than with HSV-1 (*Fig. 13.7*).[16,17] A comparison of the mean duration of symptoms and signs in patients with first-episode primary, first-episode nonprimary, and recurrent genital herpes is shown in *Fig. 13.8*.

Studies of persons who have HSV-2 antibodies but no history of genital herpes show that most of them have mild clinical disease. Most can be taught to recognize the recurrences which are infrequent and shorter than in persons with recognized genital herpes.[5,18] Some persons with undiagnosed genital herpes have atypical presentations that have been mistaken for other genital pathology.[19]

PRIMARY GENITAL INFECTION

After an incubation period of approximately 1 week (2–12 days), painful, grouped, discrete vesicles appear (*Fig. 13.9*). The vesicles usually evolve into pustules, which then erode, creating an ulcer. The remaining grayish plaques crust before healing takes place (*Fig. 13.10*). In women the lesions ulcerate rapidly, often coalescing. In men, the blisters will sometimes dry to crusts without progressing through the ulcerative stage. This process takes 15–20 days before re-epithelialization occurs. The lesions shed infectious virus for at least 10–12 days, and new lesions may appear until the 10th day. Typical lesions in men occur on the shaft of the penis, glans penis, coronal sulcus, urethra (*Fig. 13.11*), or perianal region. Less frequently, lesions occur on the scrotum, mons area, thighs, or buttocks. In women, lesions usually occur around the introitus, the urethral meatus, or the labia (*Figs 13.12* and *13.13*),

Clinical presentation	HSV-2 Serology	HSV-1 Serology	HSV culture	Terminology	Comment
First Episode	Primary Infection				
	Neg	Neg	HSV-2 +	Primary	Serologic testing must be done near the onset of symptoms prior to seroconversion to confirm primary diagnosis
	Neg	Neg	HSV-1 +	Primary	
HSV-2	Neg	Pos	HSV-2 +	Initial Non-Primary	
HSV-1	Pos	Neg	HSV-1 +	Initial Non-Primary	Non primary HSV-1 is rare
Recurrent Episode					
HSV-2	Pos	Pos/Neg	HSV-2 +	Recurrent	Once seropositivity is established, retesting not necessary.
HSV-1	Pos/Neg	Pos	HSV-1 +	Recurrent	

Table 13.2 Clinical, virologic and serologic characteristics of HSV infections

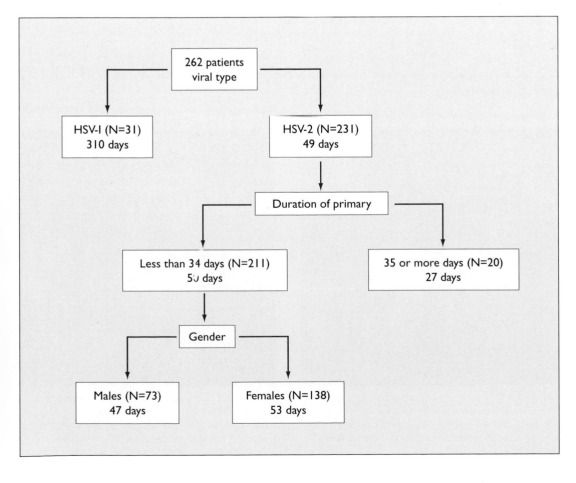

Fig. 13.7 Median time to first recurrence, in days, among patients followed after new acquisition of infection, shown by type of HSV, duration of primary episode, and gender.

but can also occur in extragenital sites, such as the perineal or perianal regions or on the thighs and buttocks. Cervicitis is common, occurring in 70–90% of women with primary genital herpes; occasionally cervical infection may occur in the absence of vulvar disease. Cervicitis occurs less often in recurrent genital herpes. The cervical mucosa may have ulcerations and appear red and friable (*Figs 13.14* and *13.15*).

The presentation of primary genital herpes may differ significantly from this classical picture. Immunosuppression resulting from either medications or disease may contribute to more severe or prolonged infections (*Fig. 13.16*). Underlying skin conditions may affect HSV infection. For example, chronic tinea cruris is characterized by scaling, vesicles or pustules, excoriations, and erosions in the folds of the groin. Exposure of this skin to fresh genital herpes lesions may lead to a super-infection with herpes (*Fig. 13.17*). Chronic eczema may also render the skin susceptible to HSV infection (eczema herpeticum) (*Figs 13.18* and *13.19*) and can involve the genitals.

Associated genitourinary symptoms in primary genital herpes include dysuria in most cases in both women and men. Vaginal discharge, urethral discharge, and tender inguinal adenopathy are also common. Pain persists for at least 1 week, occasionally for 2 weeks.

In addition, patients with primary genital herpes often have other associated systemic symptoms, including headache, fever, malaise, and myalgia. These symptoms appear more commonly in women than in men. Pharyngitis, aseptic meningitis, transverse myelitis, and radiculitis are also associated with genital herpes infections in some patients. Neurologic complications occur in about 15–30% of patients. Complaints of a stiff neck, headache, or photophobia ordinarily occur about 3–12 days after the onset of genital lesions and are more common among women and those with HSV-2 compared with HSV-1 infection. Sacral radiculitis may result in urinary retention. Even the serious neurologic complications usually resolve; persisting neurologic deficits are rare. Herpetic autoinoculation of extragenital sites — most often the

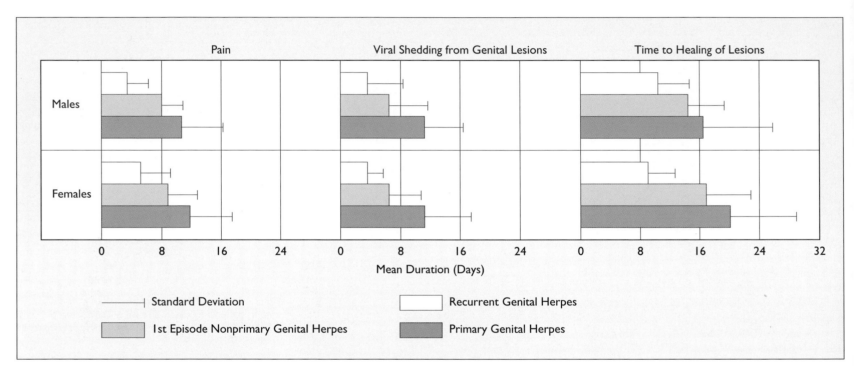

Fig. 13.8 Comparison of symptoms and signs in different types of genital herpes.

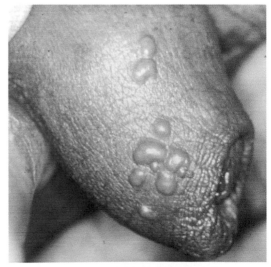

Fig. 13.9 Early lesions of primary genital herpes. Clear, grouped vesicles appear on an erythematous base. Some vesicles are discrete and some coalesce, which frequently results in a scalloped border.

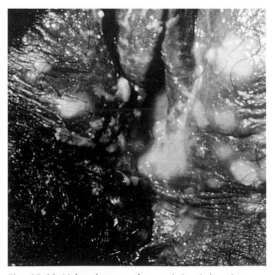

Fig. 13.10 Vulvar herpes of several days' duration. Several stages in the natural evolution of the eruption are apparent here: clear vesicles, pustules, and grayish exudate cover plaques where the roofs of blisters have eroded.

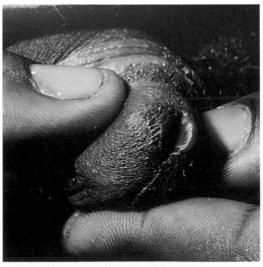

Fig. 13.11 Herpes erosion in the urethral meatus. Dysuria resulted from this erythematous and painful erosion. Urethral involvement is less common than lesions on the shaft or the foreskin of the penis.

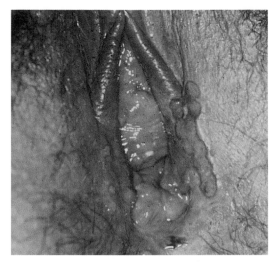

Fig. 13.12 Primary vulvar herpes. The linear appearance of these painful herpetic erosions on the labia is a result of coalescence of several closely grouped vesicles, which have subsequently shed the vesicle roof. Courtesy of Barbara Romanowski, MD.

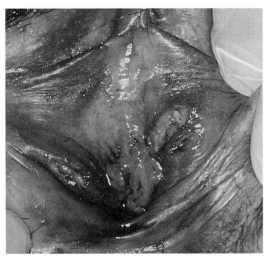

Fig. 13.13 Primary vulvar herpes. These painful ulcers were present on the vulva of the patient in Fig. 13.14. Courtesy of Barbara Romanowski, MD.

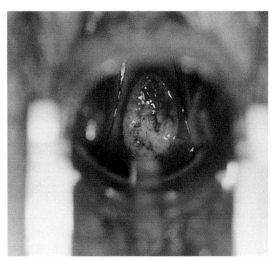

Fig. 13.14 Herpetic cervicitis. Erosive cervicitis was present in this case of primary herpes presenting with vulvar ulcers (see Fig. 13.13). Courtesy of Barbara Romanowski, MD.

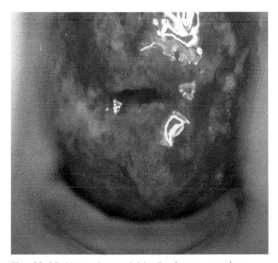

Fig. 13.15 Herpetic cervicitis. Erythema, purulent exudate, and erosions were present on the cervix of this patient with genital herpes. Courtesy of Barbara Romanowski, MD.

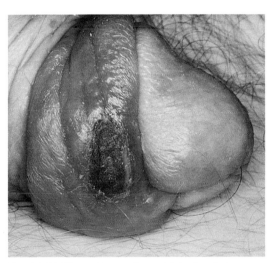

Fig. 13.16 Herpes in a patient with leukemia in whom edema is notable around a large herpetic erosion on the penis. The duration of the lesions was much longer than in healthy individuals.

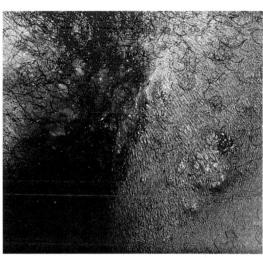

Fig. 13.17 Primary herpes arising in chronic tinea cruris infection. Hyperpigmentation and scaling in inguinal folds are signs of a chronic dermatitis.

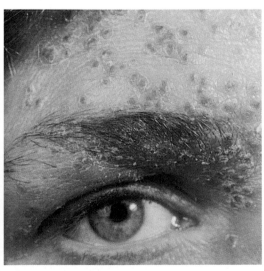

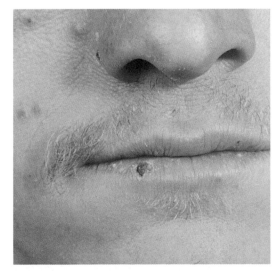

Figs 13.18 and 13.19 Eczema herpeticum. Generalized herpes simplex (13.18) in this case started with an oral lesion (13.19) in a patient with atopic dermatitis. Genital eruptions may also be the source of a generalized infection in predisposed individuals. Courtesy of David Mandeville and Peter Lane, MD.

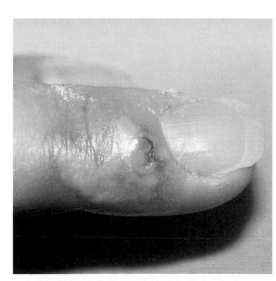

Fig. 13.20 Commonly called a herpetic whitlow, these herpes blisters are extremely painful and can be recurrent, but heal spontaneously.

fingers — is another complication of genital herpes that occurs predominantly during primary infection (*Fig. 13.20*).

RECURRENT GENITAL HERPES

The rate of recurrences is highly variable in any one individual but differs most significantly between HSV-1 and HSV-2 infection. In the first year of genital HSV-2 infection, the median number of recurrences is 4; however, 38% will have 6 or more recurrences and 20% will have more than 10 recurrences.[17] In contrast, the median number of recurrences for genital HSV-1 is one in the first year of infection, and many patients will have none. The frequency of recurrences declines over several years although the rate of decline is low and may not be clinically noticeable to the patient for a long time.[20] In addition, a minority of patients will report more frequent recurrences in the 5th year of infection than in the first year. Recurrent genital herpes symptoms vary from mild episodes (*Figs 13.21* and *13.22*) to, more rarely, severe discomfort (*Figs 13.23* and *13.24*). In most cases, however, the symptoms and signs are milder and of shorter duration than in primary infection. Often a prodrome of itching (*Fig. 13.25*), burning, or tingling occurs at the affected site a few hours to a few days before the lesions appear.[21] The dysesthesia of prodrome is often more bothersome than the genital ulcerations. Dysuria, neurologic involvement and inguinal adenopathy are less common than in primary episodes and viral shedding is shorter, lasting only about 4 days. The elapsed time until re-epithelialization is approximately 7 days in recurrent herpes. In immunocompromised patients, recurrences may be atypical in appearance or have a prolonged duration (*Fig. 13.26*). The triggers for recurrences are poorly defined. While some patients report stress, fatigue, sunlight and menses as common precipitating factors, prospective studies show no association with menstrual cycle and suggest that the recurrences cause, rather than follow, stressful events. Erythema multiforme occasionally occurs with recurrences and may become more troublesome than the herpetic lesions (*see Figs 2.52, 2.53*).

Nearly half of all individuals with recurrent genital herpes lesions will also experience prodromal symptoms without lesions.[21] Prodromes without lesions are also known as 'false' prodromes or 'aborted' prodromes, and are probably due to better immunologic control than is present when lesions develop.

Asymptomatic shedding

It appears likely that all persons with HSV-2 infection experience periodic viral shedding that is not associated with recognizable genital lesions. This has been called 'asymptomatic' or 'subclinical' shedding. The frequency appears to vary widely, but it appears highest in the first 6–12 months after acquisition of infection and in patients with frequent recurrences.[22] On average, the frequency of shedding in persons with genital HSV-2 by viral culture is 4% of the days, but it may be as high as 10% among those with recently acquired infection. The most frequent sites of asymptomatic shedding in men are the penile shaft followed by the perianal area; the latter is more common among men who have sex with men.[23] In women, the vulva and the perianal area are the most common sites of viral shedding. Of epidemiologic import is the fact that the asymptomatic shedding rate appears to be comparable in persons

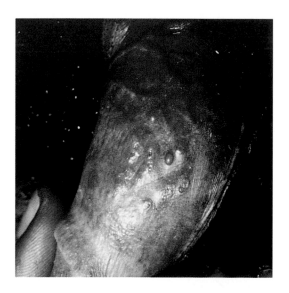

Fig. 13.21 Recurrent genital herpes. Many vesicles have eroded and are healing quickly in this mildly symptomatic case.

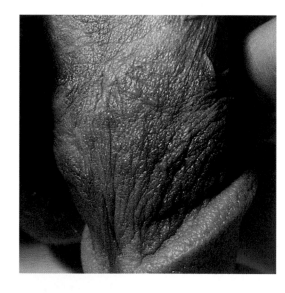

Fig. 13.22 Recurrent genital herpes. Erythema, groups of vesicles, erosions, and edema seen on the shaft of the penis.

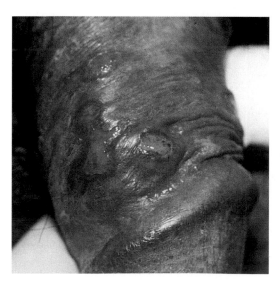

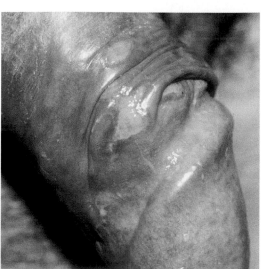

Figs 13.23 and 13.24 Recurrent penile herpes. These discrete and confluent well-demarcated shallow ulcerations on the shaft of the penis were extremely painful in this 32-year-old diabetic patient.

with diagnosed genital herpes and in those who are HSV-2 seropositive and do not have a history of genital herpes.[5] This explains the epidemiologic observation that new infections are usually acquired from persons who do not have a history of genital herpes.

It is important to note that detection of viral shedding by HSV PCR shows that mucosal replication occurs more frequently than appreciated in studies by viral cultures. In a group of women within 2 years of acquisition of genital HSV-2 infection, the overall rate of viral detection was 28%, with several women shedding on more than 50% of the days of samples.[24] While the threshold of viral amount required for sexual transmission is unknown, neonatal data show that perinatal HSV transmission can occur in women who are culture negative but PCR positive at delivery.[25]

GENITAL HERPES AND PREGNANCY

While, in general, manifestations of genital herpes do not differ between pregnant and nonpregnant women, severe first recognized episodes may be more common in pregnancy. The consequences of maternal genital herpes infection can be devastating for the neonate. Transmission to the neonate almost always occurs during parturition, but rarely can occur in utero, or from postnatal contact with a person with oral HSV. The risk of transmission depends primarily on whether the mother is experiencing primary or recurrent infection. In primary or non-primary initial maternal infection, the rate of neonatal transmission is 30–50%, compared to less than 1% in recurrent maternal disease.[26,27] The reasons for the marked discrepancy in the rate of fetal transmission between primary and recurrent maternal infection is probably the transmission of maternal HSV antibodies to the fetus in recurrent disease. In addition, primary genital herpes is associated with larger quantities of virus and a much greater likelihood of cervicitis. Despite the lower fetal transmission rate from women with recurrent genital herpes, such transmission is epidemiologically important since recurrent maternal infection is much more prevalent than newly acquired infection.

Pregnant women with a history of genital herpes should be examined under good light very carefully for genital lesions early in labor.[28] If any lesions are detected, the infant should be delivered by cesarean section, preferably before the amniotic membrane has ruptured, to prevent direct exposure of the infant to maternal virus. A small percentage of transmission occurs in utero and will not be prevented by cesarean delivery. Women with a history of genital herpes can deliver vaginally in the absence of lesions or prodromal symptoms.

NEONATAL INFECTION

Unfortunately, the majority of infants with neonatal HSV infection are born to mothers with no history of genital herpes, many of whom have recently acquired infection. Thus, no matter how carefully women with a history of genital herpes are monitored, neonatal herpes will remain problematic unless the acquisition of genital herpes in pregnancy is prevented.[29]

Neonatal HSV infection (*Figs 13.27* and *13.28*) has a high morbidity.[4] Clinical disease usually manifests at 3–30 days of age, with 71% of cases presenting with localized infections of the skin, eye, and mouth. The

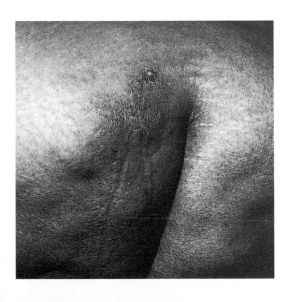

Fig. 13.25 Extragenital HSV of the buttocks. Pruritus and irritation were the first symptoms in this recurrent episode. (The black circle is the site chosen for biopsy.)

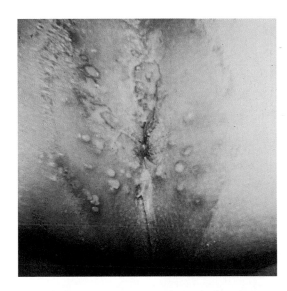

Fig. 13.26 Chronic perianal herpes in an AIDS patient. This infection was very difficult to control even with antiviral therapy.

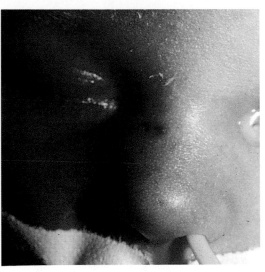

Fig. 13.27 Neonatal herpes. The crusted areas on the bridge of the nose were the only visible cutaneous lesions in this neonate with herpes who developed encephalitis and died. Courtesy of Mary Spraker, MD.

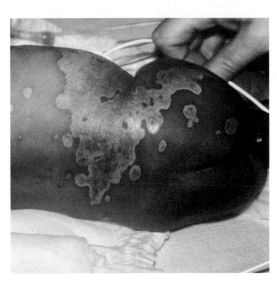

Fig. 13.28 Neonatal herpes. Extensive erosions in another case of neonatal herpes. Courtesy of Mary Spraker, MD.

diagnosis of neonatal herpes is particularly challenging when muco-cutaneous lesions are absent, as it may resemble bacterial sepsis or other congenital infections (e.g. rubella or toxoplasmosis).

While presentation with disseminated infection is less common, it is associated with considerable morbidity and mortality, despite prompt initiation of antiviral therapy. A substantial proportion of the survivors will have lasting neurologic impairment. Neonatal herpes infection should be diagnosed as early as possible since intravenous treatment with acyclovir reduces both morbidity and mortality.

Any vesicle, bulla, or erosion on the skin of a neonate should be sampled for herpes as well as for routine bacterial cultures. Rapid information can be obtained by direct immunofluorescence, but results should be confirmed by viral culture. A specimen of spinal fluid should be obtained for HSV DNA PCR to document the presence of CNS infection.

DIFFERENTIAL DIAGNOSIS OF GENITAL HERPES

When painful grouped vesicles with an erythematous base appear on the genital skin, the diagnosis is almost certainly herpes, but other STDs besides herpes can cause erosions that may be painful. Of these,

chancroid (*Figs 13.29* and *13.30*) most closely resembles herpes in the clinical presentation, frequently with multiple, painful erosions that develop an exudate similar to that seen in the postvesicular stages of genital herpes (see Chapter 3, Chancroid).

Syphilis also causes erosions on the genitals (*Figs 13.31* and *13.32*), but a primary chancre of syphilis that is not secondarily infected with bacteria is usually solitary and not painful. In primary syphilis, dark-field examination of lesion exudate is usually positive if the area has not been recently treated with topical agents and the patient has not been taking oral antibiotics. In adults, secondary syphilis is rarely erosive, but never vesicular. Serologic tests are invariably positive in secondary syphilis and should be done in any erosive genital lesions since STDs often coexist in such patients (see Chapter 2, Syphilis).

Traumatic genital ulcers are painful but are not usually multiple or grouped. They have angular borders rather than the scalloped edges seen in herpes erosions (see Chapter 1, Genital Dermatoses).

Contact dermatitis of the genitals is usually itchy and results in vesicles, crusting, and erosions. Secondary infection may result in tenderness. As contact with the offending allergen may occur up to 2 weeks before the dermatitis appears, diagnosis may be difficult. Vesicles and erosions

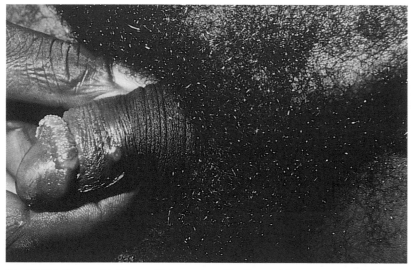

Fig. 13.29 Chancroid. The multiple erosions, like those of herpes, are painful, but blisters are not seen and the lymphadenopathy is more prominent than in comparable herpes eruptions.

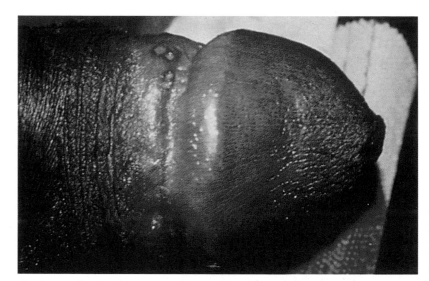

Fig. 13.30 Chancroid. Grouped ulcers resembling genital herpes; however, *Haemophilus ducreyi* was isolated by culture from these lesions. Courtesy of R.C. Ballard, PhD.

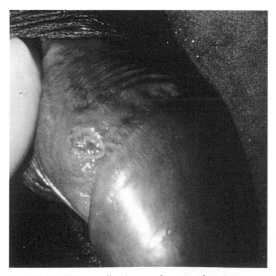

Fig. 13.31 This small primary chancre of syphilis resembles a herpetic erosion.

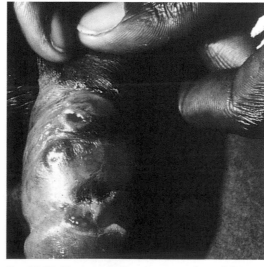

Fig. 13.32 These multiple primary penile syphilitic chancres mimic penile herpes.

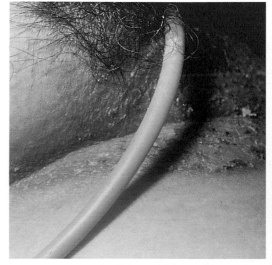

Fig. 13.33 Benign familial pemphigus (Hailey-Hailey disease). Multiple fragile vesicles and bullae are seen at the edge of these characteristic erosive plaques. The clinical history and biopsies are diagnostic.

should be sampled for viral cultures or antigen detection before the patient is treated for contact dermatitis (see Chapter 1, Genital Dermatoses). Other bullous or erosive diseases, such as impetigo, pemphigus, pemphigoid, Hailey–Hailey disease (benign familial pemphigus) (*Fig. 13.33*), Darier's disease, Behçet's disease, and Crohn's disease, may either resemble herpes because of bullae or erosions, or may become secondarily infected with the virus. Clinical history and diagnostic tests, including Gram stains, bacterial and viral cultures, usually clarify the problem, but biopsies may occasionally be necessary.

The differential diagnosis of genital herpes includes many conditions that are quite rare. Equally importantly, genital herpes can be easily mistaken for other conditions. The difficulty in clinical diagnosis has been highlighted by a recent study that showed that only 39% of new genital HSV-2 infection were diagnosed on clinical grounds.[11] At the same time the ratio of correct to incorrect diagnoses was 4:1, indicating that up to 20% of patients given a clinical diagnosis of genital herpes have another condition. These findings emphasize the pivotal role of laboratory tests in the diagnosis of genital herpes.

Laboratory Tests

The most commonly used specific techniques in the diagnosis of genital herpes involve direct examination of clinical specimens for viral antigens and the isolation of HSV by cell culture.[30] However, the recent commercial development of type-specific serologic assays for HSV-1 and HSV-2 hold promise for the diagnosis of those persons who do not present with typical lesions.

Direct Detection Methods

Samples from mucocutaneous sites or from lesion material can be obtained by firm rubbing with a dacron or cotton swab. Direct methods to detect virus include histopathology, cytopathology, electron microscopy, antigen detection by immunofluorescence (FA) or enzyme immunoassay (EIA), and the polymerase chain reaction (PCR). Histopathology and cytopathology permit the identification of nuclear-cytoplasmic inclusions and other cellular alterations by light microscopy, while electron microscopy permits the direct ultrastructural visualization of viral particles. These methods are not specific for HSV. With FA or EIA the specimen is incubated with an antibody specific for the virus (viral antigen), which is tagged with a fluorescent (FA) or enzyme that catalyzes color development following addition of substrate. PCR methods amplify a specific nucleic acid sequence which can then be detected by using a complementary labeled nucleic acid probe.

Histopathology

Early HSV infections are characterized by intracellular edema, suprabasal intraepidermal vesicles (*Fig. 13.34*), ballooning degeneration, and homogenization and margination of nuclear chromatin. Intranuclear inclusions and multinucleated giant cells are seen at the periphery of the lesions (*Fig. 13.35*). In later ulcerative stages, keratinocyte necrosis and lysis predominate. Inflammatory cells, such as polymorphonuclear leukocytes and lymphocytes, appear within the vesicle and dermis. As the lesion progresses, the epidermis sloughs, and the remaining erosion re-epithelializes as it heals. Cervical HSV infections are characterized by multinucleated giant cells and intranuclear 'ground-glass' viral inclusions visualized on Papanicolaou smears. Biopsies are not usually performed, but will show changes similar to those described above.

Cytopathology

Characteristic cytopathic effects occur in infected cells, although these are not specific for HSV. These techniques should be restricted to situations in which virus-specific testing cannot be obtained. Specimens from vesicular skin and mucosal lesions may be obtained by scraping the edge of the 'unroofed' lesion with a sterile swab or scalpel blade, smearing onto a slide and fixing the cells with 95% ethanol, Zenker's solution, or Bouin's solution (Tzanck smear). Cells are stained with Giemsa or methylene blue stain. HSV-infected cells usually exhibit a combination of virus-induced and degenerative changes. The virus predominantly infects immature epithelial cells. Early cytopathogenic characteristics of infection include: nuclear hypertrophy, disappearance of nucleoli and a distinct, homogeneous, 'ground-glass' appearance of nuclei caused by displacement of the nuclear chromatin to the periphery, which imparts a hyperchromatin appearance to the nuclear membrane (*Fig. 13.36*). Multinucleated giant cells, produced by the fusion of cytoplasmic membranes of individual infected cells, are often observed. The nuclei vary in size and shape and usually mold against one another (*Fig. 13.37*).

Later in the course of HSV infection, coarsely granular, acidophilic, intranuclear inclusions appear surrounded by a prominent halo. Degenerative changes (not HSV-specific) also occur in infected cells, including increased cytoplasmic and nuclear vacuolization, loss of normal cell shape, and in later stages of infection, breakage of cytoplasmic and nuclear membranes.

Electron Microscopy

Electron microscopy requires a concentration of viral particles greater than 10^6–10^7 particles/ml and is most applicable to biopsies or fluid and

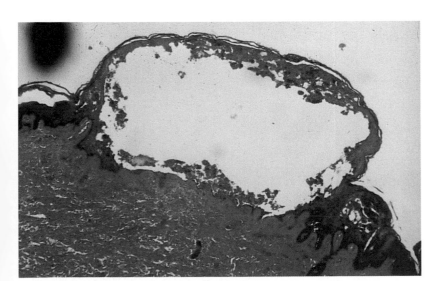

Fig. 13.34 Intraepidermal vesicle of HSV infection.

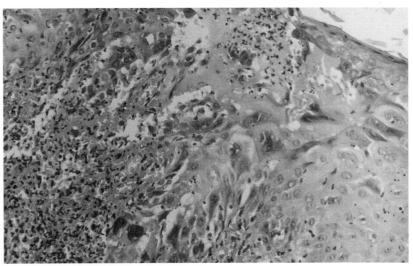

Fig. 13.35 Periphery of HSV erosion showing single and multinucleated epithelial cells with 'ground-glass' nuclei.

scrapings from vesicles (*Fig. 13.38*). In most cases, other virus detection methods are more readily available, more accurate, and less expensive than EM (*Figs 13.39* and *13.40*).

Immunofluorescence Methods

These techniques are used to detect viral antigens in clinical specimens (*Fig. 13.41*) or to confirm the presence of HSV in cell cultures inoculated with clinical materials (*Fig. 13.42*). Acceptable specimens for FA diagnosis include lesion scrapings, or resuspended cells from centrifuged vesicle fluid. Cells must be obtained in the sample; lesion exudate or mucosal secretions are unacceptable for FA. Clinical specimens or viral cultures can be evaluated for HSV by either direct (DFA) or indirect (IFA)

methods. With DFA staining, fluorescein isothiocyanate (FITC)-labeled HSV-specific immunoglobulin (anti-HSV) binds directly to HSV proteins in the infected cells present in the specimen (*Figs 13.42–13.45*). With IFA staining, the bound anti-HSV antibody is detected (*Fig. 13.46*), with a FITC-labeled antispecies immunoglobulin. Although IFA methods are more sensitive than DFA methods, DFA has several advantages over IFA, including greater specificity, (less nonspecific fluorescence), fewer necessary manipulations and reagents, and one less incubation step. Most commercially available reagents for HSV detection are monoclonal antibody products intended for use with DFA methodology (*Fig. 13.42*). Some of these products are also licensed to subtype the HSV present in clinical specimens.

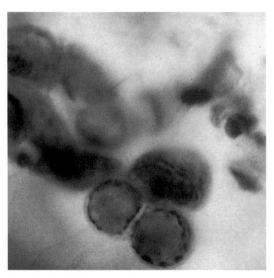

Fig. 13.36 HSV-infected cells in a cytology specimen exhibiting homogeneous, 'ground-glass'-appearing nuclei and peripheral chromatin margination imparting an irregular and more distinct appearance to the nuclear membrane.

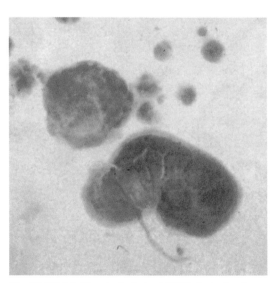

Fig. 13.37 Multinucleated giant HSV-infected cell showing variation in nuclear size and shape and the molding of individual nuclei against one another.

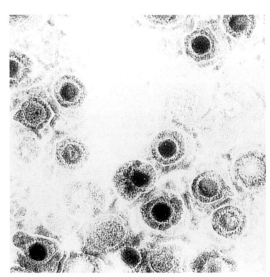

Fig. 13.38 HSV particles detected by direct electron microscopy. Defective or damaged particles have dark centers due to the penetration of phosphotungstic acid stain into the viral nucleocapsid.

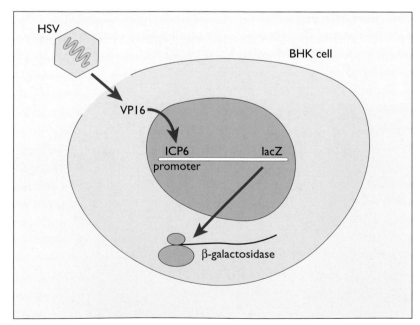

Fig. 13.39 Enzyme linked virus inducible system. A reporter gene for β-galactosidase has been inserted into HSV permissive cells behind the HSV-1 promoter. Upon entry of HSV, the viral transactivating protein binds to the promoter to switch on production of the enzyme gene product. Addition of the enzyme's substrate changes the cell's color.

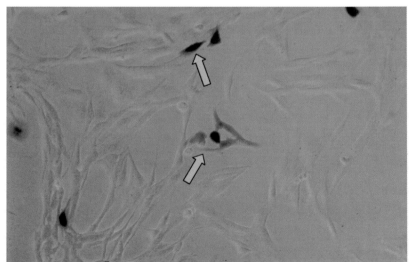

Fig. 13.40 ELVIS™ cells after incubation with HIV-2 for 4 hours. Infected cells (arrows) show distinct blue color change.

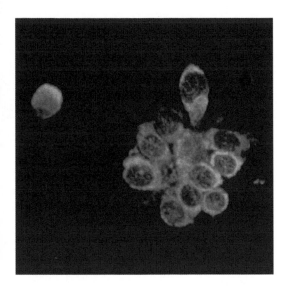

Fig. 13.41 Direct fluorescent antibody test of HSV-infected cell obtained from scraping an ulcerated genital lesion.

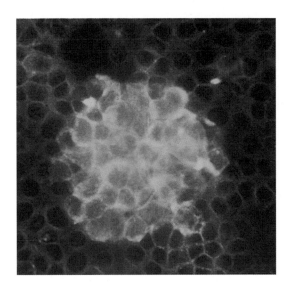

Fig. 13.42 Fluorescent antibody test of HSV-infected cells in a cell culture monolayer previously inoculated with a clinical specimen from a genital lesion.

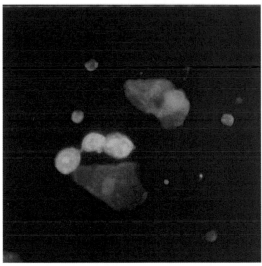

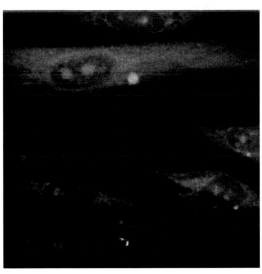

Figs 13.43 and 13.44 Direct fluorescent antibody test. (13.43) Positive result for HSV-2 with monoclonal antibody. (13.44) Negative result for HSV-2 with monoclonal antibody.

Fig. 13.43

Fig. 13.44

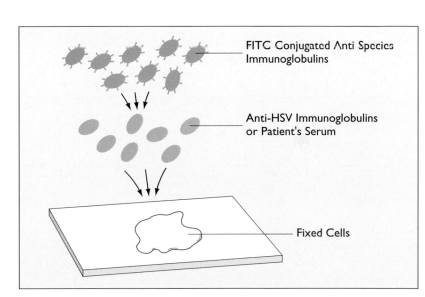

FITC-Conjugated Anti-HSV Immunoglobulins

Fixed Cells

Fig. 13.45 The direct immunofluorescence test.

FITC Conjugated Anti Species Immunoglobulins

Anti-HSV Immunoglobulins or Patient's Serum

Fixed Cells

Fig. 13.46 The indirect immunofluorescence test.

Strict criteria and appropriate positive and negative controls must be used when interpreting FA results. Fluorescence color (with FITC conjugates) is bright apple-green and should be localized to the nucleus. False-positive fluorescence can be encountered with leukocytes, mucus, and yeasts; leukocytes express immunoglobulin Fc receptors that can nonspecifically bind conjugates. False-negative tests can occur when an insufficient level of intracellular herpes antigen is present, or when inadequate numbers of infected cells are collected.

Enzyme Immunoassays

Enzyme immunoassays (ELISA or EIA), detect viral antigens by a color change resulting from a catalytic reaction with a substrate. The enzyme is linked to the specific antibody anti-HSV or, in indirect methods, to an antispecies antibody. EIA methods generally do not require intact cells. Appropriate specimens for detecting HSV antigens by EIA are swabs of lesions and vesicular fluid. Direct antigen detection by EIA can be performed within a few hours of receipt in the laboratory and does not require specialized training or experience. A commercially available EIA (HerpChek, DuPont) has comparable sensitivity to virus culture methods and also provides the results more quickly.[31]

Polymerase Chain Reaction

This biochemical process can detect a single target DNA molecule within a complex mixture of nontarget DNA, for example, a single viral genome in a milieu of thousands of uninfected cell genomes. This is accomplished by amplifying the target DNA using specific DNA primers and a thermostable DNA polymerase in a series of iterated reactions. The number of amplified segments (amplimers) increase by a factor of approximately two at each step. From a single template molecule, $2^{(n-1)}$ amplimers may be obtained after n amplification cycles. Thus, after 30 cycles, more than 500 million amplimer molecules can be generated from a single target.

The appropriate choice of primer sequences and conditions for amplification enables high specificity. This can be further enhanced by an amplimer detection system, which depends on the hybridization of a detection probe with sequences internal to the amplified segment. Although radioactive detection systems have been used in the past, these have been replaced in most laboratories by nonradioactive EIA-based detection systems. These are equally sensitive and are compatible with standard EIA plate formats found in clinical laboratories.

The exquisite sensitivity of standard PCR is its potential Achilles' heel. Even low level contamination by a target sequence can lead to a false-positive result, thus, scrupulous attention must be paid to sample acquisition, storage, shipping, and processing procedures. The amplification products themselves are substrates for the amplification reaction, requiring the physical partitioning of sample-preparation areas from areas where amplification products are processed for detection.

Semiautomated closed-system methods, such as 'TaqMan' (Perkins-Elmer) and 'Light Cycler' (Roche) have been developed to circumvent the problem of contamination. These methods are faster and less expensive than quantitative PCR with gel-based amplimer detection. The TaqMan system requires no post-PCR processing because the product is detected by Taq polymerase cleavage of a reporter fluorescent dye during the course of each round of amplification (Fig. 13.47).

PCR assays have been developed for HSV-1 and HSV-2, although none is licensed for clinical use. The greatest clinical value of these assays is the rapid detection of HSV in CSF in the diagnosis of herpes encephalitis and other CNS-related HSV diseases.[32] PCR has been of epidemiologic use in demonstrating that HSV is asymptomatically shed even more frequently than indicated by culture-based methods.

ISOLATION OF HSV IN CELL CULTURE

Culture Methods

In general, culture techniques take longer than direct methods and require special expertise. However, culture allows for amplification by viral replication, which increases sensitivity. Culture also permits recovery and identification of other viruses and provides replication-competent virus for further studies such as antiviral sensitivity. The most sensitive cell culture systems for isolating HSV cell lines derived from mink lung cells, rhabdomyosarcoma cells, and human diploid fibroblast lines such as MR5 or WI-38 (Fig. 13.48). Primary cell monolayers of guinea pig or rabbit kidney origin are sensitive but time-consuming to prepare.

The likelihood of recovery of HSV in culture relates to the clinical phase of the lesion; the yield is generally higher from vesicular (94%) than from pustular (87%), ulcerated (70%), or crusted (27%) lesions. HSV-1 and HSV-2 replicate well in many primary or established cell lines of human or primate origin.

When a specimen contains a high titer of infectious HSV, a cytopathic effect (CPE) may be detected as early as 24 hours after inoculation. Most samples require 2 to 4 days to develop visible CPE. HSV-infected cells in the monolayer develop a cytoplasmic granularity and become enlarged, ballooned, and eventually round and refractile or glassy (Fig. 13.49). Individual foci grow in size as cell-to-cell spread of virus occurs. Eventu-

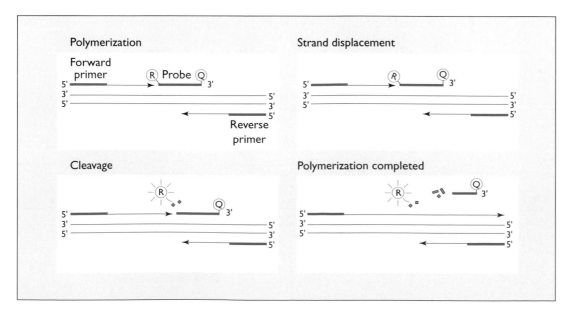

Fig 13.47 Stepwise representation of the forklike-structure-dependent, polymerization-associated, 5' to 3' nuclease activity of Taq DNA polymerase acting on a fluorogenic probe during one extension phase of PCR.

ally, the entire monolayer becomes infected. Multinucleated giant cells are usually identified. Confirmation of CPE as being HSV in origin is usually performed by antigen detection methods (FA or EIA). Subtyping of the HSV isolates can be accomplished in the same step by using subtype-specific antibodies.

Modified culture techniques

Two alternatives to cell culture that are the widely used are shell vial culture and ELVIS™ID. Both can identify HSV after a limited time of viral replication (16–72 h in culture). Shell vial or 'spin amplification' methods involve centrifuging the sample onto monolayers of cells on coverslips or on flat-bottomed wells in plastic plates (*Fig 13.50*). The centrifugal forces are likely to alter the cell membrane to make the cell more susceptible to infection. Monoclonal antibodies directed against HSV early antigens are used to visualize infected cells via direct antigen detection methods after 16–24 hours incubation. Some laboratories hold a second shell vial for additional evaluation at 48 hours. Sensitivity is usually higher for shell vial methods than for direct antigen detection alone because of the period of vial amplification in culture.

Transgenic reporter cell lines such as ELVIS cells have also been developed (*Fig. 13.39*). These cells are permissive for HSV and have been genetically altered to contain a reporter gene for β-galactosidase that is

under the control of the HSV-1 UL39 promoter, ICP6. Infection with HSV results in transactivation of the promoter and production of β galactosidase. Addition of the enzyme's substrate (ONPG or X-gal) results in a color change that is easy to read and faster (16–24 hours) than standard culture (*Fig 13.40*). The ELVIS ID version of this test subtypes HSV as part of the detection.

Serology

HSV-1 and HSV-2 are very similar genetically, with every immunogenic protein of HSV-1 virus having a closely related counterpart in HSV-2. This is the basis for the strong antigenic cross reactivity between the two HSV subtypes. The only exception is the gene that encodes glyco-protein G of HSV-1 (gG-1), which is nearly 1,500 base pairs shorter than the gene encoding HSV-2 gG (gG-2). Although some antigenic epitopes are shared between gG-1 and gG-2, human antibody responses to these proteins are functionally type-specific. Type-specific serologic assays based on gG have, until recently, been available only in research or reference laboratories.[33] Western blot, gG immunodot enzyme assays, and tests using either recombinant or purified gG have been described.

The FDA has approved tests from Diagnology (Belfast, Northern Ireland) for diagnosis of genital herpes in adults and from Focus Technologies (formerly MRL Diagnostics; Cypress CA) for diagnosis of herpes in adults, including pregnant women.[34] One other type-specific gG-based test, from Meridian Diagnostics (Cincinnati, OH) has been withdrawn from the market and is unlikely to be made available again. Other commercial tests are available for detection of HSV-2 antibodies from Roche (Cobas-HSV-2) and Trinity (CaptiaSelect-HSV-2); however, these tests are not FDA approved. These tests are based on recombinant or purified HSV gG. Focus offers two test formats, marketed under the name 'HerpeSelect'. One is an ELISA with separate test plates containing gG-1 (for HSV-1 antibody detection) and gG-2 (for HSV-2 antibody detection). The HSV-2 ELISAs are >95% sensitive and >97% specific when compared with Western blot. The second test is an immunoblot that combines gG-1 and gG-2, along with a type common antigen, on

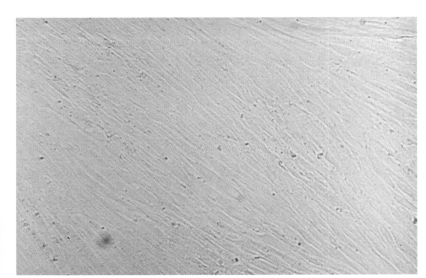

Fig. 13.48 Uninoculated human diploid fibroblast monolayer.

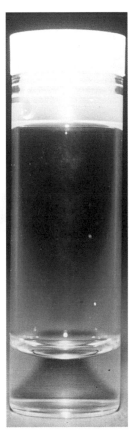

Fig. 13.50 One-dram shell vial containing cell media and coverslip with cell monolayer.

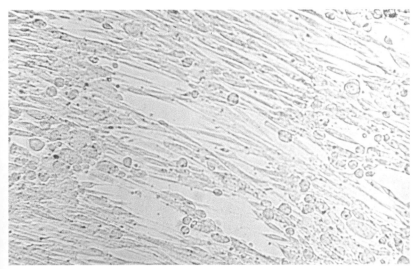

Fig. 13.49 Human diploid fibroblasts infected with HSV and showing cytopathic effects. There is extensive cell rounding, and many degenerated cells have fallen off the glass surface.

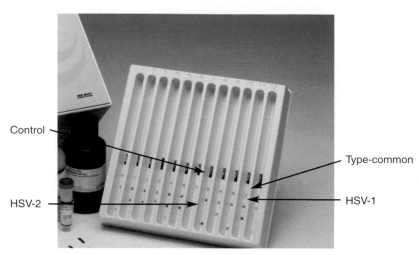

Fig. 13.51 HerpeSelect immunoblot test from Focus Technologies. Test strips each contain antihuman antibody (top band; 'control'), a type common antigen ('type common'), gG-1 ('HSV-1') and gG-2 ('HSV-2').

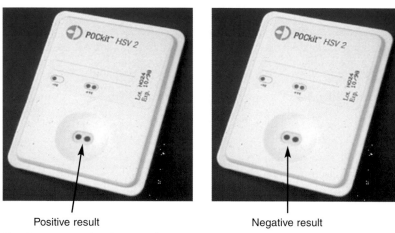

Fig. 13.52 Diagnology's Point of Care HSV-2 (POCkit-HSV-2) test. The test membrane contains a dot with lectin-purified gG-2 on the right and an anti-human antibody reagent on the left. The left panel shows a positive test with definitive red color change of both the gG-2 containing dot and the human serum control dots (arrow). The right panel shows a negative test result with only the control dot showing a red color change. If neither dot turns color, the test is invalid and must be repeated with an additional capillary blood or serum sample.

a single test strip (*Fig 13.51*). This test is similar in test performance for HSV-2 antibodies to the HerpeSelect ELISA, but is more expensive and better suited to labs that test low numbers of sera. All of the HerpeSelect tests are available in kit form for commercial laboratory use but can also be ordered by sending sera to the Focus Technologies reference lab (formerly MRL Reference Laboratory) in Cypress, CA.

The POCkit-HSV-2 test from Diagnology is a unique point of care test based on membrane-bound lectin-purified gG-2. The test requires only a small amount of blood from a fingerstick. Serum can also be used. The test can be performed in a laboratory cleared by CLIA for moderately complex laboratory work (it is not CLIA-waived) and requires 6 minutes for development of color that denotes antibodies to HSV-2 (*Fig. 13.52*). Careful training and adherence to the manufacturer's protocol is required to obtain reproducible results, as the color change is subjective. In one study of banked sera, 5–10% of tests were interpreted differently among three independent readers. POCkit has high sensitivity (93–96%) against Western blot or culture. Specificity ranges from 95–98%. Of interest, Pockit-HSV2 can detect seroconversion as fast or faster than Western blot; at a median of 2 weeks following onset of

symptoms.[35] Time to seroconversion by the Focus tests has not been determined.

Performance data from HSV-2 type-specific tests not approved by the FDA are more limited. Cobas (Roche) appears to be slightly less sensitive but equally specific as the Focus tests and Captia Select HSV-2 (Trinity) appears to be both less sensitive and specific (90–92%; 91–98%, respectively) compared with gold standard tests.

The most serious problem with HSV serology is the ongoing availability of tests that purport to be type specific but are not based on gG-1 and/or gG-2. Because of the high extent of cross reactivity between the two viruses, assays based on crude antigen preparations mainly detect type-common antibodies. Even conservative formulae for determining type-specific responses based on relative strength of reactivity against HSV-1 versus HSV-2 generate inaccurate results.[36] The problem is most severe in patients with prior HSV-1 antibodies who develop HSV-2 infections and who mount anamnestic responses to the type-common antigens. The HSV-2 responses in these patients are nearly impossible to discern without gG-2-based testing. A number of companies including Diamedix, Diasorin, Sigma, Wampole, and Zeus still market such tests as type-specific and provide kit instructions for calculating results to infer HSV-1 versus HSV-2 antibody presence. These tests are only 61–85% accurate and should not be relied on for this purpose.

Limitations of serology Even accurate gG-based type-specific testing for HSV-1 and HSV-2 antibodies has limitations. First, documenting that the infection is newly acquired can only be done by showing seroconversion from a negative test to a positive serology. Sensitive tests such as POCkit may indicate positive reactivity as early as a few days post-onset in a newly infected person. On the other hand, antibody responses to gG-2 may take up to 8 weeks to develop and a rare individual may not make such antibodies at all. Thus, a negative test does not guarantee recent infection nor does a positive result rule out primary or nonprimary first episodes.

IgM testing is not currently available in gG-based test formats. Although IgM can be useful in diagnosing a new herpes infection in patients without detectable IgG responses, as many as 35% of patients with recurrent HSV-2 episodes have IgM responses; thus, IgM is a poor marker of new infection status.

Only the Focus Technologies tests (ELISA and immunoblot) can specifically diagnose HSV-1 infection. The other type-specific commercial tests do not detect antibodies to gG-1. Type-specific serology for HSV-1 is commonly 5–10% less sensitive in culture-documented cases than is gG-2 serology in culture-documented cases. However, even accurate HSV-1 serology cannot discriminate between oral and genital infection. Seroconversion to HSV-1 around the time of new genital lesions strongly suggests genital HSV-1 but virus detection tests should be used if possible.

None of the tests on the market have been exhaustively tested for accuracy with pediatric sera. Studies using comparison with Western blot or other research-based type-specific tests suggest that some ELISA formats (particularly the Meridian product which is no longer available) appear to have high false-positive rates, and subsequently very low positive predictive values for HSV-2. Use of these tests in children under 14 years of age is not recommended.

Use of gG-based type-specific serology in medicolegal cases has several pitfalls. Virus detection methods are the best way to determine that a person has developed genital herpes. Because of the variable timing of antibody development and the highly variable presentation of genital herpes following infection, inferring a causal link between an alleged perpetrator of abuse or assault and a victim by antibody status is easily challenged. Because of high background prevalence of HSV-2, even with culture-documented infection in the victim and matching serotypes in the two individuals, one cannot conclude that the perpetrator is the source of the victim's infection. Moreover, few laboratories are equipped to handle the special chain of evidence requirements for admissibility of results in court.

TREATMENT

COUNSELING

Perhaps the most important aspect in the management of genital herpes is educating patients regarding their condition. This includes advising patients to abstain from sexual contact if prodromal symptoms or lesions are present, informing them that transmission may occur via asymptomatic shedding, and all patients, including men, should be appraised of the risk of neonatal herpes.[37] Women should be advised to inform their obstetrician and pediatrician of their condition if they are pregnant. Issues around sexuality and sexual practices emerge for most patients who are diagnosed with genital herpes, and some patients will require extensive counseling. For more information and support, patients can be referred to the National STD Hotline at 800-227-8922 or the National Herpes Hotline at 919-361-8488. American Social Health Association maintains a web site that provides excellent information for patients; the organization also supports local support groups for patients with genital herpes (http://www.ashastd.org/).

ANTIVIRAL THERAPY

Acyclovir, valacyclovir, and famciclovir are medications approved for the treatment of genital herpes.[37,38] Acyclovir is an acyclic derivative of the nucleoside guanosine (Fig. 13.53). Acyclovir is actually a 'prodrug', which must be phosphorylated by a virus-specified enzyme, thymidine kinase, to acyclovir monophosphate. Cellular enzymes further phosphorylate the compound into the active drug, acyclovir triphosphate, which inhibits the viral DNA polymerase and causes chain termination. Famciclovir, the oral prodrug of penciclovir, another nucleoside analog, and valaciclovir, the valine ester of acyclovir, are also effective in treating genital herpes. The available data from trials to compare the drugs suggest that the effectiveness in treatment of genital herpes is comparable for the three medications (Table 13.3).

Acyclovir should be used with caution in pregnancy because there is insufficient data on its safety. A pregnancy registry has followed 756 women with first trimester exposure to acyclovir.[39] The available data do not indicate an increased frequency or unusual distribution of birth defects as compared with the general population (Dr K M Stone, personal communication). More recently, use of acyclovir has increased for women near the end of pregnancy with hopes of averting recurrences at term and abdominal deliveries. However, some experts continue to be concerned about such use, as rare events may not be noted or attributed to acyclovir exposure.

Acyclovir resistance in HSV is rare, but can occur, particularly in individuals with advanced HIV disease or other causes of immunosuppression who have had prior acyclovir therapy. In most cases, acyclovir resistance is due to strains of HSV that are deficient in thymidine kinase. The treatment of choice for acyclovir-resistant HSV infection is foscarnet, which must be given intravenously.[40] The usual dosage is 60 mg/kg every 8 hours in individuals with normal renal function. Topical cidofovir is also an option.

FIRST-EPISODE GENITAL HERPES

Individuals with severe first-episode HSV infection occasionally require hospitalization, particularly when serious neurologic complications occur. This small subset of individuals should be treated with intravenous acyclovir, 5 mg/kg every 8 hours for at least 5 days. Alternatively, once improvement is noted, some clinicians have been switching to a higher than standard dose of oral valacyclovir to finish a course of

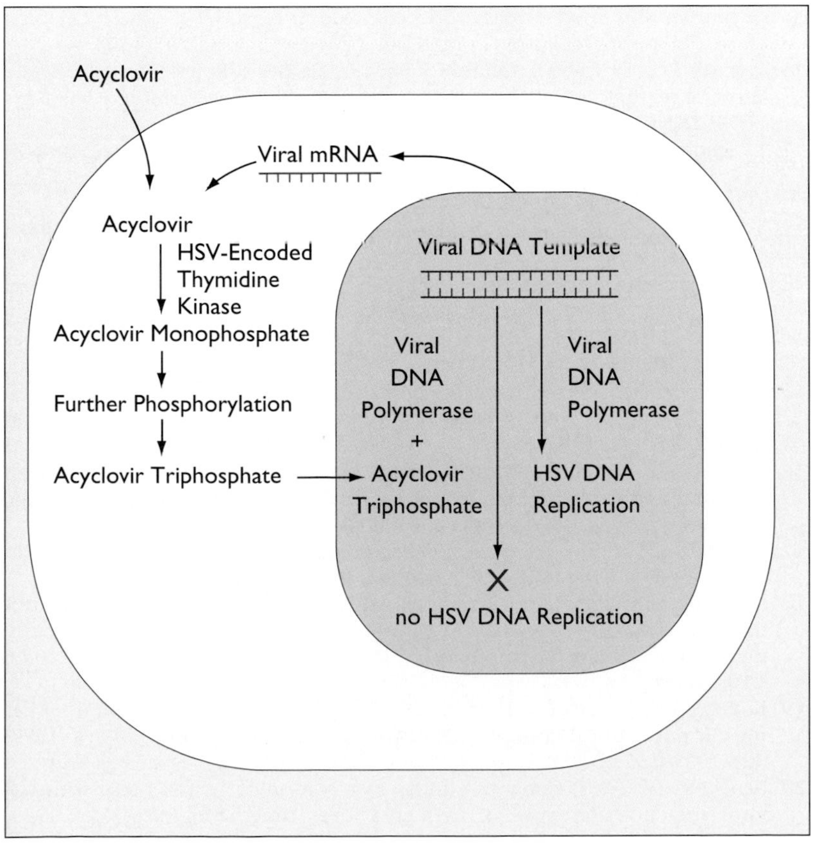

Fig. 13.53 Mechanism of action of acyclovir in infected cell. Adapted from Mertz GJ, Corey L: Genital herpes simplex virus infections in adults. Urol Clin N Am 1983; 11:107.

Recommended Antiviral Drug Regimens for Genital Herpes			
Clinical setting	Acyclovir	Famciclovir	Valacyclovir
First episode	400 mg orally tid for 7–10 days or 200 mg orally 5x daily for 7–10 days	250 mg orally tid for 7–10 days	1.0 g orally bid for 7–10 days
Recurrent episode	400 mg orally tid for 5 days or 200 mg orally 5x daily for 5 days or 800 mg orally bid for 5 days	125 mg orally bid for 5 days	500 mg orally bid for 3–5 days or 1.0 g orally QD for 5 days
Chronic suppressive therapy	400 mg orally bid	250 mg orally bid	500 mg orally QD or 1.0* g orally 1x daily
HIV+ episodic therapy	200 mg orally 5x or 400 mg orally tid for 5–10 days	500 mg bid orally for 5–10 days	1.0 g orally bid for 5–10 days
HIV+ chronic suppressive therapy	Acyclovir 400–800 mg orally bid to tid	Famciclovir 500 mg orally bid	Valaciclovir 500 mg orally bid

*In patients with > 9 recurrences.

Table 13.3 Treatment of genital herpes (adapted from CDC guidelines).

therapy. In addition to supportive care, such as analgesics, some women need urinary catheterization either for urinary retention or because voiding is extremely painful due to spillage of urine onto herpetic lesions (external dysuria).

The benefit of antiviral therapy is greatest in newly acquired genital herpes. As a result, all patients presenting with first clinical episode should be offered antiviral therapy. Not infrequently, the disease can be mild upon initial presentation, but become severe if treatment is delayed for a few days. As the risk of short-course antiviral therapy is minimal, treatment should be initiated even in atypical cases. If an alternative diagnosis becomes apparent, therapy can be discontinued. Antiviral treatment of first-episode genital herpes has no effect on the subsequent recurrence pattern.

RECURRENT GENITAL HERPES

Two strategies can be used in the treatment of recurrent genital herpes:

- Episodic oral antiviral therapy
- Chronic suppressive oral antiviral therapy

All patients should be counseled regarding the availability of antiviral therapy. While some patients with mild or infrequent recurrences may choose not to treat, even some of these patients may benefit from antiviral therapy. In our experience, patients who do not benefit will stop taking the medication.

As listed in *Table 13.3*, several regimens have been used for episodic treatment of genital herpes. More recent studies show that such episodic therapy will accelerate healing by about 30%. Episodic therapy should be started by patients at the first sign of prodrome or lesions. Earlier initiation provides more benefit and some lesions may be completely abrogated when the therapy is started during prodrome. This means that the patient should have medication available in advance.

Chronic suppressive, oral antiviral therapy is highly effective, suppressing about 90% of recurrences. Suppressive therapy with valacyclovir and famciclovir is safe and effective for at least a year. Studies with acyclovir document its safety for up to 7 years.[41] No laboratory monitoring is required for patients on daily antiviral medication. Chronic suppressive therapy is particularly suited to individuals with frequent recurrences or to those who experience significant distress with their recurrences. One study suggested that suppressive therapy results in improvement in herpes-related quality of life scores.[42] It is appropriate to assess the continuing need for therapy on an annual basis, as recurrences tend to decrease in frequency over time and many people adjust to living with genital herpes. Suppressive use of antiviral medication has not been associated with the emergence of resistant virus in immunocompetent hosts.

Topical acyclovir is ineffective in recurrent genital herpes and shows only trivial benefit in primary genital herpes. Its use is not recommended.

PREVENTION

Given the widespread prevalence of HSV-2 infection, the most rational approach to prevention would be universal vaccination prior to initiation of sexual activity. However, a vaccine that offers high-level protection remains elusive, although several candidate vaccines are in clinical or preclinical studies. A subunit vaccine with recombinant surface glycoproteins has been shown to induce levels of neutralizing antibodies that exceed those shown in natural infection. However, the vaccine failed to protect susceptible persons in clinical trials suggesting that our understanding of immunologic correlates of protection is inadequate.[43] A similar vaccine has showed partial protection against HSV-2 acquisition among seronegative women but further studies will be required to define its usefulness. Other candidate vaccines include recombinant live-virus vaccines, DISC (disabled infectious single cycle) vaccine, and DNA vaccines.[44,45]

New data suggest that condoms offer significant protection against HSV-2 acquisition. Condom use appeared especially protective for women with HSV-2 seropositive partners.[46] Whether serologic testing combined with counseling to avoid sex during lesional episodes and use condoms at other times results in a significant behavioral change remains to be seen. Chronic daily antiviral therapy has been shown to decrease the rate of viral shedding, both symptomatic and asymptomatic.[47] The role of antiviral therapy in prevention of sexual transmission of HSV-2 is currently under investigation. Even if effective, such therapy is likely to have an impact on relatively few couples and it is unlikely to have a significant public health benefit.

References

1. Fleming D, McQuillan G, Johnson R *et al*. Herpes simplex virus type 2 in the United States, 1976 to 1994. *N Engl J Med* 1997; **337**:1105–1111.
2. Nahmias A, Lee F, Beckman-Nahmias S. Sero-epidemiological and sociological patterns of herpes simplex virus infection in the world. *Scand J Infect Dis* 1990; **69**:19–36.
3. Mertz GJ, Schmidt O, Jourden JL *et al*. Frequency of acquisition of first-episode genital infection with herpes simplex virus from symptomatic and asymptomatic source contacts. *Sex Transm Dis* 1985; **12**:33–39.
4. Whitley R, Arvin A, Prober C *et al*. Predictors of morbidity and mortality in neonates with herpes simplex infections. *N Engl J Med* 1991; **324**:450–454.
5. Wald A, Zeh J, Selke S *et al*. Reactivation of genital herpes simplex virus type 2 infection in asymptomatic HSV-2 seropositive persons. *N Engl J Med* 2000; **342**:844–850.
6. DSTD – 1999 STD Surveillance Report. Department of Health and Human Services, Atlanta: Centers for Disease Control and Prevention, September 2000. http://www.cdc.gov/nchstp/dstd/Stats_Trends/1999SurvRpt.htm
7. Weiss H, Buve A, Robinson N *et al*. The epidemiology of HSV-2 infection and its association with HIV infection in four urban African populations. *AIDS* 2001; **15**(suppl 4):S97–S108.
8. Corey L, Handsfield HH. Genital herpes and public health: addressing a global problem. *JAMA* 2000; **283**:791–794.
9. Mertz KJ, Trees D, Levine WC *et al*. Etiology of genital ulcers and prevalence of human immunodeficiency virus coinfection in 10 US cities. The Genital Ulcer Disease Surveillance Group. *J Infect Dis* 1998; **178**:1795–1798.
10. Lafferty WE, Downey L, Celum C, Wald A. Herpes simplex virus type 1 as a cause of genital herpes: impact on surveillance and prevention. *J Infect Dis* 2000; **181**:1454–1457.
11. Langenberg A, Corey L, Ashley R, Leong W, Straus S. A prospective study of new infections with herpes simplex virus type 1 and type 2. *N Engl J Med* 1999; **341**:1432–1438.
12. Whitley RJ, Roizman B. Herpes simplex virus infections. *Lancet* 2001; **357**:1513–1518.
13. Mertz GJ, Benedetti J, Ashley R, Selke SA, Corey L. Risk factors for the sexual transmission of genital herpes. *Ann Intern Med* 1992; **116**:197–202.
14. Rooney JF, Felser JM, Ostrove JM, Straus SE. Acquisition of genital herpes from an asymptomatic sexual partner. *N Engl J Med* 1986; **314**:1561–1564.
15. Koelle DM, Benedetti J, Langenberg A, Corey L. Asymptomatic reactivation of herpes simplex virus in women after first episode of genital herpes. *Ann Intern Med* 1992; **116**:433–437.
16. Lafferty WE, Coombs RW, Benedetti J, Critchlow C, Corey L. Recurrences after oral and genital herpes simplex virus infection: influence of anatomic site and viral type. *N Engl J Med* 1987; **316**:1444–1449.
17. Benedetti JK, Corey L, Ashley R. Recurrence rates in genital herpes after symptomatic first-episode infection. *Ann Intern Med* 1994; **121**:847–854.
18. Langenberg A, Benedetti J, Jenkins J, Ashley R, Winter C, Corey L. Development of clinically recognizable genital lesions among women previously identified as having "asymptomatic" HSV-2 infection. *Ann Intern Med* 1989; **110**:882–887.
19. Koutsky LA, Stevens CE, Holmes KK *et al*. Underdiagnosis of genital herpes by current clinical and viral-isolation procedures. *N Engl J Med* 1992; **326**:1539–1553.
20. Benedetti JK, Zeh J, Corey L. Clinical reactivation of genital herpes simplex virus infection decreases in frequency over time. *Ann Intern Med* 1999; **131**:14–20.
21. Sacks SL. Frequency and duration of patient-observed recurrent genital herpes simplex virus infection: characterization of the nonlesional prodrome. *J Infect Dis* 1984; **150**:873–877.

22. Wald A, Zeh J, Selke S, Ashley RL, Corey L. Virologic characteristics of subclinical and symptomatic genital herpes infections. *N Engl J Med* 1995; **333**:770–775.

23. Krone MR, Wald A, Tabet SR, Paradise M, Corey L, Celum CL. Herpes simplex virus type 2 shedding in human immunodeficiency virus-negative men who have sex with men: Frequency, patterns, and risk factors. *Clin Infect Dis* 2000; **30**:261–267.

24. Wald A, Corey L, Cone R, Hobson A, Davis G, Zeh J. Frequent genital HSV-2 shedding in immunocompetent women. *J Clin Invest* 1997; **99**:1092–1097.

25. Cone R, Hobson A, Brown Z et al. Frequent detection of genital herpes simplex virus DNA by polymerase chain reaction among pregnant women. *JAMA* 1994; **272**:792–796.

26. Brown ZA, Benedetti J, Ashley R et al. Neonatal herpes simplex virus infection in relation to asymptomatic maternal infection at the time of labor. *N Engl J Med* 1991; **324**:1247–1252.

27. Prober CG, Sullender WM, Yasukawa LL, Au DS, Yeager AS, Arvin AM. Low risk of herpes simplex virus infections in neonates exposed to the virus at the time of vaginal delivery to mothers with recurrent genital HSV infections. *N Engl J Med* 1987; **316**:240–244.

28. Prober CG, Corey L, Brown ZA et al. The management of pregnancies complicated by genital infections with herpes simplex virus. *Clin Infect Dis* 1992; **15**:1031–1038.

29. Brown ZA, Selke SA, Zeh J et al. Acquisition of herpes simplex virus during pregnancy. *N Engl J Med* 1997; **337**:509–515.

30. Ashley R. Herpes viruses: type 1 and 2. In: Lennette E, ed. *Laboratory Diagnosis of Viral Infections*. New York, NY: Marcel Dekker, 1999:489–513.

31. Cone RW, Swenson PD, Hobson AC, Remington M, Corey L. Herpes simplex virus detection from genital lesions: a comparative study using antigen detection (HerpChek) and culture. *J Clin Microbiol* 1993; **31**:1774–1776.

32. Whitley R, Lakeman F. Herpes simplex virus infections of the central nervous system: therapeutic and diagnostic considerations. *Clin Inf Dis* 1995; **20**:414–420.

33. Ashley RL, Militoni J, Lee F, Nahmias A, Corey L. Comparison of Western blot (Immunoblot) and G-specific immunodot enzyme assay for detecting antibodies to herpes simplex virus types 1 and 2 in human sera. *J Clin Microbiol* 1988; **26**:662–667.

34. Ashley RL. Sorting out the new HSV type specific antibody tests. *Sex Transm Infect* 2001; **77**:232–237.

35. Ashley RL, Wald A, Eagleton M. Pre-market evaluation of the POCkitTM HSV-2 type specific serologic test in culture-documented cases of genital herpes simplex virus type 2. *Sex Transm Dis* 2000; **27**:266–269.

36. Ashley R, Cent A, Maggs V, Corey L. Inability of enzyme immunoassays to discriminate between infections with herpes simplex virus type 1 and 2. *Ann Intern Med* 1991; **115**:520–526.

37. Sexually transmitted diseases treatment guidelines 2002. Centers for Disease Control and Prevention. *MMWR Recomm Rep.* 2002; **51**:1–78.

38. Wald A. New therapies and prevention strategies for genital herpes. *Clin Infect Dis* 1999; **28**:S4–13.

39. Centers for Disease Control and Prevention. Pregnancy outcomes following systemic prenatal acyclovir exposure — June 1, 1984–June 30, 1993. *MMWR* 1993; **42**:806–809.

40. Safrin S, Crumpacker C, Chatis P et al. A controlled trial comparing foscarnet with vidarabine for acyclovir-resistant mucocutaneous herpes simplex in the acquired immunodeficiency syndrome. *N Engl J Med* 1991; **325**:551–555.

41. Fife KH, Crumpacker CS, Mertz GJ, Hill EL, Boone GS. The Acyclovir Study Group. Recurrence and resistance patterns of herpes simplex virus following cessation of > 6 years of chronic suppression with acyclovir. *J Infect Dis* 1994; **169**:1338–1341.

42. Patel R, Tyring S, Strand A et al. Impact of suppressive antiviral therapy on the health-related quality of life of patients with recurrent genital herpes infection. *Sex Transm Infect* 1999; **75**:398–402.

43. Corey L, Langenberg AG, Ashley R et al. Recombinant glycoprotein vaccine for the prevention of genital HSV-2 infection: two randomized controlled trials. Chiron HSV Vaccine Study Group [see comments]. *JAMA* 1999; **282**:331–340.

44. Stanberry L, Cunningham A, Mindel A et al. Prospects for control of herpes simplex virus disease through immunization. *Clin Infect Dis* 2000, **30**:549–566.

45. Bernstein DI, Stanberry LR. Herpes simplex virus vaccines. *Vaccine* 1999; **17**:1681–1689.

46. Wald A, Langenberg A, Link K et al. Effect of condoms on reducing the transmission of herpes simplex virus type 2 from men to women. *JAMA* 2001; **285**:3100–3106.

47. Wald A, Zeh J, Barnum G, Davis LG, Corey L. Suppression of subclinical shedding of herpes simplex virus type 2 with acyclovir. *Ann Intern Med* 1996; **124**:8–15.

Genital Human Papillomavirus Infections

14

J Douglas and A Moreland

INTRODUCTION

Genital human papillomavirus (HPV) infections are sexually transmitted infections of increasing public health importance. Known for years as the cause of genital warts, there is a growing body of evidence demonstrating the etiological association with a variety of anogenital cancers, most importantly cervical carcinoma.[1–3] Furthermore, genital HPV infections are widespread among adults who have been sexually active and are estimated to have the highest incidence of any STD in the US.[4] Genital warts and cervical squamous intraepithelial lesions (SIL), also known as cervical intraepithelial neoplasia (CIN) are the most commonly recognized manifestations of genital HPV infection, but the majority of infections are not detectable by either physical examination or cytology and are considered to be subclinical.[5]

Papillomaviruses are members of the papovaviridae family of DNA viruses, all of which are considered tumor viruses because of their ability to immortalize normal cells, and their key features are summarized in *Table 14.1*. They are non-enveloped viruses, 55 nm in diameter, with an icosahedral capsid enclosing a double-stranded, circular DNA genome (*Fig. 14.1*). The genome of HPV consists of approximately 7900 base pairs comprising three functional regions. The long control region (LCR) contains regulatory sequences which control DNA replication and transcription of early (E) and late (L) genes. Protein products of the early genes are involved in replication, transcription, and cellular proliferation, while those of late genes constitute the major and minor capsid proteins (*Fig. 14.2*).[6,7]

Papillomaviruses are species-specific and occur in a wide variety of vertebrates, where they cause benign and malignant proliferations of the skin and mucous membranes. Their life cycle begins with infection of the basal cells (stratum basale) of the epithelium, presumably as a result of microtrauma. Infection of basal cells is followed by virion uncoating and movement of the viral genome to the cell nucleus. As these cells differentiate and move to the epithelial surface, HPV replicates and is transcribed. Infectious viral particles are assembled in

- Member of papovavirus family – PApilloma, POlyoma, VAcuolating viruses (name derived from first 2 letters of each member)
- Widely distributed among mammalian species; species restricted
- Virions small (55 nm), non-enveloped
- Infection involves basal cells of epidermis, replication only in differentiated cells of upper epidermis
- Causes benign/neoplastic epithelial proliferations (warts, papillomas)
- No routine system for in vitro cultivation

Table 14.1 Summary of key characteristics of papillomaviruses.

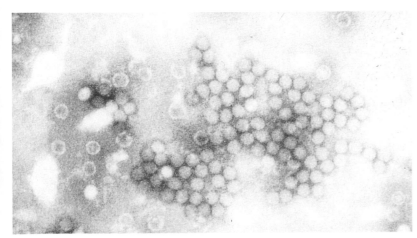

Fig. 14.1 Electron micrograph of HPV (negative stain, phosphotungstic acid). The HPV has an icosahedral capsid 55 nm in diameter.

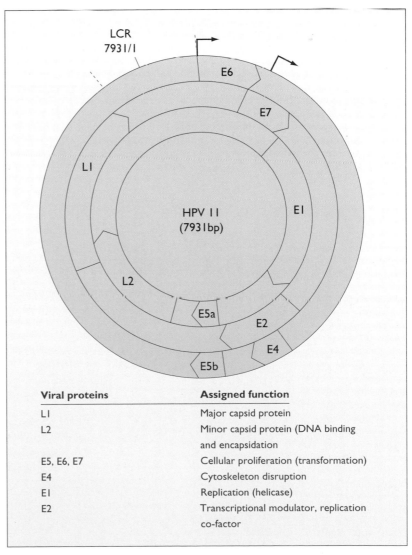

Viral proteins	Assigned function
L1	Major capsid protein
L2	Minor capsid protein (DNA binding and encapsidation
E5, E6, E7	Cellular proliferation (transformation)
E4	Cytoskeleton disruption
E1	Replication (helicase)
E2	Transcriptional modulator, replication co-factor

Fig. 14.2 Genome structure of HPV 11. A circular map of HPV 11 depicts the early (E1–E7) and late (L1–L2) open reading frames with the major transcriptional start sites indicated by arrows. The long control region (LCR) is a non-coding region containing regulatory sequences for control of replication and transcription. Functions for viral proteins encoded by the open reading frames are noted. (Modified from Phelps WC *et al. Antiviral Chem & Chemotherapy* 1998; **9**: 359–377.)

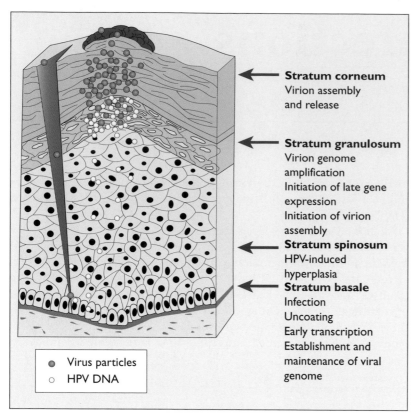

Fig. 14.3 Life cycle of HPV infection of the epidermis. Infection follows trauma to the epithelium through abrasions or friction, allowing infectious virions to reach the basal cells (stratum basale) where uncoating and early transcription and chronic maintenance of the viral genome occur. HPV persists in the basal layer and in the more differentiated stratum spinosum, where HPV-induced hyperplasia is induced. Higher levels of viral replication occur only in the more differentiated stratum granulosum and topmost layer, the stratum corneum, which is where viral capsid protein is expressed and viral particles assembled prior to their sloughing during epithelial turnover. (Modified from Phelps WC *et al. Antiviral Chem & Chemotherapy* 1998; **9**: 359–377.)

the upper layers of the stratum granulosum and stratum corneum and then released with the sloughing of dead keratinocytes during normal cell turnover (*Fig. 14.3*). Because papillomaviruses complete their life cycle only in terminally differentiated epithelial cells, they are difficult to propagate in cell culture, which has limited the study of their life cycle, immunology, transmission dynamics, diagnosis, and therapy.[6,7]

The initial lack of well-characterized viral antigens from viral culture also means that, in contrast to most other viruses, papillomavirus taxonomy is based on DNA homology rather than antigenic diversity. More than 100 different types of HIV have been identified, over 80 of which have been well-characterized by genomic sequencing, with different types defined as having ≤ 90% homology among DNA sequences of the major capsid protein, L1. Specific HPV types tend to be associated with different anatomic sites and clinical manifestations (*Table 14.2*). Approximately 30 types cause infection of genital mucosal sites, and these genital types are generally characterized as 'high-risk' types (e.g., HPV 16, 18, 31, 33, 35, 39, 45, 51, 52), which are associated with low- and high-grade squamous intraepithelial lesions (LSIL and HSIL) and invasive cancer, and 'low-risk' types (e.g., HPV 6, 11, 42, 43, 44), which are primarily associated with genital warts, LSIL, and recurrent respiratory papillomatosis (RRP).[6,7]

EPIDEMIOLOGY

MAGNITUDE OF INFECTION

Because genital HPV infection is not a reportable condition, assessments of its magnitude are based on estimates from epidemiological studies which measure current infection by detection of HPV DNA, and approximating lifetime infection by detection of HPV antibody in serologic assays. While results vary by population studied and sampling and detection methods used, overall they indicate that among sexually active women, up to 75% have been infected with one or more genital HPV types, approximately 15% have evidence of current infection, 50–75% of which are with high-risk types, and 1% have genital warts (*Fig. 14.4*).[5,8–10] These findings are supported by a recent study of incident HPV infection in young women, which documented a 36-month incidence rate of 43%.[11] Men have been less well-studied, in part because

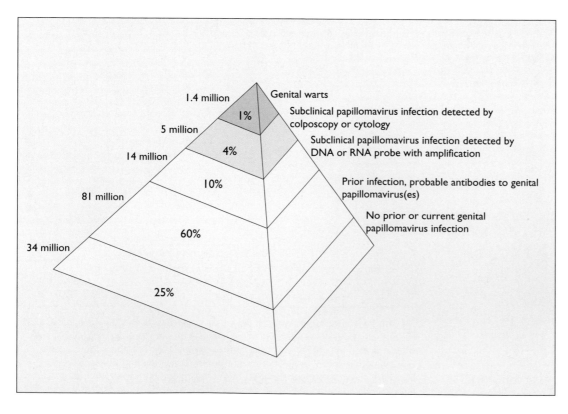

Fig. 14.4 Estimated prevalence of genital HPV infection among men and women 15–49 years of age in the U.S. in 1994. (Modified from Koutsky L. *Am J Med* 1997; **102**: 3–8.)

sites and methods of mucosal sampling are less well-standardized. In men, levels of current infection appear to be similar to women, while levels of lifetime infection are lower, possibly related to gender differences in the development of antibody after infection.[5] A recent assessment of the magnitude of various STD in the U.S. estimated an annual incidence of genital HPV infections of 5.5 million and a prevalence of 20 million (*Table 14.3*).[4] Data assessing rates of genital HPV infection over time are limited but suggest increases over the past 30 years. Trend data from private providers in the U.S. indicate that there were increased patient visits for new cases of genital warts from the early 1970s through the late 1980s, with a plateauing since then (*Fig. 14.5*). Data from public genitourinary medicine clinics in the UK over the same time period evaluating visits for both new and recurrent warts demonstrate a similar rise in the late 1970s through the mid-1980s, a subsequent plateauing, and then another rise in mid-late 1990s (*Fig. 14.6*).

RISK FACTORS FOR INFECTION

Risk factors associated with genital HPV infection have been evaluated in a large number of cross-sectional studies in women. Although smoking, pregnancy, and use of oral contraceptives have been variably associated with infection, the strongest predictors have been age, with the highest rates seen in younger women, and various parameters of sexual activity. The most consistent sexual behavior factor associated with genital HPV infection has been the lifetime number of sex partners, although some studies have noted the importance of the number of recent sex partners as well as the number of partners of the sex partner(s).[9,10,12,13] Studies in men are more limited, but suggest similar associations with age and sexual activity.[9,14,15]

A detailed understanding of the factors associated with transmission of genital HPV infection has been hindered by problems with in vitro cultivation of the virus. *Table 14.4* summarizes key features of what is currently known about transmission. While non-sexual routes of transmission of genital HPV infection via fomites, hand-to-genital contact, or vertical transmission are plausible and supported by some studies, cervical HPV infection has been rarely detected in virginal females, and it is generally accepted that most genital HPV infections are transmitted

Clinical manifestation	HPV types
Skin lesions	
Plantar warts	1, 2, 4
Common warts	2, 4, 26, 27, 29, 57
Flat warts	3, 10, 28, 49
Butcher's warts	7
Epidermodysplasia verruciformis	2, 3, 5, 8, 9, 10, 12, 14, 15, 17, 19, 20–25, 36, 37, 46, 47, 50
Genital mucosal	
Condylomata acuminata	6, 11, 42–44, 54
Squamous intraepithelial lesions	6, 11, 16, 18, 30, 31, 33, 34, 35, 39, 40, 42, 43, 51, 52, 55, 57–59, 61, 62, 64, 67–70
Carcinoma	16, 18, 31, 33, 35, 39, 45, 51, 52, 54, 56, 66, 68
Nongenital mucosal	
Mouth (focal epithelial hyperplasia)	13, 32
Recurrent respiratory papillomatosis	6, 11, 30
Carcinoma (head/neck/lung)	2, 6, 11, 16, 18, 30

Modified from Koutsky LA, Kiviat NB. Genital human papillomavirus. Holmes KK, Mardh PA, Sparling PF, et al editors. In: Sexually Transmitted Diseases, (third edition). New York: McGraw-Hill; 1999: 347–359.

Table 14.2 Clinical manifestations associated with different types of genital HPV infection.

STD	Incidence	Prevalence
Chlamydia	3 million	2 million
Gonorrhea	650,000	no estimates
Syphilis	70,000	no estimates
Herpes simplex virus type 2	1 million	45 million
Human papilloma virus	5.5 million	20 million
Hepatitis B virus	120,000	750,000
Trichomoniasis	5 million	no estimates
HIV	20,000	560,000

(Modified from Cates et al. Estimates of the incidence and prevalence of sexually transmitted diseases in the United States. Sex Transm Dis 1999; 26(supplement): S2–7.)

Table 14.3 Estimated incidence and prevalence of STDs, United States, 1996.

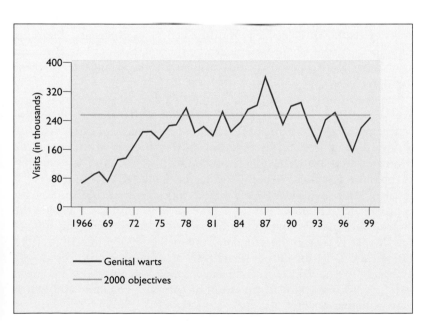

Fig. 14.5 Estimated visits to private physicians' offices for genital warts, 1966–99 and The Healthy People Year 2000 Objective. (Source: CDC Division of STD Prevention STD Surveillance Report 1999, and National Disease and Therapeutic Index, IMS America, Ltd.)

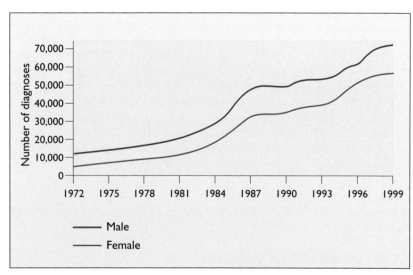

Fig. 14.6 Diagnoses of genital warts (all visits including first, recurrent, and reregistered episodes) seen in genitourinary medicine clinics in England, Scotland, and Wales, 1972–99. (Modified from Public Health Laboratory Service; www.phls.co.uk)

- Infection is virtually always sexually transmitted as a result of microtrauma to skin/mucous membranes.
- Patients with asymptomatic and subclinical infection often transmit infection.
- Role of fomite transmission unclear, probably rare.
- Incubation period unclear, probably 3–8 months for genital warts and 4–36 months for cervical SIL lesions
- Vertical transmission may very rarely result in recurrent respiratory papillomatosis in infants and young children.

Table 14.4 Transmission characteristics of genital HPV infection.

- Epidemiology of CIN and cervical cancer suggests sexually transmitted infectious etiology, with associations with
  - young age of onset of sexual activity,
  - multiple sexual partners,
  - unstable marital relationships,
  - male sexual partners with penile cancer or with prior partners with cervical cancer.
- High-risk types of genital HPV can be found in most cases of CIN and essentially all cervical cancers (and majority of anal, vulvar, vaginal, penile cancers) while other STD are rarely found
- Presence of HPV infection precedes development of CIN in prospective studies
- Odds ratios for high-risk HPV infection in cervical cancer range from 15 to ≥100
- In vitro studies support epidemiologic data
  - integration of HPV into host cell genome common in cervical cancer,
  - integration event deletes E2 regulatory gene, deregulating E6–E7 transforming genes,
  - E6–E7 of high-risk HPV types interact with cellular regulatory proteins (p53 and retinoblastoma gene product) disrupting normal cell cycle control.

Table 14.5 Association of cervical cancer and genital HPV infection.

- Smoking
- Other genital infections (*Chlamydia trachomatis*, herpes simplex virus-2)
- Prolonged hormonal exposure (multiparity, long-term oral contraceptive use)
- Vitamin A deficiency
- HLA haplotypes
- Immunodeficiency

Table 14.6 Potential co-factors of HPV infection in development of cervical cancer.

by sexual activity, often from patients who are asymptomatic or who have subclinical infections. The incubation period (the interval between exposure and development of disease) has been estimated to range from 3–8 months for genital warts and from 4–36 months for cervical SIL lesions, although the upper range has not been well-defined.[5,8,16,17] This variability means that determining the sexual source of a newly detected HPV-associated lesion is often imprecise. In contrast to genital lesions, the likely mode of transmission for RRP is upper respiratory tract exposure to infected genital mucosa. RRP is most common in young children, who are likely exposed to maternal genital infection at the time of birth. RRP in adults is likely to develop as a result of oral-genital sexual contact.[18]

ASSOCIATION WITH CANCER

The sequela of genital HPV infection of greatest public health importance is cervical cancer. For over a century, epidemiologic studies have found a relationship between cervical cancer and sexual activity, with consistent associations with age of onset of sexual activity, multiple sexual

partners, and contact to 'high-risk' males (men with multiple partners or prior partners with genital neoplasia).[2,3] During the past 50 years, there have been ongoing attempts to identify a sexually transmitted agent responsible for these observations, and associations can be found with most sexually transmitted bacteria and viruses. Over the last 15 years, however, the central role of HPV in the pathogenesis of cervical cancer has been firmly established and is based on several lines of evidence (*Table 14.5*).[19,20] High-risk types of HPV are found in 93–99% of cervical cancers worldwide, with HPV 16 present in 50% and HPV 18, 31, and 45 in another 30%,[21,22] and case-control studies from several areas have demonstrated odds ratios for HPV detection in cervical cancer of 15–≥100.[1,19,23] Furthermore, high-grade CIN precursor lesions (e.g., CIN 2 and 3) have similarly high rates of the same HPV types, and prospective studies have demonstrated a plausible temporal relationship, with infection with high-risk HPV types consistently preceding development of CIN 2/3.[16,17,19,20] Finally, the epidemiologic data are supported by laboratory studies demonstrating that high-risk HPV types contain genomic sequences with oncogenic activity, E6 and E7, which are consistently retained and expressed in cancers. Integration of HPV into cellular DNA occurs in the majority of cancers. This event generally disrupts the HPV E2 transcription regulatory gene and enhances stability of HPV mRNA by attaching it to cellular sequences. Either of these events may lead to increased expression of the E6 and E7 proteins. They, in turn, affect cell growth by binding with cellular regulatory proteins, E6 with p53 and E7 with the retinoblastoma gene product, causing their inactivation and ultimately the disruption of normal cell cycle control.[6,7,19]

This body of epidemiologic and laboratory data is sufficiently strong that the International Agency for Research on Cancer and the National Institutes of Health have concluded that high-risk genital HPV types act as carcinogens in the development of cervical cancer.[19,20] While infection with high-risk types appears to be 'necessary' for the development of cervical cancer, it is not 'sufficient' in that cancer does not develop in the vast majority of infected women, raising questions about other possible co-factors, including smoking, hormonal exposure (e.g., multiparity and prolonged oral contraceptive use), nutritional deficiency, HLA haplotypes, other genital tract infections (e.g., *Chlamydia trachomatis*, herpes simplex virus-2), and immunodeficiency, especially HIV infection (*Table 14.6*).[3,19,24,25] The data supporting the role of HPV in other anogenital cancers are more limited, although a large proportion of anal, as well as a subset of vulvar, vaginal, and penile cancers are also associated with high-risk types of genital HPV infection.[26–28] Additionally, high-risk types of genital HPV can be found in a variety of cancers of the upper aerodigestive tract (eg, oropharyngeal, laryngeal, esophageal), although an etiological association is not considered to be established at these locations.

The disease burden created by genital HPV-associated cancers is high. Worldwide, there are estimated to be 400,000–500,000 cases of cervical cancer per year.[3,29] Most cases occur in developing countries without cervical cancer prevention activities; however, even in industrialized countries, where rates have fallen by up to 75% since the introduction of Pap smear screening programs, the disease burden is still considerable.[3,30] In the US, for example, incidence rates are currently 8.3/100,000, with approximately 14,000 cases and 5000 deaths annually, despite the performance of an estimated 50 million Pap smears per year.[3] In spite of the absence of prevention programs, the incidence of other HPV-related cancers are 5–10 fold lower than that of cervical cancer,[31] with the exception of anal cancer in homosexual men, which was estimated to be 12–35/100,000 prior to the onset of the AIDS epidemic and which may be higher now.[32,33]

NATURAL HISTORY OF INFECTION

The natural history of genital HPV infection has not been fully characterized although our understanding has increased substantially over the past decade. The inverse relationship of age with infection as measured by detection of HPV DNA in cross-sectional studies has been thought to reflect the clearance of infection over time as an effective immunologic response is induced.[5,34] Recently, several prospective studies confirm that the majority of genital HPV infections are only transiently detectable by DNA detection techniques, with a median duration of incident infection of 8 months and rates of persistent infection of approximately 30% after 1 year and 9% after 2 years.[11,35] Because women with persistent infection, especially with high-risk types, are at greater risk for developing CIN and for CIN lesions which persist rather than regress, defining determinants of persistence is important in assessing which of the many women with HPV infection are at most risk of subsequent sequelae.[16,17,36,37] Studies to date suggest that infection with high-risk and multiple types of HPV, older age, and immunodeficiency are associated with persistent infection.[17,38] Questions remain as to whether HPV infection which becomes non-detectable has completely cleared or remains latent in basal cells with the potential for intermittent reactivation.[39] The possibility for reactivation from latency is supported by studies indicating increased HPV prevalence in post-menopausal women in some populations[23,40] and in HIV-infected patients with declining immunity,[41] although this issue remains unresolved.

As is the case with subclinical genital HPV infection detected by DNA testing, clinical lesions – both genital warts and SIL – may undergo clearance without treatment, presumably as a result of the development of an effective immunologic response. Spontaneous clearance rates of up to 25% have been described for genital warts.[42] The natural history of CIN has been the most intensively studied of all manifestations of genital HPV infection because of the importance of cervical cancer, although many questions remain unanswered.[3,43] Several different systems have been used to classify these lesions based on their likelihood of progression to cervical cancer. In the CIN system, lesions are generally classified as CIN 1, CIN 2, and CIN 3, which are equivalent to mild, moderate, and severe dysplasia/carcinoma in situ in an older classification system. Because of concerns over the reproducibility of the categories in the earlier systems, a new approach, the Bethesda System, was proposed in 1988 for cytologic diagnoses.[44] It uses the categories of LSIL (equivalent to CIN 1) and HSIL (equivalent to CIN 2 and CIN 3) and also categorizes cells recognized as abnormal but not clearly dysplastic or reparative as atypical squamous cells of undetermined significance (ASCUS) and atypical glandular cells of undetermined significance (AGUS). Although the Bethesda System was developed for use with cytologic diagnoses, it has been increasingly used for classification of histologic lesions as well. The most widely held view has been that the various stages of precursor lesions comprise a morphologic and biologic continuum of consecutive stages in the development of invasive cancer, with greater risk for progression and a lower chance for spontaneous regression with increasing lesion stage. Estimates for risks of progression to invasive cancer and regression are 1% and 60% for CIN 1, 5% and 40% for CIN 2, and 12% and 32% for CIN 3.[43] There are also data indicating that a subset of CIN 2 and 3 lesions may develop rapidly after the occurrence of high-risk types of genital HPV infection, bypassing an initial CIN 1 stage.[3,16] The natural history of SIL lesions of other anogenital sites (e.g., vulva, vagina, penis, anus) are less well-defined, but appear to be associated with even higher rates of regression. In patients with immunodeficiency, such as HIV infection, spontaneous clearance of genital warts and SIL occurs less frequently and rates of progression to invasive cancer appear to be higher.[3,5]

CLINICAL MANIFESTATIONS

The majority of genital HPV infections are not recognized by either physical examination or cytologic testing and are considered clinically inapparent or subclinical; they are identified only by HPV DNA testing.

- Symptoms
  - 'bumps', itching, irritation, bleeding, often none
- Occur at sites of sexual friction
  - men: foreskin, coronal sulcus, shaft, urethral meatus; less commonly perianal
  - women: vaginal introitus, labia minora and majora, perineal/perianal area; less commonly vagina and cervix
  - intraanal: if receptive anal intercourse
  - oral: occasionally if oral–genital sex
- Types of lesions:
  - condylomata acuminata
  - smooth, papular
  - keratotic warts
  - flat-topped papules

Table 14.7 Genital warts: clinical manifestations.

The spectrum of clinically apparent conditions ranges from genital warts, which are primarily recognized by physical examination, and SIL, most commonly detected by cytologic screening of the cervix, to the HPV-associated anogenital malignancies. Additional clinically apparent conditions associated with genital types of HPV include condyloma of the oral and upper respiratory mucosa.

GENITAL WARTS

Genital warts are benign papillomatous, pedunculated, or sessile growths which occur throughout the anogenital area, including the vulva, vagina, cervix, penis, scrotum, urethra, perineum, perianal skin, and anal canal.[5,42] They are generally associated with low-risk types of genital HPV infection, especially HPV 6 and 11, although warts with high-risk types do occur, especially in immunocompromised patients. They are usually asymptomatic, either noticed by the patient simply as 'bumps' on the anogenital skin or detected inadvertently by a clinician during a genital examination, and many likely never come to attention at all (Table 14.7). When symptoms do occur the most common are itching, burning, pain, or bleeding. Genital warts typically occur in areas that have been traumatized by sexual intercourse. In uncircumcised men, lesions occur most commonly on the inner aspect of the foreskin, the glans penis, frenulum, and coronal sulcus, while in circumcised men, the coronal sulcus and shaft are more commonly involved (Figs 14.7–14.9). In females, lesions are most frequently seen around the vaginal introitus, labia minora and majora and less commonly in the vaginal canal and on the cervix (Figs 14.10–14.12). The urethral meatus is involved in men more often than women, presumably because of greater sexual friction. In contrast, perineal and perianal warts are more common in women than men, again presumably because of differences in sexual contact and friction (Figs 14.13, 14.14). Perianal warts are more common in persons practicing receptive anal intercourse, but can occur in both men and women who deny such contact, while intra-anal warts occur almost exclusively in those with a history of anal intercourse. Less common locations include the groin, pubic area, and, among those practicing oral-genital intercourse, the lips and oral cavity (Figs 14.15, 14.16).[5,42]

Genital warts are usually flesh- to gray-colored but may be hyperpigmented or erythematous, and they usually occur in groups of from 5 to ≥15 lesions.[5,42,45] Individual lesions usually range from 1 to 4 mm in diameter and from 2 to 15 mm in height, and groups of lesions may become confluent, plaquelike, or multilobed masses. Four morphologic types of genital warts have been described: condyloma acuminata, smooth papular warts, keratotic warts, and flat macular-papular lesions. Condyloma acuminata (condylomata, knuckles; acuminata, pointed) have a rough cauliflower-like appearance and represent the most classic manifestation of genital warts. They occur most commonly on moist, non hair-bearing anogenital skin (*Figs 14.7, 14.8, 14.10–14.14*). Smooth papular warts are flesh-colored, dome-shaped papules 1–4 mm in diameter more commonly occurring on thicker hair-bearing skin (lateral labia majora, penile shaft, scrotum, pubic area) (*Figs 14.9, 14.17*); papular lesions which are pigmented are more likely to represent SIL (bowenoid papulosis). Keratotic warts have a thick horny surface, resembling common skin warts and like papular warts, occur on fully keratinized skin (*Fig. 14.18*). Finally, small papular warts known as 'flat warts' or condylomata plana can occur on either moist or keratinized skin, and because they are small and not easily noticed, are the most commonly asymptomatic. They have the least specific clinical appearance and their recognition can be enhanced by the use of acetic acid (*Figs 14.19–14.21*).

Physical complications from genital warts are uncommon (*Table 14.8*).[5,42,45] Obstruction by urethral meatal warts can cause hematuria and abnormalities of the urinary stream in males. In pregnancy, presumably because of either transient changes in cell-mediated immunity or increased levels of estrogen and progesterone, warts can increase dramatically in size, occasionally necessitating a Caesarian section because of obstruction of the birth canal. Similar dramatic increases in size can occur in patients with profound defects in cell-mediated immunity, such as patients with AIDS (*Figs 14.22–14.24*). In some cases, large plaques or masses may reach several centimeters in size, and genital

warts may become so large as to cause the deformity of normal structures. These large lesions are sometimes called giant condylomata of Buschke and Löwenstein (*Fig. 14.25*) and are associated with downgrowth into underlying dermal tissue. Finally, there are case reports of longstanding genital warts transforming into invasive squamous cell carcinoma (SCC), although this complication is extremely rare. Because genital warts are typically small and asymptomatic, the most common complication is psychosocial rather than physical, with feelings of anxiety, guilt, and anger, largely related to concerns over transmission and risk for cancer and these concerns often require the greatest clinical attention.[46]

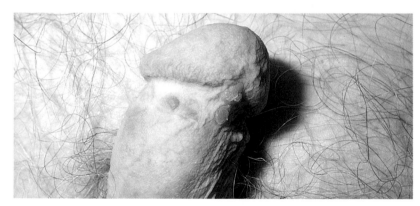

- Most common is psychosocial (anger, guilt, anxiety)
- Occasionally urethral obstruction
- Rarely local invasion (giant condyloma)
- Pregnancy:
  - enlargement with birth canal obstruction
  - perinatal transmission leading to recurrent respiratory papillomatosis
- Immunodeficiency
  - enlargement, rarely malignant transformation

Table 14.8 Complications of genital warts.

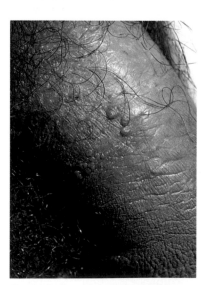

Fig. 14.7 Condylomata acuminata – preputial borders. These lesions had become secondarily infected due to occlusion of the foreskin.

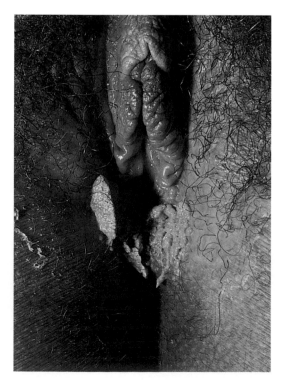

Fig. 14.8 Condylomata acuminata – penile. Asymptomatic, flesh-colored papules are present on the shaft of the penis.

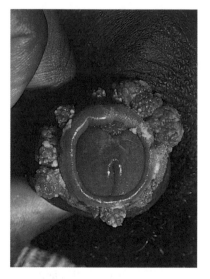

Fig. 14.9 Condylomata acuminata – penile shaft. Very early lesions may be difficult to see.

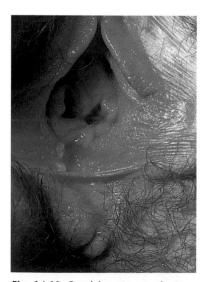

Fig. 14.10 Condylomata acuminata – vulvar introitus. These small papules seen at the fourchette are nearly invisible to the examiner and asymptomatic to the patient.

Fig. 14.11 Condyloma acuminata – vulvar. The rough, corrugated surface is characteristic and papillary projections may form as seen here.

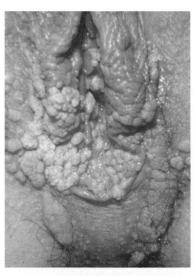

Fig. 14.12 Condylomata acuminata – vulvar and perineal. This patient has extensive involvement around the introitus and the labia with extension onto the perineum and perianal region. Courtesy of Woodruff JD, Parmley TH: Atlas of Gynecologic Pathology. New York, Gower Medical Publishing, 1988.

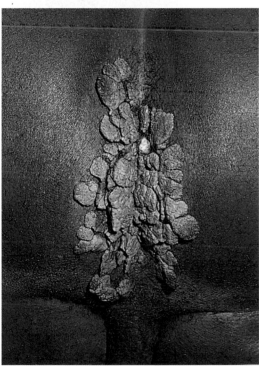

Fig. 14.13 Condylomata acuminata – perianal. Treatment of these large, recurrent warts was made more difficult by the patient's poor compliance with office follow-up visits.

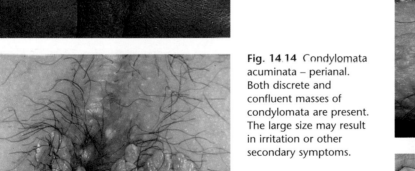

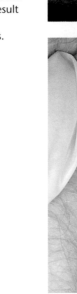

Fig. 14.14 Condylomata acuminata – perianal. Both discrete and confluent masses of condylomata are present. The large size may result in irritation or other secondary symptoms.

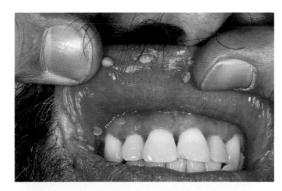

Fig. 14.15 Condylomata acuminata-orolabial. This patient developed characteristic genital wart lesions of the oral mucosa, likely as a result of orogenital sexual contact. Courtesy of C.A.M. Rietmeijer, MD.

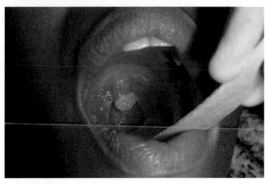

Fig. 14.16 Condylomata acuminata-oropharyngeal. This large typical condylomatous lesion was asymptomatic and was noted by this HIV+ patient as a 'bump'. Courtesy of C.A.M. Rietmeijer, MD.

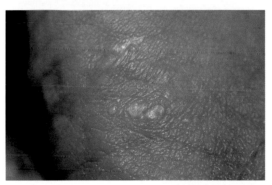

Fig. 14.17 Genital wart – penile shaft. These smooth papular warts are generally found on keratinized skin and are usually asymptomatic. Courtesy of Karl Beutner MD.

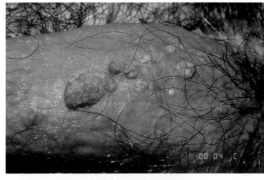
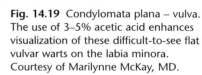

Fig. 14.18 Genital wart-penile shaft. These keratotic genital warts, occurring with more typical condylomata acuminata, resemble common warts, and are generally found on more heavily keratinized genital skin. Courtesy of Karl Beutner MD.

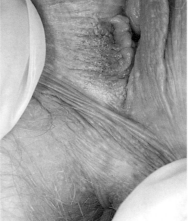

Fig. 14.19 Condylomata plana – vulva. The use of 3–5% acetic acid enhances visualization of these difficult-to-see flat vulvar warts on the labia minora. Courtesy of Marilynne McKay, MD.

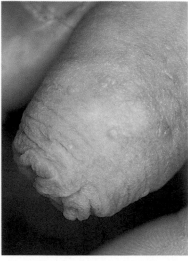

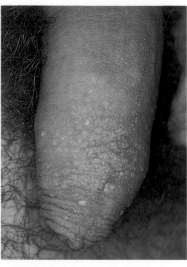

Figs 14.20 and 14.21 Condylomata plana – penile. Acetowhite penile lesions. Penile skin showing areas of 'acetowhitening' after the application of 3–5% acetic acid in a patient with very small and recent condylomata positive for HPV 6/11. Without the use of acetic acid and a magnifying lens, these lesions were not clinically apparent. Note the area of nonspecific acetowhitening adjacent to the separate acetowhite condylomatous papules.

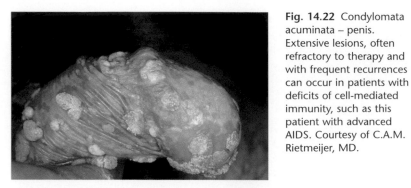

Fig. 14.22 Condylomata acuminata – penis. Extensive lesions, often refractory to therapy and with frequent recurrences can occur in patients with deficits of cell-mediated immunity, such as this patient with advanced AIDS. Courtesy of C.A.M. Rietmeijer, MD.

Fig. 14.23 Condylomata acuminata – perianal. Large, perianal lesions in patients with AIDS are most commonly seen in homosexual men. Courtesy of C.A.M. Rietmeijer, MD.

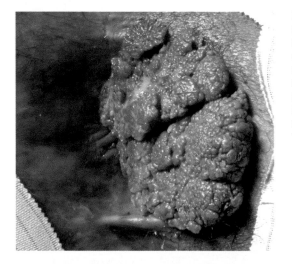

Fig. 14.24 Condylomata acuminata/high-grade SIL-perianal. This large, condylomatous lesion in a man with AIDS was refractory to cryotherapy and was found to have HSIL on biopsy. Courtesy of Jeff Johnson MD.

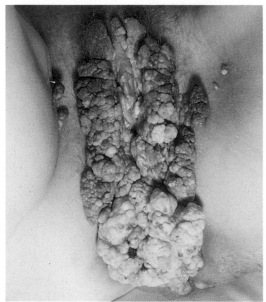

Fig. 14.25 Condylomata acumina – vulva and perineum. The clinical diagnosis was giant condyloma of Buschke and Löwenstein. Such large and confluent lesions should be carefully examined and multiple biopsies obtained to rule out underlying malignancy.

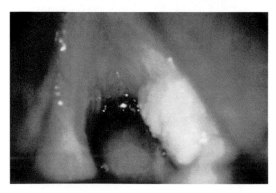

Fig. 14.26 Recurrent respiratory papillomatosis – larynx. This adult developed a solitary laryngeal papilloma. These HPV 6/11-induced lesions typically present with hoarseness and are particularly problematic in children, in whom repetitive surgical procedures are often required. Courtesy of Renzo Barrasso, MD.

Fig. 14.27 Squamous intraepithelial lesion – cervix. These lesions are usually detected by abnormal cervical cytology and are usually clearly defined after the application of 3–5% acetic acid, allowing targeted biopsy of the most abnormal appearing areas.

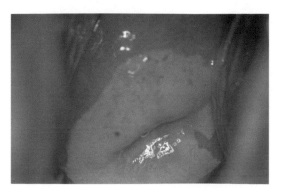

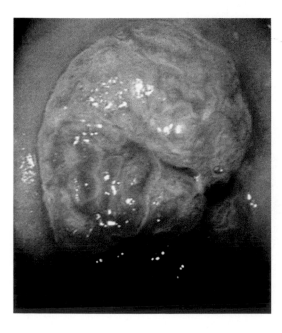

Fig. 14.28 Invasive squamous cell carcinoma – cervix. Exophytic cervical cancers often have raised edges, an irregular contour around the cervical os, ulcerations, and easily induced bleeding. These lesions are often asymptomatic. Courtesy of Renzo Barrasso, MD.

Because of the occurrence of genital warts at sites of sexual trauma and the potential for irritation during the friction of intercourse, questions have been raised as to whether, like several other STD, genital HPV infection could enhance HIV transmission. Although plausible, there are presently no data to support this premise.

Recurrent respiratory papillomatosis is a condition resulting from the development of HPV 6/11-associated papillomatous lesions in the upper respiratory tract (*Fig. 14.26*). Lesions occur most commonly in the larynx, usually presenting with hoarseness, but occasionally leading to respiratory obstruction, especially in young children due to the small diameter of the airways. Lesions often recur after treatment, necessitating repeat invasive procedures; can spread to previously uninvolved sites of the tracheobronchial tree and even the lung; and can rarely undergo malignant transformation into squamous cell carcinoma.[18]

SQUAMOUS INTRAEPITHELIAL LESIONS

The other commonly recognized manifestation of genital HPV infection is cervical SIL or CIN, detected through cytologic screening and generally confirmed by colposcopy and directed biopsy. It is estimated that 2.5 million Pap smears with low-grade abnormalities (e.g., ASCUS and LSIL) are detected annually in the US and that HPV-associated CIN 2/3 is present in 10–20% of these women. There are an additional 200,000–300,000 women annually in the US whose Pap smears have findings of HSIL, the vast majority of whom have CIN 2/3 on biopsy.[47] CIN 1 lesions can be caused by any of the genital HPV types, both low-risk and high-risk, while CIN 2 and 3 are caused primarily by high-risk types.[3,8] For the most part, these lesions are asymptomatic and are clinically visible only following application of 3–5% acetic acid and magnification via colposcopy (*Fig. 14.27*). In contrast, the lesions of invasive cervical cancer, while also usually asymptomatic, are commonly raised and exophytic in nature (*Fig. 14.28*).

SIL lesions commonly occur at other anogenital locations including the vulva, vagina, penis, and anal canal. Similar to the cervix, these have been categorized as either various stages of intraepithelial neoplasia (e.g, vulva – VIN, vagina – VAIN, penis – PIN, anus – AIN) or as LSIL/HSIL. They are usually caused by high-risk types of genital HPV infection. Most lesions at these sites are not visible on routine physical exam and can be detected only with diagnostic aids such as colposcopy and biopsy. The most commonly recognized clinical manifestation of external genital SIL is bowenoid papulosis, dome-shaped or flat papules that are often hyperpigmented (*Figs 14.29, 14.30*).[48] These lesions can sometimes be flesh-colored and clinically indistinguishable from genital warts, but on biopsy demonstrate HSIL. As for genital warts, their recognition can be enhanced by the application of acetic acid (*Fig. 14.31*). Progression to invasive squamous cell carcinoma occasionally may occur, especially in immunocompromised patients; however, because the likelihood of regression in immunocompetent hosts appears to be high and the incidence of malignancies at these sites is low, the role of diagnosis and treatment has not been well-established.[3] When carcinomas do occur, it is generally at the site of slowly evolving progressive lesions, often associated with induration and ulceration (*Fig. 14.32*).

An area of particular controversy is SIL of the anal canal in persons with HIV infection. There is a growing body of data linking anal cancer to anal intercourse as well as HPV infection in both men and women,[26,41,49] and the risk of both anal SIL and cancer appear to be further increased in persons with HIV infection.[50,51] These observations have led to consideration of the value of cytologic screening for detection of precursor SIL lesions in HIV+ homosexual men in order to prevent subsequent anal cancer, analogous to cervical cancer prevention,[52,53] although at present there are insufficient data to recommend this approach routinely.[54,55] As with the cervix, application of 3–5% acetic acid and magnification via colposcopy can enhance detection and characterization of anal SIL lesions (*Fig. 14.33*).

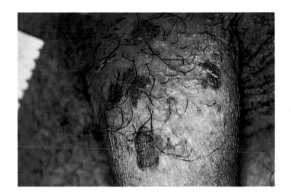

Fig. 14.29 Bowenoid papulosis – penis. These large, hyperpigmented, flat papules on the shaft of the penis were asymptomatic. A biopsy to rule out carcinoma in situ is recommended in such cases. Courtesy of Heidi Watts, PA-C.

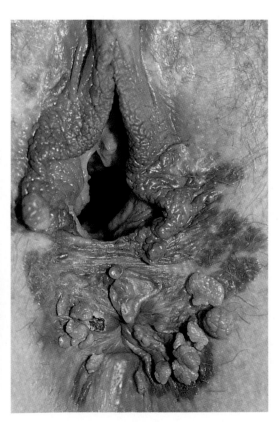

Fig. 14.30 Bowenoid papulosis – vulvar and perineal. Although these lesions resemble condylomata clinically, the presence of multiple pigmented papular lesions in a young woman should raise the possibility of bowenoid papulosis or carcinoma in situ and biopsies should be obtained. Courtesy of D.R. Popkin, MD.

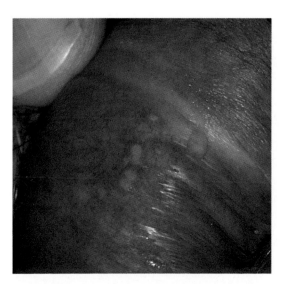

Fig. 14.31 Carcinoma in situ – penis. These flat penile papules appeared white after acetic acid application and biopsy showed carcinoma in situ. Courtesy of Michael Campion, MD.

DIFFERENTIAL DIAGNOSIS

Genital warts, especially condylomata acuminata, ordinarily present a distinct and easily recognized clinical picture. However, the clinician should be familiar with other common papular entities in the differential diagnosis as described below. Less common differential diagnostic considerations include flat erythematous lesions in the genital area due to psoriasis, seborrheic dermatitis, and circinate balanitis of Reiter's syndrome. For a more detailed discussion of other genital dermatologic considerations, the reader is referred to Chapter 1.

Verruca vulgaris

Verruca vulgaris (usually caused by HPV types 2, 3, and 4) may occur in or near the genital region, especially on the skin of the lower abdomen, upper thigh, or buttocks (*Fig. 14.34*). A thickened, dry, hyperkeratotic appearance is more typical of verruca vulgaris; differentation from keratotic genital warts may require histopathologic examination or other diagnostic tests to differentiate viral type, although a clear distinction is rarely indicated clinically since treatment is similar to that for genital warts.

Molluscum contagiosum

The umbilicated papules of molluscum contagiosum infection can resemble genital warts and appear in the genital region in sexually active patients (*Fig. 14.35*). The umbilication of the papules helps to distinguish them from condylomata acuminata, but crusting or other secondary changes may obscure this helpful feature. This pox virus infection is transmitted by both sexual and nonsexual routes. It is usually self-limited but may be progressive in immunocompromised patients. Although usually distinguishable by careful physical examination, it can be definitively diagnosed by characteristic inclusions seen on cytologic or histologic examination. Treatment modalities are similar to those for genital warts.

Seborrheic keratoses

Seborrheic keratoses are rough, usually brown or black hyperpigmented, flat, broad papules. They have a waxy texture and minute puncta on the surface. These benign tumors may be multiple and are treated only for cosmetic reasons.

Condylomata lata

Condylomata lata lesions of secondary syphilis must always be considered when condylomata acuminata-like lesions are present (*Fig. 14.36*). The two entities may not only look remarkably similar but may coexist, as patients with multiple sexual partners are often exposed to and become infected with more than one STD at a time. Condylomata lata, however, are typically more moist than condylomata acuminata and may even be ulcerated. In condylomata lata, dark-field examination almost always demonstrates spirochetes and syphilis serology is invariably reactive. The distinction is important both for treatment as well as rapid partner evaluation in the case of syphilis.

Lichen planus

Lichen planus is a chronic inflammatory process of skin and mucous membranes characterized by flat-topped, shiny, well-demarcated papules (*Fig. 14.37*). Lesions are usually white-pink in color often with white lines (Wickham's striae) across the surface. They occasionally occur on the genital skin where they can mimic papular and flat-topped warts; other common locations include the oral mucosa, shins, scalp, and flexor wrists. Lesions generally respond to topical or systemic corticosteroids.

Other

Skin tags (acrochordons) and syringomas may also be confused with condylomata acuminata, as can pearly penile papules (*Fig. 14.38*). They can be differentiated from genital warts based on their surface texture,

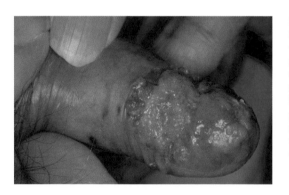

Fig. 14.32 Invasive squamous cell carcinoma – penis. Related to the same high-risk types which cause cervical cancer, penile carcinoma is much less common and generally seen in uncircumcised men. Courtesy of www.dermis.net/doia

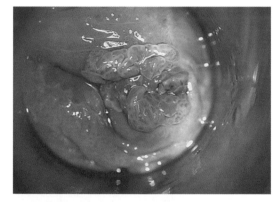

Fig. 14.33 Anal intrapithelial neoplasia. This condylomatous-appearing lesion was detected in an asymptomatic HIV+ homosexual man and revealed AIN 3 on biopsy. Courtesy of Joel Palefsky, MD.

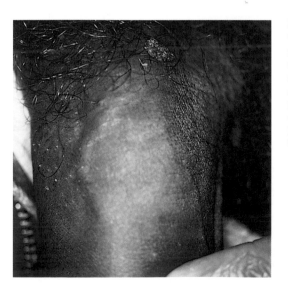

Fig. 14.34 Verruca vulgaris – penis. This raised, rough papule at the base of the penis appeared similar to condylomata acuminata but proved to be a verruca vulgaris on biopsy. Courtesy of Heidi Watts, PA-C.

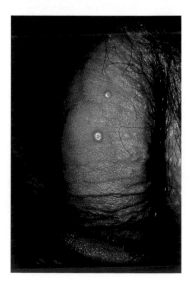

Fig. 14.35 Molluscum contagiosum – penile shaft. The characteristic smooth, umbilicated papules caused by the molluscum contagiosum virus are typically asymptomatic, but may become secondarily infected, crusted, or pruritic. Courtesy of C.A.M. Rietmeijer, MD.

which is smooth rather than rough, and their arrangement in rows for part or much of the circumference of the glans penis. Similar normal anatomic variants, vestibular papillae, can be found around the vaginal introitus. They can be distinguished from genital warts by their bases, which are discrete rather than fused, and their tips, which are rounded and non-keratotic.

DIAGNOSIS

Most cases of genital warts can be diagnosed by physical examination, assisted by good illumination and the magnification provided by a hand-held lens. Because HPV-associated lesions usually turn grayish-white after application of 3–5% acetic acid, the use of the acetic acid (or acetowhite) test can improve lesion assessment and help target lesions for biopsy (*Figs 14.19, 14.21, 14.31*). However, because acetowhitening may occur in other conditions, such as lichen planus, nonspecific inflam-

mation, eczema, post-traumatic scar tissue, and seborrheic dermatitis (*Figs 14.39, 14.40*), the test is not recommended for screening, and should be used only by clinicians familiar with its use.[42,45,54] Biopsy provides the most definitive diagnostic information but is not needed to supplement the physical exam in typical cases of condylomata acuminata. Biopsies may be helpful with atypical lesions, those suggestive of HSIL or malignancy (e.g, lesions which are pigmented, indurated or fixed to underlying tissue, nonresponsive to therapy), or in immunocompromised patients. HPV testing of mucosal swabs or biopsies has not been shown to affect clinical management of genital warts and is not presently recommended.[42,45] Women with genital warts should have a vaginal speculum exam to search for vaginal and cervical warts and undergo Pap smear screening at the same interval as other women. It has also been suggested that for patients with perianal warts who have engaged in receptive anal intercourse, routine anoscopy be considered because of the high proportion who will also have warts of the anal canal,[5,45] although the clinical benefit of this approach has not been established.

LABORATORY TESTS

The principal laboratory procedures in the diagnosis of genital HPV-related conditions have been cytologic screening for cervical lesions and histopathologic evaluation of tissue samples for diagnostic confirmation.[56] Although viral culture in routine laboratory cell lines remains unavailable, a variety of virologic techniques for the detection of HPV

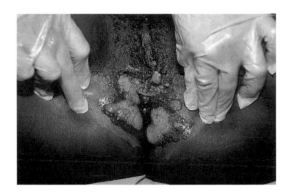

Fig. 14.36 Condylomata lata – bilateral labia minora. The exophytic nature of these well-demarcated lesions mimics condylomata acuminata, although these manifestations of secondary syphilis tend to be moister and often in a 'kissing lesion' pattern. Dark-field examination and serology were positive. Courtesy of David Cohn, MD.

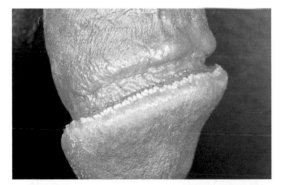

Fig. 14.38 Pearly penile papules (hirsutoid papillomatosis) – glans penis. These dome-shaped, regularly arrayed papules are a normal anatomic variant, largely important because they can be confused with genital warts; they do not require treatment. Courtesy of C.A.M. Rietmeijer, MD.

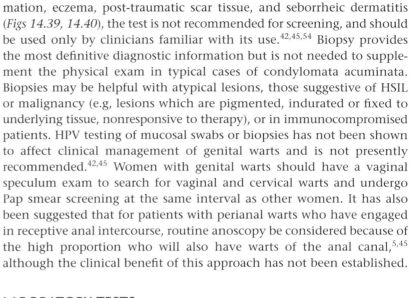

Fig. 14.37 Lichen planus – glans penis. This chronic inflammatory process can resemble papular warts, although genital lesions are commonly accompanied by lesions in the mouth and flexor wrists. Courtesy of C.A.M. Rietmeijer, MD.

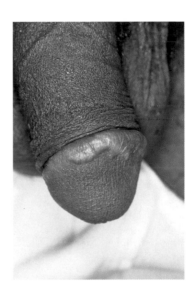

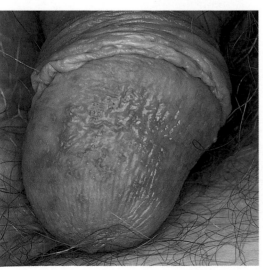

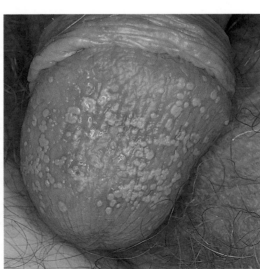

Figs 14.39 and 14.40 Seborrheic dermatitis also acetowhitens. Pre- (14.39) and post-3% acetic acid (14.40) of a biopsy-proven HPV-negative penile seborrheic dermatitis.

Fig. 14.39

Fig. 14.40

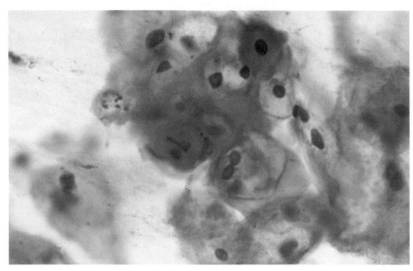

Fig. 14.41 Koilocyte and superficial desquamated epithelial cells on a Papanicolaou smear. The koilocyte is the cell with the perinuclear halo. It is a relatively specific yet insensitive diagnostic indicator of HPV infection.

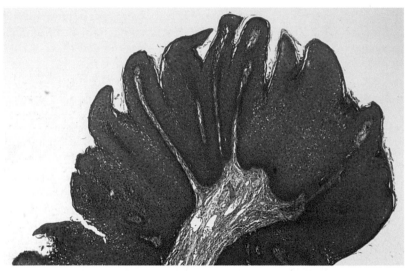

Fig. 14.42 Anogenital condyloma. Histologic preparation of condyloma showing hyperkeratotic squamous epithelium with multiple papillary fronds. Courtesy of J. Michael Hall, DSS.

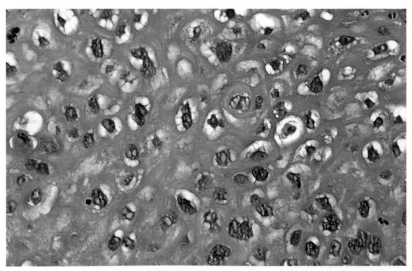

Fig. 14.43 Anogenital condyloma. Histologic examination shows multiple large cells with clear cytoplasm and atypical wrinkled nuclei (koilocytes), which are highly suggestive of HPV infection. Courtesy of J. Michael Hall, DSS.

has been in use over the past two decades, including electron microscopy for the detection of viral particles, immunohistochemical detection of viral antigens, both amplified and non-amplified tests for detection of viral DNA, and serologic assays for detection of HPV antibody. Up until the present, they have been primarily useful in research settings, although there are emerging data indicating the potential usefulness of HPV DNA testing for several situations including the triage of women with low-grade cytologic abnormalities, the follow-up of women with CIN, and as a primary screening modality for cervical cancer.[57]

CYTOLOGY

The Papanicolaou smear is the most commonly used means of detecting asymptomatic cervical HPV infection, but it is relatively insensitive and subject to sampling error. Viral atypia and koilocytosis are characteristic cytologic features of cervical HPV infection. Koilocytosis is considered fairly specific for HPV infection although relatively insensitive. Koilocytes have an irregular, hyperchromatic nucleus surrounded by a clear, cytoplasmic perinuclear halo, which, in turn, is surrounded by peripherally located dense cytoplasm (*Fig. 14.41*). The halo is a result of cytoplasmic organelles congregating at the periphery of the cell, leaving the remainder of the cytoplasm clear. The diagnosis of HPV infection is further suggested by other cytologic findings, such as dyskeratocytosis, multinucleation, anucleation, and parakeratosis.

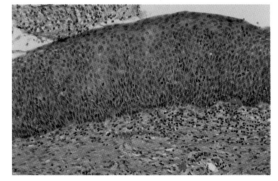

Fig. 14.44 High-grade SIL of the cervix. Colposcopically targeted biopsy demonstrating atypical cells with multiple mitotic figures extending the full thickness of the epithelium, consistent with CIN 3/carcinoma in situ. Courtesy of Dr Loretta Gaido, MD.

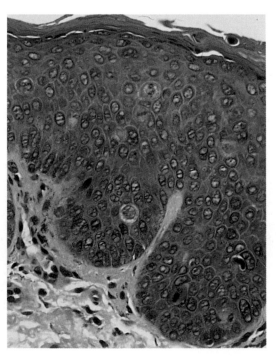

Fig. 14.45 High-grade SIL of the vulva. Histologic examination shows the presence of hyperchromatic nuclei, multiple mitoses, and disruption of the maturation sequence involving the full thickness of the epithelium, consistent with VIN 3 Courtesy of J. Michael Hall, DSS.

HISTOPATHOLOGY

Genital warts

The most obvious histologic changes are epithelial papillomatosis and acanthosis. The dermal papillae are usually elongated, narrow, and branching, forming a pattern of pseudoepitheliomatous hyperplasia (*Fig. 14.42*). The most characteristic feature is the presence of koilocytes in the upper stratum spinosum, stratum granulosum, and stratum corneum (*Fig. 14.43*). Hyperplasia of the parabasal cells may be present beneath the atypical cells, and orthokeratosis and parakeratosis are common. Chronic inflammatory cells and dilated capillaries and edema are usually present in the dermis.

Squamous Intraepithelial Lesions

Hyperkeratosis, parakeratosis, and psoriasiform epidermal hyperplasia with a focally prominent granular zone are accompanied by crowding of epidermal nuclei, increased mitotic figures in the upper half of the epidermis, atypical mitotic figures, and keratinocytes with hyperchromatic and pleomorphic nuclei. Koilocytosis may be present, but is less prominent than in classic forms of condyloma, although it is common to see features of both condyloma and intraepithelial neoplasia in contiguous parts of the same tissue sample. The grade of intraepithelial neoplastic lesions is based on the proportion of the epithelium involved by the process, from CIN 1 (lesions with basaloid, undifferentiated cells occupying the lower one-third of the epithelium) to CIN 2 (with undifferentiated cells comprising the lower one-third to two-thirds of the epithelium) and CIN 3/carcinoma in situ (with undifferentiated cells across the full thickness of the epithelium) (*Figs 14.44–14.46*). Invasive carcinoma is considered to have occurred when the the underlying stroma is invaded by cells which have penetrated the basement membrane; it is characterized by sheets of flat squamoid cells with nuclear atypia and prominent mitotic figures (*Fig. 14.47*).

ELECTRON MICROSCOPY

Electron microscopy was the first laboratory method to detect evidence of HPV in clinical lesions (*Fig. 14.1*). However, the procedure is extremely time-consuming and insensitive compared with other diagnostic methods. Genital wart tissues contain only 1/10,000 as many virions as common skin warts, and electron microscopy is therefore not a practical diagnostic procedure.

IMMUNOHISTOCHEMICAL STAINING

Immunoperoxidase staining of cells or tissues directly detects HPV capsid antigen. In this technique, commercially prepared antibodies (directed against disrupted virions) are attached to an enzyme (peroxidase) that will yield a colored reaction product. Immunoperoxidase stains may be performed on tissues or cytologic smears (*Fig. 14.48*). However, this method is substantially less sensitive than DNA detection and even routine cytologic examination. The likelihood of detecting capsid antigen decreases with an increasing severity of dysplasia, and tests for capsid antigen are invariably negative in genital cancers that contain HPV DNA.

DNA DETECTION TESTS

Several approaches exist for the detection and typing of HPV DNA.[57] They are all based on nucleic acid hybridization reactions in which a specific type of HPV DNA is identified by association with a diagnostic probe (e.g., a molecule of HPV DNA or RNA made from a known type of HPV which is labeled with a radioisotope or chemically reactive ligand to allow recognition of the hybridized product). This reaction can either be carried out on cytologic smears or fixed tissue as a tissue *in situ* hybridization procedure, which preserves cellular detail and allows localization of HPV within the infected tissue, or by extracting nucleic acid from the specimen and carrying out the hybridization reaction on a solid surface (e.g., a nylon membrane for blotting procedures) or in a liquid suspension. HPV DNA testing can be carried out on both biopsy samples as well as swabs of exfoliated cells. The sensitivity of the reaction can be enhanced by amplification of the target DNA through procedures such as the polymerase chain reaction

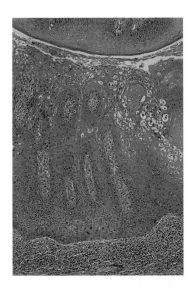

Fig. 14.46 High-grade SIL of the perianal skin. Histologic exam of the lesion seen in Figure 14.24 reveals koilocytes in the superficial layers of the epithelium, with undifferentiated cells occupying the lower half of the epithelium, consistent with AIN 2, including cells with mitotic activity at the basal layer. Courtesy of Loretta Gaido, MD.

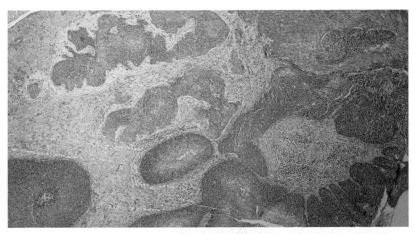

Fig. 14.47 Carcinoma of the cervix. Histopathologic specimen demonstrating that some of the abnormal epithelial cells have breached the basement membrane and invaded the cervical stroma; this is invasive carcinoma.

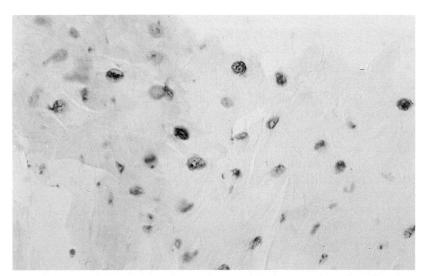

Fig. 14.48 Immunoperoxidase stain. Tissue section containing HPV identified by an immunoperoxidase method, which stains the intranuclear capsid antigen brown. Capsid antigen is generally found only in the superficial layers of the epidermis, correlating with the assembly of infectious viral particles.

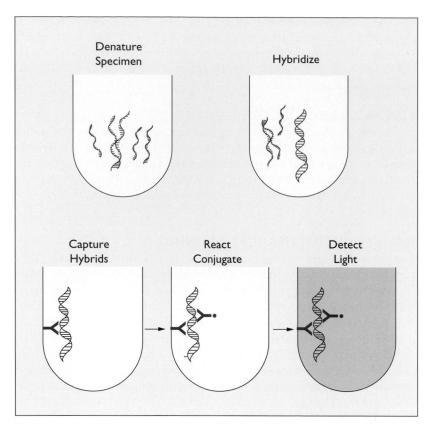

Fig. 14.49 Hybrid Capture-II assay. This microplate-based technique uses two pools of HPV RNA probes (one of high-risk types and one of low-risk types) that are hybridized in solution with denatured target DNA from a specimen. The resulting RNA:DNA hybrids are captured on the surface of the microwell by an anti-hybrid antibody. The captured RNA-DNA hybrids are then reacted with an alkaline phosphatase antibody conjugate. Detection is accomplished by addition of a chemiluminescent substrate and measurement of the light emitted, after cleavage of the substrate by the bound alkaline phosphatase conjugate in a luminometer. The emitted light intensity is proportional to the amount of target DNA in the specimen. Courtesy of Attila Lörincz, PhD.

Assay performance	ALTS study*		Manos study**	
	HPV Testing	Repeat Pap Smear	HPV Testing	Repeat Pap Smear
Sensitivity	96%	85%	89%	76%
Specificity	na	na	64%	64%
Positive predictive value	20%	17%	15%	13%
Negative predictive value	99%	96%	99%	97%
Percent referred for colposcopy	56%	58%	40%	39%

*Modified from Solomon D et al. JNCI 2001: 93:293–9.
**Modified from Manos MM et al. JAMA 1999; 281:1605–10.

Table 14.9 Performance of HPV testing by the Hybrid Capture-II assay versus repeat pap smear in the detection of CIN 2/3 among women with ASCUS pap smears.

(PCR), which is currently considered to be the most sensitive available method for detection of genital HPV infection. Two widely used 'consensus' PCR assays (the GP5+/6+ primer pair and the MY 09/11 degenerate primers) amplify highly conserved sequences in the L1 region and are capable of detecting most or all of the recognized genital types of HPV.

The most widely available HPV DNA detection assay and the only one which is commercially available in the US is the Hybrid Capture-II assay (Digene Diagnostics) (*Fig. 14.49*).[57,58] The assay is available in microplate format and is designed to detect HPV DNA from exfoliated cervical cells collected with a dacron swab or by cervicovaginal lavage. It uses pools of RNA from multiple types of HPV as probes, and the resulting RNA probe:target DNA hybrids are captured by an antibody specific for such hybrids and which is then recognized by a signal amplification assay, using an anti-hybrid antibody conjugated to alkaline phosphatase which is detected after addition of a chemiluminescent substrate in a luminometer. The two probe pools can detect the presence of 13 high-risk types (types 16, 18, 31, 33, 35, 39, 45, 51, 52, 56, 58, 59, 68) and five low-risk types (types 6, 11, 42, 43, 44), although the assay does not allow identification of specific HPV types. Sensitivity is estimated to be similar to that of PCR.[59]

The most immediately promising use of HPV testing is for triage of women with low-grade ASCUS Pap smear abnormalities. Although the majority of women with these cytologic findings have normal histology or lesions which are likely to regress (CIN 1), a minority (5–20%) will have CIN2/3, representing the majority of women with high-grade

lesions in some settings.[60] Current management recommendations for women with ASCUS offer several options, including immediate colposcopy for all women or follow-up Pap smear evaluation, with colposcopy only for those with persistent abnormalities.[47] Neither approach is ideal since routine colposcopy is costly and generates a large number of unnecessary procedures, while the follow-up Pap smear approach may result in women being lost to follow-up and lower cost-effectiveness. Emerging data indicate that HPV testing, with colposcopy only for those with high-risk types identified, may be a useful management strategy.[57] Two recently published trials of large numbers of women with ASCUS demonstrate that such an approach can maintain high sensitivity (approximately 90%) and acceptable specificity (40–65%) and positive predictive value (15–20%) while reducing the number of women referred for colposcopy by approximately half (*Table 14.9*).[61,62] Test specificity and positive predictive value for detecting CIN2/3 appear to be lower in settings where the prevalence of HPV infection is higher, as in younger women or those with LSIL.[63] Obtaining a sample with the initial Pap smear to save for possible HPV testing (using either liquid-based cytology media or a vial of sample transport media specific for HPV testing) allows 'reflex testing' of only the samples from women with ASCUS without the need for a return visit to collect additional samples. The use of HPV testing for triage is being further evaluated in two large ongoing randomized trials in the US and the UK, which are comparing the three management strategies and which should provide even more information on their relative clinical value and cost-effectiveness.[57,62]

HPV testing for primary cervical cancer screening is a more difficult issue to assess, but one with potentially greater benefit. Used together with the Pap smear, it may increase sensitivity and specificity of primary screening and enhance cost-effectiveness by lengthening the screening interval and determining the point at which screening can be stopped, especially among older women.[57] Of even greater importance is potential use as an alternative to the Pap smear for accessing women not currently being screened. In developing countries without screening programs, intermittent or even once in a lifetime HPV testing might be more feasible and cost-effective than Pap smear screening. Several studies have reported enhanced screening sensitivity for detection of CIN2/3 when HPV testing is combined with cytology in comparison to cytology alone[64,65] and others have reported sensitivities of HPV testing alone for detection of CIN 2/3 of ≥ 85%.[66,67] However, specificity is an added concern, especially in younger women with their higher rates of incident and usually transient infection, and additional data about positive and negative predictive value and optimal age for HPV testing are needed to determine its value in primary screening.[57]

- Primary goal is removal of symptomatic warts
- No data to suggest that currently available treatment eradicates infection, and treatment may/may not decrease infectivity and transmission risk
- No evidence that treatment affects development of cancer
- No treatment is ideal and choice should be guided by patient preference, resources, and provider experience
- Provider should have access to/experience with at least one type of self-applied and provider-applied therapy
- Multiple treatments are often required: treatment can achieve clearance in 1–6 months in most patients, multiple treatments are required in up to one-third of patients and recurrences develop in 20–50%
- Complications are rare with proper treatment, patients should be advised about rare cosmetic sequelae (e.g., scarring, pigmentation, etc.)

Table 14.10 Basic approach to the treatment of genital warts.

- Patient-applied
  - Podophyllotoxin (Podofilox) 0.5% solution or gel; to be applied in 4–6 weekly cycles (bid for 3 days, followed by 4 days without treatment)
  - Imiquimod 5% cream; to be applied 3 times per week for 6–10 hours for up to 12–16 weeks
- Provider-administered
  - Cryotherapy with liquid nitrogen or cryoprobe; to be applied once weekly*
  - Podophyllin resin 10–25% in compound tincture of benzoin; to be applied once weekly
  - Trichloroacetic or bichloroacetic acid 80–90% solution; to be applied once weekly*
  - Office surgery* (excision, electrocautery, curettage

*Safe for use in pregnancy.

Table 14.11 Recommended treatments for genital warts.

Lastly, there is interest in the potential use of HPV testing to manage women who have already developed CIN, both in monitoring those who have not been treated as well as in following those who have. First, since the majority of CIN 1 lesions regress spontaneously, many women with these lesions are observed without treatment.[68,69] Studies which indicate that persistent high-risk HPV infection predicts subsequent development of CIN 2/3[16,36,70] suggest that in women with CIN 1, determination of whether high-risk HPV types are present, and if so, whether they persist, may help select a group in whom closer follow-up and/or treatment would be most useful. Recent data suggest that quantitation of high-risk types of HPV DNA may be useful in defining the likelihood of progression and thus may also have clinical value.[37,71] Second, following ablative treatment of CIN, approximately 10–15% of women will experience a recurrence.[72,73] Presence of high-risk types of HPV DNA is associated with recurrences, and follow-up HPV testing could enhance identification of those most likely to recur, allowing more intensive follow-up.[72,74,75] These remain areas of active evaluation.

SEROLOGY

Analogous to other viral infections, a reliable type-specific assay to measure serum antibody to genital HPV proteins could provide a method of determining past or persistent infection. The development of such an assay has been hindered by difficulties with in vitro cultivation and thus limited availability of conformationally intact type-specific viral protein. Recent success with the production in various expression systems (e.g., vaccinia virus, baculovirus) of large quantities of major capsid antigen in native conformation on the surface of virus-like particles (VLPs) has led to the development of serologic assays which appear to provide type-specific results. These have proven increasingly valuable in epidemiologic analyses, although further studies to better define sensitivity and specificity and clinical meaning of a positive serologic test are needed before such assays could be useful for clinical management.[9,10,57]

TREATMENT

The therapy of genital HPV-associated disease is based on local therapy of involved tissue since there are currently no virus-specific drug therapies available.[7] Treatment approaches generally include removal of lesions by surgical excision; lesion ablation by destructive modalities such as cryotherapy, electrocautery, or laser; or topical therapy with cytotoxic or immunomodulating agents. Because treatment may not eradicate HPV from surrounding tissues, recurrences of lesions are common. Additionally, the benefit of treatment in reducing infectivity and preventing transmission, one of the basic rationales of STD treatment in general, is unknown.[54]

GENITAL WARTS

The primary goal of the treatment of genital warts is amelioration of symptoms including those related to cosmetics (*Table 14.10*).[42,45,54] Although treatment can result in clearance of genital warts in most patients, approximately 30% may fail to clear with recommended first-line treatments, and recurrences after clearance are common, occurring in 20–50% of patients. Given the lack of evidence that treatment prevents future transmission, aggressive efforts to identify and treat small warts is of unclear clinical value. Likewise, there is no evidence that treatment of warts affects the subsequent development of cancer. Because no treatment is ideal, the choice of therapeutic regimen should be guided by patient preference, provider experience, and available resources. Indeed, given that the goal of therapy is relief of symptoms, that preventing transmission by treatment is uncertain, and that some warts will resolve spontaneously, an acceptable approach for some patients is to defer treatment and observe their warts. Although complications are rare if treatments are used properly, patients should be advised about the uncommon cosmetic sequelae of scarring or pigmentation changes.[54]

Currently available first-line treatment options for warts on the external genital skin include patient-applied topical therapies (podophyllotoxin 0.5% solution or gel and imiquimod 5% cream) and provider-administered therapies (cryotherapy, trichloroacetic and bichloracetic acid 80–90% solution, and office surgical techniques) (*Table 14.11*). The patient-applied therapies generally are more efficacious for warts on moist skin surfaces (labia minora, inner foreskin) than for warts on drier, more keratinized skin. Podophyllotoxin is an antimitotic agent which results in necrosis of proliferating wart tissue. It is available as either a 0.5% solution or gel in the US as well as a 0.15% cream in the UK; the more viscous gel and cream preparations facilitate application on sites not easily visualized, such as the perianal area. Imiquimod is a topically active immunomodulating agent which enhances in vivo production of interferon and other cytokines and appears to stimulate an immune-induced regression of genital warts. For both agents, the most common adverse events are self-limited erythema and burning and occasional transient problems in retracting the foreskin in uncircumcised men; neither is approved for use in pregnancy.[42,45,54]

Provider-administered treatments are appropriate for patients who are uncomfortable with self-applied therapy, who have genital warts at poorly accessible sites or those which have not responded to self-applied therapy, or who have only a few small lesions which may be treatable in a single session. Cryotherapy destroys warts by thermally induced cell necrosis. It is relatively simple and can be learned with less training than surgical techniques, although it requires basic equipment (either a cannister of liquid nitrogen or a closed cryoprobe system) and application techniques can be difficult to standardize, often necessitating repeat treatment sessions. Podophyllin resin contains several antimitotic agents including podophyllotoxin. Although inexpensive, various preparations of podophyllin resin vary in the concentrations of active components resulting in variable efficacy and toxicity, and thus its use has diminished over time. Like podofilox, podophyllin is not considered to be safe for use in pregnancy. Trichloroacetic and bichloracetic acid (TCA/BCA) induce tissue necrosis through protein coagulation; because of their low viscosity, run-off onto normal tissue can induce chemical burns. A variety of office surgical procedures have been used for genital wart treatment. Although they can sometimes accomplish wart removal in a single visit, all require substantial training, the use of local anesthesia, and specialized equipment. Additional provider-administered treatments include ablation by carbon dioxide laser or full surgical excision, which are most appropriate for treatment of extensive or refractory warts because of their expense. Intralesional injections of interferon have effectiveness similar to other modalities, but are not recommended for routine use because of the inconvenient route of administration, high cost, and frequent systemic side effects.[42,45,54]

Fewer options are available for the treatment of genital warts at internal sites and referral to a specialist is often required. Warts of the urethral meatus can be treated with cryotherapy, podophyllin, podofilox, or imiquimod, although lesions which extend proximally require urologic management. Treatment options for vaginal and anal warts include cryotherapy, TCA/BCA, laser ablation, and surgical excision. Oral warts can be treated with cryotherapy or surgical excision. Patients with cervical warts should undergo colposcopy and biopsy to rule out HSIL.[45,54]

Genital warts in pregnant women should be treated with TCA/BCA or surgical removal, both to ameliorate symptoms as well as to prevent their growth and occasional problems with obstruction of the birth canal. The value of treatment in preventing transmission to neonates is plausible but unproven. Likewise, the preventive value of cesarian delivery is unknown and thus this procedure is not recommended solely for the prevention of transmission.[54] Genital warts in children are problematic because of the potential for sexual abuse, and although non-sexual routes of transmission are possible, it is recommended that such children be referred for evaluation of sexual abuse.[54] HPV testing of genital warts in children is not recommended since this generally requires a biopsy procedure and since the finding of a genital type does not prove sexual transmission nor does the finding of a non-genital type rule out transmission due to manual-genital fondling.[76]

Because of the potentially chronic nature of genital HPV infection and the commonly associated psychological morbidity, education and counseling are important aspects of clinical management.[45,54,77] Although such counseling can be time-consuming, it may be assisted by the use of written informational materials and referral to a growing number of helpful websites (e.g. www.ashastd.org). Attempts should be made to cover the key messages outlined in *Table 14.12*.

SQUAMOUS INTRAEPITHELIAL LESIONS

Recommendations for management approaches for women with abnormal cervical cytology depend on the degree of the abnormality.[3,47,68] For Pap smears with ASCUS, recommended options include follow-up Pap smears (every 4–6 months for 2 years until there have been three consecutive negative smears), immediate colposcopy, or triage by HPV testing, with referral to colposcopy for those positive for high-risk types of HPV infection and a return to a routine Pap smear screening interval for those who are negative. For LSIL Pap smears, either follow-up cytology or colposcopy are recommended. Women with Pap smears with findings of HSIL should have immediate colposcopy. Similarly, treatment decisions depend on the results of colposcopy and histopathologic staging. Because the majority of CIN 1 lesions regress spontaneously, conservative management with close observational follow-up and treatment only for those which persist is considered a clinically appropriate option.

- Genital HPV is a viral STD which is highly prevalent in sexually active persons
- Because of the variable incubation period, it is often difficult to determine the source of infection, and current partners are likely already infected by the time of the diagnosis, although they may have no signs or symptoms
- Natural history is usually benign: although treatment may require several months and recurrences are common, complete clearance virtually always occurs
- The HPV types usually found in genital warts are not cancer-associated
- Infectivity to sexual partners likely decreases over time, but its duration is unknown
- There are limited data supporting the benefit of long-term condom use to prevent genital HPV infection; however, condoms should be used with future sex partners to prevent other STD
- Because genital HPV infection is so common among sexually active persons, and because the duration of infectivity is unknown, the value of disclosing a past diagnosis to future partners is unknown. Candid discussions about past STD should be encouraged and attempted whenever possible

Table 14.12 Counseling for patients with genital warts: key points (modified from 2001 CDC STD Treatment Guidelines).

Alternatively, to avoid the need for compliance with follow-up visits, some patients and providers prefer to treat CIN 1 lesions. Treatment is generally recommended for all CIN2/3 lesions. Treatment options include cryocautery, laser vaporization, and loop electrosurgical excision procedure (LEEP).[68] A recent randomized clinical trial comparing the three approaches found similar rates of post-treatment complications (2–8%) and treatment failure due to persistence (3–5%) and recurrence (13–19%); risk factors for persistence were large lesion size and predictors of recurrence were older age, presence of HPV16 or 18, and prior history of treatment.[72]

The treatment of bowenoid papulosis or other clinical forms of HPV-associated SIL at genital locations should be referred to dermatologists or gynecologists familiar with these entities.[45] Superficial destruction with cryotherapy or laser excision is frequently curative. Extensive surgical procedures are not recommended because of the high probability of spontaneous remission;[3] however, follow-up to assess lesion clearance, with biopsies of residual or recurrent areas, is important because of the occasionally progressive nature of genital SIL.

Education and counseling about HPV infection may be important for persons with SIL, especially if the association with HPV infection is raised due to HPV testing. Apart from the disease management issues noted above, the transmission issues relevant for patients with genital warts are relevant for patients with genital HPV-associated SIL as well.

PREVENTION

In contrast to bacterial STD, examination of sex partners is not considered necessary for the management of patients with genital warts or SIL because there are no data indicating that reinfection plays a role in recurrences. However, sex partners may benefit from an examination to assess the presence of genital warts and to undergo STD screening and Pap smears (for women) as well as to understand their own transmission potential with future sexual partners.[54]

There are currently few data on the benefit of condoms in preventing sexual transmission of HPV.[78] Theoretically, condoms are less likely to be effective in preventing epithelial infections such as genital HPV than they are for infections which are limited to specific mucosal areas or spread by semen and cervicovaginal secretions, such as gonorrhea or HIV. Studies evaluating the benefit of condoms for preventing HPV infection in women have generally found little evidence of protection;[11–13,79] however, there are limited data suggesting a benefit of condoms for men,[14,15] and some reports have suggested a benefit in prevention of HPV-related disease (e.g., genital warts, SIL, cervical cancer),[14,25,80–82] possibly by reducing viral inoculum, repeated viral exposure, or exposure to other co-factors which might be involved in development of disease. A better understanding of the benefit of condoms for prevention is an important research priority.

Ultimately, prophylactic vaccines are likely to have the greatest benefit in preventing genital HPV transmission and its sequelae.[83] Despite difficulties with in vitro cultivation of HPV and the absence of animal models for HPV infection and disease, several potential approaches are under investigation. The most promising use capsid protein-containing VLPs, which preserve the native conformation of viral proteins without the presence of viral DNA and which have successfully prevented species-specific papillomavirus infection in three different animal models. A number of human trials of monovalent and polyvalent vaccines containing one or more of HPV 6, 11, 16 and 18 are in progress. The most useful vaccines would have value in the therapy of early infections allowing them to be used in young adults who may already be infected, as well as having prophylactic benefit.[83–85]

References

1. Munoz N, Bosch F. The causal link between HPV and cervical cancer and its implications for prevention of cervical cancer. *Bulletin of PAHO* 1996; **30**:362–377.
2. Schiffman M, Bauer H, Hoover R *et al*. Epidemiologic evidence showing that human papillomavirus infection causes most cervical intraepithelial neoplasia. *J Natl Cancer Inst* 1993; **85**:958–964.
3. Kiviat N, Koutsky L, Paavonen J. Cervical neoplasia and other STD-related genital tract neoplasias. In: Holmes K, Mardh P, Sparling P, *et al.*, eds. *Sexually Transmitted Diseases*. New York: McGraw-Hill, 1999:811–832.
4. Cates W, American Social Health Association Panel. Estimates of the incidence and prevalence of sexually transmitted diseases in the United States. *Sex Transm Dis* 1999; **26**(suppl):S2–S7.
5. Koutsky L, Kiviat NB. Genital Human Papillomaviruses. In: Holmes K, Mardh P, Sparling P, *et al.*, eds. *Sexually Transmitted Diseases*. New York: McGraw-Hill, 1999:347–360.
6. Galloway DA. Biology of Human Papillomaviruses. In: Holmes K, Mardh P, Sparling P, *et al.*, eds. *Sexually Transmitted Diseases*. New York: McGraw-Hill, 1999: 335–346.
7. Phelps WC, Barnes JA, Lobe DC. Molecular targets for human papillomaviruses: prospects for antiviral therapy. *Antivir Chem Chemother* 1998; **9**:359–377.
8. Koutsky L. Epidemiology of genital human papillomavirus infection. *Am J Med* 1997; **102**(5A):3–8.
9. Svare EK, Kjaer SK, Nonnenmacher B, Worm AM *et al*. Seroactivity to human papillomavirus type 16 virus-like particles is lower in high-risk men than in high-risk women. *J Infect Dis* 1997; **176**:876–883.
10. Wideroff L, Schiffman M, Hoover R *et al*. Epidemiologic determinants of seroactivity to human papillomavirus (HPV) type 16 virus-like particles in cervical HPV-16 DNA-positive and -negative women. *J Infect Dis* 1996; **174**:937–943.
11. Ho G, Bierman R, Beardsley L, Chang C, Burk R. Natural history of cervicovaginal papillomavirus infection in young women. *N Engl J Med* 1998; **338**:423–428.
12. Burk RD, Kelly P, Feldman J *et al*. Declining prevalence of cervicovaginal human papillomavirus infection with age is independent of other risk factors. *Sex Transm Dis* 1996; **23**:333–341.
13. Burk RD, Ho GYF, Beardsley L *et al*. Sexual behavior and partner characteristics are the predominant risk factors for genital human papillomavirus infection in young women. *J Infect Dis* 1996; **174**:679–689.
14. Hippelainen M, Syrjanen S, Hippelainen M *et al*. Prevalence and risk factors of genital human papillomavirus (HPV) infections in healthy males: a study on Finnish conscripts. *Sex Transm Dis* 1993; **20**: 328.
15. Strickler H, Kirk G, Figueroa J *et al*. HPV 16 antibody prevalence in Jamaica and the United States reflects differences in cervical cancer rates. *Int J Cancer* 1999; **80**:339–344.
16. Koutsky L, Holmes K, Critchlow M *et al*. A cohort study of the risk of cervical intraepithelial neoplasia grade 2 or 3 in relation to papillomavirus infection. *N Engl J Med* 1992; **327**:1272–1278.
17. Ho G, Burk R, Klein S *et al*. Persistent genital human papillomavirus infection as a risk factor for persistent cervical dysplasia. *J Natl Cancer Inst* 1995; **87**:1365–1371.
18. Kashima HKS, Mounts P. Recurrent respiratory papillomatosis. In: Holmes K, Mardh P, Sparling P, eds. *Sexually Transmitted Diseases*. McGraw-Hill, 1999:1213–1218.
19. World Health Organization. IARC Monograph on the Evaluation of Carcinogenic Risks to Humans: Human Papillomaviruses. Vol. 64. Lyons: IARC, 1995.
20. National Institutes of Health. *Cervical Cancer*. NIH Consensus Statement 1996; **14**:1–38.
21. Bosch FX, Manos MM *et al*. Prevalence of human papillomavirus in cervical cancer: a worldwide perspective. *J Natl Cancer Inst* 1995; **87**:796–802.
22. Walboomers J, Jacobs M, Manos M *et al*. Human papillomavirus is a necessary cause of invasive cervical cancer worldwide. *J Pathol* 1999; **189**:12–19.
23. Herrero R, Hildesheim A, Bratti C *et al*. Population-based study of human papillomavirus infection and cervical neoplasia in rural Costa Rica. *J Natl Cancer Inst* 2000; **92**:464–474.
24. Anttila T, Saikku P, Koskela P *et al*. Serotypes of *Chlamydia trachomatis* and risk for development of cervical squamous cell carcinoma. *JAMA* 2001; **285**:47–51.
25. Hildesheim A, Herrero R, Castle PE *et al*. HPV co-factors related to the development of cervical cancer: results from a population-based study in Costa Rica. *Br J Cancer* 2001; **84**:1219–1226.
26. Frisch M, Glimelius B, van den Brule J *et al*. Sexually transmitted infection as a cause of anal cancer. *N Engl J Med* 1997; **337**:1350–1358.
27. Bjorge T, Dillner J, Anttila T *et al*. A prospective seroepidemiological study of the role of human papillomavirus in non-cervical anogenital cancers. *Br Med J* 1997; **15**:646–649.
28. Maden C, Sherman K, Beckmann A *et al*. History of circumcision, medical conditions, and sexual activity and risk of penile cancer. *J Natl Cancer Inst* 1993; **85**:19–24.
29. Pisani P, Parkin D, Munoz N, Ferlay J. Cancer and infection: estimates of the attributable fraction in 1990. *Cancer Epidemiol Biomarkers Prev* 1997; **6**:387–400.
30. Eddy D. Screening for cervical cancer. *Ann Intern Med* 1990; **113**:214–226.
31. Ries L, Kosery C, Hankey B *et al*. SEER Cancer Statistics Review 1973–1996 Vol. NIH Pub. No. 99–2789. Bethesda, MD: National Cancer Institute, 1999.
32. Daling J, Weiss N, Klopfenstein L *et al*. Correlates of homosexual behavior and the incidence of anal cancer. *JAMA* 1982; **247**:1988–1990.
33. Melbye M, Rabkin C, Frisch M, Biggar R. Changing patterns of anal cancer incidence in the United States, 1940–1989. *Am J Epidemiol* 1994; **139**:772–780.
34. Schiffman M. Recent progress in defining the epidemiology of human papillomavirus infection and cervical neoplasia. *J Natl Cancer Inst* 1992; **84**:394–398.
35. Franco EL, Villa LL, Sobrinho JP *et al*. Epidemiology of acquisition and clearance of cervical human papillomavirus infection in women from a high-risk area for cervical cancer. *J Infect Dis* 1999; **180**:1415–1423.
36. Nobbenhuis M, Walboomers J, Helmerhorst T *et al*. Relation of human papillomavirus status to cervical lesions and consequences for cervical-cancer screening: a prospective study. *Lancet* 1999; **354**:20–25.
37. Ylitalo N, Sorensen P, Josefsson AM *et al*. Consistent high viral load of human papillomavirus 16 and risk of cervical carcinoma in situ: a nested case-control study. *Lancet* 2000; **355**:2194–2198.
38. Hildesheim A, Schiffman M, Gravitt P *et al*. Persistence of type-specific human papillomavirus infection among cytologically normal women. *J Infect Dis* 1994; **169**:235–240.
39. Wheeler C, Greer C, Becker T *et al*. Short-term fluctuations in the detection of cervical human papillomavirus DNA. *Obstet Gynecol* 1996; **88**:261–268.
40. Lazcano-Ponce E, Herrero R, Munoz N *et al*. Epidemiology of HPV infection among Mexican women with normal cervical cytology. *Int J Cancer* 2001; **91**:412–420.
41. Palefsky J. Anal human papillomavirus infection and anal cancer in HIV-positive individuals: an emerging problem. *AIDS* 1994; **8**:283–295.
42. Beutner KR, Richwald GA, Wiley DJ, Reitano MV, AMA Expert Panel on External Genital Warts. External genital warts: report of the American Medical Association Consensus Conference. *Clin Infect Dis* 1998; **27**:796–806.
43. Ostor AG. Natural history of cervical intraepithelial neoplasia: a critical review. *Int J Gynecol Pathol* 1993; **12**: 86–192.
44. The 1988 Bethesda System for reporting cervical/vaginal cytologic diagnoses: National Cancer Institute Workshop. *JAMA* 1989; **262**:931–934.
45. von Krogh G, Lacey CJ, Gross G *et al*. European course on HPV associated pathology: guidelines for primary care physicians for the diagnosis and management of anogenital warts. *Sex Transm Infect* 2000; **76**:162–168.
46. Clarke P, Ebel C, Catotti DN, Stewart S. The psychosocial impact of human papillomavirus infection: implications for health care providers. *Int J STD AIDS* 1996; **7**:197–200.
47. Kurman R, Henson D, Herbst A *et al*. Interim guidelines for management of abnormal cervical cytology. *JAMA* 1994; **271**:1866–1869.

48. Schwartz RA, Janniger CK. Bowenoid papulosis. *J Am Acad Dermatol* 1991; **24**:261–264.

49. Daling J, Weiss N, Hislop T *et al*. Sexual practices, sexually transmitted diseases, and the incidence of anal cancer. *N Engl J Med* 1987; **317**:973–977.

50. Palefsky J, Holly E, Ralston M *et al*. High incidence of anal high-grade squamous intra-epithelial lesions among HIV-positive and HIV-negative homosexual and bisexual men. *AIDS* 1998; **12**:495–503.

51. Melbye M, Cote T, Kessler L *et al*. High incidence of anal cancer among AIDS patients. *Lancet* 1994; **343**:636–639.

52. Palefsky J, Holly E, Hogeboom C *et al*. Anal cytology as a screening tool for anal squamous intraepithelial lesions. *Lancet* 1997; **351**:1833–1839.

53. Goldie S, Kuntz K, Weinstein M *et al*. The clinical effectiveness and cost-effectiveness of screening for anal squamous intraepithelial lesions in homosexual and bisexual HIV-positive men. *JAMA* 1999; **281**:1822–1829.

54. Centers for Disease Control and Prevention. Sexually Transmitted Diseases Treatment Guidelines 2002. *MMWR* 2002; **51**:1–78.

55. Centers for Disease Control. 1999 USPHS/IDSA guidelines for the prevention of opportunistic infections in persons infected with human immunodeficiency virus. *MMWR* 1999; **48**:1–87.

56. Trofatter KF, Jr. Diagnosis of human papillomavirus genital tract infection. *Am J Med* 1997; **102**:21–27.

57. Jenkins D. Diagnosing human papillomaviruses: recent advances. *Curr Opin Infect Dis* 2001; **14**:53–62.

58. Lorincz AT. Hybrid Capture method for detection of human papillomavirus DNA in clinical specimens. *Papillomavirus Report* 1996; **7**:1–5.

59. Peyton C, Schiffman M, Lorincz A *et al*. Comparison of PCR- and hybrid capture-based human papillomavirus detection systems using multiple cervical specimen collection strategies. *J Clin Micro* 1998; **36**:3248–3254.

60. Kinney W, Manos M, Hurley L, Ransley J. Where's the high-grade cervical neoplasia? The importance of minimally abnormal Papanicolaou diagnoses. *Obstet Gynecol* 1998; **85**:202–210.

61. Manos M, Kinney W, Hurley L *et al*. Identifying women with cervical neoplasia: using human papillomavirus DNA testing for equivocal Papanicolaou results. *JAMA* 1999; **281**:1605–1610.

62. Solomon D, Schiffman M, Tarone R. Comparison of three management strategies for patients with atypical squamous cells of undetermined significance: baseline results from a randomized trial. *J Natl Cancer Inst* 2001; **93**:293–299.

63. The Atypical Squamous Cells of Undetermined Significance/Low-Grade Squamous Intraepithelial Lesions Triage Study (ALTS) Group. Human papillomavirus testing for triage of women with cytologic evidence of low-grade squamous intraepithelial lesions: baseline data from a randomized trial. *J Natl Cancer Inst* 2000; **92**:397–402.

64. Schneider A, Zahm D, Kirchmayr R, Schneider V. Screening for cervical intraepithelial neoplasia grade 2/3: validity of cytologic study, cervicography, and human papillomavirus detection. *Am J Obstet Gynecol* 1999; **174**:1534–1541.

65. Cuzick J, Terry G, Ho L *et al*. The value of HPV testing in primary screening of older women. *Br J Cancer* 1998; **81**:554–558.

66. Schiffman M, Herrero R, Hildesheim A *et al*. HPV DNA testing in cervical cancer screening: results from women in a high-risk province of Costa Rica. *JAMA* 2000; **283**:87–93.

67. Clavel C, Masure M, Bory JP *et al*. Hybrid Capture II-based human papillomavirus detection, a sensitive test to detect in routine high grade cervical lesions: a preliminary study on 1518 women. *Br J Cancer* 1999; **80**:1306–1311.

68. American College of Obstetrics and Gynecology. Cervical Cytology: Evaluation and management of abnormalities. *ACOG Technical Bulletin* 1993; **183**:1–8.

69. Cox J. Clinical role of HPV testing. *Obstet Gynecol Clin North Am* 1996; **23**:811–851.

70. Remmink A, Walboomers J, Helmerhorst TJ *et al*. The presence of persistent high-risk HPV genotypes in dysplastic cervical lesions is associated with progressive disease: natural history up to 36 months. *Int J Cancer* 1995; **61**:306–311.

71. Josefsson AM, Magnusson PK, Ylitalo N *et al*. Viral load of human papilloma virus 16 as a determinant for development of cervical carcinoma in situ: a nested case-control study. *Lancet* 2000; **355**:2189–2193.

72. Mitchell M, Tortolero-Luna G, Cook E *et al*. A randomized clinical trial of cryotherapy, laser vaporization, and loop electrosurgical excision for treatment of squamous intraepithelial lesions of the cervix. *Obstet Gynecol* 1998; **92**:737–744.

73. Cox J. Management of cervical intraepithelial neoplasia. *Lancet* 1999; **353**:857–859.

74. Elfgren K, Bistoletti P, Dillner L *et al*. Conization for cervical intraepithelial neoplasia is followed by disappearance of human papillomavirus deoxyribonucleic acid and a decline in serum and cervical mucus antibodies against human papillomavirus antigens. *Am J Obstet Gynecol* 1996; **174**:937–942.

75. Bollen L, Tjong-a-Hung S, van der Velden J *et al*. Prediction of recurrent and residual dysplasia by human papillomavirus detection among patients with abnormal cytology. *Gynecol Oncol* 1999; **72**:199–201.

76. Armstrong DK, Handley JM. Anogenital warts in prepubertal children: pathogenesis, HPV typing and management. *Int J STD AIDS* 1997; **8**:78–81.

77. Reitano M. Counseling patients with genital warts. *Am J Med* 1997; **102**(5A):38–43.

78. Division of STD Prevention. *Prevention of Genital HPV Infection and Sequelae: Report of an External Consultants' Meeting*. Department of Health and Human Services, Atlanta: Centers for Disease Control and Prevention, 1999:1–33.

79. Svare E, Kjaer S, Worm AM *et al*. Risk factors for HPV infection in women from sexually transmitted disease clinics: comparison between two areas with different cervical cancer incidence. *Cancer* 1998; **75**: 1–8.

80. Peters R, Thomas D, Hagan D, Mack T, Henderson B. Risk factors for invasive cervical cancer among Latinas and Non-Latinas in Los Angeles County. *J Natl Cancer Inst* 1986; **77**:1063–1077.

81. Slattery M, Overall Jr J, Abbott T *et al*. Sexual activity, contraception, genital infections, and cervical cancer: support for a sexually transmitted disease hypothesis. *Am J Epidemiol* 1989; **130**:248–258.

82. Wen LM, Estcourt CS, Simpson JM, Mindel A. Risk factors for the acquisition of genital warts: are condoms protective? *Sex Transm Infect* 1999; **75**:312–316.

83. World Health Organization. The current status of development of prophylactic vaccines against human papillomavirus infection. Report of a technical meeting, Geneva, 16–18 February, 1999:1–18.

84. Galloway D. Is vaccination against human papillomavirus a possibility? *Lancet* 1998; **351**(suppl III):22–24.

85. Hines J, Ghim S, Jenson A. Prospects for human papillomavirus vaccine development: emerging HPV vaccines. *Curr Opin Infect Dis* 1998; **11**:57–61.

Viral Hepatitis

W Bower and C Shapiro

15

INTRODUCTION

Five human hepatitis viruses — hepatitis viruses A through E — have been characterized to date. The corresponding clinical entities caused by each of these viruses are referred to as hepatitis A, B, C, delta, and E, respectively (*Table 15.1*). Hepatitis A virus (HAV) is transmitted predominantly by the fecal–oral route and can be transmitted between sexual partners. Hepatitis B virus (HBV), hepatitis C virus (HCV), and hepatitis D virus (HDV) are bloodborne viruses, and both parenteral and sexual transmission of these viruses occurs. Hepatitis E virus (HEV) is transmitted by the fecal–oral route; however, unlike HAV sexual transmission has not been documented. Other viruses have been recently described (e.g., 'hepatitis G virus', TTV, SEN-V), but their role in causing liver disease and their epidemiologic features need to be determined.

In the USA, an estimated 55% of acute viral hepatitis is due to hepatitis A; 32%, hepatitis B; 12% hepatitis C; and 1%, other possible viral agents (*Fig. 15.1*). United States population-based studies indicate that 40–60% of chronic liver disease is related to viral hepatitis, resulting in an estimated 10,000–15,000 deaths each year due to complications of chronic liver disease (CDC, unpublished data) (*Table 15.2*).

The clinical presentation of acute infection with each of these viruses is similar (*Table 15.3*), with jaundice (*Fig. 15.2*) and elevation of alanine aminotransferase (ALT) and other liver enzymes as manifestations of hepatitis. Diagnosis therefore depends on the use of specific tests for serologic markers (*Tables 15.4* and *15.5*). The epidemiology of these viruses is determined by a variety of factors, including their modes of transmission, which are in turn determined by the body fluids in which each virus is found in infected persons. With the availability of vaccines to prevent HAV, HBV, and (indirectly) HDV transmission, specific interventions exist to protect persons who are at risk of acquiring these viruses through sexual activity.

	Hepatitis A	Hepatitis B	Hepatitis C	Delta hepatitis	Hepatitis E
Incubation period	15–50 days (mean 28)	60–180 days (mean 120)	15–180 days (mean 42)	15–60 days	15–60 days (mean 42)
Transmission	Fecal–oral	Bloodborne Sexual	Bloodborne Sexual	Bloodborne Sexual	Fecal-oral
Progression to chronicity	No	Occasionally Varies by age	Usually	Coinfection – Occasionally Super infection – Usually	No
Etiologic agent	Hepatitis A virus (HAV): a nonenveloped single-stranded RNA virus (picornavirus)	Hepatitis B virus (HBV): an enveloped double-stranded DNA virus (hepadnavirus)	Hepatitis C virus (HCV): an enveloped single-stranded RNA virus (flavivirus)	Hepatitis D virus (HDV): a single-stranded RNA virus (deltavirus)	Hepatitis E virus (HEV): a nonenveloped single-stranded (currently unclassified)
Comments	Vaccine available	Vaccine available		Occurs only as coinfection with HBV or as superinfection of chronic hepatitic B	Rarely occurs in the United States

Table 15.1 Basic features of viral hepatitis.

	HAV	HBV	HCV
Acute infections (× 1000)/year*	181–373	79–232	36–179
Fulminant deaths/year	100	150	?
Chronic infections	No chronic infection	1.25 million	2.7 million
Chronic liver disease deaths/year	No chronic infection	5,000	8–10,000

*Range based on estimated annual incidence, 1990–1999; 1990–1997 for HCV.

Table 15.2 1990–1999 estimates of acute and chronic disease burden for hepatitis types A, B, and C, USA. Courtesy of Centers for Disease Control and Prevention.

Symptoms of acute viral hepatitis
• Malaise
• Anorexia
• Nausea
• Abdominal pain
• Jaundice
• Dark urine
• Fever, rash, arthralgias
• Pruritus

Table 15.3 Symptoms of acute viral hepatitis. The clinical symptoms of acute viral hepatitis caused by the various hepatitis viruses are similar. Serologic tests are necessary to establish a diagnosis.

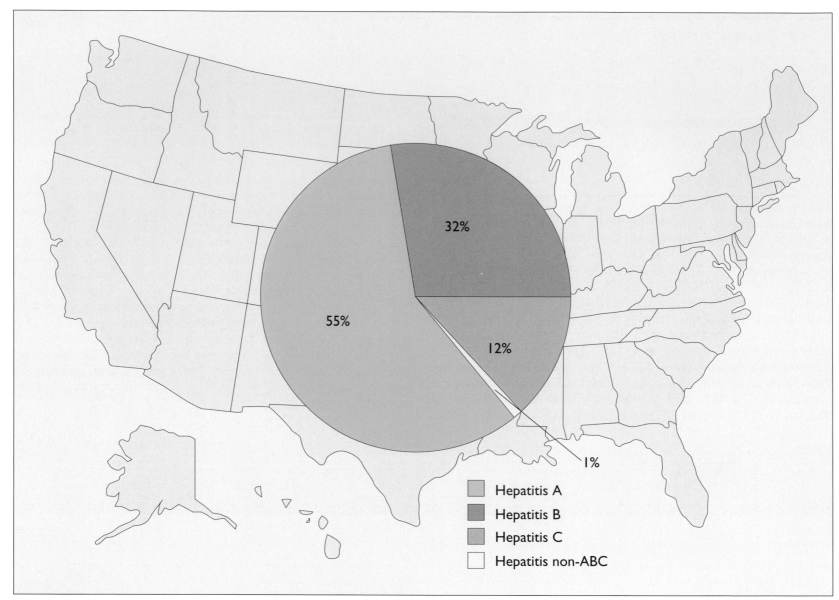

Fig. 15.1 Relative proportions of acute viral hepatitis by type, in the USA, 1991–1998. Courtesy of Sentinel Counties Study, Centers for Disease Control and Prevention.

32%

55%

12%

1%

Hepatitis A

Hepatitis B

Hepatitis C

Hepatitis non-ABC

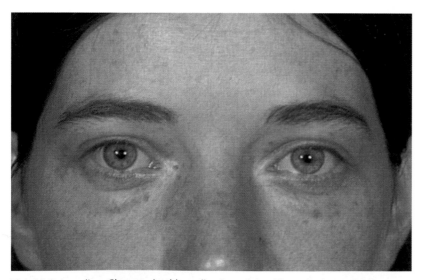

Fig. 15.2 Jaundice. Characterized by yellowing of the skin and sclerae. Other findings in patients with hepatitis may include abdominal pain under the right costal margin, hepatomegaly, dark urine, and pale stools.

Among adolescents and adults, sexual transmission of HAV, HBV, HCV, and HDV is an important route of transmission. Therefore, this chapter will focus on these hepatitis viruses.

HEPATITIS A

EPIDEMIOLOGY

Hepatitis A is caused by infection with HAV, a nonenveloped single-stranded RNA virus, which is classified as a picornavirus. HAV replicates in the liver, is shed in the feces, and peak titers occur during the 2 weeks before and 1 week after the onset of illness.[1] Virus is also present in serum and saliva during this period, though in concentrations several orders of magnitude less than in feces. Thus, the most common mode of HAV transmission is fecal–oral, with the virus being transmitted from person-to-person between household contacts or sex partners, or via contaminated food or water (*Table 15.6*). The transmission between sex partners occurs through oral–anal contact, and can occur both between heterosexuals and same-sex contacts. Since viremia occurs in acute infection,[2] bloodborne HAV transmission can occur, but it has been infrequently reported. Although HAV is present in low concentrations in the saliva of infected persons, it has not been shown that saliva plays a role in transmission.

Hepatitis A	
HAV	Hepatitis A virus, etiologic agent of hepatitis A, also known as infectious hepatitis; a picornavirus with a single serotype.
anti-HAV	Total antibody to HAV; detectable at onset of symptoms; lifetime persistence.
IgM anti-HAV	IgM-class antibody indicating recent infection with HAV.
Hepatitis B	
HBV	Hepatitis B virus; etiologic agent of hepatitis B, also known as serum hepatitis; agent also known as Dane particle.
HBsAg	Hepatitis B surface antigen; produced in large quantities in serum both as whole virus and as smaller surface antigen particles; originally known as Australian antigen; several serotypes. Indicates present infection with HBV.
HBeAg	Hepatitis B e antigen; soluble antigen that correlates with HBV replication and infectivity; conformational antigen of HBcAg.
HBcAg	Hepatitis B core antigen; found within the core of the virus; no commercial test available.
anti-HBs	Antibody to hepatitis B surface antigen; indicates immune response to HBV infection, due either to passive acquisition, immune response to infection, or vaccination.
anti-HBc	Antibody to hepatitis B core antigen; indicates past or present infection with HBV; not present in vaccine-induced immunity.
IgM anti-HBc	IgM-class antibody to HBcAg; indicates recent infection with HBV.
Delta hepatitis	
HDV	Delta virus; etiologic agent of delta hepatitis; only causes infection in the presence of HBV.
HDAg	Delta antigen; detectable in early acute infection. No commercial test available in US
anti-HDV	Total antibody to delta antigen; indicates past or present infection.
IgM anti-HDV	IgM-class antibody to HDV; indicates recent infection with HDV. No commercial test available in US
Hepatitis C	
HCV	Hepatitis C virus; etiologic agent of most parenterally transmitted non-A, non-B hepatitis; single stranded RNA virus classified in the family Flaviviridae.
anti-HCV	Antibody to hepatitis C virus; does not distinguish between acute and chronic infection. Detectable in 90 percent of patients with hepatitis C; interval between onset of disease and seroconversion may be prolonged.
RIBA	Recombinant immunoblot assay; supplemental confirmatory test for anti-HCV screening assay.
HCV RT-PCR	Reverse transcription polymerase chain reaction for hepatitic C virus; defects virus in blood and indicates present infection with HCV
Hepatitis E	
HEV	Hepatitis E virus; etiologic agent of hepatitis E; single stranded RNA virus that is currently unclassified because it has molecular similarities to both calicivirus and alphavirus
anti-HEV	Total antibody to HEV; detectable during convalesence from the disease; indicates past or present infection with HEV
IgM anti-HEV	IgM-class antibody to HEV; indicates recent infection with HEV

Source: Adapted from Centers for Disease Control and Prevention. Hepatitis B virus infection. A comprehensive strategy for eliminating transmission in the United States through immunization. MMWR, in press

Table 15.4 Markers of viral hepatitis infection.

HAV infection is distributed globally, and geographic areas can be characterized with respect to the prevalence of antibodies to HAV (anti-HAV), indicating prior HAV infection in the general population (*Fig. 15.3*). Disease patterns differ in areas of differing endemicity, and correlate with the hygienic and sanitary conditions of a given geographic region. In countries with very poor sanitary and hygienic conditions, most persons are infected as young children, at an age when HAV infection is often asymptomatic; reported disease rates in these areas are low and outbreaks are rare. In countries with variable sanitary conditions, transmission can predominate in children, adolescents, or adults, depending on the geographic region. Paradoxically, because transmission in these areas often occurs in age groups when infection is symptomatic, but conditions which promote transmission are common, disease rates can be higher than in countries with very poor sanitary conditions. Community-wide epidemics contribute significantly to the burden of disease in regions with variable sanitation. In countries with very good sanitation and hygienic conditions, infection rates in children are generally low. In these countries, disease tends to occur in circumscribed groups, such as travellers to hepatitis A endemic areas, or as outbreaks among specific risk groups, such as intravenous drug users (IDU) or men who have sex with men (MSM).[3]

In the USA, hepatitis A has occurred in large nationwide epidemics approximately every 10 years, with the last increase in cases in 1996

(*Fig. 15.4*). The highest disease rates are in young adults aged 25–39 years old (*Fig. 15.5*). Many children have unrecognized, asymptomatic infection and can be the source of infection for others. In 1999, an estimated 180,000 persons in the USA were infected with HAV. Among cases reported to the CDC, the most frequently reported risk factor was household or sexual contact with a person with hepatitis, followed by MSM, recent international travel, and IDU; however, recently MSM has replaced contact with a known HAV case as the most frequently reported risk factor (*Fig. 15.6*). Many persons with hepatitis A do not identify risk factors; their source of infection may be other infected persons who are asymptomatic. Based on testing from the Third National Health and Nutrition Examination Survey (NHANES III) survey, conducted in 1988–1994, the prevalence of total anti-HAV is 33% among the general population in the USA (CDC, unpublished data, 1998).

Although, in the USA, the percentage of males with hepatitis A who report a history of MSM is approximately 10%, over the past three decades hepatitis A outbreaks among MSM have been reported in urban areas, in the USA, Canada, Europe and Australia.[4–10] Seroprevalence and case-control studies have suggested that the number of years of homosexual activity and number of sex partners, history of a sexually transmitted infection, as well as specific sexual practices, such as oral–anal or digital–anal sex, are associated with infection (*Table 15.7*).[10–15]

Virus	Diagnostic Test Result			Interpretation
HAV				
Anti-HAV	IgM anti-HAV			
+/–	+			Recent HAV infection
+	–			Old HAV infection
HBV				
HBsAg	Anti-HBs	IgM anti HBc	Anti-HBc	
+/–	–	+	+/–	Recent HBV infection
–	+	–	+	Old resolved HBV infection. Immune to HBV infection
+	–	–	+	Chronic HBV infection[1]
–	+	–	–	Immune for vaccination or passive transfer
–	–	–	+	Four possible interpretations[2]
HCV				
Anti-HCV	RIBA	HCV RT-PCR		
–	–	+		Possible acute HCV infection
+	+	+		Chronic HCV infection
+	+	–		Resolved HCV infection[3]
+	–	–		False positive anti-HCV
Delta hepatitis				
HBsAg	IgM anti-HBc	Anti-HBc	Anti-HDV	
+/–	+	+/–	+	HBV-HDV coinfection
+	–	+	+	HBV-HDV superinfection
HEV				
Anti-HEV	IgM anti-HEV			
+/–	+			Recent HEV infection
+	–			Old HEV infection

[1] < 1% of persons with chronic HBV infection can have HBsAg and anti-HBs present simultaneously.
[2] May be recovering from acute HBV infection; may be distantly immune and test not sensitive enough to detect very low level of anti-HBs in serum; may be susceptible with a false positive anti-HBc; may have undetectable level of HBsAg present in the serum and the person is actually a carrier.
[3] Some chronically HCV-infected persons might be only intermittently HCV RNA-positive, particularly those with acute hepatitis C.

Table 15.5 Diagnostic patterns and interpretation of test results.

CLOSE PERSONAL CONTACT
  Household contact
  Sexual contact
  Day care centers

CONTAMINATED FOOD/WATER
  Infected foodhandlers
  Shellfish

BLOOD EXPOSURES (RARE)
  Injecting drug users
  Blood transfusion

Table 15.6 Modes of transmission of hepatitis A virus (HAV).

CROSS-SECTIONAL STUDIES		ANTI-HAV
LOCATION	GROUP	PREVALENCE
Amsterdam,	Homosexual men	30%
Netherlands	Heterosexual men	12%
(Couthino et al.)		
Seattle,	Homosexual men	42%
Washington	Heterosexual men	16%
(Corey et al.)		
Nova Scotia,	Homosexual men	42%
Canada	Heterosexual men	39%
(McFarlane et al.)		

PROSPECTIVE STUDIES		LENGTH OF	ANTI-HAV
LOCATION	GROUP	FOLLOW-UP	SEROCONVERSION (%)
Amsterdam,	Homosexual men	1.9 years	14%*
Netherlands	Heterosexual men	0.5 years	0%
(Couthino et al.)			
Seattle,	Homosexual men	1 year	22%
Washington	Heterosexual men	1 year	0%
(Corey et al.)			

*Attack rate calculated by the product limit method.

Table 15.7 Cross-sectional and prospective studies evaluating the risk of hepatitis A among MSM.

CLINICAL MANIFESTATIONS

The incubation period of hepatitis A is 15–50 days, with an average of 28 days. The illness caused by HAV infection typically has an abrupt onset of signs and symptoms that include fever, malaise, anorexia, nausea, abdominal discomfort, dark urine and jaundice (*Table 15.3*). Hepatitis A usually does not last longer than 2 months, though some individuals may have prolonged or relapsing signs and symptoms for up to 6 months. The likelihood of having symptoms with HAV infection is directly related to age. In children younger than 6 years of age, most infections are asymptomatic; among older children and adults, infection is usually symptomatic (*Table 15.8*).[16]

HAV infection causes acute inflammation of the liver with varying degrees of necrosis (*Fig. 15.7*). HAV infection does not result in chronic infection or chronic liver disease. However, HAV infection occasionally results in acute liver failure associated with massive hepatonecrosis. The case-fatality rate among reported cases of all ages is approximately 0.3%, but can be higher among older persons (approximately 2% among patients of more than 40 years of age).

DIAGNOSIS

Virtually all patients with acute hepatitis A have detectable IgM antibodies to hepatitis A virus (IgM anti-HAV). The diagnosis of acute HAV infection is therefore confirmed during the acute or early convalescent phase of infection by the presence of IgM anti-HAV (*Fig. 15.8*). In most persons, IgM anti-HAV becomes detectable 5–10 days before the onset of symptoms and can persist for 6 months or more after infection.[2,7,17] IgG anti-HAV, which appears in the convalescent phase of infection, remains detectable in serum for the lifetime of the individual and confers enduring protection against disease.[18] Commercial diagnostic tests are available for the detection of IgM and total anti-HAV in serum.

TREATMENT

As HAV infection is self-limited and does not result in chronic infection or chronic liver disease, treatment is generally supportive. Hospitalization may be necessary for patients who are dehydrated from nausea and vomiting, or who have fulminant hepatitis A. Medications that might cause liver damage, or that are metabolized by the liver, should be used with caution. No specific restrictions on diet or activity are necessary. In patients with acute liver failure due to hepatitis A, liver transplantation has been successful in some patients.[19]

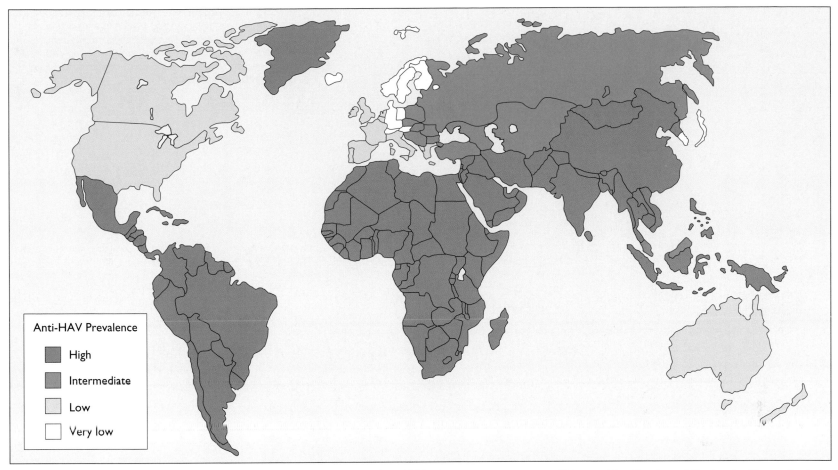

Fig. 15.3 Global prevalence of antibody to HAV. This map generalizes currently available data; patterns may vary within countries. Courtesy of Centers for Disease Control and Prevention.

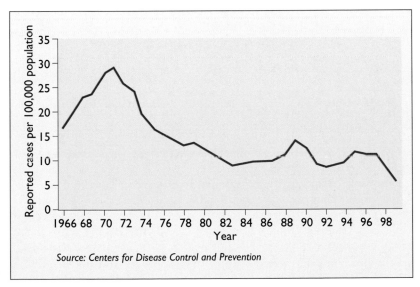

Source: Centers for Disease Control and Prevention

Fig. 15.4 Reported hepatitis A cases (per 100,000 population) USA, 1966–1999. Courtesy of National Notifiable Disease Surveillance System, Centers for Disease Control and Prevention and Viral Hepatitis Surveillance Program, Centers for Disease Control and Prevention.

Less than 3 years of age	< 5%
4 to 6 years of age	5%–10%
6 years of age and above	75%

Table 15.8 Frequency of symptoms with acute hepatitis A by age.

Good hygiene and sanitation
Immune globulin for postexposure prophylaxis
Hepatitis A vaccine for pre-exposure protection

*Adapted from Centers for Disease Control and Prevention: Prevention of hepatitis A through active or passive immunization: recommendations of the Advisory Committee on Immunization Practices (ACIP). MMWR 1999; **48**(No. RR-12): 1–37.*

Table 15.9 Measures for the prevention of hepatitis A.

PREVENTION

General measures for the prevention of hepatitis A include the maintenance of good personal hygiene, with attention to handwashing before preparing food; provision of safe drinking water; and adequate disposal of sanitary waste (*Table 15.9*). To help control and prevent hepatitis A in communities experiencing hepatitis A outbreaks among homosexual and bisexual men, health education messages should stress the modes of HAV transmission and the measures which can be taken to reduce the risk of transmission of any STD, including enterically transmitted agents such as HAV.

Two types of products are available for the prevention of hepatitis A, immune globulin (IG) and hepatitis A vaccine. IG is a sterile preparation of concentrated antibodies prepared from pooled human plasma processed by cold ethanol fractionation.[20] In the United States, only plasma that has tested negative for hepatitis B surface antigen (HBsAg), antibody to human immunodeficiency virus (HIV), and antibody to HCV is used to produce IG. In addition, the process used to produce IG includes a viral inactivation step or the final product is tested for HCV RNA by the

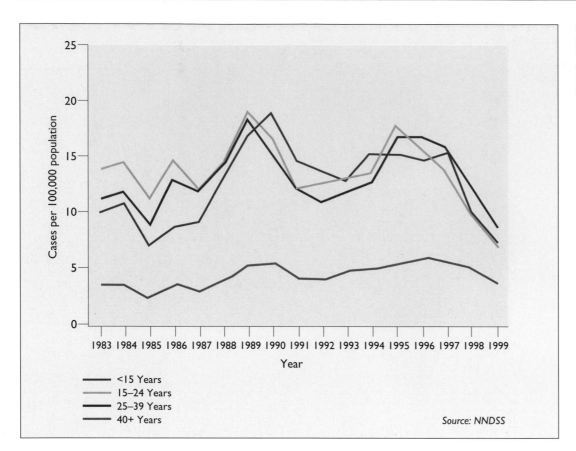

Fig. 15.5 Reported hepatitis A cases (per 100,000 population) by age, USA, 1983–1999. Courtesy of National Notifiable Disease Surveillance System, Centers for Disease Control and Prevention and Viral Hepatitis Surveillance Program, Centers for Disease Control and Prevention.

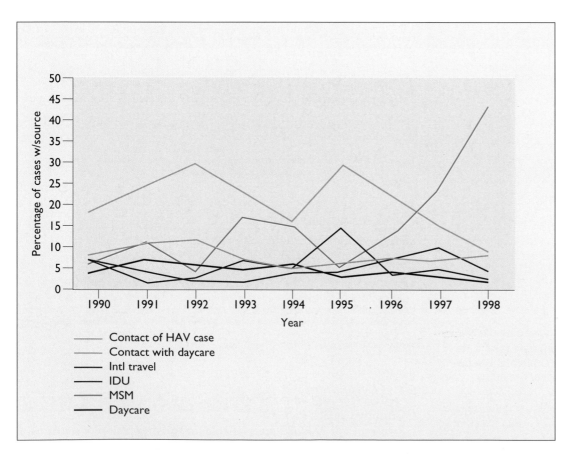

Fig. 15.6 Risk factors reported for hepatitis A by mutually exclusive groups, USA, 1990–1999. (Source: Centers for Disease Control and Prevention.) Courtesy of Sentinel Counties Study, Centers for Disease Control and Prevention.

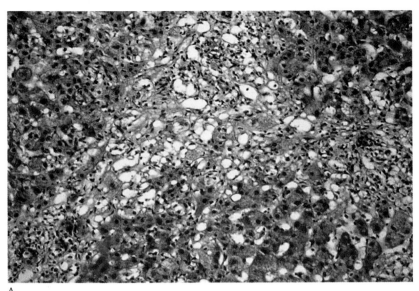
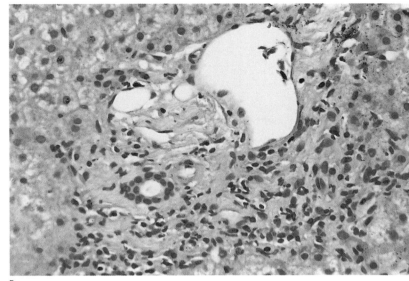

A   B

Fig. 15.7 (A) Acute hepatitis A. There is spotty parenchymal necrosis with a predominance of periportal injury. **(B)** Normal hepatic portal triad. H and E stain. Courtesy of the Armed Forces Institute of Pathology.

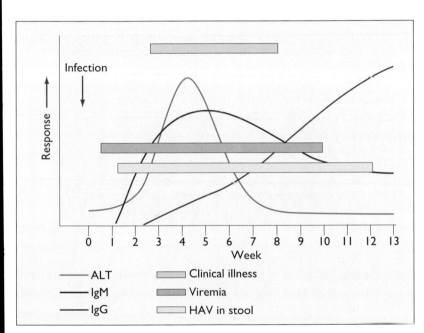

Fig. 15.8 Typical serologic profile of acute hepatitis A infection.

POSTEXPOSURE
- Household and sexual contacts of hepatitis A cases
- Staff and children at a day care center where a child or employee is recognized to have acute hepatitis A
- Patrons of food establishments with an infected foodhandler with poor hygiene who handled uncooked foods or foods after cooking
- Selected settings where HAV transmission is occurring (hospitals, institutions)

PRE-EXPOSURE
- Travelers who elect not to receive hepatitis A vaccine

Adapted from Centers for Disease Control and Prevention: Prevention of hepatitis A through active or passive immunization: recommendations of the Advisory Committee on Immunization Practices (ACIP). MMWR 1999; 48(No. RR-12): 1–37.

Table 15.10 Indications for immune globulin administration for prophylaxis of hepatitis A.

SETTING	DURATION OF COVERAGE	IMMUNE GLOBULIN DOSE*
Pre-exposure	Short term (1–3 months)	0.02 ml/kg
	Long-term (3–5 months)	0.06 ml/kg Repeat every 5 months if continued exposure
Postexposure		0.02 ml/kg

*IG is to be given by intramuscular injection in the deltoid muscle or the buttocks. For children < 24 months of age, it can be given in the anterolateral thigh muscle.
†Infants and pregnant women should receive a preparation that does not include thimerosal.
Adapted from Centers for Disease Control and Prevention: Prevention of hepatitis A through active or passive immunization: Recommendations of the Advisory Committee on Immunization Practices (ACIP). MMWR 1999; 48(No. RR-12): 1–37.

Table 15.11 Recommended doses of immune globulin for hepatitis A pre-exposure and postexposure prophylaxis†.

polymerase chain reaction. No transmission of HBV, HIV, HCV, or other viruses has been reported from IG for intramuscular administration (IMIG).[21,22]

When administered prior to exposure to HAV, or within 2 weeks after exposure, IMIG is more than 85% effective in preventing hepatitis A.[23–25] Efficacy is greatest when IMIG is administered early in the incubation period; when administered later in the incubation period, IMIG often only attenuates the clinical expression of HAV infection.[25] IMIG administration is recommended for a variety of exposure situations, including persons who are sexual or household contacts of persons with hepatitis A (*Table 15.10*). IMIG may also be used for pre-exposure prophylaxis, e.g. individuals traveling to countries with endemic hepatitis A. The duration of protection is dependent on dose (*Table 15.11*).

Inactivated hepatitis A vaccines provide long-term protection against hepatitis A. These vaccines have been shown to be safe, highly immunogenic and highly efficacious. Immunogenicity studies indicate that between 97–100% of persons aged 2–18 years and 94–100% of adults

Vaccine	Age (yrs)	Dose	Volume (mL)	Dose schedule (months)†
Havrix®	2–18	720 EL.U.	0.5	0,6–12
	> 18	1,440 EL.U.	1.0	0,6–12
Vaqta®	2–18	25 U	0.5	0,6–18
	> 18	50 U	1.0	0,6–12
Twinrix®‡	> 18	720 EL.U (HAV)	1.0	0,1,6
		20 mcg (HBsAG)		

†0 months represents timing of the initial dose; subsequent numbers represent months after the initial dose.

‡Twinrix is a bivalent vaccine containing inactivated hepatitis A virus and recombinant surface antigen of the hepatitis B virus.

Adapted from Centers for Disease Control and Prevention: Prevention of hepatitis A through active or passive immunization: Recommendations of the Advisory Committee on Immunization Practices (ACIP). MMWR 1999; **48**(No. RR-12): 1–37.

Table 15.12 Recommended doses of inactivated hepatitis A vaccine. (Use of trade names is for identification purposes only and does not imply endorsement by the US Public Health Service).

Persons traveling or working in countries with high or intermediate endemicity of infection

Children living in states or communities with high rates of HAV infection and periodic hepatitis A outbreaks

Men who have sex with men

Drug users

Persons who work with experimentally HAV-infected non-human primates or with HAV in a laboratory setting

Persons with chronic liver disease

Adapted from Centers for Disease Control and Prevention: Prevention of hepatitis A through active or passive immunization: Recommendations of the Advisory Committee on Immunization Practices (ACIP). MMWR 1999; **48**(No. RR-12): 1–37.

Table 15.13 Groups recommended for hepatitis A vaccination.

HIGH	MODERATE	LOW/NONE
Blood	Semen	Urine
Serum	Vaginal fluid	Feces
Wound exudates	Saliva	Sweat
		Tears
		Breast milk

Table 15.14 Relative concentration of hepatitis B virus (HBV) in various body fluids.

develop protective antibodies 1 month after the first dose, and all persons develop protective antibodies after the second dose.[26–30] Long-term protective efficacy studies indicate that > 99% of persons had protective antibody levels 5–6 years after receiving vaccine.[31,32] Efficacy studies show that inactivated hepatitis A vaccines are 94–100% effective in preventing hepatitis A.[33,34] Table 15.12 lists the recommended doses and schedule for inactivated hepatitis A vaccines licensed in the USA.[35] Recently, a bivalent vaccine (combination inactivated HAV and recombinant HBsAg vaccine) has been licensed for use in adults that offers the advantage of providing protection for groups at risk for both HAV and HBV infection, such as IDU and MSM.[36] Prevaccination screening may be advisable, depending on the anti-HAV seroprevalence among potential vaccine recipients and the costs for screening and vaccination.

Recommendations for use of hepatitis A vaccine were first issued by the Advisory Committee on Immunization Practices (ACIP) of the US Public Health Service, the American Academy of Pediatrics (AAP), and other groups in 1996, and updated in 1999 (Table 15.13).[35,37] To achieve a sustained reduction in the national incidence of hepatitis A, widespread routine vaccination is needed. Therefore, these recommendations call for routine vaccination of children, beginning at or after two years of age, living in states or communities where rates of hepatitis A have been consistently elevated. Vaccination of successive cohorts of young children should significantly lower the incidence of hepatitis A in the United States over time and eventually provide the opportunity to eliminate HAV transmission. To achieve this goal, children throughout the United States will need to be vaccinated.

The targeted use of hepatitis A vaccine in specific groups experiencing hepatitis A outbreaks (e.g., MSM) should help protect such individuals. However, vaccinating adults in high-risk groups for vaccine-preventable diseases has proven difficult.[5] Vaccination programs targeted to persons in age groups other than infants historically have been difficult to implement because many adolescents and adults do not visit health-care providers for preventive health care, or they may not perceive themselves to be at high risk. In addition, health-care providers often do not ask about risk behaviors during health-care visits, resulting in missed opportunities for vaccination. Hepatitis A vaccine should be offered at multiple sites that provide health care to MSM, including primary-care clinics, specialty clinics, sexually transmitted diseases clinics, and human immunodeficiency virus testing and counseling sites. In addition, innovative approaches to reach high-risk adult populations, such as vaccination using mobile health vans or at bars, may be effective.

HEPATITIS B

EPIDEMIOLOGY

HBV is a DNA virus, with an outer envelope consisting of HBsAg and an inner core consisting of HBcAg, double-stranded DNA, and DNA polymerase. HBV is present in high titers in blood and exudates (e.g. skin lesions) of acutely and chronically infected persons. Moderate viral titers are found in semen, vaginal secretions and saliva. Other body fluids that do not contain blood or serous fluid, such as feces or urine, are not a source of HBV (Table 15.14). Thus, the three principal modes of HBV transmission are:[38]

- Percutaneous (injecting drug use, blood or body fluid exposures among health-care workers, and blood transfusions)
- Sexual (heterosexual or male homosexual)
- Perinatal (from infected mothers to infants through blood exposure at the time of birth).

Transmission between siblings and other household contacts readily occurs, through contact with skin lesions such as eczema or impetigo; sharing of potentially blood-contaminated objects such as toothbrushes and razor blades; and occasionally through bites.[39] Nosocomial outbreaks, although rare, have occurred because of the improper use or disinfection of medical devices (e.g. fingerstick devices, acupuncture needles), or from infected health-care workers to patients during invasive procedures. HBV infection occurs worldwide. Approximately 45% of the world's population live in geographic areas with high HBV endemicity (≥8% of the general population are chronically infected); 43% in areas of moderate endemicity (2–7% are chronically infected); and 12% in areas of low endemicity (<2% are chronically infected) (Fig. 15.9). Overall, an estimated 300 million persons worldwide are HBV carriers. Based on the NHANES III survey, the overall prevalence of chronic HBV infection among the general US population is 0.3%, with 0.1% among Whites and 1.1% among Blacks. Other seroprevalence studies conducted over

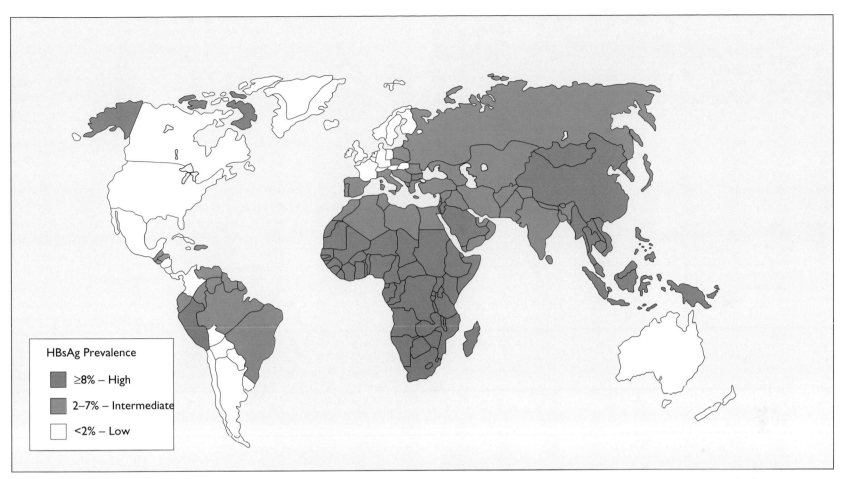

Fig. 15.9 Global prevalence of chronic HBV infection (determined by the percentage of the population positive for hepatitis B surface antigen or HBsAg). This map generalizes currently available data; patterns may vary within countries. Courtesy of Centers for Disease Control and Prevention.

the past several decades have identified a variety of groups at increased risk of HBV infection (*Table 15.15*).[40]

The risk of sexual transmission among MSM and between heterosexual partners is well documented.[41] Historically, HBV infection has been endemic among MSM. Studies among patients attending STD clinics have shown the prevalence of HBV infection among MSM to be several times higher compared with heterosexual patients (*Table 15.16*).[42–49] From these studies, factors associated with a higher prevalence of HBV infection include a history of multiple episodes of STDs; large numbers of sexual partners; long duration of homosexual activity; and receptive anal intercourse. The presumed mechanisms of transmission include transfer of HBV in semen or in exudates from genital lesions to open mucous membrane and skin lesions from infections or trauma.

Heterosexual partners of persons with acute or chronic HBV infection are also at substantial risk of HBV infection. In several studies, susceptible heterosexual partners of persons with acute hepatitis B followed for 3–12 months had a risk of infection of 20–27% (*Table 15.17*).[50–52] The prevalence of serologic markers indicating past or present HBV infection (HBsAg or antibody to HBsAg [anti-HBs]) among household (including sexual) contacts of persons with chronic HBV infection was two to 10 times higher compared with household contacts of noninfected persons. Spouses had higher rates than other household members (*Table 15.18*).[44,53,54]

As with MSM, a history of multiple episodes of STDs, duration of sexual activity, and large numbers of sexual partners, are associated with an increased risk of HBV infection among heterosexual men and women (*Table 15.19*).[42,44,47,55,56] For example, in a US study of an STD clinic's patients and a university student population, after controlling for age, gender and race, the number of lifetime sexual partners in both populations was directly associated with the prevalence of HBV infection

POPULATION GROUP	PREVALENCE OF SEROLOGIC MARKERS OF HBV INFECTION	
	HBsAg (%)	ANY MARKER (%)
Immigrants/refugees from areas of high HBV endemicity	13	70–85
Alaska Natives/Pacific Islanders	5–15	40–70
Clients in institutions for the developmentally disabled	10–20	35–80
Users of illicit injection drugs	7	60–80
Sexually active homosexual men	6	35–80
Household contacts of HBV carriers	3–6	30–60
Hemodialysis patients	3–10	20–80
Health care workers — frequent blood contact	1–2	15–30
Prisoners (male)	1–8	10–80
Staff of institutions for the developmentally disabled	1	10–25
Heterosexuals with multiple partners	0.5	5–20
Health care workers — no or infrequent blood contact	0.3	3–10
Blood donors (per donation)	0.3	2
General population (NHANES III)*		
Blacks	1.1	11.6
Whites	0.1	3.2

*Adapted from McQuillan et al: *NHANES: Viral hepatitis. In: Everhart JE (ed): Digestive diseases in the United States: Epidemiology and impact. NIH Publication 94–1447, 1994.*

Table 15.15 Prevalence of HBV serologic markers in various population groups.

Group	HBsAg (%)	Any marker (%)	Year	Reference Number
MSM	3.2	21.7	1973	42
Heterosexual men	2.6	5.1		
MSM	3.9	ND*	1974	43
Heterosexual men	0.2	ND		
MSM	4.3	48.1	1975	44
Heterosexual men	1.3	17.9		
MSM	5.6	39.6	1977	45
Heterosexual men	0.9	4.5		
MSM	0.9	18	1994	46
Heterosexual men	0.0	5		
MSM	4.2	38.7	1998	47
Heterosexual men	0.6	5.9		
Heterosexual women	0.4	3.5		
MSM	ND	2–17	1994–1998	48
MSM	ND	37	1998	49
Heterosexual men	ND	14		

*ND = Not done or reported.

Table 15.16 Prevalence of HBV infection among groups with different sexual behaviors.

TYPE OF CONTACT	OBSERVATION PERIOD	NO. INFECTED/ NO. FOLLOWED (%)	REFERENCE NUMBER
Heterosexual partners	5 months	9/33 (27.3)	50
Heterosexual partners	12 months	3/13 (23.1)	51
Other household contacts		0/68 (0.0)	
Heterosexual partners	3–12 months	2/10 (20.0)	52
Household children		4/41 (9.8)	
Adults		3/60 (5.0)	

Table 15.17 Incidence of HBV infection in contacts of persons with acute hepatitis B.

STUDY	NUMBER OF SUBJECTS	POSITIVE (%) HBsAg+	POSITIVE (%) ANTI-HBs+	REFERENCE NUMBER
Heterosexual women				42
0–2 sex partners within 6 mos.	339	ND*	1.4	
> 3 sex partners within 6 mos.	22	ND	18.2	
Heterosexual STD clinic patients	597	1.3	16.6	44
Healthy adult blood donors	700	0.3	7.0	
Female prostitutes	293	4.4	56.7	55
Pregnant women	397	3.4	24.5	
Female prostitutes	272	5	20	56
Nuns	30	10	23	
MSM	441			47
≥ 2 lifetimes STDs		ND	72.2	
< 2 lifetime STDs		ND	28.9	
≥ 2 sex partners in past 12 months		ND	51.9	
< 2 sex partners in past 12 months		ND	40.5	
Heterosexual men	527			
≥ 2 lifetime STDs		ND	6.0	
< 2 lifetime STDs		ND	6.3	
≥ 2 sex partners in past 12 months		ND	4.5	
< 2 sex partners in past 12 months		ND	9.6	
Heterosexual women	821			
≥ 2 lifetime STDs		ND	4.5	
< 2 lifetime STDs		ND	4.6	
≥ 2 sex partners in past 12 months		ND	4.7	
< 2 sex partners in past 12 months		ND	4.1	

*ND = not done or reported

Table 15.19 Prevalence of HBsAg or anti-HBs in study groups which differ according to sexual behavior.

TYPE OF CONTACT	CONTACTS OF HBsAg CARRIERS (%) HBsAg +	CONTACTS OF HBsAg CARRIERS (%) ANTI-HBs +	CONTROLS (%) HBsAg +	CONTROLS (%) ANTI-HBs +	REFERENCE NUMBER
Spouses	0	58.8	0	18.2	53
Children	5.7	11.4	0	4.5	
Sexual partners	9.1	36.4			54
Others	3.1	18.7	0	1.6	
Spouses	3.4	36.4			44
Children	3.6	8.9			
Parents	8.2	34.2			
Siblings	19.7	22.9			
Total	6.7	23.4	0.8	7.3	

Table 15.18 Prevalence of HBV infection in household contacts of HBsAg positive compared with HBsAg negative persons.

(*Fig. 15.10*).[57] Population-based serosurveys have also found an association between sexual activity and HBV infection. In the NHANES II serosurvey, conducted between 1976 and 1980, the prevalence of HBV infection among persons who were sero-positive for syphilis by the fluorescent treponemal antibody (FTA) test was 49%, compared with 5% among persons who were FTA-negative.[58]

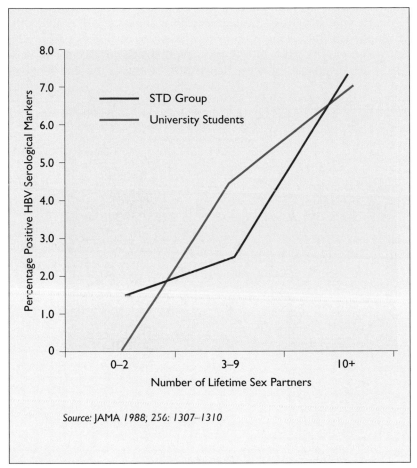

Fig. 15.10 Prevalence of HBV infection by sexual activity for white heterosexuals 18–25 years of age, with more than 12 years of education.

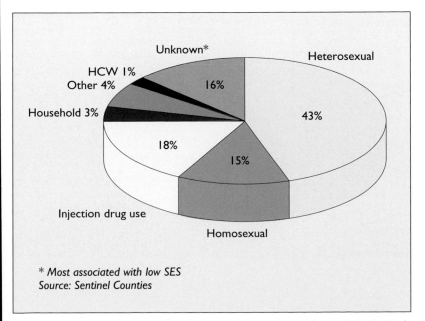

Fig. 15.11 Risk factors associated with reported cases of acute hepatitis B, Sentinel Counties, USA, 1990–1998. Note that heterosexual and homosexual sexual activity together account for 50% of all reported hepatitis B cases. Courtesy of Sentinel Counties Study, Centers for Disease Control and Prevention.

Among cases reported during 1991–1998 in the Sentinel Counties Study, a surveillance system operated by CDC in four US counties, the most frequently identified risk factor was heterosexual exposure to a contact with hepatitis or to multiple partners (43%), followed by injecting drug use (18%), homosexual activity (15%), household contact (3%), and health-care employment (1%) (*Fig. 15.11*). Changes in sexual practices and other risk behaviors in response to the AIDS epidemic have resulted in substantial changes in the distribution of hepatitis B cases during the past decade. Nevertheless, sexual transmission currently accounts for more reported cases than any other mode of transmission. After correcting for under-reporting and asymptomatic infections, an estimated 100,000–200,000 new HBV infections have occurred annually in the USA during the past 10 years (*Fig. 15.12*). Since the mid 1980s, however, the estimated number of acute HBV infections occurring each year has decreased by approximately 75% (*Fig. 15.13*). Based upon risk-factor data collected by CDC, this decrease is believed to be due to behavior changes among MSM and drug users (*Fig. 15.14*). In more recent years, hepatitis B vaccination may also have had an impact in lowering disease rates (CDC, unpublished data)

CLINICAL MANIFESTATIONS

The incubation period of hepatitis B ranges from 2 months to 6 months (average 4 months). The onset of symptoms is gradual, and may include skin rashes and arthralgias, in addition to the usual symptoms of viral hepatitis (*Table 15.3*). Symptoms of acute hepatitis generally last 2–4 weeks, but fatigue and other symptoms may persist for several months. The clinical manifestations of hepatitis B are highly age-dependent. Infection rarely produces symptoms in infants; produces typical illness in only 5–15% of young children; and is symptomatic in 33–50% of

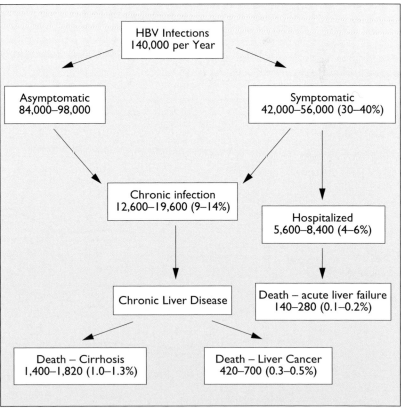

Fig. 15.12 Disease burden of acute and chronic HBV infection, showing the average annual number in all age groups, USA, 1990–1999 estimates. Overall, about 30–40% of HBV infections are symptomatic. In children and adults, about 9–14% of acute HBV infection will progress to chronic infection, and of these, 15–25% may result in premature deaths from either cirrhosis or liver cancer. Courtesy of Centers for Disease Control and Prevention.

adolescents and adults (*Fig. 15.15*).[59] Acute HBV infection resulting in acute liver failure (*Fig. 15.16*) is uncommon (≥1%) but frequently fatal.[60]

Acute HBV infection (*Figs 15.17* and *15.18*) usually resolves with the development of protective antibodies, but may develop into chronic infection. Among the most serious consequences of hepatitis B are the sequelae associated with chronic HBV infection (*Fig. 15.19*), including chronic hepatitis, cirrhosis, and liver cancer (*Fig. 15.20*). The risk of developing chronic HBV infection is inversely associated with the age at which infection is acquired (*Fig. 15.15*).[59] Children less than 5 years old have a 20–50% risk of becoming carriers of the virus after acute infection, while older children and adults have a 5–10% risk of becoming carriers after acute infection. Persons with chronic infection have an estimated

15–25% lifetime risk of dying prematurely from cirrhosis or liver cancer.

A number of other clinical entities are associated with chronic hepatitis B. These include polyarteritis nodosa and glomerulonephritis. The pathogenesis of these diseases is thought to be due to the deposition of circulating HBsAg-antibody complexes in affected organs.

DIAGNOSIS

As the clinical manifestations of acute hepatitis B are similar to other types of viral hepatitis, serologic testing is necessary to establish the diagnosis (*see Table 15.5*). Commercial assays to distinguish acute HBV infection, chronic HBV infection, susceptibility, and vaccine response are widely available. In acute hepatitis B, HBsAg is the first serologic

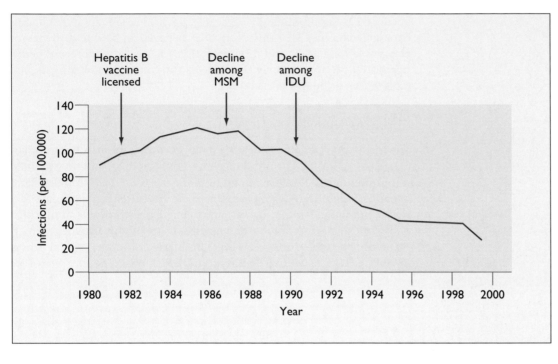

Fig. 15.13 Estimated incidence of acute hepatitis B infections, USA, 1980–1999. Courtesy of Centers for Disease Control and Prevention.

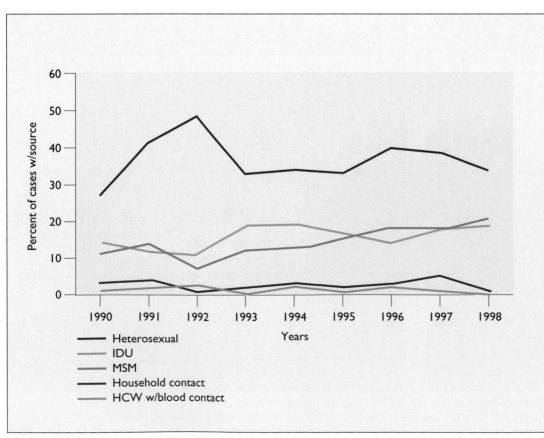

Fig. 15.14 Percentage of reported cases of acute hepatitis B by selected risk factors, Sentinel Counties, USA, 1990–1998. Courtesy of Sentinel Counties Study, Centers for Disease Control and Prevention.

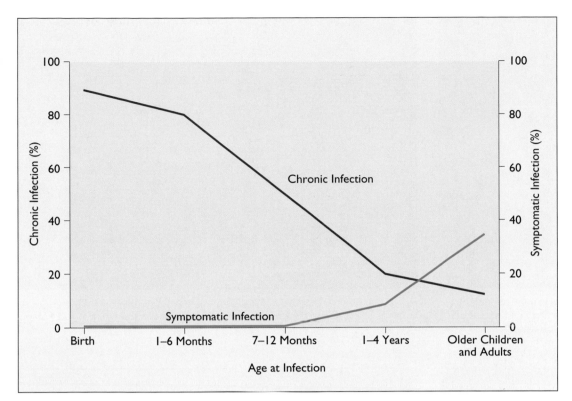

Fig. 15.15 Outcome of HBV infection by age. The frequency of symptoms with acute HBV infection is directly related to the age of acquisition. The risk of acute infection developing into chronic infection is inversely associated with age.

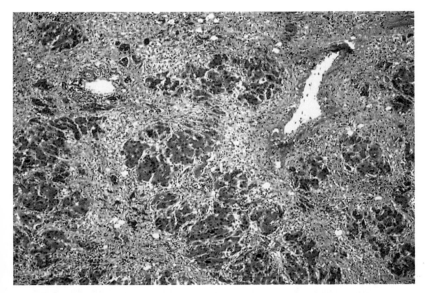

Fig. 15.16 Acute liver failure with submassive necrosis. In this case of fulminant hepatitis B, there is loss of most of the hepatocytes and collapse of the supporting stroma. H and E stain. Courtesy of the Armed Forces Institute of Pathology.

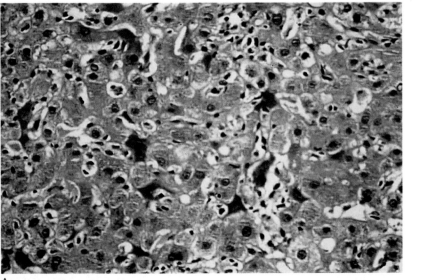

A

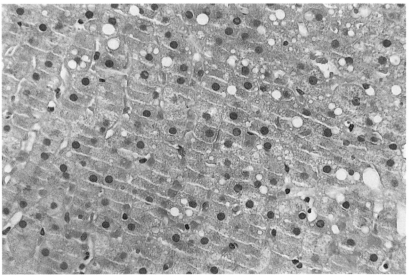

B

Fig. 15.17 (A) Acute hepatitis B. There is apoptosis of hepatocytes and a lymphocytic inflammatory cell infiltrate. (B) Normal hepatocytes. H and E stain. Courtesy of the Armed Forces Institute of Pathology.

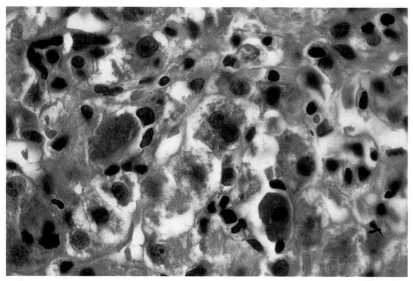

Fig. 15.18 Acute hepatitis B (high magnification). This case demonstrates injured hepatotocytes, apoptotic bodies, and a lymphocytic inflammatory infiltrate. H and E stain. Courtesy of the Armed Forces Institute of Pathology.

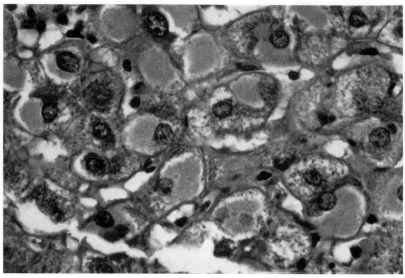

Fig. 15.19 Chronic hepatitis B. 'Ground-glass' hepatocytes with uniformly eosinophilic cytoplasm contain abundant hepatitis B surface antigen. H and E stain. Courtesy of the Armed Forces Institute of Pathology.

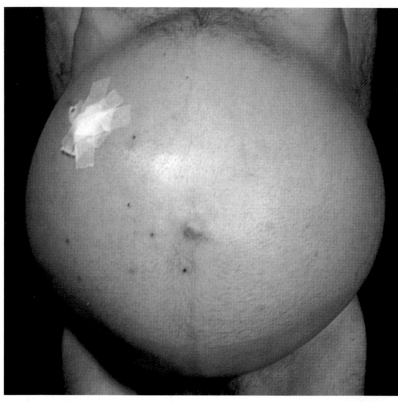

Fig. 15.20 Cirrhosis with ascites – an outcome of chronic hepatitis B, associated with high mortality.

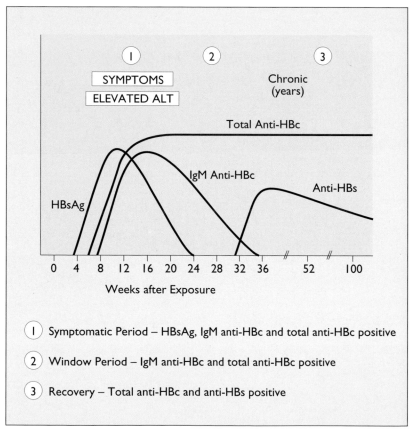

Fig. 15.21 Typical serologic profile of acute HBV infection with recovery. HBsAg usually appears 1–3 months after exposure. In acute HBV infection with recovery, HBsAg disappears within 6 months, while anti-HBs and total anti-HBc persists for lifetime.

marker to become detectable, usually between 2–11 weeks after exposure. IgM antibody to hepatitis B core antigen (IgM anti-HBc) and IgG anti-HBc (measured as total anti-HBc) appear shortly after HBsAg, as does hepatitis B e antigen (HBeAg). In persons who recover from infection, HBsAg and HBeAg persist for up to several months, and then gradually become undetectable (*Fig. 15.21*). Subsequently, IgM anti-HBc gradually disappears, after which antibody to HBsAg (anti-HBs) develops, indicating recovery with lifelong immunity to reinfection. IgG anti-HBc persists for life. In some persons with acute HBV infection, there is a period referred to as 'the window', between the disappearance of HBsAg and the appearance of anti-HBs, when only IgM and total anti-HBc are detectable.

In patients with chronic HBV infection, HBsAg remains detectable, and can persist for life (*Fig. 15.22*). The diagnosis of chronic HBV infection

is made by detecting HBsAg in two serum specimens at least 6 months apart, or by the presence of HBsAg and IgG anti-HBc in the absence of IgM. In chronic HBV infection, total anti-HBc is detectable, but IgM anti-HBc and anti-HBs are generally not detectable. HBeAg may be present, and is associated with active viral replication and higher circulating viral titers. The presence of HBsAg in persons with acute infection and with chronic infection indicates that the person is infectious, regardless of the HBeAg status. Since anti-HBs, but not anti-HBc, is elicited in persons who receive hepatitis B vaccine, immunity from hepatitis B vaccine can be distinguished from immunity due to natural infection by the presence of anti-HBs in the absence of total anti-HBc.

In vaccination programs targeting persons with high risk of HBV infection, it may be cost-effective to pre-screen for the presence of prior immunity due to natural infection. In this situation, the appropriate screening test is total anti-HBc.[61]

TREATMENT

As with hepatitis A, symptoms of acute hepatitis B are generally self-limited, and initial treatment of acutely infected patients is supportive. Liver transplantation has been used to treat patients who have fulminant acute hepatitis B, with favorable survival rates (>50%).

For chronically infected persons, treatment resulting in clearance of HBV is expected to reduce the risk of developing cirrhosis and liver cancer and of transmitting HBV to others. Two agents, interferon alpha and lamivudine, are licensed in the United States for the treatment of chronic HBV infection in adults, and other agents are being evaluated. The treatment course for interferon alpha is 5 million units (MU) daily or 10 MU three times a week subcutaneously for 16 weeks, with monitoring of HBsAg, HBeAg, HBV DNA, and ALT before and after therapy to assess response. With this regimen, approximately 40% of persons have loss of viral replication (as measured by disappearance of HBeAg and/or HBV DNA), and 10–20% lose HBsAg. The response is sustained after treatment, with a relapse of hepatitis occurring in less than 10% of patients within a year of treatment.[62–66] Among those in whom treatment results in loss of HBeAg, many will eventually also lose HbsAg.[67] A meta-analysis of 15 prospective, randomized, controlled trials estimated that adults treated with interferon alpha lose detectable HBsAg 6% more often and detectable HBV DNA 20% more often than untreated controls.[68] The most important factors associated with a favorable response to interferon alpha include high pretreatment serum ALT levels, low pretreatment serum HBV DNA levels, HBeAg-positivity, and adult-acquired HBV infection.[62–65,68] Clearance of HBeAg is advantageous; both treated patient and untreated patients who clear HBeAg have reductions in mortality and clinical complications of cirrhosis.[69]

Lamivudine has emerged as an alternative treatment for adults with chronic HBeAg-positive hepatitis B, as it is easier to administer (orally vs. subcutaneously for interferon) and has fewer side effects compared to interferon alpha therapy. Adults with chronic hepatitis treated with lamivudine for 1 year were more likely to have a histological response and undergo HBeAg seroconversion compared to untreated patients.[70] However, stopping lamivudine at one year often leads to relapse, while continuing lamivudine treatment indefinitely often selects for mutations in the HBV polymerase ('YMDD mutants') which may limit clinical response.[71] Thus, lamivudine therapy for HBeAg-positive patients should be limited to 52 weeks. Lamivudine is administered orally at 100 mg per day. For patients coinfected with human immunodeficiency virus (HIV), lamivudine should be used only in combination with other antiretrovirals and at a dose of 150 mg twice daily. The combination of interferon alpha and lamivudine has not been proven to be more effective than either alone.

Patients with chronic hepatitis B should be counseled to limit alcohol consumption, as this may accelerate progression of disease.[72,73] Hepatitis A vaccination is recommended for HBV-infected patients with chronic liver disease.[35]

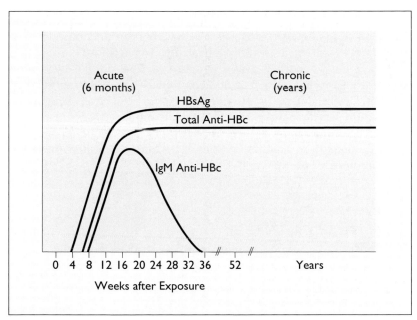

Fig. 15.22 Typical serologic profile of acute HBV infection with progression to chronic infection. HBsAg persists indefinitely and anti-HBs does not develop.

Age at vaccination	Vaccine[a]	n	Years of follow-up	Anti-HBs positive	HBsAg positive	Anti-HBc positive	Reference Number
Infants of HBsAg positive mothers							
Taiwan	P	805	10	85%	0.4%	14%	74
Taiwan	R	118	10	67%	0	12%	75
Italy	R	53	10	68%	0	0	76
China	P	33	9	51%	0	21%	77
USA	P/R	104	4–9	96%	0	7%	78
Infants and children							
China	P	52	15	50%	2%	6%	79
Hong Kong	P/R	148	12	74%	0	1%	80
Senegal	P	41	9–12	68%	2%	27%	81
Gambia	P	675	9	–	1%	13%	82
Italy	P	474	10	68%	0	1%	83
Adolescents							
China	P	95	5	73%	0	8%	84
Adults							
USA[b]	P	1194	9–10	65–84%	0	1%	85
USA	P	634	7–9	48%	<1%	7%	86

[a]P = plasma derived vaccine; R = recombinant vaccine.
[b]Includes children.

Table 15.20 Long-term protection from hepatitis B vaccination

PREVENTION

The prevention of sexually transmitted HBV infection relies upon three general measures:

- Behavior modification to reduce the risk of infection, including using condoms and decreasing the number of sexual partners
- Postexposure prophylaxis of contacts of acutely infected persons with hepatitis B vaccine and hepatitis B immune globulin (HBIG)
- Pre-exposure immunization with hepatitis B vaccine

Hepatitis B vaccine is safe and highly effective. Three doses of vaccine induce protective levels of antibody in 90% or greater of vaccine recipients, and studies of long-term protection indicate that protective efficacy lasts at least 12 years (Table 15.20).[74–86] The recommended doses and schedules for the hepatitis B vaccines available in the United States are given in Table 15.21. The vaccines are considered equivalent in their immunogenicity and effectiveness.

In specific exposure situations, timely post-exposure administration of HBIG and hepatitis B vaccine is effective (>75%) in preventing HBV infection. Unvaccinated sexual partners of persons with acute HBV infection should receive a single dose of HBIG (0.06 ml/kg) followed by the hepatitis B vaccine series, if prophylaxis can be started within 14 days of the last sexual contact. Sexual partners of persons found to be HBV carriers should be vaccinated.

The most effective measure for preventing HBV infection is pre-exposure immunization with hepatitis B vaccine. The World Health Organization recommends that all countries integrate hepatitis B vaccination into their routine infant immunization program, and as of 2001, more than 100 countries have initiated routine infant hepatitis B immunization. However, the relatively high cost of hepatitis B vaccine, and competing health priorities, have been major impediments in less developed countries to implement vaccination. Recent initiatives, such as the Global Alliance for Vaccines and Immunizations, are focused on extending routine infant hepatitis B immunization to all countries.

Over the past two decades a comprehensive immunization strategy in the United States has been developed that includes the following four components: 1) prevention of perinatal HBV infection through routine screening of all pregnant women and appropriate treatment of children born to HbsAg-positive women; 2) routine vaccination of infants; 3) routine vaccination of adolescents who have not previously been vaccinated; and 4) vaccination of children, adolescents, and adults at increased risk of infection (Table 15.22).[61]

It has proved difficult to prevent transmission of HBV between adults in the United States. Immunization programs targeted to adults have been limited in scope and have inadequate resources, and some persons with high-risk behaviors may not seek preventive care. In STD clinics vaccination programs in Birmingham, Alabama, and San Francisco, California, in which hepatitis B vaccine was offered to patients, only 14% of the susceptible target population received two doses of vaccine, and only 4% completed the three-dose series (Fig. 15.23)[87] Among young adult MSM surveyed in 7 US metropolitan areas between 1994–1998, only 9% had received hepatitis B vaccine.[48] In a survey of STD clinic managers in the United States in 1997, while 45% reported that their clinics had implemented policies recommending hepatitis B vaccination, managers reported lack of funding to cover vaccine cost and lack of resources to administer vaccine and track clients for vaccine series completed as major barriers to implementation of programs.[88] Nevertheless, studies of persons with acute hepatitis B indicate missed opportunities to be vaccinated, such as having been previously seen in an STD clinic or in a correctional facility. Furthermore, vaccination programs have reported relatively high vaccination coverage after intensified efforts in targeting adults at high risk.[89] To improve vaccination coverage levels among adults with high-risk behavior, hepatitis B vaccination services must be better integrated into settings where such persons seek health care, such as STD clinics, correctional facilities (juvenile detention facilities, prisons, jails), drug treatment facilities, and community-base HIV prevention sites.[49]

Vaccine	Groups	Dose	Dose schedule (months)[†]
Recombivax®	0–19 years of age	5 μg/0.5ml	0,1,6
	11–15 years of age*	10 μg/0.5ml	0,4–6
	> 19 years of age	10 μg/0.5ml	0,1,6
	Dialysis patients[£]	40 μg/1.0ml	0,1,6
Engerix-B®	0–19 years of age	10 μg/0.5ml	0,1,6
	> 19 years of age	20 μg/1.0ml	0,1,6
	Dialysis patients[¶]	40 μg/2.0ml	0,1,2,6
Twinrix®[‡]	> 18 years of age	729 EL.U (HAV) 20 μg (HBsAg)	0,1,6

[†]0 months represents timing of the initial dose; subsequent numbers represent months after the initial dose

*Alternate two-dose regimen for routine vaccination of adolescents (11 to 15 years of age).

[£]Special 1.0 ml formulation for dialysis patients.

[¶]Two 1.0 ml doses given at one sight given in a 4 dose schedule.

[‡]Twinrix is a bivalent vaccine containing inactivated hepatitis A virus and recombinant surface antigen of the hepatitis B virus.

Adapted with permission from Centers for Disease Control and Prevention: Hepatitis B virus infection. A comprehensive strategy for eliminating transmission in the United States through universal childhood vaccination. MMWR 1991; **40**(No. RR-13): 1–25.

Table 15.21 Recommended doses of currently licensed hepatitis B vaccines.

Routine vaccination
- Infants
- Adolescents, 11–12 years old, not previously vaccinated
- Catch-up vaccination of children and adolescents through 18 years of age

Selective vaccination of high-risk children, adolescents, and adults
- Sexually active heterosexual persons at risk of HBV infection as evidenced by having more than one sex partner in the previous 6 months, a recently acquired sexually transmitted disease, or being treated for a sexually transmitted disease
- Household contacts and sex partners of HBsAg-positive persons
- Men who have sex with men
- Injection drug users
- Persons at occupational risk of infection through exposure to blood or blood-contaminated body fluid (e.g., health care workers, public safety workers), including trainees in schools of medicine, dentistry, nursing, laboratory technology, and other allied health professions
- Clients and staff of institutions for the developmentally disabled
- Hemodialysis patients and patients with early renal failure before they require hemodialysis
- Persons who receive clotting-factor concentrates
- Members of households with adoptees from countries where HBV infection is endemic should be tested for HBsAg and for those found to be HBsAg positive, all family members should be vaccinated. Those found to be HBsAg-negative should be vaccinated
- International travelers who will be in areas with high or intermediate rates of HBV infection for > 6 months, or who will be in these areas for any time period and have close contact with the local population, have contact with blood (e.g., in a medical setting) or have sexual contact with residents
- Inmates in correctional facilities

Adapted with permission from Centers for Disease Control and Prevention: Hepatitis B virus infection. A comprehensive strategy for eliminating transmission in the United States through universal childhood vaccination. MMWR 1991; **40**(No. RR-13): 1–25.

Table 15.22 Strategy for elimination of HBV transmission in the USA.

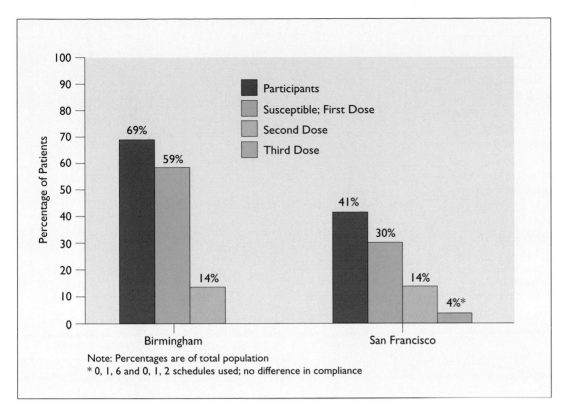

Fig. 15.23 Results of hepatitis B vaccination program: coverage among first-time patients attending STD clinics in Birmingham, Alabama, and San Francisco, California, 1990–1991. Among attendees, 41–69% enrolled, and only 4–14% received a full vaccine series (three doses).

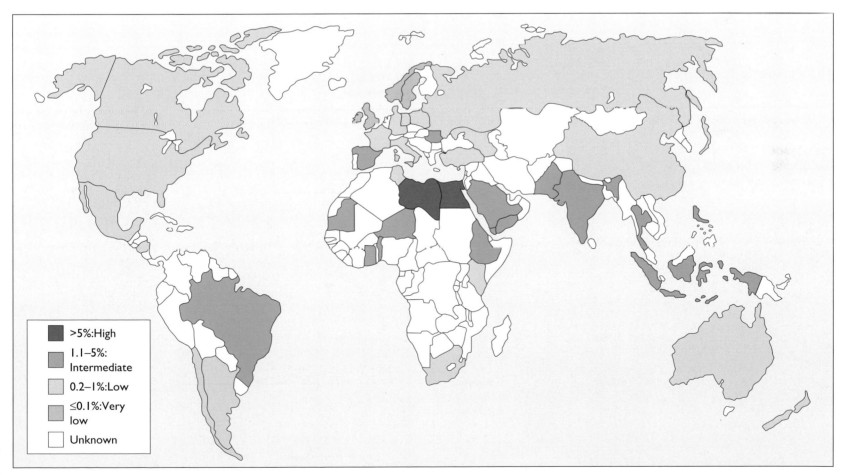

Fig. 15.24 Global prevalence of chronic HCV infection (determined by the percentage of the population positive for antibody to HCV). This map generalizes currently available data; patterns may vary within countries. Courtesy of Centers for Disease Control and Prevention.

HEPATITIS C

EPIDEMIOLOGY

Hepatitis C virus (HCV) is a bloodborne pathogen that appears to be endemic in most parts of the world (*Fig. 15.24*). HCV is the most common cause of posttransfusion hepatitis worldwide. As chronic infection with HCV can ultimately result in cirrhosis and liver cancer, HCV is one of the leading causes of chronic liver disease and end-stage liver disease requiring liver transplantation.

HCV was discovered in 1989. It is an RNA virus, and has been classified as a separate genus in the family Flaviviridae. Although transmission via parenteral, sexual, and perinatal exposures has been identified (*Table 15.23*), many patients with hepatitis C do not report such exposures. The most efficient mode of HCV transmission is direct percutaneous blood exposure, such as via transfusion of blood or blood products or through needle-sharing among drug users. The risk of HCV transmission

Transfusion or transplant (prior to 1992)
Injecting drug use
Hemodialysis (years of treatment)
Accidental injuries with needlestick/sharps
Sexual or household exposure to anti-HCV positive contact
Multiple sexual partners
Infants born to HCV-infected women

*Adapted from Centers for Disease Control and Prevention. Recommendations for the prevention and control of hepatitis C virus (HCV) infection and HCV-related chronic disease. MMWR 1998; **47**(No. RR-19): 1–39.*

Table 15.23 Risk factors associated with the transmission of HCV.

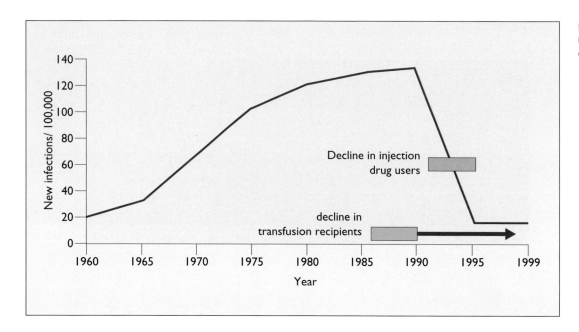

Fig. 15.25 Estimated incidence of acute hepatitis C, USA, 1960–1999. Courtesy of Sentinel Counties Study, Centers for Disease Control and Prevention.

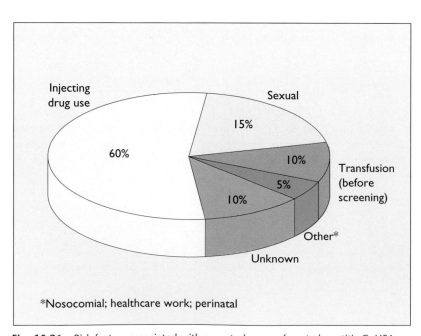

Fig. 15.26 Risk factors associated with reported cases of acute hepatitis C, USA, 1990–1998. Courtesy of Sentinel Counties Study, Centers for Disease Control and Prevention.

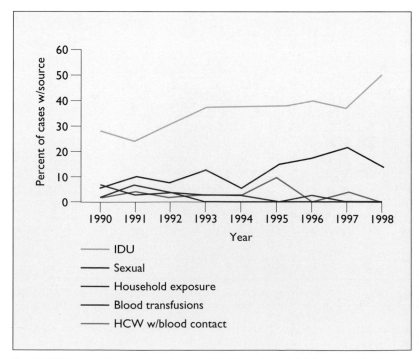

Fig. 15.27 Reported cases of acute hepatitis C by selected risk factors, United States, 1983–1998. Data from 1983–1990 based on non-A, non-B hepatitis. Courtesy of Sentinel Counties Study, Centers for Disease Control and Prevention.

- Evidence supporting sexual transmission
  - Case–control, cross sectional studies indicate that sex with an infected partner, multiple partners, sex at an early age, non-use of condoms, other STDs, and sex with trauma are risk factors of HCV infection
  - Seroprevalence studies indicate male to female transmission more efficient
- Evidence against sexual transmission
  - In case–control studies MSM are at no higher risk than heterosexuals for infection with HCV
  - Anti-HCV seroprevalence among long-term sexual partners of HCV infected person (1.5%) is no greater than the general population (1.8%)

Adapted from Centers for Disease Control and Prevention. Recommendations for the prevention and control of hepatitis C virus (HCV) infection and HCV-related chronic disease. MMWR 1998; 47(No. RR-19): 1–39.

Table 15.24 Evidence in support of and against sexual/household transmission of HCV.

GROUP	ANTI-HCV PREVALENCE	RISK FACTORS
Homosexual men	1% to 4%	No. of partners
Heterosexual STD patients	1% to 10%	No. of partners Non-use of condoms
Prostitutes	4% to 19%	No. of partners Others STDs Non-use of condoms Sex with trauma

Table 15.25 HCV infection in populations with different sexual behaviors.

following a needlestick exposure to blood from a source positive for antibody to HCV (anti-HCV) is 1.8% (range: 0–7%).[90–93]

The number of cases of acute hepatitis C has declined dramatically since 1989, due largely to a decrease in cases among IDU (*Fig. 15.25*). However, IDU is still the most commonly identified risk factor associated with acute IICV infection in surveillance studies (*Fig. 15.26*).[94, 95] IDU also currently accounts for most HCV transmission in the United States, and has accounted for a substantial proportion of HCV infections during past decades (*Fig. 15.27*).[96–98] Middle-aged or older persons may have acquired their infection decades earlier as a result of limited or occasional illegal drug injecting. Injecting-drug use leads to HCV transmission in a manner similar to that for other blood-borne pathogens, i.e., through transfer of HCV-infected blood by sharing syringes and needles either directly or through contamination of drug preparation equipment.[99,100] However, HCV infection is acquired more rapidly after initiation of injecting than other viral infections, and rates of HCV infection among younger injecting-drug users are four times higher than rates of human immunodeficiency virus (HIV) infection.[101] After 5 years of injecting, as many as 90% of users are infected with HCV. More rapid acquisition of HCV infection compared with other viral infections among injecting-drug users is likely caused by high prevalence of chronic HCV infection among injecting-drug users, which results in a greater likelihood of exposure to an HCV-infected person.

Studies examining the risk of sexual HCV transmission have provided conflicting results (*Table 15.24*). Case-control studies have reported an association between exposure to a sex contact with a history of hepatitis or exposure to multiple sex partners and acquiring hepatitis C.[102] In addition, 15–20% of patients with acute hepatitis C reported to CDC's Sentinel Counties surveillance system have a history of sexual exposures in the absence of percutaneous risk factors. Two-thirds of these have an anti-HCV-positive sex partner, and one-third reported more than two partners in the 6 months prior to illness.[98] In contrast, a low prevalence of HCV infection has been reported in studies of long-term spouses of patients with chronic HCV infection who had no other risk factors for infection. Five of these studies have been conducted in the United States, involving 30–85 partners each, in which the average prevalence of HCV infection was 1.5% (range, 0–4.4%).[103–106] Among the partners of persons with hemophilia coinfected with HCV and HIV, two studies have reported a relatively low average prevalence of HCV infection of 3%.[106,107] Among persons with evidence of high-risk sexual practices (e.g., patients attending STD clinics and female prostitutes) who denied a history of injecting-drug use, the prevalence of anti-HCV has been found to average 6% (range, 1–10%).[108–111] Specific factors associated with anti-HCV positivity for both heterosexuals and homosexual men included greater numbers of sex partners, a history of prior STDs, and

failure to use a condom (*Table 15.25*). Only one study has found an association between HCV infection and MSM activity,[112] and at least in STD clinic settings, the prevalence rate of HCV infection among MSM men generally has been similar to that of heterosexuals.

Because sexual transmission of bloodborne viruses is recognized to be more efficient among MSM compared with heterosexual men and women, why HCV infection rates are not substantially higher among MSM compared with heterosexuals is unclear. This observation and the low prevalence of HCV infection observed among the long-term sex partners of persons with chronic HCV infection have raised doubts about the importance of sexual activity in the transmission of HCV. Unacknowledged percutaneous risk factors (i.e., illegal injecting-drug use) might contribute to increased risk for HCV infection among persons with high-risk sexual practices. Although there are considerable inconsistencies between studies, overall, the data suggest that sexual transmission of HCV may occur, but that the virus appears to be inefficiently spread in this manner.

Studies of infants born to HCV-infected HIV-negative women have found the risk of transmission is 5–6% (range 0–25%), based on detection of anti-HCV and HCV RNA, respectively.[113–125] The average infection rate for infants born to women coinfected with HCV and HIV is higher at 14% (range: 5–36%) and 17%, based on detection of anti-HCV and HCV RNA, respectively.[113–116,119,124,126–128] The only factor consistently found to be associated with transmission has been the presence of HCV RNA in the mother at the time of birth. Two studies of infants born to HCV-positive, HIV-negative women reported an association with titer of HCV RNA.[121,122] However, studies of HCV/HIV-coinfected women more consistently have indicated an association between virus titer and transmission of HCV.[126]

Case-control studies also have reported an association between non-sexual household contact and acquiring hepatitis C.[129,130] The presumed mechanism of transmission is inapparent percutaneous or permucosal exposure to infectious blood or body fluids containing blood. Although the prevalence of HCV infection among non-sexual household contacts of persons with chronic HCV infection in the United States is unknown, it is likely that HCV transmission to such contacts is very uncommon. In studies from other countries of non-sexual household contacts of patients with chronic hepatitis C, the average anti-HCV prevalence was 4%.[131] Although the infected contacts in these studies reported no other commonly recognized risk factors for hepatitis C, most of these studies were done in countries where it has been suggested that the clustering of HCV infections in families may be associated with exposures commonly experienced in the past from contaminated equipment used in traditional and nontraditional medical procedures

Results from the Third National Health and Nutrition Examination Survey (NHANES III) conducted during 1988–1994 have indicated that the prevalence of anti-HCV among the general US population is 1.8%, which corresponds to 3.9 million anti-HCV-positive individuals nationwide, the majority of which (2.7 million) have chronic infection.[132]

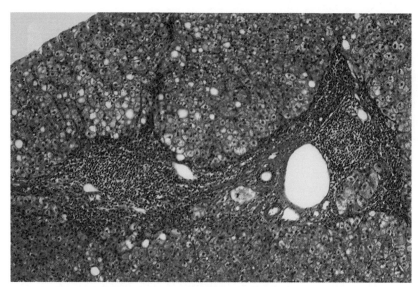

Fig. 15.28 Chronic hepatitis C. This relatively mild case has portal lymphoid aggregates and local interface hepatitis ('piecemeal necrosis'). H and E stain. Courtesy of the Armed Forces Institute of Pathology.

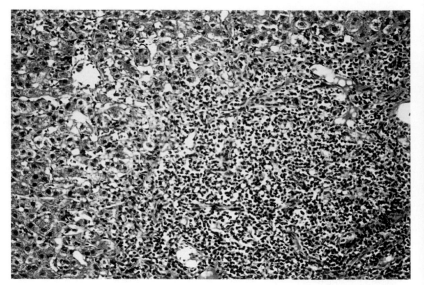

Fig. 15.29 Chronic hepatitis C. In this severe case, the portal area (lower right) has severe chronic inflammation and a marked degree of interface hepatitis as well as spotty parenchymal inflammation and hepatocyte dropout. H and E stain. Courtesy of the Armed Forces Institute of Pathology.

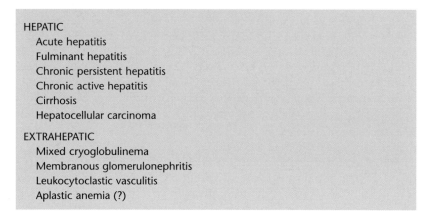

HEPATIC
  Acute hepatitis
  Fulminant hepatitis
  Chronic persistent hepatitis
  Chronic active hepatitis
  Cirrhosis
  Hepatocellular carcinoma

EXTRAHEPATIC
  Mixed cryoglobulinema
  Membranous glomerulonephritis
  Leukocytoclastic vasculitis
  Aplastic anemia (?)

Table 15.26 Hepatic and extrahepatic manifestations associated with HCV infection.

Population-based studies indicate that 40–60% of chronic liver disease is HCV-related, resulting in an estimated 8,000–10,000 deaths each year (CDC, unpublished data) (*Table 15.2*).

CLINICAL MANIFESTATIONS

Acute HCV infection is generally mild, with 25% or fewer of infected persons having a recognized illness. When symptoms do occur with acute HCV infection, the incubation period ranges from 14–180 days (average 6–7 weeks), and the symptoms are indistinguishable from those of other types of viral hepatitis (*Table 15.3*).[133–135]

An important feature of hepatitis C is the high frequency with which acute disease progresses to chronic infection. After acute infection, 15–25% of persons with normal immune status appear to resolve their infection without sequelae as defined by sustained absence of HCV RNA in serum and normalization of ALT levels.[136,137] Chronic HCV infection (*Figs 15.28* and *15.29*) develops in most persons (75–85%),[137–140] with persistent or fluctuating ALT elevations indicating active liver disease developing in 60–70% of chronically infected persons.[138,140–143]

No clinical or epidemiologic features among patients with acute infection have been found to be predictive of either persistent infection or chronic liver disease. Most studies have reported that cirrhosis develops in 10–20% of persons with chronic hepatitis C over a period of 20–30 years, and hepatocellular carcinoma in 1–5%.[140,144,145] Extrahepatic manifestations of chronic HCV infection (*Table 15.26*) are considered to be of immunologic origin, and include cryoglobulinemia, membranoproliferative glomerulonephritis, and porphyria cutanea tarda.[146]

DIAGNOSIS

Assays are available for detection of both antibody to HCV (anti-HCV) and HCV RNA (*Table 15.27*).[147] Anti-HCV can be detected in 80% of patients within 15 weeks after exposure, in ≥90% within 5 months after exposure, and in ≥97% by 6 months after exposure (*Figs 15.30* and *15.31*).[138,148] Enzyme immunoassays (EIAs) measure anti-HCV but do not distinguish between acute, chronic, or resolved infection. As with any screening test, the positive predictive value varies depending on the prevalence of infection in the population, and is low in populations with an HCV infection prevalence of <10%.[149,150] To prevent the reporting of false-positive results, particularly in settings where asymptomatic persons are being tested, the currently recommended HCV testing algorithm (*Fig. 15.32*) includes supplemental testing with a more specific

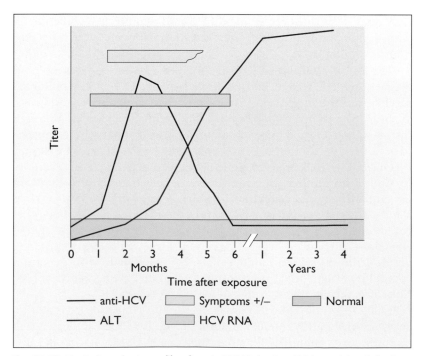

Fig. 15.30 Typical serologic profile of acute HCV infection. With resolving infection, alanine aminotransferase (ALT) levels normalize and HCV RNA is not detectable.

Tests for Hepatitis C

Test/Type	Application	Comments
ANTI-HCV (ANTIBODY)		
• EIA (enzyme immunoassay) and supplemental assay [i.e., recombinant immunoblot assay (RIBA)].	– indicates past or present infection, but does not differentiate between acute, chronic or resolved infection – All positive EIA results should be verified with a supplemental assay.	– Sensitivity ≥ 97%. – EIA alone has low positive predictive value in low prevalence populations.
HCV RNA (VIRUS) **Qualitative tests***		
• Reverse transcription polymerase chain reaction (RT-PCR) amplification of HCV RNA by in-house or commercial assays (e.g., Amplicor HCV™).	– Detects presence of circulating HCV RNA. – Monitor patients on antiviral therapy.	– Detects virus as early as 1–2 weeks after exposure. – Detection of HCV RNA during course of infection may be intermittent. A single negative RT-PCR is not conclusive. – False-positive and false-negative results may occur.
Quantitative tests*		
• RT-PCR amplification of HCV RNA by in-house or commercial assays [e.g., Amplicor HCV Monitor™]. • Branched chain DNA (bDNA) assays (e.g., Quantiplex™ HCV RNA Assay).	– Determines concentration of HCV RNA. – May be useful for assessing the likelihood of response to antiviral therapy, but clinical utility has not been standardized.	– Less sensitive than qualitative RT-PCR. – Should not be used to exclude the diagnosis of HCV infection or to determine treatment endpoint.
Genotype*		
• Several methodologies available (e.g., hybridization, sequencing).	– Groups isolates of HCV based on genetic differences into 6 genotypes and > 90 subtypes. – With new therapies, length of treatment may vary based on genotype.	– Genotype 1 (subtypes 1a and 1b) most common in US and associated with lower response to antiviral therapy

*Samples require special handling (e.g., serum must be separated within 2–4 hours of collection and stored frozen (≤ 20°C); samples should be shipped on dry ice).
Adapted from Centers for Disease Control and Prevention. Recommendations for the prevention and control of hepatitis C virus (HCV) infection and HCV-related chronic disease. MMWR 1998; **47**(No. RR-19): 1–39.

Table 15.27 Tests for hepatitis C virus infection.

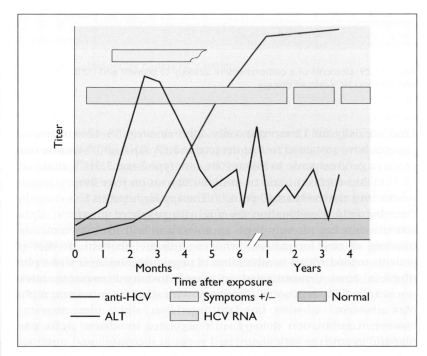

Fig. 15.31 Typical serologic profile of acute HCV infection progressing to chronic HCV infection. In chronic HCV infection, alanine aminotransferase (ALT) levels continue to fluctuate, and HCV RNA can be detected intermittently. Approximately two-thirds of individuals with acute HCV infection develop chronic hepatitis.

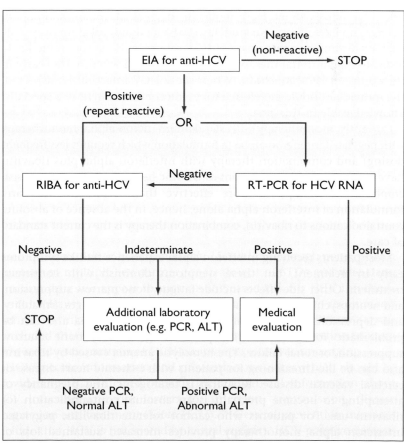

Fig. 15.32 HCV infection testing algorithm for diagnosis of asymptomatic persons. Adapted from Centers for Disease Control and Prevention. Recommendations for the prevention and control of hepatitis C virus (HCV) infection and HCV-related chronic disease. *MMWR* 1998; 47(No. RR-19): 1–39.

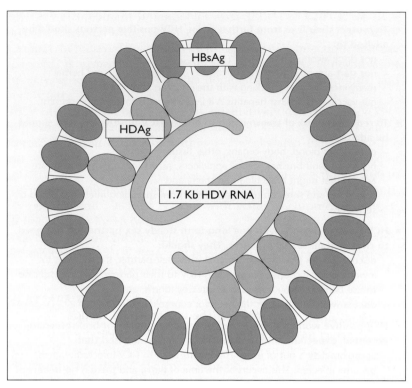

Fig. 15.33 Hepatitis D (delta) virus.

HEPATITIS DELTA

EPIDEMIOLOGY

The virus HDV was discovered in 1977. It is molecularly distinct from other hepatitis viruses and is classified as a satellite virus or subviral agent because of its inability to encode its own envelope protein.[161,162] The delta viral particle has a core of delta-specific proteins (HDAg) and RNA, with an envelope of HBsAg that is contributed by the host HBV infection (*Fig 15.33*). Because of the unique situation in which HBV must be present for transmission of HDV, infections with HDV occur in two forms – HBV-HDV coinfection and HDV superinfection. In HBV-HDV coinfection, there is simultaneous transmission of HBV and HDV to an individual who is susceptible to infection with HBV. Individuals who are immune to HBV infection either through prior infection or adequate hepatitis B vaccination response cannot be infected with HDV. In HDV superinfection, HDV is transmitted to an individual with a pre-existing chronic HBV infection. The pre-existing HBV infection provides the HBsAg needed to establish the HDV infection.

Since HDV infection is dependent on HBV infection, the epidemiology of HDV infection is similar to that of HBV infection (*Table 15.32*). Percutaneous transmission of HDV is highly efficient, as evidenced by the high prevalence of HDV among persons who have frequent percutaneous exposures such as injection drug users.[163,164] Sexual and perinatal transmission of HDV is much less efficient than that of HBV.[165–168] Worldwide, the endemicity of HDV infection varies, with areas of high endemicity including southern Italy, several countries in Africa, and the Amazon basin in South America (*Fig. 15.34*). In areas of

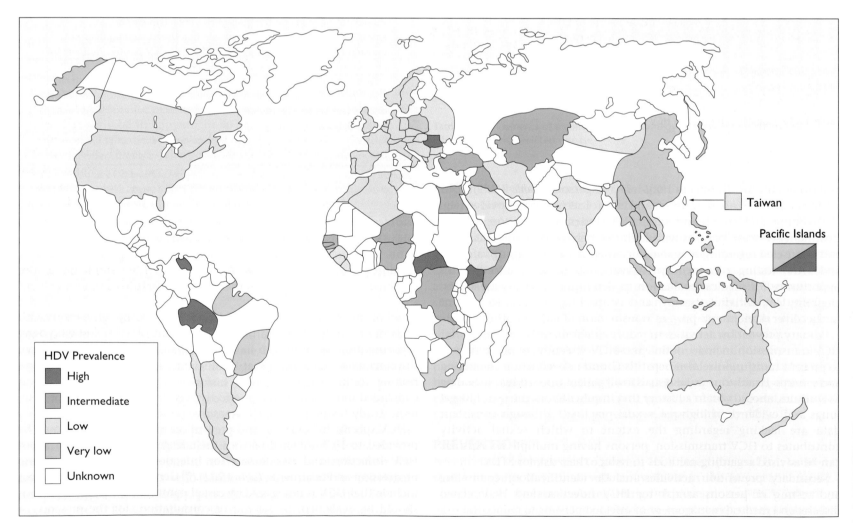

Fig. 15.34 Prevalence of HDV infection worldwide. Very low: 0–2% HDV prevalence in HBV carriers. Low: 3–9% HDV prevalence in HBV carriers. Moderate: 10–19% HDV prevalence in HBV carriers. High: >20% HDV prevalence in HBV carriers. White: no data available. This map generalizes currently available data; patterns may vary within counties. Courtesy of Centers for Disease Control and Prevention.

high endemicity, transmission occurs predominantly from person-to-person contact, whereas in areas of low endemicity, transmission occurs within well-defined high-risk groups with frequent percutaneous exposures such as injecting drug users, hemophiliacs, and less frequently among persons with high-risk sexual practices such as homosexual men and prostitutes.[169,170]

In the United States, the prevalence of HDV in the general population is low – only 4% of HbsAg-positive blood donors were anti-HDV positive (Table 15.33).[171] In contrast, the prevalence of HDV among HbsAg-positive injection drug users ranged from 42% to 73%.[163,164] The prevalence of HDV among HbsAg-positive persons with high-risk sexual behaviors, hemophiliacs, and persons in institutions for the developmentally disabled was intermediate, ranging from 6% to 30%.[172–174] Among MSM, the prevalence of HDV ranged from 0 to 15% depending on city, and the risk of infection increases with an increasing number of sexual partners and the frequency of rectal intercourse.[173]

In the United States, HBV-HDV coinfection is responsible for an estimated 4% of cases of acute viral hepatitis, corresponding to 7,500 infections annually and 5% of cases of chronic viral hepatitis.[173,175] There are approximately 850 deaths from HDV infection annually: 800 from chronic infection and 50 from fulminant hepatitis D.[169]

CLINICAL MANIFESTATIONS

In general, the symptoms of acute HBV-HDV coinfection or HDV superinfection are similar to those of acute hepatitis due to other viruses (Table 15.3). One feature that may distinguish HBV-HDV coinfection from other viral hepatitides is a biphasic course of illness, with two peaks of liver cell damage (increased serum liver enzymes and bilirubin). The first peak in liver enzymes is related to appearance of

HBV antigens in the liver while the second is related to appearance of HDV antigens.[176]

For HBV-HDV coinfection, the incubation period ranges from 6 to 24 weeks.[177] Coinfection with HBV and HDV results in fulminant hepatitis more often than does infection with HBV alone. Studies have shown that the prevalence of HDV markers in patients with acute fulminant hepatitis B is as high as 50%.[178–181] Following acute HBV-HDV coinfection, approximately 2% of individuals will become chronically infected,[182,183] whereas the risk of developing chronic HBV infection after acute infection with HBV alone is 2–10% among adults.[184,185]

The incubation period for HDV superinfection ranges from 2 to 8 weeks.[177] Similar to HBV-HDV coinfection, fulminant hepatitis occurs more often with HDV superinfection than with acute HBV infection alone. Studies have shown that up to 30% of HDV superinfections will develop a fulminant course.[180,186,187] In contrast to HBV-HDV coinfection, HDV superinfection results in chronic HDV infection (Fig. 15.35) in up to 90% of patients.[188–190]

Throughout the world, the prevalence of HDV is higher among persons with chronic liver disease compared to persons chronically infected with HBV alone.[186,191,192] The rate at which cirrhosis develops once chronic HDV infection is established also appears to be greater than with HBV infection alone.[193–197] However, persons with long-term chronic HDV infection have been described without elevated serum hepatic enzymes or histopathologic changes on liver biopsy. The spectrum of HDV disease ranges from a rapidly progressive course that leads to liver failure in several months to a few years[198,199] to a disease that runs a benign nonprogressive course.[165,200] The majority of persons with chronic HDV infection progress to cirrhosis within a few years; but once established, cirrhosis may remain clinically stable for several years.[201] Although there is a well-documented association between chronic HBV infection and development of hepatocellular carcinoma, none has been documented with chronic HDV infection.[201,202]

DIAGNOSIS

Persons with HDV infection produce both IgM and IgG antibodies to the hepatitis delta antigen (anti-HDV). During acute coinfection, antibodies are produced to both HBV and HDV antigens, yet the anti-HDV, including the IgM class of anti-HDV, response is often weak and may be delayed by several months. Since anti-HDV may not be present until several weeks after onset of illness, testing of acute and con-valescent sera may be required to make the diagnosis of HDV infection. The anti-HDV produced often does not persist making diagnosis of past

MODE	GROUPS AT RISK
Parenteral	Injecting drug users
	Persons with multiple blood transfusions
Indirect parenteral	Persons living in communities with endemic infection
	Developmentally disabled
Sexual	Heterosexual and homosexual contacts of persons with HBV–HDV coinfection or chronic HBV–HDV carriers

Table 15.32 Modes of transmission of hepatitis delta virus (HDV).

Group	Prevalence HBsAg (%)	Prevalence Anti-HD (%)*
Blood donors	0.1–0.5	1–12
Injection drug users	5–19	42–73
Men who have sex with men	5–10	0–15
Female prostitutes (injection drug users)	74	21
Female prostitutes (non-injection drug users)	38	6
Developmentally disabled	5–15	30
Hemophiliacs	8	19
Southeast Asian refugees	5–15	2–8
Alaskan Eskimos	5–15	0.6
Pacific Islanders	5–15	0–9

*Among HBsAg positive persons.

Table 15.33 Prevalence of HDV infection among HBsAg carriers in certain groups in North America.

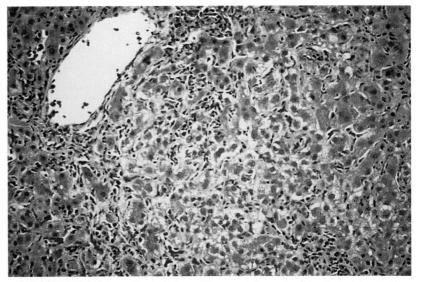

Fig. 15.35 Chronic hepatitis D. This case demonstrates severe intraparenchymal inflammation. H and E stain. Courtesy of the Armed Forces Institute of Pathology.

coinfection difficult (*Fig.15.36*). HDV superinfection, by contrast, produces a brisk anti-HDV response that persists throughout the chronic infection (*Fig. 15.37*).[203,204] In persons with acute hepatitis, HDV-HBV coinfection can usually be distinguished from HDV superinfection by the presence or absence, respectively, of IgM antiHBc. The IgM anti-HDV response is not useful for distinguishing acute from chronic HDV infection, as IgM anti-HDV production persists throughout chronic infection.[205] Availability of assays for detection of IgM and IgG anti-HDV for clinical purposes vary country to country. In the United States, tests for detecting IgM anti-HDV are not commercially available for clinical use.

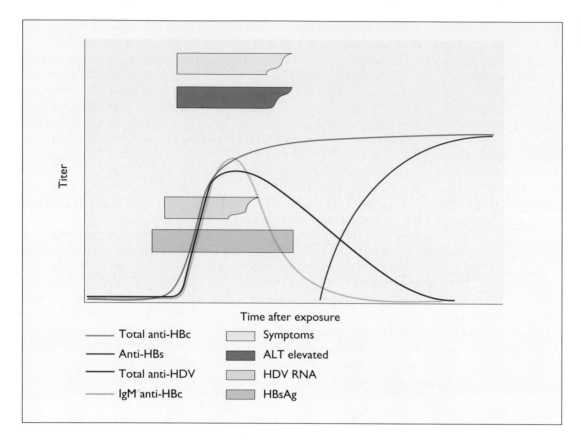

Fig. 15.36 Typical serologic profile of HBV–HDV coinfection.

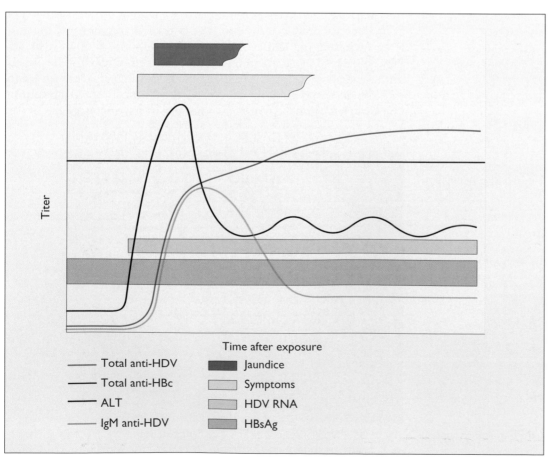

Fig. 15.37 Typical serologic profile of HBV–HDV superinfection.

HDV infection can also be diagnosed by the presence of hepatitis D antigen (HDAg) in serum and liver tissue;[206] however serum HDAg is bound by immunocomplexes early in the course of infection leading to false-negative results.[207] Detection of HDV RNA by reverse transcription polymerase chain reaction (RT-PCR) may provide a more sensitive assay for diagnosis of HDV infection, especially in the early phase of the disease. HDV RNA detection by RT-PCR has been shown to be positive in 93% of patients with HBV-HDV coinfection and in 100% with superinfection.[208] In general, however, assays for the detection of HDAg and HDV RNA are not available in the United States outside the research setting.

Testing for HDV infection should be considered in patients with acute and chronic hepatitis B, particularly in patients with fulminant hepatitis. Knowledge of patient's HDV infection status may help in counseling about prognosis and the prevention of transmission to others.

TREATMENT

Interferon alpha is the only approved therapy for chronic hepatitis D. Randomized trials using low-dose interferon alpha found that 25% to 60% of patients respond with normalization of ALT values after 12 to 16 weeks of treatment; however, almost all persons relapse when treatment is stopped.[209–213] Better responses rates have been reported using higher doses of interferon alpha (9 million units three times a week) for 48 weeks with significant improvement in liver histology and sustained normalization of ALT in 36% of patients; however, none maintained clearance of viremia after treatment was stopped.[214]

Liver transplantation for end stage chronic hepatitis D has a 5-year survival rate as a high as 88%.[215] The success of liver transplantation for chronic hepatitis D is believed due to the suppressive effect of HDV on HBV replication, which greatly reduces the post-transplant HBV reinfection rate in the grafted liver. When hepatitis B immunoglobulin is used for prophylaxis prior to liver transplantation for end-stage chronic hepatitis D, the HBV/HDV reinfection rate is approximately 10%, compared to a HBV reinfection of close to 100% following liver transplantation for end-stage liver disease due to HBV alone.[215,216]

PREVENTION

Hepatitis B vaccine is the single most important tool to prevent HBV-HDV coinfection since persons immune from HBV infection cannot become infected with HDV. Safer sexual and injection practices are also important as they reduce exposure to HDV-contaminated body fluids. Post-exposure prophylaxis with hepatitis B vaccine and hepatitis B immunoglobulin, when indicated, will prevent HBV-HDV coinfection.[61]

No vaccine exists to prevent HDV superinfection in persons who are chronically infected with HBV. In the short term, prevention depends on modification of behaviors to avoid contact with HDV-infected blood and body fluid. In the United States this primarily means safer sexual and injection practices. Prevention of HDV superinfection in less-developed countries is more difficult since household transmission is thought to play an important role. In the long term, routine infant hepatitis B vaccination programs will have a substantial impact on HBV-HDV coinfection and HBV-HDV superinfection by decreasing the number of new and chronic HBV infections, respectively. Over the past decade, such a decrease in incidence and prevalence of HDV infection has been documented in Italy, Hong Kong, and Taiwan.[217–221] These decreases have been attributed to hepatitis B vaccination, and safer sexual and injection practices.[222]

References

1. Cohen JI, Feinstone S, Purcell RH. Hepatitis A virus infection in a chimpanzee: duration of viremia and detection of virus in saliva and throat swabs. *J Infect Dis* 1989; **160**:887–890.

2. Bower WA, Nainan OV, Han X, Margolis HS. Duration of viremia in hepatitis A virus infection. *J Infect Dis* 2000; **182**:12–17.

3. Shapiro CN, Margolis HS. Worldwide epidemiology of hepatitis A virus infection. *J Hepatol* 1993; **18**(Suppl 2):S11–S14.

4. Anonymous. Hepatitis A among homosexual men – United States, Canada, and Australia. *MMWR* 1992; **41**:155–154.

5. Anonymous. Hepatitis A vaccination of men who have sex with men – Atlanta, Georgia, 1996–1997. *MMWR* 1998; **47**:708–711.

6. Christenson B, Brostrom C, Bottiger M *et al.* An epidemic outbreak of hepatitis A among homosexual men in Stockholm. Hepatitis A, a special hazard for the male homosexual subpopulation in Sweden. *Am J Epidemiol* 1982; **116**:599–607.

7. Leentvaar-Kuijpers A, Kool JL, Veugelers, PJ, Coutinho RA, van Griensven GJ. An outbreak of hepatitis A among homosexual men in Amsterdam, 1991–1993. *Int J Epidemiol* 1995; **24**:218–222.

8. Stokes ML, Ferson MJ, Young LC. Outbreak of hepatitis A among homosexual men in Sydney. *Am J Public Health* 1997; **87**:2039–2041.

9. Sundkvist T, Aitken C, Duckworth G, Jeffries D. Outbreak of acute hepatitis A among homosexual men in East London. *Scand J Infect Dis* 1997; **29**:211–212.

10. Henning KJ, Bell E, Braun J, Barker ND. A community-wide outbreak of hepatitis A: risk factors for infection among homosexual and bisexual men. *Am J Med* 1995; **99**:132–136.

11. Coutinho RA, Albrecht-van Lent P, Lelie N, Nagelkerke N, Kuipers H, Rijsdijk T. Prevalence and incidence of hepatitis A among male homosexuals. *Br Med J (Clin Res Ed)* 1983; **287**:1743–1745.

12. Kryger P, Pedersen NS, Mathiesen L, Nielsen JO. Increased risk of infection with hepatitis A and B viruses in men with a history of syphilis: relation to sexual contacts. *J Infect Dis* 1982; **145**:23–26.

13. McFarlane ES, Embil JA, Manuel FR, Thiebaux HJ. Antibodies to hepatitis A antigen in relation to the number of lifetime sexual partners in patients attending an STD clinic. *Br J Vener Dis* 1981; **57**:58–61.

14. Corey L, Holmes KK. Sexual transmission of hepatitis A in homosexual men: incidence and mechanism. *N Engl J Med* 1980; **302**:435–438.

15. Katz MH, Hsu L, Wong E, Liska S, Anderson L, Janssen RS. Seroprevalence of and risk factors for hepatitis A infection among young homosexual and bisexual men. *J Infect Dis* 1997; **175**:1225–1229.

16. Lednar WM, Lemon SM, Kirkpatrick JW, Redfield RR, Fields ML, Kelley PW. Frequency of illness associated with epidemic hepatitis A virus infections in adults. *Am J Epidemiol* 1985; **122**:226–233.

17. Liaw YF, Yang CY, Chu, CM, Huang MJ. Appearance and persistence of hepatitis A IgM antibody in acute clinical hepatitis A observed in an outbreak. *Infection* 1986; **14**:156–158.

18. Stapleton JT. Host immune response to hepatitis A virus. *J Infect Dis* 1995; **171**(Suppl 1):S9–14.

19. O'Grady J. Management of acute and fulminant hepatitis A. *Vaccine* 1992; **10**(Suppl 1):S21–S23.

20. Cohen EJ, Oncley JL, Strong LE, Hughes WLJ, Armstrong SH. Chemical, clinical, and immunological studies on the products of human plasma fraction. I. The characterization of the protein fractions of human plasma. *J Clin Invest* 1944; **23**:417–432.

21. Anonymous. Safety of therapeutic immune globulin preparations with respect to transmission of human T-lymphotropic virus type III/lymphadenopathy-associated virus infection. *MMWR* 1986; **35**:231–233.

22. Bresee JS, Mast EE, Coleman PJ *et al.* Hepatitis C virus infection associated with administration of intravenous immune globulin. A cohort study. *JAMA* 1996; **276**:1563–1567.

23. Kluge T. Gamma-globulin in the prevention of viral hepatiits: A study on the effect of medium-size doses. *Acta Med Scand* 1963; **174**:469–477.

24. Mosley JW, Reisler DM, Brachott D, Roth, D, Weiser J. Comparison of two lots of immune serum globulin for prophylaxis of infectious hepatitis. *Am J Epidemiol* 1968; **87**:539–550.

25. Stokes J, Neefe JR. The prevention and attenuation of infectious hepatitis by gamma globulin: Preliminary note. *JAMA* 1945; **127**:144–145.

26. Ashur Y, Adler R, Rowe M, Shouval D. Comparison of immunogenicity of two hepatitis A vaccines – VAQTA and HAVRIX – in young adults. *Vaccine* 1999; **17**:2290–2296.

27. Chen XQ, Bulbul M, de Gast GC, van Loon AM, Nalin DR, van Hattum J. Immunogenicity of two versus three injections of inactivated hepatitis A vaccine in adults. *J Hepatol* 1997; **26**:260–264.

28. Clemens R, Safary A, Hepburn A, Roche C, Stanbury WJ, Andre FE. Clinical experience with an inactivated hepatitis A vaccine. *J Infect Dis* 1995; **171**(Suppl 1):S44–S49.

29. McMahon BJ, Williams J, Bulkow L *et al.* Immunogenicity of an inactivated hepatitis A vaccine in Alaska Native children and Native and non-Native adults. *J Infect Dis* 1995; **171**:676–679.

30. Nalin DR, Kuter BJ, Brown L *et al.* Worldwide experience with the CR326F-derived inactivated hepatitis A virus vaccine in pediatric and adult populations: an overview. *J Hepatol* 1993; **18**(Suppl 2):S51–S55.

31. Van Herck K, Van Damme P. Inactivated hepatitis A vaccine-induced antibodies: follow-up and estimates of long-term persistence. *J Med Virol* 2001; **63**:1–7.

32. Werzberger A, Kuter B, Nalin D. Six years' follow-up after hepatitis A vaccination [letter]. *N Engl J Med* 1998; **338**:1160.

33. Innis BL, Snitbhan R, Kunasol P *et al.* Protection against hepatitis A by an inactivated vaccine. *JAMA* 1994; **271**:1328–1334.

34. Werzberger A, Mensch B, Kuter B *et al.* A controlled trial of a formalin-inactivated hepatitis A vaccine in healthy children. *N Engl J Med* 1992; **327**:453–457.

35. Anonymous. Prevention of hepatitis A through active or passive immunization: Recommendations of the Advisory Committee on Immunization Practices (ACIP). *MMWR* 1999; **48**:1–37.

36. Thoelen S, Van Damme P, Leentvaar-Kuypers A *et al.* The first combined vaccine against hepatitis A and B: an overview. *Vaccine* 1999; **17**:1657–1662.

37. Anonymous. Prevention of hepatitis A through active or passive immunization: Recommendations of the Advisory Committee on Immunization Practices (ACIP). *MMWR* 1996; **45**:1–30.

38. Francis DP, Favero MS, Maynard JE. Transmission of hepatitis B virus. *Semin Liver Dis* 1981; **1**:27–32.

39. Davis LG, Weber DJ, Lemon SM. Horizontal transmission of hepatitis B virus. *Lancet* 1989; **1**:889–893.

40. McQuillan GM, Coleman PJ, Kruzon-Moran D, Moyer LA, Lambert SB, Margolis HS. Prevalence of hepatitis B virus infection in the United States: the National Health and Nutrition Examination Surveys, 1976 through 1994. *Am J Public Health* 1999; **89**:14–18.

41. Alter MJ, Margolis HS. The emergence of hepatitis B as a sexually transmitted disease. *Med Clin North Am* 1990; **74**:1529–1541.

42. Fulford KW, Dane DS, Catterall RD, Woof R, Denning JV. Australia antigen and antibody among patients attending a clinic for sexually transmitted diseases. *Lancet* 1973; **1**:1470–1473.

43. Jeffries DJ, James WH, Jefferiss FJ, MacLeod KG, Willcox RR. Australia (hepatitis-associated) antigen in patients attending a venereal disease clinic. *Br Med J* 1973; **2**:455–456.

44. Szmuness W, Harley EJ, Prince AM. Intrafamilial spread of asymptomatic hepatitis B. *Am J Med Sci* 1975; **270**:293–304.

45. Dietzman DE, Harnisch JP, Ray CG, Alexander ER, Holmes KK. Hepatitis B surface antigen (HBsAg) and antibody to HBsAg. Prevalence in homosexual and heterosexual men. *JAMA* 1977; **238**:2625–2626.

46. Yuan L, Robinson G. Hepatitis B vaccination and screening for markers at a sexually transmitted disease clinic for men. *Can J Public Health* 1994; Revue Canadienne de Sante Publique **85**:338–341.

47. Gilson RJ, de Ruiter A, Waite J *et al.* Hepatitis B virus infection in patients attending a genitourinary medicine clinic: risk factors and vaccine coverage. *Sex Transm Infect* 1998; **74**:110–115.

48. MacKellar DA, Valleroy LA, Secura GM *et al.* Two decades after vaccine license: hepatitis B immunization and infection among young men who have sex with men. *Am J Public Health* 2001; **91**:965–971.

49. Gunn RA, Murray PJ, Ackers ML, Hardison WG, Margolis HS. Screening for chronic hepatitis B and C virus infections in an urban sexually transmitted disease clinic: rationale for integrating services. *Sex Transm Dis* 2001; **28**:166–170.

50. Redeker AG, Mosley JW, Gocke DJ, McKee AP, Pollack W. Hepatitis B immune globulin as a prophylactic measure for spouses exposed to acute type B hepatitis. *N Engl J Med* 1975; **293**:1055–1059.

51. Koff RS, Slavin MM, Connelly JD, Rosen DR. Contagiousness of acute hepatitis B. Secondary attack rates in household contacts. *Gastroenterology* 1977; **72**:297–300.

52. Peters CJ, Purcell RH, Lander JJ, Johnson KM. Radioimmunoassay for antibody to hepatitis B surface antigen shows transmission of hepatitis B virus among household contacts. *J Infect Dis* 1976; **134**:218–223.

53. Irwin GR, Allen AM, Bancroft WH *et al.* Hepatitis B antigen and antibody. Occurrence in families of asymptomatic HB AG carriers. *JAMA* 1974; **227**:1042–1043.

54. Heathcote J, Gateau P, Sherlock S. Role of hepatitis-B antigen carriers in non-parenteral transmission of the hepatitis-B virus. *Lancet* 1974; **2**:370–371.

55. Papaevangelou G, Trichopoulos D, Kremastinou T, Papoutsakis G. Prevalence of hepatitis B antigen and antibody in prostitutes. *Br Med J* 1974; **2**:256–258.

56. Adam E, Hollinger FB, Melnick JL, Duenas A, Rawls WE. Type B hepatitis antigen and antibody among prostitutes and nuns: a study of possible venereal transmission. *J Infect Dis* 1974; **129**:317–321.

57. Alter MJ, Ahtone J, Weisfuse I, Starko K, Vacalis TD, Maynard JE. Hepatitis B virus transmission between heterosexuals. *JAMA* 1986; **256**:1307–1310.

58. McQuillan GM, Townsend TR, Fields HA, Carroll M, Leahy M, Polk BF. Seroepidemiology of hepatitis B virus infection in the United States. 1976 to 1980. *Am J Med* 1989; **87**:5S–10S.

59. McMahon BJ, Alward WL, Hall DB *et al.* Acute hepatitis B virus infection: relation of age to the clinical expression of disease and subsequent development of the carrier state. *J Infect Dis* 1985; **151**:599–603.

60. Pappas SC. Fulminant viral hepatitis. *Gastroenterol Clin North Am* 1995; **24**:161–173.

61. Anonymous. Hepatitis B virus: a comprehensive strategy for eliminating transmission in the United States through universal childhood vaccination. Recommendations of the Immunization Practices Advisory Committee (ACIP). *MMWR* 1991; **40**:1–25.

62. Perrillo RP, Schiff ER, Davis GL *et al.* A randomized, controlled trial of interferon alfa-2b alone and after prednisone withdrawal for the treatment of chronic hepatitis B. The Hepatitis Interventional Therapy Group. *N Engl J Med* 1990; **323**:295–301.

63. Di Bisceglie AM, Fong TL, Fried MW *et al.* A randomized, controlled trial of recombinant alpha-interferon therapy for chronic hepatitis B. *Am J Gastroenterol* 1993; **88**:1887–1892.

64. Lok AS, Wu PC, Lai CL *et al.* A controlled trial of interferon with or without prednisone priming for chronic hepatitis B. *Gastroenterology* 1992; **102**:2091–2097.

65. Hoofnagle JH, Peters M, Mullen KD *et al.* Randomized, controlled trial of recombinant human alpha-interferon in patients with chronic hepatitis B. *Gastroenterology* 1988; **95**:1318–1325.

66. Alexander GJ, Brahm J, Fagan EA *et al.* Loss of HBsAg with interferon therapy in chronic hepatitis B virus infection. *Lancet* 1987; **2**:66–69.

67. Lau DT, Everhart J, Kleiner DE *et al.* Long-term follow-up of patients with chronic hepatitis B treated with interferon alfa. *Gastroenterology* 1997; **113**:1660–1667.

68. Wong DK, Cheung AM, O'Rourke K *et al.* Effect of alpha-interferon treatment in patients with hepatitis B e antigen-positive chronic hepatitis B. A meta-analysis. *Ann Intern Med* 1993; **119**:312–323.

69. Niederau C, Heintges T, Lange S *et al.* Long-term follow-up of HBeAg-positive patients treated with interferon alfa for chronic hepatitis B. *N Engl J Med* 1996; **334**:1422–1427.

70. Dienstag JL, Schiff ER, Wright TL *et al.* Lamivudine as initial treatment for chronic hepatitis B in the United States. *N Engl J Med* 1999; **341**:1256–1263.

71. Lai CL, Chien RN, Leung NW *et al.* A one-year trial of lamivudine for chronic hepatitis B. Asia Hepatitis Lamivudine Study Group. *N Engl J Med* 1998; **339**:61–68.

72. Ikeda K, Saitoh S, Koida, I *et al.* A multivariate analysis of risk factors for hepatocellular carcinogenesis: a prospective observation of 795 patients with viral and alcoholic cirrhosis. *Hepatology* 1993; **18**:47–53.

73. Sokal EM, Bortolotti F. Update on prevention and treatment of viral hepatitis in children. *Curr Opin Pediatr* 1999; **11**:384–389.

74. Wu JS, Hwang LY, Goodman KJ, Beasley RP. Hepatitis B vaccination in high-risk infants: 10-year follow-up. *J Infect Dis* 1999; **179**:1319–1325.

75. Huang LM, Chiang BL, Lee CY, Lee PI, Chi WK, Chang MH. Long-term response to hepatitis B vaccination and response to booster in children born to mothers with hepatitis B e antigen. *Hepatology* 1999; **29**:954–959.

76. Resti M, Azzari C, Mannelli F, Rossi ME, Lionetti P, Vierucci A. Ten-year follow-up study of neonatal hepatitis B immunization: are booster injections indicated? *Vaccine* 1997; **15**:1338–1340.

77. Ding L, Zhang M, Wang Y, Zhou S, Kong W, Smego RA, Jr. A 9-year follow-up study of the immunogenicity and long-term efficacy of plasma-derived hepatitis B vaccine in high-risk Chinese neonates. *Clin Infect Dis* 1993; **17**:475–479.

78. Stevens CE, Toy PT, Taylor PE, Lee T, Yip HY. Prospects for control of hepatitis B virus infection: implications of childhood vaccination and long-term protection. *Pediatrics* 1992; **90**:170–173.

79. Liao SS, Li RC, Li H, Yang JY *et al.* Long-term efficacy of plasma-derived hepatitis B vaccine: a 15-year follow-up study among Chinese children. *Vaccine* 1999; **17**:2661–2666.

80. Yuen MF, Lim WL, Cheng CC, Lam SK, Lai CL. Twelve-year follow-up of a prospective randomized trial of hepatitis B recombinant DNA yeast vaccine versus plasma-derived vaccine without booster doses in children. *Hepatology* 1999; **29**:924–927.

81. Coursaget P, Leboulleux D, Soumare M *et al.* Twelve-year follow-up study of hepatitis B immunization of Senegalese infants. *J Hepatol* 1994; **21**:250–254.

82. Viviani S, Jack A, Hall AJ *et al.* Hepatitis B vaccination in infancy in The Gambia: protection against carriage at 9 years of age. *Vaccine* 1999; **17**:2946–2950.

83. Da Villa G, Peluso F, Picciotto L, Bencivenga M, Elia S, Pelliccia MG. Persistence of anti-HBs in children vaccinated against viral hepatitis B in the first year of life: follow-up at 5 and 10 years. *Vaccine* 1996; **14**:1503–1505.

84. Mintai Z, Kezhou L, Lieming D, Smego RA, Jr. Duration and efficacy of immune response to hepatitis B vaccine in high-risk Chinese adolescents. *Clin Infect Dis* 1993; **16**:165–167.

85. Wainwright RB, Bulkow LR, Parkinson AJ, Zanis C, McMahon, BJ. Protection provided by hepatitis B vaccine in a Yupik Eskimo population – results of a 10-year study. *J Infect Dis* 1997; **175**:674–677.

86. Hadler SC, Coleman PJ, O'Malley P, Judson FN, Altman N. Evaluation of long-term protection by hepatitis B vaccine for seven to nine years in homosexual men. In: Hollinger FB, Lemon SM, Margolis HS, eds. *Viral Hepatitis and Liver Disease*. Baltimore: Williams and Williams, 1991:766–768.

87. Moran JS, Peterman TA, Weinstock HS et al. Hepatitis B vaccination trials in sexually transmitted disease clinics: Implications for program development. Presented at the 26th National Immunization Conference, 1–6 June 1992, St. Louis, Missori.

88. Wilson BC, Moyer L, Schmid G et al. Hepatitis B vaccination in sexually transmitted disease (STD) clinics: a survey of STD programs. *Sex Transm Dis* 2001;**28**: 148–152.

89. Savage RB, Hussey MJ, Hurie MB. A successful approach to immunizing men who have sex with men against hepatitis B. *Public Health Nurs* 2000; **17**:202–206.

90. Alter MJ. Occupational exposure to hepatitis C virus: a dilemma. *Infect Control Hosp Epidemiol* 1994; **15**:742–744.

91. Lanphear BP, Linnemann CC, Jr., Cannon CG, DeRonde MM, Pendy L, Kerley LM. Hepatitis C virus infection in healthcare workers: risk of exposure and infection. *Infect Control Hosp Epidemiol* 1994; **15**:745–750.

92. Puro V, Petrosillo N, Ippolito G. Risk of hepatitis C seroconversion after occupational exposures in health care workers. Italian Study Group on Occupational Risk of HIV and Other Bloodborne Infections. *Am J Infect Control* 1995; **23**:273–277.

93. Mitsui T, Iwano K, Masuko K et al. Hepatitis C virus infection in medical personnel after needlestick accident. *Hepatology* 1992; **16**:1109–1114.

94. Villano SA, Vlahov D, Nelson KE et al. Incidence and risk factors for hepatitis C among injection drug users in Baltimore, Maryland. *J Clin Microbiol* 1997; **35**:3274–3277.

95. Garfein RS, Doherty MC, Monterroso ER et al. Prevalence and incidence of hepatitis C virus infection among young adult injection drug users. *J Acquir Immune Defic Syndr Hum Retrovirol* 1998; **18**(Suppl 1):S11–S19.

96. Alter MJ, Hadler SC, Judson FN et al. Risk factors for acute non-A, non-B hepatitis in the United States and association with hepatitis C virus infection. *JAMA* 1990; **264**:2231–2235.

97. Alter MJ. The epidemiology of acute and chronic hepatitis C. *Clinics in Liver Disease* 1997; **1**(3):559–567.

98. Alter MJ. Epidemiology of hepatitis C. *Hepatology* 1997; **26**:62S–65S.

99. Heimer R, Khoshnood K, Jariwala-Freeman B, Duncan B, Harima Y. Hepatitis in used syringes: the limits of sensitivity of techniques to detect hepatitis B virus (HBV) DNA, hepatitis C virus (HCV) RNA, and antibodies to HBV core and HCV antigens. *J Infect Dis* 1996; **173**:997–1000.

100. Koester SK, Hoffer L. "Indirect sharing": additional HIV risks associated with drug injection. *AIDS & Pub Policy J* 1994; **9**:100–105.

101. Garfein RS, Vlahov D, Galai N, Doherty MC, Nelson KE. Viral infections in short-term injection drug users: the prevalence of the hepatitis C, hepatitis B, human immunodeficiency, and human T-lymphotropic viruses. *Am J Public Health* 1996; **86**:655–661.

102. Alter MJ, Gerety RJ, Smallwood LA et al. Sporadic non-A, non-B hepatitis: Frequency and epidemiology in an urban U.S. population. *J Infect Dis* 1982; **145**:886–892.

103. Conry-Cantilena C, VanRaden M, Gibble J et al. Routes of infection, viremia, and liver disease in blood donors found to have hepatitis C virus infection. *N Engl J Med* 1996; **334**:1691–1696.

104. Everhart JE, Di Bisceglie AM, Murray LM et al. Risk for non-A, non-B (type C) hepatitis through sexual or household contact with chronic carriers. *Ann Intern Med* 1990; **112**:544–545.

105. Gordon SC, Patel AH, Kulesza GW, Barnes RE, Silverman AL. Lack of evidence for the heterosexual transmission of hepatitis C. *Am J Gastroenterol* 1992; **87**:1849–1851.

106. Eyster ME, Alter HJ, Aledort LM, Quan S, Hatzakis A, Goedert JJ. Hetero-sexual co-transmission of hepatitis C virus (HCV) and human immuno-deficiency virus (HIV). *Ann Intern Med* 1991; **115**:764–768.

107. Brettler DB, Mannucci PM, Gringeri A et al. The low risk of hepatitis C virus transmission among sexual partners of hepatitis C-infected hemophilic males: an international, multicenter study. *Blood* 1992; **80**:540–543.

108. Thomas DL, Cannon RO, Shapiro CN, Hook EW, III, Alter MJ, Quinn TC. Hepatitis C, hepatitis B, and human immunodeficiency virus infections among non-intravenous drug-using patients attending clinics for sexually transmitted diseases. *J Infect Dis* 1994; **169**:990–995.

109. Buchbinder SP, Katz MH, Hessol NA, Liu J, O'Malley PM, Alter MJ. Hepatitis C virus infection in sexually active homosexual men. *J Infect* 1994; **29**: 263–269.

110. Weinstock HS, Bolan G, Reingold AL, Polish LB. Hepatitis C virus infection among patients attending a clinic for sexually transmitted diseases. *JAMA* 1993; **269**:392–394.

111. Osmond DH, Charlebois E, Sheppard HW et al. Comparison of risk factors for hepatitis C and hepatitis B virus infection in homosexual men. *J Infect Dis* 1993; **167**:66–71.

112. Thomas DL, Zenilman JM, Alter HJ et al. Sexual transmission of hepatitis C virus among patients attending sexually transmitted diseases clinics in Baltimore—an analysis of 309 sex partnerships. *J Infect Dis* 1995; **171**:768–775.

113. Granovsky MO, Minkoff HL, Tess BH et al. Hepatitis C virus infection in the mothers and infants cohort study. *Pediatrics* 1998; **102**:355–359.

114. Paccagnini S, Principi N, Massironi E et al. Perinatal transmission and manifestation of hepatitis C virus infection in a high risk population. *Pediatr Infect Dis J* 1995; **14**:195–199.

115. Manzini P, Saracco G, Cerchier A et al. Human immunodeficiency virus infection as risk factor for mother-to-child hepatitis C virus transmission; persistence of anti-hepatitis C virus in children is associated with the mother's anti-hepatitis C virus immunoblotting pattern. *Hepatology* 1995; **21**:328–332.

116. Zuccotti GV, Ribero ML, Giovannini M et al. Effect of hepatitis C genotype on mother-to-infant transmission of virus. *J Pediatr* 1995; **127**:278–280.

117. Resti M, Azzari C, Lega L et al. Mother-to-infant transmission of hepatitis C virus. *Acta Paediatr* 1995; **84**:251–255.

118. Giacchino R, Picciotto A, Tasso L, Timitilli A, Sinelli N. Vertical transmission of hepatitis C [letter]. *Lancet* 1995; **345**:1122–1123.

119. Zanetti AR, Tanzi E, Paccagnini S et al. Mother-to-infant transmission of hepatitis C virus. Lombardy Study Group on Vertical HCV Transmission. *Lancet* 1995; **345**:289–291.

120. Ni YH, Lin HH, Chen PJ, Hsu HY, Chen DS, Chang MH. Temporal profile of hepatitis C virus antibody and genome in infants born to mothers infected with hepatitis C virus but without human immunodeficiency virus coinfection. *J Hepatol* 1994; **20**:641–645.

121. Ohto H, Terazawa S, Sasaki N et al. Transmission of hepatitis C virus from mothers to infants. The Vertical Transmission of Hepatitis C Virus Collaborative Study Group. *N Engl J Med* 1994; **330**:744–750.

122. Lin HH, Kao JH, Hsu HY et al. Possible role of high-titer maternal viremia in perinatal transmission of hepatitis C virus. *J Infect Dis* 1994; **169**:638–641.

123. Roudot-Thoraval F, Pawlotsky JM, Thiers V et al. Lack of mother-to-infant transmission of hepatitis C virus in human immunodeficiency virus-seronegative women: a prospective study with hepatitis C virus RNA testing. *Hepatology* 1993; **17**:772–777.

124. Lam JP, McOmish F, Burns SM, Yap PL, Mok JY, Simmonds P. Infrequent vertical transmission of hepatitis C virus. *J Infect Dis* 1993; **167**:572–576.

125. Wejstal R, Widell A, Mansson AS, Hermodsson S, Norkrans G. Mother-to-infant transmission of hepatitis C virus. *Ann Intern Med* 1992; **117**:887–890.

126. Thomas DL, Villano SA, Riester KA et al. Perinatal transmission of hepatitis C virus from human immunodeficiency virus type 1-infected mothers. Women and Infants Transmission Study. *J Infect Dis* 1998; **177**:1480–1488.

127. Cilla G, Perez-Trallero E, Iturriza M, Carcedo A, Echeverria J. Maternal-infant transmission of hepatitis C virus infection. *Pediatr Infect Dis J* 1992; **11**:417.

128. Novati R, Thiers V, Monforte AD et al. Mother-to-child transmission of hepatitis C virus detected by nested polymerase chain reaction. *J Infect Dis* 1992; **165**:720–723.

129. Alter MJ, Gerety RJ, Smallwood LA et al. Sporadic non-A, non-B hepatitis: frequency and epidemiology in an urban U.S. population. *J Infect Dis* 1982; **145**:886–893.

130. Alter MJ, Coleman PJ, Alexander WJ et al. Importance of heterosexual activity in the transmission of hepatitis B and non-A, non-B hepatitis *JAMA* 1989; **262**:1201–1205.

131. Alter MJ. Epidemiology of hepatitis C in the West. *Semin Liver Dis* 1995; **15**:5–14.

132. Alter MJ, Kruszon-Moran D, Nainan OV et al. The prevalence of hepatitis C virus infection in the United States, 1988 through 1994. *N Engl J Med* 1999; **341**:556–562.

133. Koretz RL, Brezina M, Polito AJ et al. Non-A, non-B posttransfusion hepatitis: comparing C and non-C hepatitis. *Hepatology* 1993; **17**:361–365.

134. Marranconi F, Mecenero V, Pellizzer GP et al. HCV infection after accidental needlestick injury in health-care workers. *Infection* 1992; **20**:111.

Sexually Transmitted Infections in Infants, Children and Adolescents

16

C Beck-Sague, K Dominguez and A Robinson

INTRODUCTION

Sexually transmitted diseases (STDs) can affect children's health at three stages in their development:

- During infancy, as a result of maternal–neonatal transmission
- During childhood, as a result of sexual abuse, and
- During adolescence, as a result of sexual assault or consensual sexual activity.

PERINATALLY TRANSMITTED INFECTIONS

Vertical transmission of many recognized sexually transmissible pathogens, including *Treponema pallidum*, *Neisseria gonorrhoeae*, *Chlamydia trachomatis*, herpes simplex virus (HSV), human immunodeficiency virus (HIV), and human papilloma virus (HPV), is well documented. Although clinical manifestations of perinatally acquired STDs are distinct, there are certain similarities among these diseases, and similarities to other infectious diseases, particularly other TORCH syndromes (congenital toxoplasmosis, rubella, cytomegalovirus, herpes), which should be considered (*Table 16.1*).

CONGENITAL SYPHILIS

EPIDEMIOLOGY

The incidence of congenital syphilis closely reflects the incidence of primary and secondary syphilis in women (*Fig. 16.1*), as well as the effectiveness of prenatal interventions to prevent vertical transmission.[1] The CDC surveillance definition for congenital syphilis was revised in 1996 (*Table 16.2*).[2] The incidence of congenital syphilis in the US among infants less than one year of age peaked during the nationwide syphilis epidemic in 1991 at 107.3 cases per 100,000 live births, and has since declined by 87% to 14.3.[3] However, the US rate remains many times that of other developed countries.[3]

						Symptoms during infancy							
Infectious agent	Type of transmission	Perinatal mortality	Pre-maturity	Intrauterine growth retardation	Occular findings	Hepatospleno-megaly	Jaundice	Anemia	Other	Bone lesions	Sepsis	CNS involve-ment
Bacterial												
Treponema pallidium	Transplacental	+	+	+	Chorioretinitis, glaucoma	+	+	+	Vesiculobullous rashes	Osteitis, periostitis, metaphysitis	+	+
Neisseria qonorrhoeae	Intrapartum	+	+	+	Conjunctive	–	–	–	–	Arthritis	+	Rare
Chlamydia trachomatis	Intrapartum	–	+	?	Conjunctivitis	–	–	–	Pneumonitis	–	–	–
Viral												
Human papillomavirus	Intrapartum	–	–	–	–	–	–	–	Laryngeal papilloma; laryngeal cancer; oral, genital warts	–	–	–
Human immuno-deficiency virus	Intrapartum (Can be trans-placental & postpartum)	+/–	+/–	+/–	Keratitis Keratoconjunc-junctivitis CMV retinitis Herpes retinopathy Optic neuropathy Bacterial, fungal, parasitic infections	+	–	+	Diarrhea failure to thrive, opportunistic and other infections, parotitis, AIDS	–	+	+
Herpes simplex virus	Intrapartum (can be trans-placental & postpartum)	+	+	–	Chorioretinitis, keratitis	+	+	–	Vesicles, erosions	–	+	+

Table 16.1 Perinatal transmission of selected sexually transmitted pathogens.

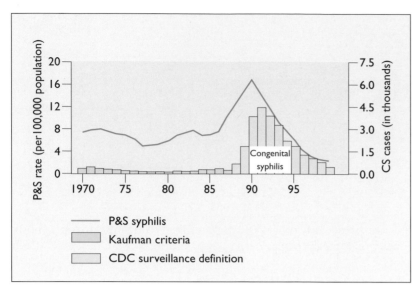

Fig. 16.1 Congenital syphilis. Reported cases in infants < 1 year of age and rates of primary and secondary (P&S) syphilis among women, USA, 1970–1999. Courtesy of DSTDP STD Surveillance 1999, CDC Atlanta, GA, 2000.

Syphilitic stillbirth

A fetal death that occurs after a 20-week gestation or in which the fetus weighs greater than 500 g and the mother had untreated or inadequately treated syphilis at delivery.

Syphilis, congenital

Clinical description

An infant or child (<2 years) may have signs such as hepatosplenomegaly, rash, condyloma lata, snuffles, jaundice (non-viral hepatitis), pseudoparalysis, anemia, or edema (nephrotic syndrome and/or malnutrition). An older child may have stigmata (e.g., interstitial keratitis, nerve deafness, anterior bowing of shins, frontal bossing, mulberry molars, Hutchinson teeth, saddle nose, rhagades, or Clutton joints).

Laboratory criteria for diagnosis

- Demonstration of *T. pallidum* by darkfield microscopy, fluorescent antibody, or other specific stains in specimens from lesions, placenta, umbilical cord, or autopsy material

Probable: a condition affecting an infant whose mother had untreated or inadequately treated syphilis at delivery, regardless of signs in the infant, or an infant or child who has a reactive treponemal test for syphilis and any one of the following:

- Any evidence of congenital syphilis on physical examination
- Any evidence of congenital syphilis on radiographs of long bones
- A reactive cerebrospinal fluid (CSF) Venereal Disease Research Laboratory (VDRL)
- An elevated CSF cell count or protein (without other cause)
- A reactive fluorescent treponemal antibody absorbed – 19S-IgM antibody test or IgM enzyme-linked immunosorbent assay

Confirmed: a case that is laboratory confirmed.

Source: CDC MMWR: *1997 46 1–55.*

Table 16.2 Congenital Syphilis Case Definition.

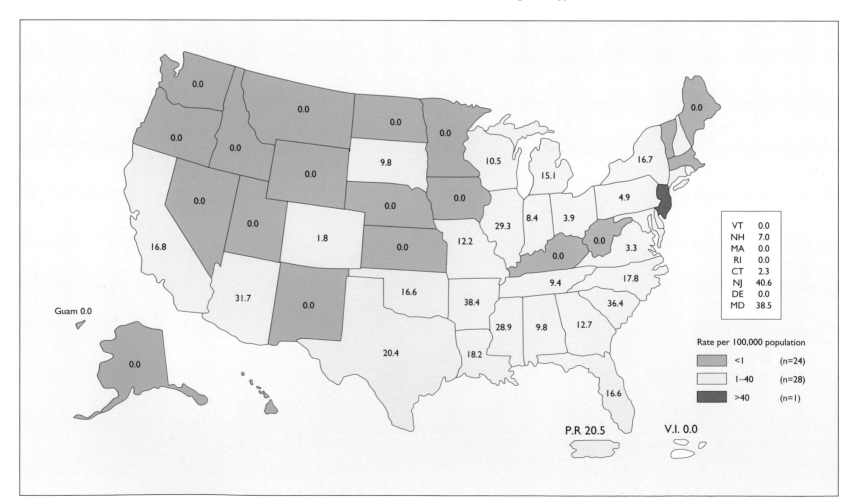

Fig. 16.2 Congenital syphilis cases USA, 1999; 68.5% are reported by seven states (New York, California, Florida, Illinois, Texas, Maryland, New Jersey), and rates are highest in the Southeast. Courtesy of DSTDP STD Surveillance 1999, CDC Atlanta, GA, 2000.

Congenital syphilis in the US is concentrated where the incidence of primary and secondary syphilis among women is high (*Fig. 16.2*).[3] The prevalence of reactive prenatal serologic tests for syphilis tends to be high in some developing countries, particularly in Sub-Saharan Africa, where it is sometimes exceeded only by HIV seroprevalence (*Fig. 16.3*).[4-16]

VERTICAL TRANSMISSION

The risk of congenital syphilis varies with stage of untreated maternal syphilis; it is over 80% in primary and secondary syphilis, somewhat less in early latent, and very low during late latent and tertiary syphilis. Prenatal treatment failures to prevent vertical transmission are more common in primary and secondary syphilis and in the third trimester.[17,18]

PREVENTION

Congenital syphilis is almost entirely preventable, or curable before the birth of the infant if the mother is diagnosed and treated before the infant has been irreversibly affected. Prenatal diagnosis and treatment with long-acting penicillin is highly effective.[19] Most missed opportunities to prevent congenital syphilis occur because pregnant women enrolled in prenatal care do not receive penicillin treatment as indicated (*Table 16.3*).[20] Prenatal screening should be conducted in the first prenatal visit, and repeated in the third trimester in high prevalence areas and seropositive women should be treated with a long-acting penicillin preparation (*Table 16.4*).

CLINICAL MANIFESTATIONS

Vasculitis and its consequences — necrosis and fibrosis — are the fundamental histologic lesions of congenital syphilis. Placental changes associated with congenital syphilis include proliferative vascular changes, chronic and sometimes acute villitis, and villous immaturity (*Figs 16.4* and *16.5*). *T. pallidum* can also be demonstrated in the amniotic fluid and histologically normal umbilical cord or placental tissue of asymptomatic seropositive newborns, confirming that they are infected (*Fig. 16.6*). About 5.6% of infants reported with congenital syphilis in the US are stillborn (*Fig. 16.7*).[20] Maceration is often associated with stillbirth due to congenital syphilis, but *T. pallidum* can be demonstrated even in fetuses with advanced autolysis (*Fig. 16.8*).

• Failure to receive prenatal care	29.1%
• Non-penicillin or other inadequate maternal treatment	52.2%
• Maternal treatment status unknown or equivocal	11.4%
• Inappropriate maternal serologic response to therapy, reinfection, treatment failure, other reasons	7.4%

Source: CDC. MMWR 1999: 48 757–761.

Table 16.3 Reasons for occurrence of congenital syphilis among US infants reported in 1998 (*n* = 801).

- Primary, secondary, early latent: Benzathine penicillin G 2.4 million units (MU) intramuscularly (IM) in a single dose. Late latent syphilis, latent syphilis of unknown duration, or tertiary syphilis (not neurosyphilis): Benzathine penicillin G 7.2 (MU) total, administered as three doses of 2.4 MU IM each at 1 week intervals
- Neurosyphilis: aqueous crystalline penicillin G 18–24 MU a day, administered as 3–4 MU intravenously every 4 hours for 10–14 days OR procaine penicillin 2.4 MU IM a day PLUS probenecid 500 mg orally four times a day, both for 10–14 days.

If patient is penicillin allergic, desensitize, and then treat with penicillin.

*Some experts recommend a second dose of benzathine penicillin 2.4 MU IM 1 week after the initial dose for women who have primary, secondary, or early latent syphilis. Ultrasonographic signs of fetal syphilis suggest greater risk for fetal treatment failure. Women with such signs should be managed in consultation with obstetric specialists. All persons with syphilis, and all pregnant women, should be offered testing for HIV infection.
Source: CDC 2002 STD Treatment Guidelines.

Table 16.4 Treatment of syphilis during pregnancy.

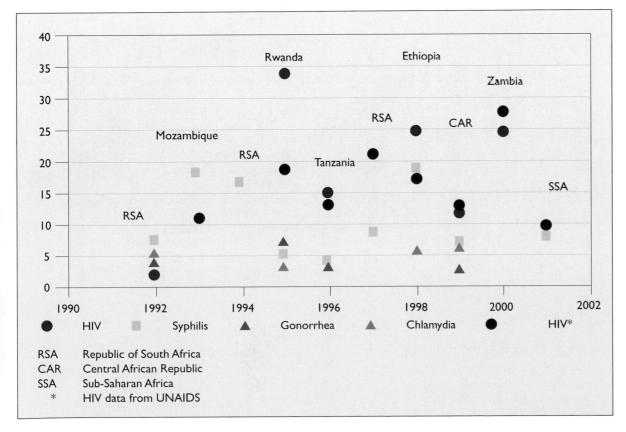

Fig. 16.3 Proportion of women enrolled in prenatal care in Africa with syphilis, gonorrhea, HIV or chlamydia, 1992–2001. Compiled from: Asseffa A, Ishak A, Stevens R *et al. Epidemiol & Infect* 1998; **120**: 171 177.

RSA	Republic of South Africa
CAR	Central African Republic
SSA	Sub-Saharan Africa
*	HIV data from UNAIDS

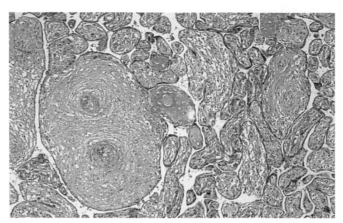

Fig. 16.4 Placental changes associated with congenital syphilis. Villi are enlarged and hypercellular, a typical finding of villous immaturity. Chronic villitis and proliferative vascular changes are also evident. Dense connective tissue almost obliterates the vessel lumen. Note villous immaturity, hypercellularity, chronic villitis, and vascular proliferation. Courtesy of F Qureshi, MD and S Jacques, MD.

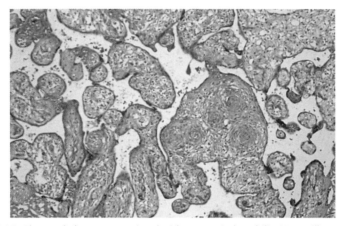

Fig. 16.5 Placental changes associated with congenital syphilis. Note villous immaturity, hypercellularity, chronic villitis, vascular proliferation, and compression of capillaries. Courtesy of F Qureshi, MD and S Jacques, MD.

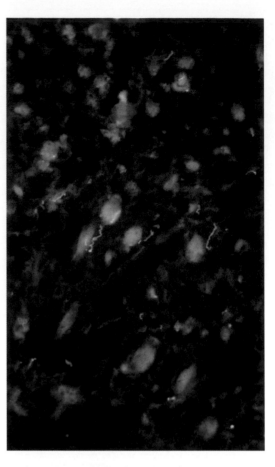

Fig. 16.6 Demonstration by direct fluorescent antibody technique of *Treponema pallidum* in histologically normal umbilical cord tissue from infant of a reactive mother diagnosed at delivery. Courtesy of D. Schwartz, MD.

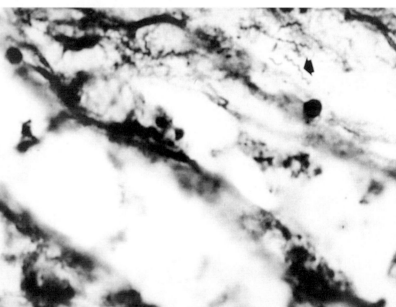

Fig. 16.8 Spirochetes (arrow) demonstrated by Warthin–Starry silver staining in autolyzed liver tissue of macerated stillbirth (x 1,000). Courtesy of Young SA, Crocker DW. *Arch Patha Lab Med* 1994; **118**: 44–47.

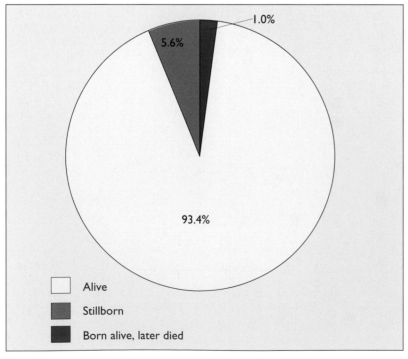

1.0%

5.6%

93.4%

- ☐ Alive
- Stillborn
- Born alive, later died

Fig. 16.7 Proportion of infants reported with congenital syphilis (CS), 1998, by whether the infant was alive or dead at time of report (*N*=801). Possible under-reporting of CS stillbirths may account for the low proportion of stillborn cases, relative to the natural history of CS. CDC. *MMWR* 1999; **48**: 757–761*.

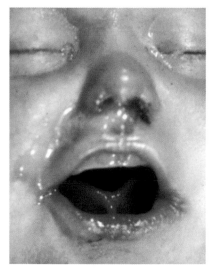
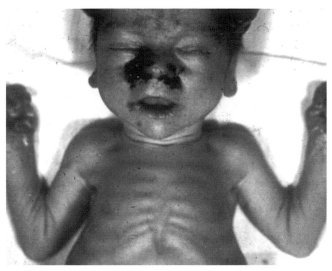

Fig. 16.9 and 16.10 Congenital syphilis. (**16.9**) Mucopurulent nasal discharge and (**16.10**) sanguinous nasal discharge in infants with snuffles. Courtesy of CDC Still Pictures Archives.

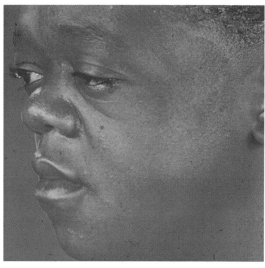

Fig. 16.11 Nasal deformity, 'saddle nose', typical of late congenital syphilis. Courtesy of CDC Still Pictures Archives.

Fig. 16.12 Proportion of infants with congenital syphilis (CS) exhibiting selected findings on physical examination, 1983-1986. Mean age of infants at time of report loas 1.6 months.

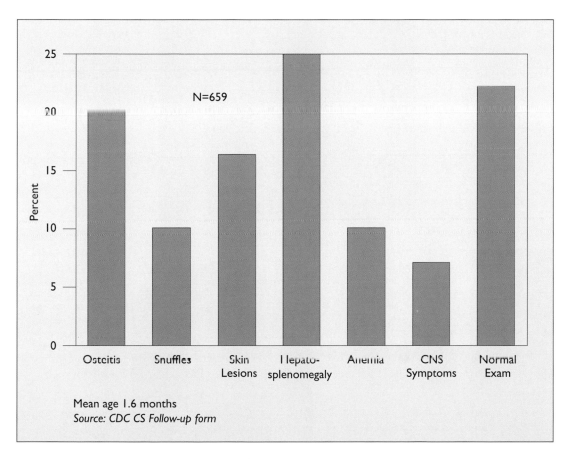

N=659

Mean age 1.6 months
Source: CDC CS Follow-up form

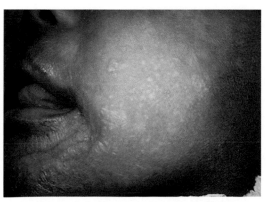
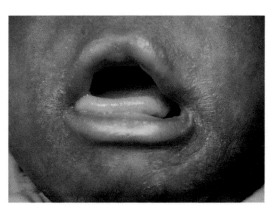
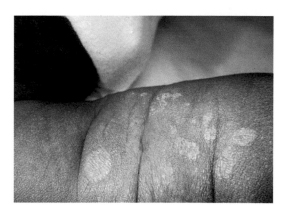

Figs 16.13–16.15 Congenital syphilis. (**16.13**) Lesions on cheeks and (**16.14**) perioral region, and ovoid and annular lesions (**16.15**) on upper legs of 6-week-old infant with congenital syphilis, who presented with upper respiratory tract symptoms, irritability, and rash. Courtesy of Tunnessen WW. *AJDC* 1992; **146**: 115–116.

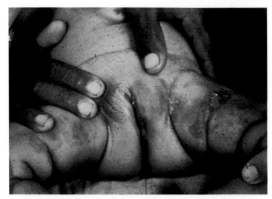

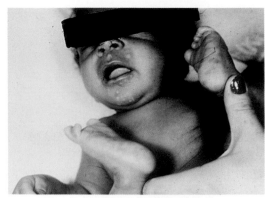

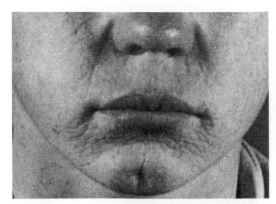

Fig. 16.16 Desquamative lesion on the thigh of an infant with dermal lesions due to congenital syphilis. Courtesy of Wood VD. *J Fam Pract* 1992; **35**: 327–329.

Fig. 16.17 Macular plantar rash in 2-month-old infant with congenital syphilis. Courtesy of CDC Still Pictures Archives.

Fig. 16.18 Radiating scars (rhagades) due to healing of fissures of mucous membranes at the mucocutaneous junction around the mouth. Courtesy of CDC Still Pictures Archives.

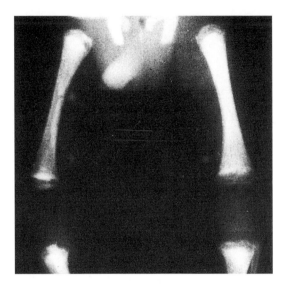

Fig. 16.19 Syphilitic metaphysitis in an infant. Note diminished density in the ends of the shaft and destruction at the proximal end of the tibia (right); this is known as the 'Wimberger sign'. Courtesy of Ilagan NB, Weyhing B, Liang KC, Womack SJ, Shankaran S. *Clin Pediatr* 1993; **32**:312–313.

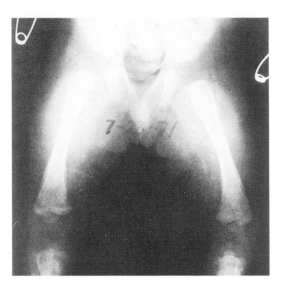

Fig. 16.20 Diaphyseal periostitis in long bones, presenting as a single-layered periosteal calcification, is the most characteristic feature of congenital syphilis in an infant. Courtesy of Ikeda MK, Jenson HB. *J Peds* 1990; **117**: 843–852.

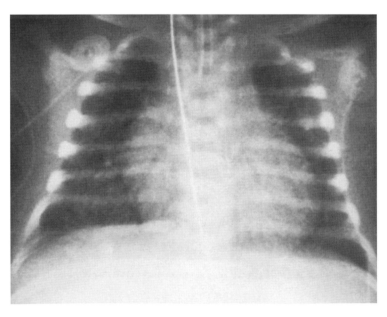

Fig. 16.21 Bilateral diffuse lung opacities in a newborn with pneumonia due to congenital syphilis. Courtesy of Edell DS, Davidson JJ, Mulvilhill DM, Majure M. *Ped Pulmon* 1993; **15**: 376–379.

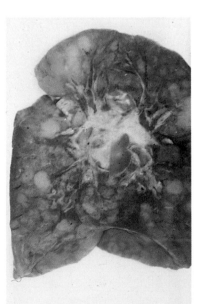

Fig. 16.22 Gross pathology of pneumonia alba in congenital syphilis. Lungs are enlarged, firm, and yellowish white in color. Courtesy of CDC Still Pictures Archives.

Most infants with early congenital syphilis are asymptomatic at birth.[1] If infection is not diagnosed by serologic testing at the time of delivery, the first signs of disease appear within the first 3–4 months – generally between 3–9 weeks of life. The earliest sign, occurring up to 14 days before cutaneous lesions, is an initially watery nasal discharge, which becomes mucopurulent, crusting, and sanguinous (*Figs 16.9* and *16.10*). This discharge, 'snuffles', may be teeming with spirochetes and can result in ulceration, chondritis, septal perforation, or formation of the saddle-nose deformity, which is typical of late congenital syphilis (*Fig. 16.11*). Mucocutaneous lesions occur in over 50% of infants in most series, and in 17% of US cases, most of whom are diagnosed as newborns (*Fig. 16.12*). The most common mucocutaneous lesions are large, round or ovoid, maculopapular or papulosquamous lesions, on the face, arms, and legs, which resolve over a period of 1–3 months with the formation of hyperpigmented patches (*Figs 16.13–16.15*). Vesicles, macular rashes and scaling may occur on the palms and soles with

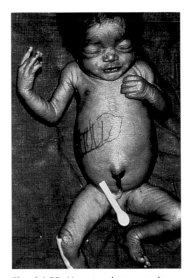

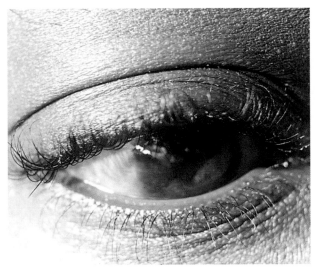

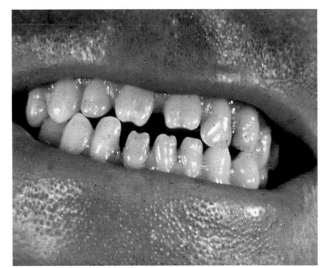

Fig. 16.23 Hepatosplenomegaly and jaundice in an infant with congenital syphilis. Courtesy of Jennifer Flood, MD.

Figs 16.24 and 16.25 Hutchinson's triad of late congenital syphilis: (**16.24**) interstitial keratitis; (**16.25**) Hutchinson's notched incisors; and deafness. Courtesy of CDC Still Pictures Archives.

NONTREPONEMAL	TREPONEMAL
Standard diagnostic tests	
Venereal Disease Research Laboratory (VDRL)	Fluorescent treponemal antibody (FTA)
	Fluorescent treponemal antibody absorbed (FTA-ABS)
Rapid plasma reagin (RPR)	Particle agglutination assay for antibody to *Treponema pallidum* (TP-PA)
	T. pallidum ELISA for IgG and IgM
Provisional and research tests	
VDRL ELISA for IqG and IgM	19S-IgM FTA-ABS
	T. pallidum Western blot
	Rabbit infectivity test (RIT)
	T. pallidum polymerase chain reaction (PCR)
	T. pallidum antigen-capture ELISA

Table 16.5 Serologic tests used for the diagnosis of congenital syphilis.

desquamation (*Figs 16.16–16.17*). Lesions on the lips, nostrils, and anus may become fissured and hemorrhagic and heal into radial scars, 'rhagades' (*Fig. 16.18*).

Symptomatic bone lesions with pseudoparalysis are uncommon. However, radiologic evidence of bone involvement is present in more than 90% of infants with confirmed congenital syphilis[21] (*Figs 16.19–16.20*). Pneumonia alba, so-called because of the whitish appearance of the lung at autopsy, is rare and typically presents as diffuse, patchy lung densities and respiratory distress (*Figs 16.21–16.22*). Hepatosplenomegaly and jaundice are common but nonspecific findings (*Fig. 16.23*). Late congenital syphilis may present with deafness, interstitial keratitis, and/or notched incisors (*Figs 16.24–16.25*).

The evaluation of newborns whose mothers may have had syphilis during pregnancy requires careful documentation of maternal and infant history, physical examination, and laboratory findings (*Fig. 16.26*). Currently used serologic tests for syphilis detect both IgG and IgM antibodies (*Table 16.5*)[22] During the third trimester, transplacental transfer of IgG into the fetal circulation may cause an uninfected newborn to become seroreactive by both nontreponemal tests, such as the Venereal Disease Research Laboratory (VDRL) and Rapid Plasma Reagin (RPR) tests, and/or treponemal tests, such as the fluorescent treponemal

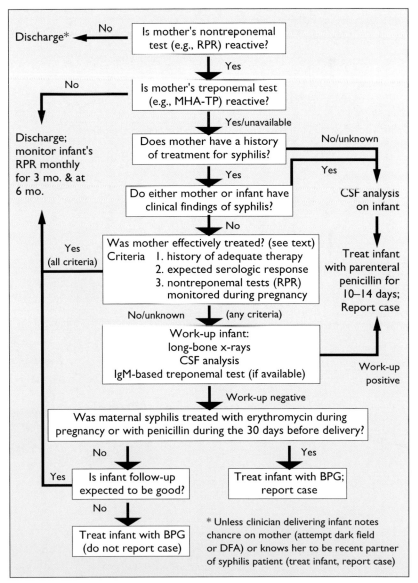

Fig. 16.26 Algorithm for evaluation of seropositive newborns. Courtesy of Zenker PN, Berman SM. Ped Infect Dis J 1991; **10**:516–522.

Aqueous crystalline penicillin G 100,000–150,000 units/kg/day, administered as 50,000 units/kg/dose IV every 12 hours during the 7 days of life, and every 8 hours thereafter for a total of 10 days;

OR

Procaine penicillin G 50,000 units/kg/dose IM a day in a single dose for 10 days.

Benzathine penicillin G 50,000 units/kg (single dose IM) if the infant's evaluation (i.e., CSF examination, long-bone radiographs, and CBC with platelets) is normal and follow-up is certain. If any part of the infant's evaluation is abnormal or not done, or the CSF analysis is uninterpretable, 10-day course of penicillin is required.

If the infant's nontreponemal test is nonreactive and the likelihood of the infant being infected is low, some experts recommend no evaluation but treatment of the infant with

Benzathine penicillin G 50,000 units/kg (single dose IM) for possible incubating syphilis, after which the infant should have close serologic follow-up.

Evaluation is unnecessary if the maternal treatment a) was during pregnancy, appropriate for the stage of infection, and >4 weeks before delivery; b) was for early syphilis and the nontreponemal serologic titers decreased fourfold after appropriate therapy; or c) was for late latent infection, the nontreponemal titers remained stable and low, and there is no evidence of maternal reinfection or relapse, recommend treatment with:

Benzathine penicillin G 50,000 units/kg single dose IM

(Note: Some experts would not treat the infant but would provide close observation)

Source: CDC 2001 STD Treatment Guidelines.

Table 16.6 Treatment of congenital syphilis in the newborn or infant.

antibody absorption (FTA-ABS) test, *T. pallidum* assay hemagglutination (TPHA) or the *T. pallidum* particle agglutination assay (TP-PA).

TREATMENT

The recommended treatment for congenital syphilis in the neonate is aqueous penicillin G, 50,000 units/kg per dose intravenously every 12 hours during the first 7 days of life and every 8 hours thereafter for a total of 10 days intravenously (*Table 16.6*).[19] Procaine penicillin G, 50,000 units/kg/dose in a single daily dose intramuscularly for 10 days is considered equivalent. Benzathine penicillin G should be used only for asymptomatic infants with a low likelihood of being infected, and only if follow-up can be ensured, because treatment failures with the use of this regimen for asymptomatic newborns with congenital syphilis have been reported (*Table 16.6*).[18]

GONOCOCCAL INFECTIONS

EPIDEMIOLOGY

The incidence of gonorrhea among pregnant US women aged 15–24 years screened in 1999 ranged from less than 0.1% to 4.1% (*Fig. 16.27*).[3] In some prenatal populations in developing countries in the 1990s, incidence rates as high as 7.0% have been recorded (*Fig. 16.3*).

VERTICAL TRANSMISSION

Gonococcal infection is rarely transmitted through intact placental membranes. Contact with an infected birth canal is the most common way in which infection is transmitted to the child. The risk of trans-

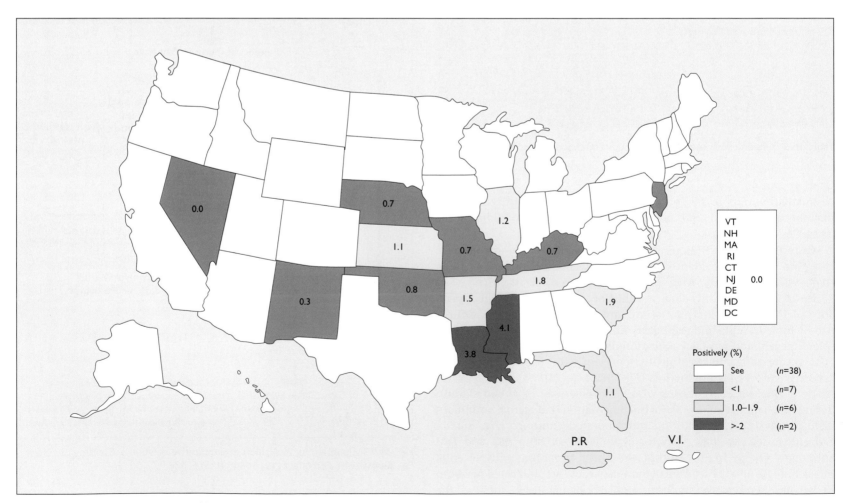

Fig. 16.27 Proportion of 15–24-year-old women in prenatal clinics in the US tested for gonorrhea whose tests were positive. Courtesy of DSTDP STD Surveillance 1999, CDC Atlanta, GA, 2000.

mission in the absence of prophylaxis is estimated at 30–50%. The vertical transmission rate is higher among mothers with concomitant chlamydial infection (68% versus 31%), endometritis, prolonged rupture of membranes, and possibly, when application of ocular prophylaxis is delayed.

PREVENTION

PRENATAL SCREENING
The most important strategy in the prevention of vertical transmission is screening of pregnant women by culture and treatment of all those found positive at their first prenatal visit, or at other opportunities, if not enrolled in prenatal care.[19] Nucleic-acid amplification tests may offer increased sensitivity for detecting the presence of *N. gonorrhoeae* in anogenital specimens.

TREATMENT OF PREGNANT WOMEN WITH GONORRHEA
Pregnant women who are diagnosed with uncomplicated gonococcal infections, or who are the sexual partners of men with gonorrhea, should be treated with a β-lactamase stable cephalosporin as a single dose[19,23] (*Table 16.7*). All recommended cephalosporins are generally effective against pharyngeal gonorrhea, which is important because pharyngeal infection may be more frequent in pregnant women than in other women. Women who cannot tolerate cephalosporins should be treated with spectinomycin, and should have a pharyngeal culture 3–5 days after treatment, as this regimen is only 52% effective in eradicating pharyngeal infections. Women with gonorrhea should also be treated presumptively for *C. trachomatis* (*Table 16.7*).

OCULAR PROPHYLAXIS AT BIRTH
The use of neonatal silver nitrate ocular prophylaxis has resulted in a dramatic reduction in neonatal gonococcal disease.[24,25] Ocular prophylaxis should be performed as soon after birth as possible in the delivery room, ideally before the infant opens her/his eyes (*Table 16.8*).

CLINICAL MANIFESTATIONS

GONOCOCCAL OPHTHALMIA NEONATORUM
The most common manifestation of infant gonococcal infection is ophthalmia neonatorum.[26,27] Arthritis, sepsis and meningitis are far less common. Before the introduction of silver nitrate prophylaxis in 1880, the incidence of gonococcal ophthalmia neonatorum varied from 1–4%, while up to 79% of children in institutions for the blind had a history of gonococcal ophthalmia. A seasonal incidence of the disease has been reported (*Fig. 16.28*).

The severity of gonococcal ophthalmia ranges from a mild conjunctivitis similar to chemical conjunctivitis, to corneal ulceration, perforation and blindness. Gonococcal ophthalmia neonatorum is most often seen 4–7 days after birth (range 1–28 days) (*Fig. 16.29*).[23–27] Typically, the disease is bilateral and the discharge purulent (*Figs 16.30* and *16.31*). Gonococcal ophthalmia tends to be more severe in terms of palpebral edema, conjunctival injection, and purulent discharge than ophthalmia caused by *C. trachomatis* and ophthalmia not attributable to either pathogen. If Gram-negative diplococci are found in the conjunctival exudate, the likelihood of gonococcal opthalmia is very high, justifying presumptive treatment for gonorrhea after appropriate cultures for *N. gonorrhoeae* are obtained.

The severe inflammation of the conjunctivae may be associated with a serosanguinous exudate and may produce inflammatory membranes; these membranes are replaced by scar tissue in the conjunctivae as the disease resolves (*Fig. 16.32*). Corneal involvement presents initially as a diffuse epithelial edema, giving the cornea a hazy, smoky-gray appearance, and often results in blindness due to involvement of the

---

Pregnant women should not be treated with quinolones or tetracyclines. They should be treated with a recommended or alternate cephalosporin. Women who cannot tolerate a cephalosporin should be administered a single 2-g dose of spectinomycin IM. Either erythromycin or amoxicillin is recommended for treatment of presumptive or diagnosed *C. trachomatis* infection during pregnancy.

Cefixime 400 mg orally in a single dose,

OR

Ceftriaxone 125 mg IM in a single dose,

PLUS

Erythromycin base 500 mg orally four times a day for 7 days,

OR

Amoxicillin 500 mg orally three times a day for 7 days.

OR

Erythromycin base 250 mg orally four times a day for 14 days,

OR

Erythromycin ethylsuccinate 800 mg orally four times a day for 7 days,

OR

Erythromycin ethylsuccinate 400 mg orally four times a day for 14 days,

OR

Azithromycin 1 g orally in a single dose.

Note: Erythromycin estolate is contraindicated during pregnancy because of drug-related hepatotoxicity. Preliminary data indicate that azithromycin may be safe and effective. However, data are insufficient to recommend the routine use of azithromycin in pregnant women.

Source: CDC 2002 Treatment Guidelines.

Table 16.7 Treatment of gonorrhea during pregnancy.

Silver nitrate (1%) aqueous solution in a single application,

OR

Erythromycin (0.5%) ophthalmic ointment in a single application,

OR

Tetracycline ophthalmic ointment (1%) in a single application.

One of these recommended preparations should be instilled into both eyes of every neonate as soon as possible after delivery. If prophylaxis is delayed (i.e., not administered in the delivery room), a monitoring system should be established to ensure that all infants receive prophylaxis. All infants should be administered ocular prophylaxis, regardless of whether delivery is vaginal or cesarian. Single-use tubes or ampules are preferable to multiple-use tubes. Bacitracin is not effective. Povidone iodine has not been studied adequately.

CDC 2002 STD Treatment Guidelines.

Table 16.8 Ocular prophylaxis for the prevention of opthalmia neonatorum.

central cornea (*Fig. 16.33*). The prevalence of corneal involvement with residual scarring in neonates has been reported to be as high as 16%, but in other series and case reports, no evidence of corneal involvement has been noted.

DISSEMINATED GONOCOCCAL INFECTION
In most cases, gonococcal infection in newborns is localized, though cough, irritability or poor feeding may accompany gonococcal

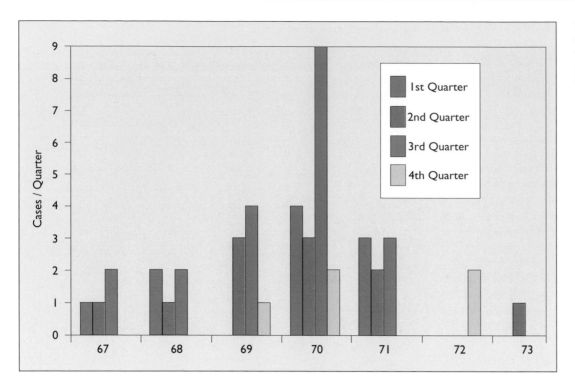

Fig. 16.28 Seasonal incidence of gonococcal ophthalmia neonatorum, showing peak occurrence in the third quarter of the year, Grady Memorial Hospital, Atlanta, GA, 1967–1973. Control measures were instituted in 1971. Courtesy of Armstrong JH, Zacarias F, Rein MF. *Pediatrics* 1976; **57**: 884–892.

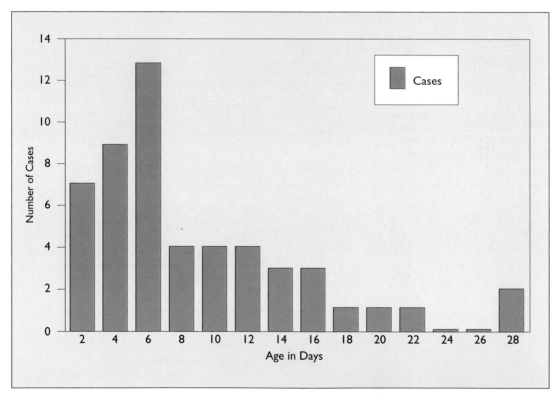

Fig. 16.29 Cases of neonatal gonococcal ophthalmia, by age in days at diagnosis, National Gonococcal Study, Florida, 1984–1988. Note that most are diagnosed in the first week of life. Courtesy of Desenclos JCA, Garrity D, Scaggs M, Wroten JE. *Sex Transm Dis* 1992; **19**: 10539.

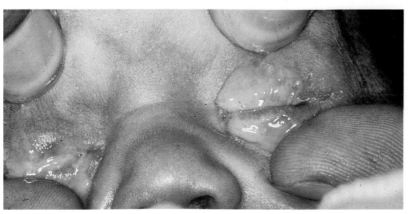
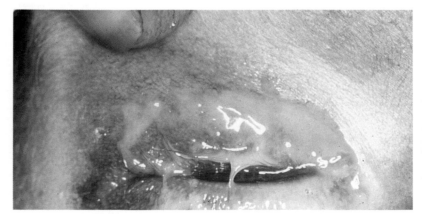

Figs. 16.30 and 16.31 Gonococcal ophthalmia. (**16.30**) Bilateral gonococcal ophthalmia in a 5-day-old infant. (**16.31**) Note purulent discharge. Courtesy of CDC Still Pictures Archives.

conjunctivitis.[23] Nonspecific symptoms commencing within 1–2 weeks of birth, including fever, irritability, and poor feeding, however, often herald the onset of dissemination. Sepsis, arthritis, meningitis or any combination of these are rare complications of neonatal gonococcal infection. Localized gonococcal infection of the scalp might result from fetal monitoring through scalp electrodes. Detection of gonococcal infection in neonates who have sepsis, arthritis, meningitis, or scalp abscesses requires cultures of blood, cerebrospinal fluid (CSF) and synovial or abscess fluid on chocolate agar.

TREATMENT

Infants born to mothers with untreated gonorrhea are at substantial risk of infection, even if ocular prophylaxis is applied, and should be evaluated with orogastric, vaginal, rectal, and blood cultures if they have signs suggestive of sepsis. If there is no evidence of gonococcal infection, such infants should be treated with ceftriaxone, 25–50 mg/kg intravenously or intramuscularly in a single dose[19] (Table 16.9).

Infants with conjunctivitis should have specimens taken from the conjunctivae, for Gram stain, culture on chocolate agar for *N. gonorrhoeae* and for detection of *C. trachomatis*. Culture is essential to confirm in vitro susceptibility to antimicrobials used, and the laboratory should perform confirmatory testing to differentiate *N. gonorrhoeae* from *Branhamella catarrhalis* and other *Neisseria* species that can mimic *N. gonorrhoeae* on Gram staining (*see Ch. 6*).[19,23] Patients with corneal involvement should have corneal cultures and Gram stains and be managed promptly in consultation with an ophthalmologist.

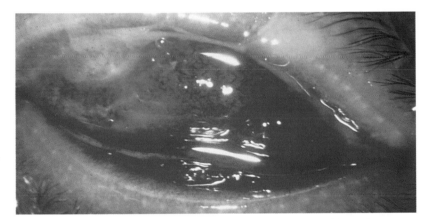

Fig. 16.32 Inflammation of the conjunctiva, with sanguinous exudate and inflammatory membrane which bleeds in response to attempts to remove it. Courtesy of CDC Still Pictures Archives.

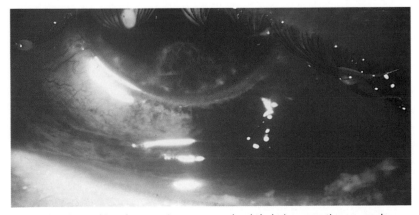

Fig. 16.33 Corneal involvement in gonococcal ophthalmia presenting as smoky, grey haziness in the peripheral cornea, resulting in partial blindness. Courtesy of CDC Still Pictures Archives.

CHLAMYDIAL INFECTIONS

EPIDEMIOLOGY

C. trachomatis is probably the most common sexually transmitted bacterial pathogen in US prenatal populations, ranging from 4.5–14.4% of women tested[3] (*Fig. 16.34*). In some developing countries, the prevalence appears to be lower than the prevalence of gonorrhea, syphilis and HIV (*Fig. 16.3*), possibly related to the use of less-sensitive tests, or other factors. Cervical gonorrhea is a significant predictor for endocervical *C. trachomatis* infection among women. Core groups, such as have been described for gonorrhea, have not been described for chlamydial infections;

Prophylactic treatment for infants whose mothers have gonococcal infection in the absence of signs of gonococcal Infection in the infant:

Ceftriaxone 25–50 mg/kg IV or IM, not to exceed 125 mg, in a single dose.

Neonatal gonococcal conjunctivitis:

Ceftriaxone 25–50 mg/kg IV or IM in a single dose, not to exceed 125 mg.

Disseminated gonococcal infection, gonococcal scalp abscess in newborns recommended regimens:

Ceftriaxone 25–50 mg/kg/day IV or IM in a single daily dose for 7 days, with a duration of 10–14 days if meningitis is documented;

OR

Cefotaxime 25 mg/kg IV or IM every 12 hours for 7 days, with a duration of 10–14 days if meningitis is documented.

Source: CDC 2002 STD Treatment Guidelines.

Table 16.9 Recommended treatment for infants exposed to or diagnosed with *Neisseria gonorrhoeae* infection.

Doxycycline and ofloxacin are contraindicated for pregnant women. Data are insufficient to recommend the routine use of azithromycin in pregnant women. However, clinical experience of some experts and preliminary data suggest that azithromycin is safe and effective. Repeat testing, preferably by culture, 3 weeks after completion of therapy with the following regimens is recommended, because a) these regimens may not be highly efficacious and b) the frequent side effects of erythromycin might discourage patient adherence to this regimen.

Erythromycin base 500 mg orally four times a day for 7 days,

OR

Amoxicillin 500 mg orally three times a day for 7 days.

Alternative regimens for pregnant women

Erythromycin base 250 mg orally four times a day for 14 days,

OR

Erythromycin ethylsuccinate 800 mg orally four times a day for 7 days,

OR

Erythromycin ethylsuccinate 400 mg orally four times a day for 14 days,

OR

Azithromycin 1 g orally in a single dose.

Note: Erythromycin estolate is contraindicated during pregnancy because of drug-related hepatotoxicity.

Source: CDC 2002 STD Treatment Guidelines.

Table 16.10 Recommended regimens for pregnant women infected with *Chlamydia trachomatis*.

these infections are broadly dispersed geographically and socio-economically. Adolescents and young adults tend to have the highest prevalence, as high as 37% of women screened.[28] Those serovars of *C. trachomatis* associated with sexually transmitted cervicitis and urethritis in sexually active adults are also associated with perinatally transmitted conjunctivitis, pneumonia, and other chlamydial syndromes. Maternal chlamydial infection may be associated with adverse pregnancy outcomes.

VERTICAL TRANSMISSION

Neonates often acquire *C. trachomatis* during delivery through an infected birth canal, occurring in approximately 50% of infants born vaginally to infected mothers, and in a few delivered by cesarean section. The risk of conjunctivitis is 25–50% and that of pneumonia is 5% to 20% in infants who acquire *C. trachomatis*.[28–30] Symptoms in the mother may tend to increase the risk of vertical transmission. Women with recent chlamydial infections are at higher risk of delivering low-birthweight infants than women with chronic infections. Infection can persist in the conjunctivae, nasopharynx, and oropharynx for over 2 years; up to 70% of infants have some evidence of infection, including rhinitis, pharyngitis, and possibly, otitis media. Asymptomatic anogenital infection occurs in up to 15% of infants born to infected mothers.

PREVENTION

Prenatal care, particularly for those populations at highest risk (including adolescent and other women < 25 years of age), should include screening for cervical chlamydial infection. Cervical screening with nucleic acid amplification tests (NAATs), such as polymerase chain reaction (PCR)[30] or ligase chain reaction (LCR), should be performed during the third trimester, to reduce chances for reinfection and to ensure treatment before delivery. NAATs are more sensitive than cell culture, and are more sensitive and specific than non-amplified DNA probes and other non-culture tests. Maternal treatment with an erythromycin base is recommended, though amoxicillin may be administered to those unable to tolerate erythromycin base[19] (*Table 16.10*).

Silver nitrate prophylaxis is not as effective in preventing chlamydial conjunctivitis as it is in preventing gonococcal conjunctivitis. Studies on the clinical efficacy of erythromycin and of tetracycline ointment of prophylaxis have been conflicting. However, prophylaxis effective for gonococcal ophthalmia is recommended[19] (*Table 16.8*).

CLINICAL MANIFESTATIONS

CONJUNCTIVITIS AND OPHTHALMIA NEONATORUM

C. trachomatis is the most common infectious cause of neonatal conjunctivitis, and conjunctivitis is the most common presentation of symptomatic perinatal *C. trachomatis* infection in infants.[28] Although a wide range of severity exists, chlamydial conjunctivitis tends to be milder than gonococcal conjunctivitis, and does not progress to corneal scarring or blindness, or present with adenopathy. It is more likely to be unilateral, at least initially. Chlamydial conjunctivitis generally presents in the second to third week of life, commonly with pseudomembrane formation and a diffuse matte infection of the tarsal conjunctiva (*Fig. 16.35*). A seasonal variation has been reported (*Fig. 16.36*).

All infants who present with conjunctivitis in the first 30 days of life should be evaluated for chlamydial conjunctivitis.[19,28] Specimens for

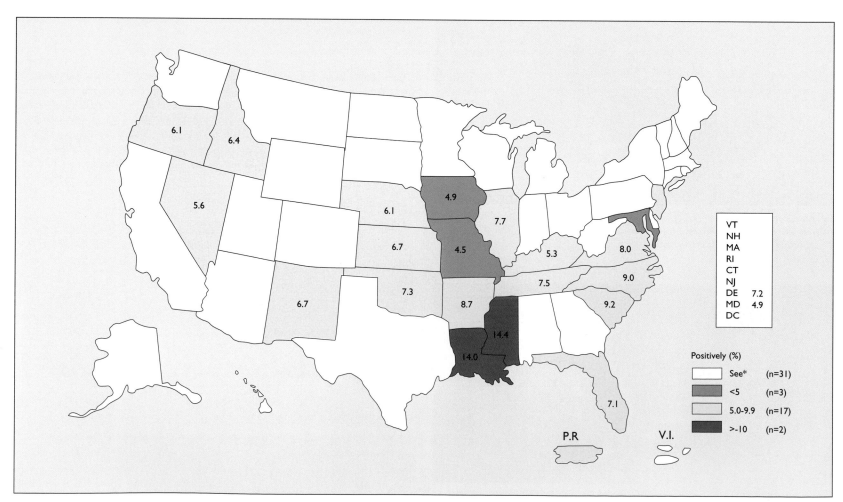

Fig. 16.34 Proportion of 15–24-year-old women in prenatal clinics in the US tested for *Chlamydia trachomatis* whose tests were positive. Courtesy of DSTDP STD Surveillance 1999, CDC Atlanta, GA, 2000.

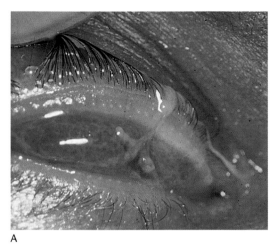
A

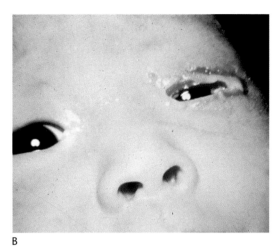
B

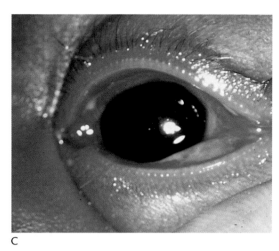
C

Fig. 16.35 Chlamydial conjunctivitis presenting with pseudomembrane formation and diffuse matte injection of the conjunctivae (left), with purulent conjunctivitis clinically indistinguishable from gonococcal conjunctivitis (center), and more typical mucopurulent ocular discharge (right). Courtesy of J. Schachter.

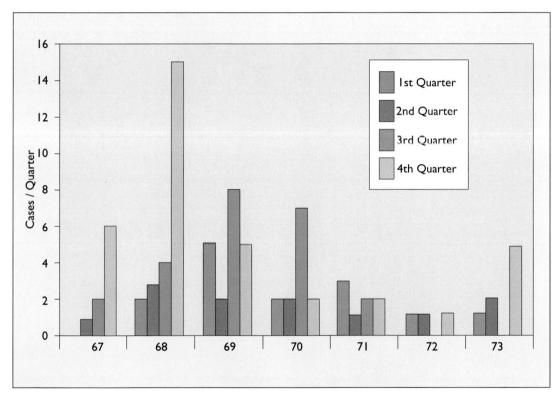

Fig. 16.36 Seasonal variation chlamydial ophthalmia neonatorum, Grady Memorial Hospital, Atlanta, GA, 1967–1973, before institution of control measures. Courtesy of Armstrong JH, Zacarias F, Rein MF. *Pediatrics* 1976; **57**: 884–892.

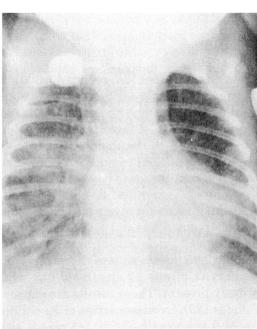

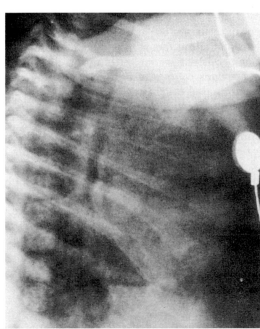

Fig. 16.37 Hyperinflation with flattening of the diaphragm and diffuse interstitial infiltrates in the anteroposterior (left) and lateral (right) views of a chest radiograph of a severely ill newborn with chlamydial pneumonia. Courtesy of Harrison HR, Alexander ER. In: Holmes KK, Mardh PA, Sparling PF, Wiesner PJ (eds): *Sexually Transmitted Diseases*. McGraw Hill Book Co., New York, pp 270–280, 1984.

diagnosis by culture should contain conjunctival cells, not exudate alone, and should be obtained from the everted eyelid using a dacron-tipped swab. Tests for detection of chlamydial antigen or specific nucleic acid sequences can also be used to test conjunctival specimens (*see Chapter 4*).

PNEUMONIA

Chlamydial neonatal pneumonia typically presents at 3–11 weeks of age with a history of prolonged congestion and cough.[28,30–32] Generally, infants are afebrile and do not show signs of significant systemic illness. Tachypnea and rales are common physical findings. Although con-

junctivitis and a pertussis-like staccato cough are not usually part of the typical presentation, these findings should alert the physician to the possibility of *C. trachomatis* pneumonia; hyperinflation with diffuse interstitial infiltrates are frequently seen (*Fig. 16.37*). An eosinophilia and elevations of serum IgG and IgM are common non-specific signs of *C. trachomatis* pneumonia.

C. trachomatis pneumonia should be considered in all cases of pneumonia in the first 3 months of life (*Table 16.11*). Nasopharyngeal and tracheal aspirates or lung biopsy specimens, if collected, should be cultured for *C. trachomatis*, since non-culture tests have not been evaluated extensively for detection of *C. trachomatis* in nasopharyngeal specimens, and some may be falsely negative. However, a positive non-culture test in the presence of a compatible clinical picture can be used to make a specific diagnosis.[28] *C. trachomatis* specific IgM at a titer of ≥ 1:32 is strongly suggestive of chlamydial neonatal pneumonia.

	CHLAMYDIA-POSITIVE	CHLAMYDIA-NEGATIVE
Presentation at 3–11 weeks	53/57 (93%)	19/42 (45%)
Prodrome more than 1 week	45/57 (79%)	17/42 (40%)
Conjunctivitis	26/57 (46%)	5/39 (13%)
Ear abnormalities	24/41 (59%)	0/15 (0%)
Staccato cough	24/41 (59%)	4/15 (27%)
Wheeze	9/57 (16%)	14/32 (44%)
Rales	14/16 (88%)	14/27 (52%)

Table 16.11 Characteristics of *C. trachomatis* pneumonia including short prodrome, rales, and early presentation.

Erythromycin base or ethyl succinate 50 mg/kg/day orally divided into four doses daily for 14 days.

Follow-up of infants is recommended to determine whether the pneumonia has resolved.

Source: CDC 2002 STD Treatment Guidelines.

Table 16.12 Recommended treatments for perinatally acquired infant *Chlamydia trachomatis* infection, including ophthalmia, pneumonia, and others.

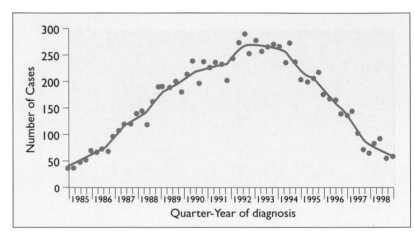

Fig. 16.38 Cases of perinatally acquired immunodeficiency syndrome (AIDS) among infants and children, by quarter of report, 1985–1999. Courtesy of DHAP, CDC, Pediatric HIV Surveillance.

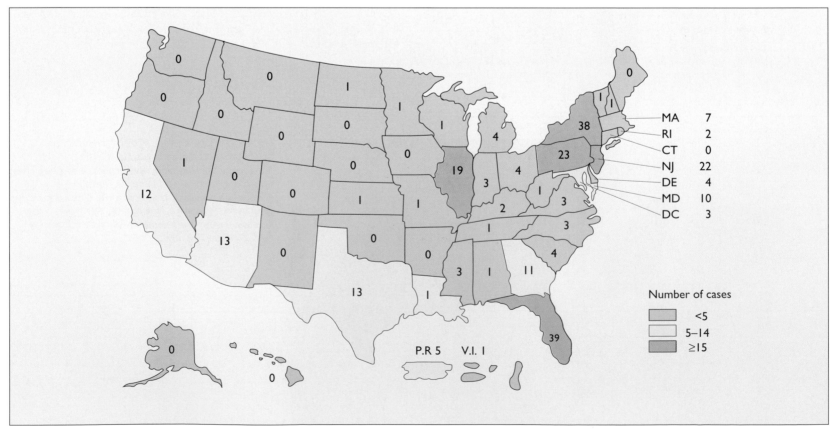

Fig. 16.39 Cases of pediatric AIDS reported, by state, USA, 1999. N=263 Note the marked geographic variation. Courtesy of Division of HIV AIDS Prevention, CDC, Pediatric HIV Surveillance.

OTHER CLINICAL MANIFESTATIONS

Chronic respiratory disease characterized by chronic cough, wheezing, and abnormal functional residual capacity occurs in a small proportion of infected infants. Otitis media, rhinitis, and upper respiratory infections due to *C. trachomatis* can also occur in the first year of life.

TREATMENT

Systemic erythromycin should be used to treat chlamydial conjunctivitis and pneumonia, and other infections due to *C. trachomatis* in infants; prophylactic antibiotic treatment is not indicated[19,28] (*Table 16.12*). There appears to be an increased risk of hypertrophic pyloric stenosis associated with use of erythromycin in infancy; a high index of suspicion is indicated. The effectiveness of systemic treatment for *C. trachomatis* infection in infants is approximately 80%, and a second course may be needed. Topical antibiotic therapy alone is inadequate to treat chlamydial ophthalmic infections and is unnecessary when systemic treatment is given.

HUMAN IMMUNODEFICIENCY VIRUS (HIV)

EPIDEMIOLOGY

Acquired immunodeficiency syndrome (AIDS) cases among infants and children have accounted for as many as 2% of all reported cases in the US.[33] Since the beginning of the AIDS epidemic, 8,718 children have been reported with AIDS; the majority of these children (91%) were infected perinatally. In 1999, 263 children were reported to CDC with AIDS, a marked decrease from 382 in 1998.[34-37] The number of cases due to perinatally acquired HIV infection had increased much more rapidly than cases due to other causes. However, since the introduction of prenatal and perinatal maternal treatment, and treatment of the newborn,[34] the number of perinatally infected infants born each year, and of infected infants progressing to AIDS, has declined by 75% in the years from 1993 to 1999[37] (*Fig. 16.38*). Of children reported in 1999, 88% acquired HIV perinatally; 4% from a blood or blood product transfusion, 3% because of blood product exposure due to hemophilia and 2% due to 'other or not reported exposure'. Of 147 due to other or not reported exposures, 12 (8%) had sexual contact with an adult with HIV infection.[37] The geographic distribution of pediatric AIDS cases in the USA (*Fig. 16.39*) closely reflects the distribution of HIV infection among child-bearing women. Three states (New York, New Jersey, Florida) have reported 50% of all pediatric AIDS cases.[37] In 1994, the prevalence of HIV infection was 1.6/1000 US women delivering live-born infants. In Florida, the prevalence was 4.6 and in Washington D.C., 6.9. In Sub-Saharan Africa, HIV seroprevalence in pregnant women has risen quickly from very low levels to >30% in some areas. (*Fig. 16.3, Fig. 16.40*).[12] In these same areas, over 50% of infant mortality is related to perinatally acquired HIV infection.

VERTICAL TRANSMISSION

The prevalence of HIV infection among infants born to infected mothers ranges from 13–39%.[33] The exact timing of transmission is uncertain; probably, 20–30% occuring before birth, and about 70% occuring during delivery. About 66% of transmissions before birth occur within 14 days of delivery. Breast-feeding has been demonstrated to have a risk of over 16%, and in some populations may account for over 40% of all transmissions. Breast feeding may be associated with a higher risk of mortality among HIV-infected women.[38] A number of maternal factors are associated with increased risk of perinatal HIV transmission. The highest transmission risk appears to be associated with advanced maternal disease, typically with repeatedly positive blood cultures, high viral loads and low CD4+ lymphocyte counts. Infants born after prolonged rupture of maternal membranes, vaginal delivery, complicated deliveries, or the first born of twins are more likely to be infected.[33,39,40] There is evidence that intrauterine infection does occur; HIV has been isolated from fetal and placental tissue as early as the first trimester as well as from cord blood of infants.

PREVENTION

In 1994, zidovudine was demonstrated to substantially reduce perinatal transmission of HIV. Guidelines regarding the use of zidovudine to reduce transmission (*Table 16.13*) and regarding counseling and testing of pregnant women were issued in 1994 and 1995, respectively (*Table 16.14*). The widespread implementation of recommendations to offer testing to all pregnant women, and to offer prophylaxis as needed, has resulted in marked declines in the number of infected infants, but over 200 cases still occur yearly in the US.

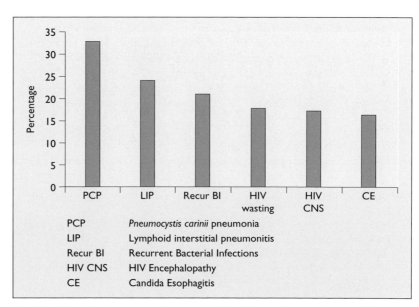

Fig. 16.40 HIV seroprevalence among STD clinic attenders (Johannesburg), and antenatal clinic attenders (South Africa). Courtesy R.C. Ballard, PhD.

PCP	*Pneumocystis carinii* pneumonia
LIP	Lymphoid interstitial pneumonitis
Recur BI	Recurrent Bacterial Infections
HIV CNS	HIV Encephalopathy
CE	Candida Esophagitis

Fig. 16.41 Relative frequency of selected AIDS-defining illnesses in perinatally acquired HIV infection reported through June 1993, USA (*N* = 4,004). Courtesy of Division of HIV AIDS Prevention, CDC, Pediatric HIV Surveillance, 1999.

- Oral administration of 100 mg of zidovudine (ZDV) five times daily, initiated at 14–34 weeks of gestation and continued throughout the pregnancy.
- During labor, intravenous administration of ZDV in a 1-hour loading dose 2 mg per kg of body weight, followed by a continuous infusion of 1 mg per kg of body weight per hour until delivery.
- Oral administration of ZDV syrup to the newborn at 2 mg per kg of body weight per dose every 6 hours for the first 6 weeks of life, beginning 8–12 hours after birth.

CDC. MMWR 1994; 43: 1–2.

Table 16.13 Zidovudine regimen used in the AIDS Clinical Trials Group Protocol 076 and recommended for prevention of HIV mother to child transmission in the United States.

Pre-Test Counseling
1. HIV testing of pregnant women and their infants should be voluntary.
2. Health-care providers should counsel and offer HIV testing to women as early in pregnancy as possible.
3. The prevalence of HIV infection may be higher in women who have not received prenatal care. These women should be assessed promptly for HIV infection.
4. Pregnant women should be provided access to other HIV prevention and treatment.

Interpretation of HIV Test Results
1. HIV antibody testing should be performed according to the recommended algorithm
2. HIV infection (as indicated by the presence of antibody to HIV) is defined as a repeatedly reactive EIA and a positive confirmatory supplemental test.
3. Confirmation or exclusion of HIV infection in a person with indeterminate test results should be made not only on the basis of HIV antibody test results, but with consideration of a) the person's medical and behavioral history, b) results from additional virologic and immunologic tests when performed, and c) clinical follow-up
4. Pregnant women who have repeatedly reactive EIA and indeterminate supplemental tests should be retested immediately for HIV antibody to distinguish between recent seroconversion and a negative test result.

Recommendations for HIV-Infected Pregnant Women
1. HIV-infected pregnant women should receive counseling services.
2. HIV-infected pregnant women should be evaluated to assess their need for antiretroviral therapy, antimicrobial prophylaxis, and treatment of other conditions. Medical management of HIV infection is essentially the same for pregnant and nonpregnant women.
3. HIV-infected women should be provided information concerning ZDV therapy to reduce the risk for perinatal HIV transmission.
4. HIV-infected pregnant women should receive information about all reproductive options.
5. HIV-infected women should be advised against breastfeeding.
6. To optimize medical management, HIV test results should be available in her and her infant's confidential medical file.
7. Counseling for HIV-infected pregnant women should include an assessment of the potential for negative effects resulting from HIV infection
8. HIV testing for any of their children born after they became infected or after 1977.

Recommendations for Follow-up of Infected Women and Perinatally Exposed Children
1. Following pregnancy, HIV-infected women should be provided ongoing HIV-related medical care.
2. Follow-up for their children
3. Medical and social services to focus on the needs of the entire family.

CDC. MMWR 1995; 44: 1–15.

Table 16.14 Recommendations for HIV counseling and voluntary testing for pregnant women.

DIAGNOSIS: HIV INFECTED
a. A child <18 months of age who is known to be HIV seropositive or born to an HIV-infected mother and has positive results on two separate determinations (excluding cord blood) from one or more of the following HIV detection tests: HIV culture, HIV polymerase chain reaction, HIV antigen (p24), or meets criteria for acquired immunodeficiency syndrome (AIDS) diagnosis based on the 1987 AIDS surveillance case definition.
b. A child ≥18 months of age born to an HIV-infected mother or any child infected by blood, blood products, or other known mode of transmission (e.g., sexual contact) who is HIV-antibody positive by repeatedly reactive enzyme immunoassay (EIA) and confirmatory test (e.g., Western blot or immunofluorescence assay {IFA}); or meets any of the criteria in a) above.

DIAGNOSIS: PERINATALLY EXPOSED
A child who does not meet the criteria above who:
a. is HIV seropositive by EIA and confirmatory test (e.g., Western blot or IFA) and
b. is <18 months of age at the time of test; or
c. has unknown antibody status, but was born to a mother known to be infected with HIV.

DIAGNOSIS: SEROREVERTER
A child who is born to an HIV-infected mother and who has been documented as HIV-antibody negative (i.e., two or more negative EIA tests performed at 6–18 months of age or one negative EIA test after 18 months of age); and has had no other laboratory evidence of infection (has not had two positive viral detection tests, if performed); and has not had an AIDS-defining condition.

*Source: CDC. MMWR 1994; 43(RR12):1–10. *This definition of HIV infection replaces the definition published in the 1987 AIDS surveillance case definition.*

Table 16.15 Diagnosis of human immunodeficiency virus (HIV) infection in children*.

CLINICAL MANIFESTATIONS

Although some studies in the United States and Europe suggest more spontaneous abortions among women with HIV infection, in general, studies in developed countries do not consistently show an association between HIV and adverse outcomes of pregnancy (*Table 16.1*). However, in developing countries, preterm birth, low birthweight, and premature rupture of membranes have all been associated with maternal HIV infection. The failure to detect an association in developed countries may be the result of the recruitment of HIV un-infected mothers from among women with exposures such as gestational drug abuse, poor nutrition and other infections or the ability to identify appropriate control groups. These exposures may have increased the risk of prematurity. In high-HIV prevalence countries, uninfected women were not likely to be substance abusers.

HIV infection in children under 18 months of age is defined for reporting purposes as definitive or presumptive (*Table 16.15*). If individuals cannot be classified thus, they are categorized as 'exposed'.[36] HIV infection in children >18 months of age, adolescents and adults is defined as positive results on serologic or virologic tests, or on conditions that meet criteria in the case definition of AIDS (*Table 16.16*). The manifestations of HIV infection include generalized lymphadenopathy, hepato-splenomegaly, failure to thrive, HIV wasting syndrome, oral candidiasis and *Candida* esophagitis, recurrent diarrhea, invasive bacterial infections, parotitis, and opportunistic infections. The most common is *Pneumocystis carinii* pneumonia (PCP) (*Fig. 16.41*).[37] HIV encephalopathy, central nervous system disease is believed to be due to HIV infection of macrophages, microglia and multinucleated giant cells.[41,42] It includes developmental delay, which can be progressive. HIV encephalopathy affects 20–50% of children, and is more likely to occur in those with more severe immune suppression.

	Clinical categories			
Immunologic categories	N: No signs/ symptoms	A: Mild signs/ symptoms	B: Moderate signs/ symptoms	C: Severe signs/ symptoms
1: No evidence of suppression	N1	A1	B1	C1
2: Evidence of moderate suppression	N2	A2	B2	C2
3: Severe suppression	N3	A3	B3	C3

Clinical Categories for Children with HIV Infection, by Symptom Severity

CATEGORY N: NOT SYMPTOMATIC
Children who have no signs or symptoms considered to be the result of HIV infection or who have only one of the conditions listed in Category A.

CATEGORY A; MILDLY SYMPTOMATIC
Children with two or more of the conditions listed below but none of the conditions listed in Categories B and C.
- Lymphadenopathy (>=0.5 cm at more than two sites; bilateral = one site)
- Hepatomegaly
- Splenomegaly
- Dermatitis
- Parotitis
- Recurrent or persistent upper respiratory infection, sinusitis, or otitis media

CATEGORY B: MODERATELY SYMPTOMATIC
Children who have symptomatic conditions other than those listed for Category A or C that are attributed to HIV infection. Examples of conditions in clinical Category B include but are not limited to:
- Anemia (<8 gm/dL), neutropenia (<1,000/mm^3), or thrombocytopenia (<100,000/mm^3) persisting≥30 days
- Bacterial meningitis, pneumonia, or sepsis (single episode)
- Candidiasis, oropharyngeal (thrush), persisting (>2 months) in children >6 months of age
- Cardiomyopathy
- Cytomegalovirus infection, with onset before 1 month of age
- Diarrhea, recurrent or chronic
- Hepatitis
- Herpes simplex virus (HSV) stomatitis, recurrent (more than two episodes within 1 year)
- HSV bronchitis, pneumonitis, or esophagitis with onset before 1 month of age
- Herpes zoster (shingles) involving at least two distinct episodes or more than one dermatome
- Leiomyosarcoma
- Lymphoid interstitial pneumonia (LIP) or pulmonary lymphoid hyperplasia complex
- Nephropathy
- Nocardiosis
- Persistent fever (lasting >1 month)
- Toxoplasmosis, onset before 1 month of age
- Varicella, disseminated (complicated chickenpox)

CATEGORY C: SEVERELY SYMPTOMATIC
- Serious bacterial infections, multiple or recurrent (i.e., any combination of at least two culture-confirmed infections within a 2-year period), of the following types: septicemia, pneumonia, meningitis, bone or joint infection, or abscess of an internal organ or body cavity (excluding otitis media, superficial skin or mucosal abscesses, and indwelling catheter-related infections)
- Candidiasis, esophageal or pulmonary (bronchi, trachea, lungs)
- Coccidioidomycosis, disseminated (at site other than or in addition to lungs or cervical or hilar lymph nodes)
- Cryptococcosis, extrapulmonary
- Cryptosporidiosis or isosporiasis with diarrhea persisting >1 month
- Cytomegalovirus disease with onset of symptoms at age >1 month (at a site other than liver, spleen, or lymph nodes)

(Cont'd)

- Encephalopathy (at least one of the following progressive findings present for at least 2 months in the absence of a concurrent illness other than HIV infection that could explain the findings): a) failure to attain or loss of development milestones or loss of intellectual ability, verified by standard developmental scale or neuropsychological tests; b) impaired brain growth or acquired microcephaly demonstrated by head circumference measurements or brain atrophy demonstrated by computerized tomography or magnetic resonance imaging (serial imaging is required for children <2 years of age); c) acquired symmetric motor deficit manifested by two or more of the following: paresis, pathologic reflexes, ataxia, or gait disturbance Herpes simplex virus infection causing a mucocutaneous ulcer that persists for >1 month; or bronchitis, pneumonitis, or esophagitis for any duration affecting a child >1 month of age
- Histoplasmosis, disseminated (at a site other than or in addition to lungs or cervical or hilar lymph nodes)
- Kaposi's sarcoma
- Lymphoma, primary, in brain
- Lymphoma, small, noncleaved cell (Burkitt's), or immunoblastic or large cell lymphoma of B-cell or unknown immunologic phenotype
- *Mycobacterium tuberculosis*, disseminated or extrapulmonary
- *Mycobacterium*, other species or unidentified species, disseminated (at a site other than or in addition to lungs, skin, or cervical or hilar lymph nodes)
- *Mycobacterium avium* complex or *Mycobacterium kansasii*, disseminated (at site other than or in addition to lungs, skin, or cervical or hilar lymph nodes)
- *Pneumocystis carinii* pneumonia
- Progressive multifocal leukoencephalopathy
- *Salmonella* (nontyphoid) septicemia, recurrent
- Toxoplasmosis of the brain with onset at >1 month of age
- Wasting syndrome in the absence of a concurrent illness other than HIV infection that could explain the following findings: a) persistent weight loss >10% of baseline OR b) downward crossing of at least two of the following percentile lines on the weight-for-age chart (e.g., 95th, 75th, 50th, 25th, 5th) in a child >=1 year of age OR c) <5th percentile on weight-for-height chart on two consecutive measurements, ≥30 days apart PLUS a) chronic diarrhea (i.e., at least two loose stools per day for >30 days) OR b) documented fever (for >=30 days, intermittent or constant)

*Children whose HIV infection status is not confirmed are classified by using the above grid with a letter E (for perinatally exposed) placed before the appropriate classification code (e.g., EN2).
+Both Category C and lymphoid interstitial pneumonitis in Category B are reportable to state and local health departments as acquired immunodeficiency syndrome.
*See the 1987 AIDS surveillance case definition for diagnosis criteria.

Immunologic categories based on age-specific CD4+ T-lymphocyte counts and percent of total lymphocytes

	Age of child		
Immunologic category	<12 mos uL (%)	1–5 yrs uL (%)	6–12 yrs uL (%)
1: No evidence of suppression	≥1,500 (≥25)	≥1,000 (≥25)	≥500 (≥25)
2: Evidence of moderate suppression	750–1,499 (15–24)	500–999 (15–24)	200–499 (15–24)
3: Severe suppression	<750 (<15)	<500 (<15)	<200 (<15)

Source: CDC. MMWR 1994; *43*(RR12) 1–10.

Table 16.16 Pediatric human immunodeficiency virus (HIV) classification by clinical and immunologic categories.

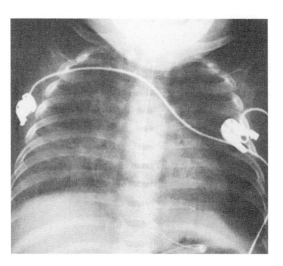

Fig. 16.42 *Pneumocystis carinii* pneumonia in a 3-month-old infant with HIV infection. Note the bilateral confluent interstitial pulmonary densities associated with hyperinflation of the lungs. Courtesy of Marquis JR, Bardeguez AD. *Clin Perinatol* 1994; 1: 125–147.

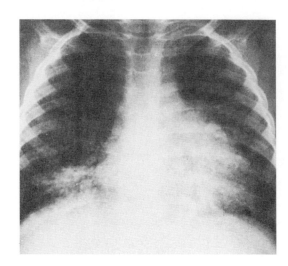

Fig. 16.43 Diffuse nodules throughout the lungs of a 20-month-old infant with HIV infection typical of lymphocytic interstitial pneumonia and pulmonary lymphoid hyperplasia. Courtesy of Marquis JR, Bardeguez AD. *Clin Perinatol* 1994; 1: 125–147.

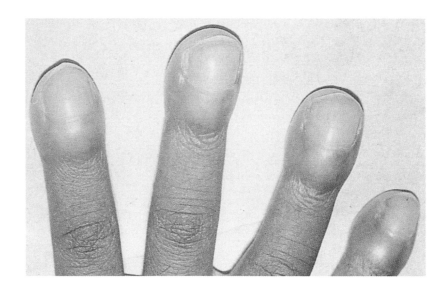

Fig. 16.44 Clubbing in a child with AIDS and lymphocytic interstitial pneumonia. Courtesy of Gwendolyn B. Scott, University of Miami School of Medicine, and Skoner DP, Urbach AH, Fireman P. Pediatric Allergy and Immunology. In: Zitelli BJ, Davis HW (eds). *Atlas of Pediatric Physical Diagnosis*. 2nd edn. Gower Medical Publishing, 1992.

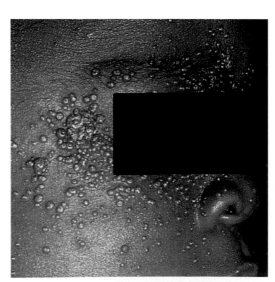

Fig. 16.45 Severe molluscum contagiosum in a child with AIDS. Courtesy of Gwendolyn B. Scott, University of Miami School of Medicine, and Skoner DP, Urbach AH, Fireman P. Pediatric Allergy and Immunology. In: Zitelli BJ, Davis HW (eds). *Atlas of Pediatric Physical Diagnosis*. 2nd edn. Gower Medical Publishing, 1992;

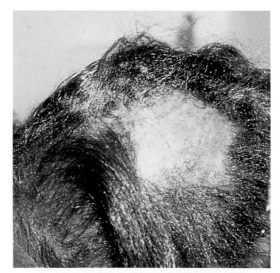

Fig. 16.46 Severe tinea capitis due to *Trichophyton tonsurans* in a child with HIV infection. Courtesy of Prose NS. *Dermatol Clin* 1991; **9**: 543–550.

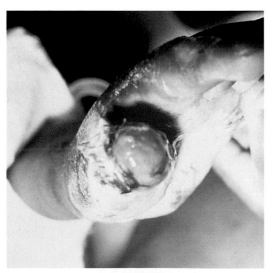

Fig. 16.47 Severe herpetic whitlow of the hand in a child with AIDS. Courtesy of Prose NS. *Dermatol Clin* 1991; **9**: 543–550.

PNEUMOCYSTIS CARINII PNEUMONIA

Most infants diagnosed with AIDS in infancy have PCP.[33] Although improvements in PCP prophylaxis and in the management of pediatric HIV infection have led to a decrease in the incidence of PCP, the proportion of AIDS cases among children defined by PCP remains about 33%. About 57% of cases of PCP in children occur among those <1 year of age, and the majority of these occur between 3 and 6 months. PCP presents with abrupt onset of increasing dyspnea and respiratory distress, fever, tachypnea, and cough. On physical examination, hypoxia, bibasilar rales and respiratory distress are typical. The radiologic picture generally shows interstitial infiltrates, and rapidly advances to diffuse bilateral airspace involvement (*Fig. 16.42*). Often, lactate dehydrogenase may be increased, but this finding is neither specific nor particularly sensitive. Serum total protein and albumin are often depressed.

PULMONARY INTERSTITIAL DISEASES

After 1 year of age, PCP becomes less common, and diffuse interstitial processes in the lungs, due to a variety of interstitial diseases, become more common. Lymphoid lesions, including lymphocytic interstitial pneumonia (LIP) and pulmonary lymphoid hyperplasia, cause diffuse nodular or reticulonodular patterns in the lung (*Fig. 16.43*). Frequently, hypoxia, hepatosplenomegaly, bronchospasm, and clubbing, accompany lymphoid interstitial processes (*Fig. 16.44*). Lymphoid lesions can progress to neoplastic lymphoproliferative diseases. LIP may be associated with improved survival. LIP involves the diffuse lymphoid infiltration of the lung parenchyma. LIP can range from asymptomatic disease with isolated radiologically observed abnormalities to severe pulmonary insufficiency, usually presenting in the second or third year of life with the insidious onset of dyspnea, fatiguability, tachypnea, cough, and occasionally fever, accompanied by generalized lymphadenopathy and salivary gland enlargement.

RECURRENT SEVERE INFECTIONS

Severe bacterial infections occur commonly in children with HIV infection, particularly those with perinatally acquired infections. Over a third of infants with HIV infection have at least one episode of bacteremia. The organisms causing severe infections most commonly among HIV-infected children include *Streptococcus pneumoniae*, *Salmonella* species, *Staphylococcus aureus* and *Haemophilus influenzae* type b. *Mycobacterium tuberculosis*, *M. avium*, and cytomegalovirus infections occur less commonly. Chronic, severe skin infections, including molluscum contagiosum, tinea capitis, and herpetic skin disease are common (*Figs 16.45–16.47*).

HIV-WASTING SYNDROME

A nonspecific syndrome characterized by chronic diarrhea, weight loss, failure to thrive, and/or refusal to feed, is very common among HIV-infected infants and young children.[43] Frequently, no causative organisms can be found. Mucosal edema and malabsorption patterns can be seen. Most radiographic changes are nonspecific (*Fig. 16.48*). As immune function deteriorates, intestinal function declines more than would be expected from opportunistic infections alone. Manifestations of gastro-intestinal dysfunction in these children include growth retardation, increased caloric requirements, and/or diarrhea and malabsorption.

CANDIDA ESOPHAGITIS, ORAL CANDIDIASIS AND DIAPER DERMATITIS

Oral candidiasis, generally severe, is seen in most children with HIV infection. It can present as punctate or diffuse mucosal erythema, angular cheilitis and the more commonly recognized white-beige plaques on the oropharyngeal mucosa (*Figs 16.49–16.50*). Cutaneous candidiasis

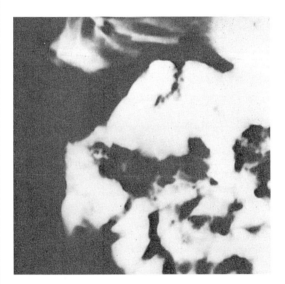

Fig. 16.48 Edema of mucosal folds in the proximal small bowel and malabsorption patterns, with nonspecific thickening of mucosal folds in the proximal small bowel of a 6-month-old HIV-positive infant hospitalized for failure to thrive. Stool was negative for pathogenic organisms. Courtesy of Marquis JR, Bardeguez AD. *Clin Perinatol* 1994; 1: 125–147.

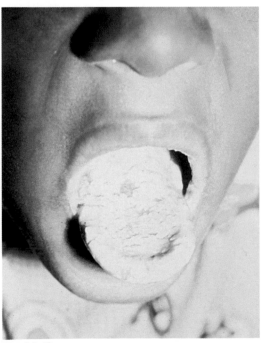

Fig. 16.49

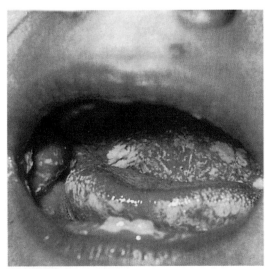

Fig. 16.50

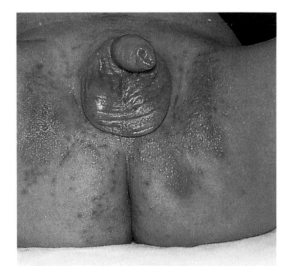

Fig. 16.51

Figs 16.49–16.51 Oral candidiasis (**16.49**, **16.50**) and *Candida* diaper dermatitis (**16.51**) in children with AIDS. Courtesy of Gwendolyn B. Scott, University of Miami School of Medicine, and Skoner DP, Urbach AH, Fireman P. Pediatric Allergy and Immunology. In: Zitelli BJ, Davis HW (eds). *Atlas of Pediatric Physical Diagnosis*. 2nd edn. Gower Medical Publishing, 1992 and courtesy of Prose NS. *Dermatol Clin* 1991; **9**: 543–550.

may develop as a diaper dermatitis or generalized eruption, and is characterized by erythema bordered by scales with satellite papules and pustules (*Fig. 16.51*). *Candida* esophagitis is less common, and may occur with or without oropharyngeal candidiasis. Symptoms include odynophagia, dysphagia, or substernal pain. Although esophagoscopy with mucosal biopsy is the best method for establishing a definitive diagnosis of esophageal candidiasis, this practice may not be feasible or safe in many children. An empiric approach based on clinical presentation and a positive barium swallow with the typical 'moth-eaten' appearance on esophagram consistent with ulceration and mucosal irregularities is often warranted (*Figs 16.52* and *16.53*).[44]

HIV ENCEPHALOPATHY

Most children with HIV infection have developmental delay. Central nervous system (CNS) abnormalities are a frequent and important complication of HIV disease, causing significant morbidity and mortality; it is estimated that 20–50% of children with HIV infection have HIV CNS disease. Infants have higher rates of CNS disease than older children, and those with more severe degrees of immunosuppression tend to

have higher rates. HIV encephalopathy, the fifth most common AIDS-defining condition in children, occurred in 17%, and presents typically with loss of developmental milestones, progressive motor and oromotor dysfunction, hypertonicity, microcephaly due to failure of brain growth, cognitive deterioration and apathy. Rarely, movement disorders, cerebellar signs or seizures may be seen. A computerized tomographic (CT) scan typically shows changes consistent with cerebral atrophy and multifocal leukoencephalopathy, and less commonly, basal ganglion calcification (*Figs 16.54* and *16.55*). MRI scans typically show cerebral/cerebellar atrophy, and abnormal signal in basal ganglia and white matter.

CARDIAC MORBIDITY

Dysrhythmias, hemodynamic abnormalities, congestive heart failure and sudden cardiovascular events, including cardiac arrest, are among the most serious complications of HIV infection in children.[45] These cardiac events may be due to HIV-related disease of the cardiac tissue or the nervous system. Myocarditis, pericarditis and inflammatory processes of the cardiac conduction tissues seen in HIV-infected children and

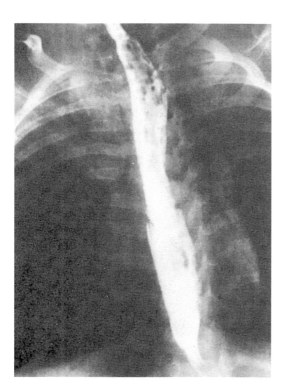

Fig. 16.52 Barium esophagram of 6-month-old infant with Candida esophagitis, showing mucosal irregularities and ulcerations. Courtesy of Marquis JR, Bardeguez AD. *Clin Perinatol* 1994; **1**: 125–147.

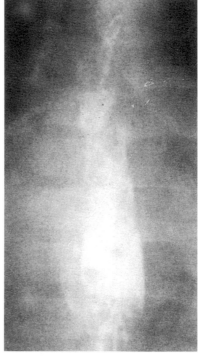

Fig. 16.53 Barium esophagram of child with AIDS, showing irregular plaques on walls of distal esophagus, and cobblestone appearance. Courtesy of Haller JO, Cohen HL. *AJR* 1994; **162**: 387–393.

Fig. 16.54 Nonenhanced CT scan of a 3-month-old infant with HIV infection. Ventricles are dilated and the interhemispheric fissure is widened, consistent with cerebral atrophy. Periventricular hypodensity, suggestive of progressive multifocal leukoencephalopathy, is present at the anterior horns. Courtesy of Marquis JR, Bardeguez AD. *Clin Perinatol* 1994; **1**: 125–147.

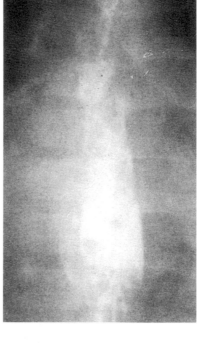

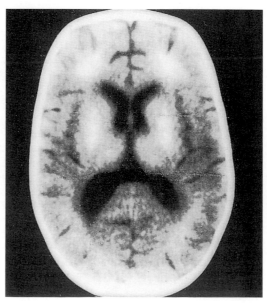

Fig. 16.55 Infant with AIDS, showing frontal lobe and basal ganglia calcification and ventricular dilation. Courtesy of Gwendolyn B. Scott, University of Miami School of Medicine, and Skoner DP, Urbach AH, Fireman P. Pediatric Allergy and Immunology. In: Zitelli BJ, Davis HW (eds). *Atlas of Pediatric Physical Diagnosis*. 2nd edn. Gower Medical Publishing, 1992.

adults may lead to dysrhythmias and other hemodynamic problems. Dysrhythmias and cardiorespiratory arrests have also been described with autonomic neuropathy. The most common adverse cardiac event in one series of children with HIV infection was sinus tachycardia.

OTHER

Ophthalmologic problems, including keratoconjunctivitis, keratitis, and multiple other lesions related to opportunistic infections and malignancies, are common in infants with HIV infection.[46]

TREATMENT

Antiretroviral therapy is indicated for most HIV-infected children. Initiation of antiretroviral therapy depends on various virologic, immunologic and clinical criteria.[47] This is one of the most rapidly changing areas of knowledge in pediatrics. Diagnostic and therapeutic strategies are evolving so rapidly that it is essential to frequently consult the most current recommendations (http://www.hivatis.org). Management of pediatric HIV infection should be conducted in consultation with an expert.

Antiretroviral therapy should probably be initiated for all HIV-infected children younger than 12 months of age, or those with more than 100,000 copies of HIV RNA per milliliter of plasma regardless of age. Most experts recommend therapy for all treated infants and children with at least three antiretrovirals (Table 16.17). Monotherapy with zidovudine is reserved only for newborns classified as 'exposed.' The goals of therapy are suppression of virus to undetectable levels, immunologic and clinical restoration, and preventing the progression of HIV disease.

Because PCP is a common early complication of perinatally acquired HIV infection, and has very high mortality, PCP chemoprophylaxis should be administered beginning at 4–6 weeks of age and continued for the first year of life unless HIV infection is excluded.[48] Guidelines for prevention and treatment of other opportunistic infections provide indications and protocols for administration of drugs for cytomegalovirus, toxoplasmosis, *Mycobacterium avium* complex, and other organisms (Table 16.18).[48]

HERPES SIMPLEX VIRUS (HSV)

EPIDEMIOLOGY

From 1,500–2,000 cases of neonatal herpes (200–500 cases/100,000 live births) occur yearly in the USA. Approximately 67–80% are caused by HSV type 2 (HSV-2), and the rest by HSV-1. Most are acquired through contact with the birth canal intrapartum, but some are due to postnatal or intrauterine HSV infection.[49,50] The overall incidence of asymptomatic infection at delivery is 0.3%; viral shedding may be as likely in women with clinically inapparent genital HSV-2 infections as those known to have genital herpes. Primary maternal infection before 20 weeks of gestation is associated with an increased incidence of abortion, stillbirth, hydroencephaly, and chorioretinitis (*Figs 16.56* and *16.57*)

VERTICAL TRANSMISSION

Neonatal disease can result from primary or recurrent maternal infection. The HSV infection rate in vaginally delivered infants is influenced by the type of genital herpes in the mother or factors such as instrumentation (*Table 16.19*).[49–51]

PREVENTION

Prevention of neonatal herpes should emphasize prevention of acquisition of genital herpes during late pregnancy. Susceptible women whose partners have oral or genital HSV or whose infection status is unknown should be counseled to avoid genital- and oro-genital contact during late pregnancy. Viral cultures during pregnancy do not predict viral shedding at delivery, and are not indicated. Careful questioning and examination of all women, regardless of history of genital herpes, for symptoms and physical findings suggestive of genital herpes or its

Strongly Recommended
- One protease inhibitor plus two nucleoside analogue reverse transcriptase inhibitors (NRTIs)

Alternative
- Nevirapine and two NRTIs

Only in Special Circumstances
- Two NRTIs

NOT RECOMMENDED because of overlapping toxicity and/or because may be virologically contraindicated
- Any monotherapy
- d4T and ZDV
- ddC and ddI
- ddC and d4T
- ddC and 3TC

Sources: CDC. MMWR 1998: 47(RR-4) 1–43.
Mostenton LM. Handbook of Pediatric Care. Lippincot Williams & Wilkins 1999, pp 273–293.

Table 16.17 Recommended antiretroviral therapy regimen for initial therapy for HIV-1 infection in children.

<1 Year	1–2 Years	2–5 Years	>5 Years	Regardless of age, CD4+ cell count
PCP;	PCP;	PCP; Toxo*	PCP; Toxo*	PCP (After PCP episode)
all children	<750 CD4+/μL	<500 CD4+/μL	<200 CD4+/μL	Toxo (After Toxo episode)
Toxo*, MAC	Toxo*, MAC	MAC	MAC:	TB (After close contact with person with active TB)
<750 CD4+/μL	<500 CD4+/μL	<75 CD4+/μL	<75 CD4+/μ MAC[a], CMV[b]	Bacterial respiratory infections (if hypogamma globulinemic)
				Bacterial enteric infections (after *Salmonella* sepsis)
				HSV disease if severe or frequent
				VZV infection (if close contact with chickenpox or shingles)

PCP = Pneumocystic carinii pneumonia; Toxo = toxoplasmosis; MAC = Mycobacterium avium complex; CMV = Cytomegalovirus; TB = tuberculosis.
If seropositive for Toxoplasma gondii.
[a]*If >6 years old.*
[b]*If >12 years old.*
Source: Orejas G, Simonds RJ. In: Handbook of Pediatric HIV Care. SL Zeichner, JS Read, Eds., 1999.

Table 16.18 Indications for opportunistic infection prophylaxis among HIV-infected children in relation to age and to CD4 cell counts.

prodrome should be performed at onset of labor. Cesarean section should be confined to those who have evidence of genital herpes, or its prodrome, at that time. Cesarean section greatly reduces, but does not completely eliminate the risk of transmission. Infants of mothers with active primary genital herpes at delivery that are delivered vaginally have a risk of ~50% of infection, compared to 15–20% if delivered by cesarean section within 24 hours of membrane rupture.

CLINICAL MANIFESTATIONS

Perinatal HSV infection tends to produce three categories of disease:[49]

- Skin, eye, and mucous membrane involvement, generally appearing after the first 24 hours (42%)
- A nonspecific disseminated disease resembling sepsis, involving hepatic dysfunction, pneumonitis, adrenal involvement, and coagulopathy, presenting 7–10 days after birth (23%)
- Encephalitis, presenting 10–30 days after birth (35%).

The prognosis of all these categories, except localized eye, skin, and mucous membrane involvement, is poor. Without antiviral treatment, over 70% of infants with localized HSV involvement will progress to disseminated infection; even after completing antiviral treatment, some infants with localized infection have recurrences of skin vesicles and long-term neurologic sequelae. Infants with neonatal HSV encephalitis present with fever, poor feeding, irritability, and lethargy. In approximately 67% of these infants, a rash develops.

Risk factor		Possible mechanism
Primary lesion	(30%–59%) US	Higher viral titer in
Recurrent lesion	(3%–5%)	primary lesions
Recurrent lesion, symptomatic	(3%–5%) vs.	Higher viral titer in recurrent lesions
Shedding, asymptomatic	(<3%)	
Cervical lesion* vs. lesions on vulva, buttocks, etc.		Higher viral titer in vaginal secretions
Prolonged rupture of membranes*		Longer duration of fetal exposure
Use of fetal scalp electrodes*		Provides site of entry for virus
Multiple lesions vs. single lesion		More virus from several lesions

*May be associated with higher risk
Adapted from: Overall JC. Herpes simplex virus infection of the fetus and newborn. *Pediatric Annals* 1994; **23**:131–136

Table 16.19 Risk factors for neonatal HSV infection should be considered in management of infants whose mothers are noted postpartum to have genital herpes.

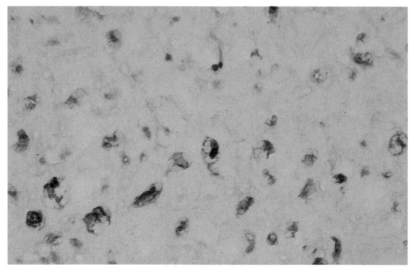
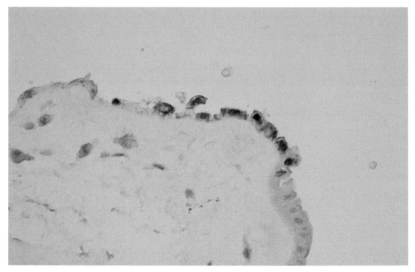

Figs 16.56 and 16.57 Amniotic membrane from placenta of an infant with congenital HSV infection whose membranes were intact before cesarean delivery, documenting chorioamnionitis and ascending route of infection with intact membranes. (**16.56**) Section of umbilical cord (x 400) shows antigen staining pattern of inclusion consistent with HSV within mesenchymal cells. (**16.57**) Section of amniotic membrane demonstrating immunostaining pattern of cells. Cells are bordered on the right by antigen-negative cells with normal cytoarchitecture. On the left, they are bordered by debris of cells sloughed off the basement membrane. Fig 16.56 courtesy of Hyde SR, Giacoia GP. *Obstet Gynecol* 1993; **81**: 852–855.

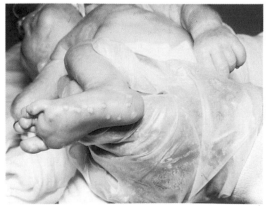
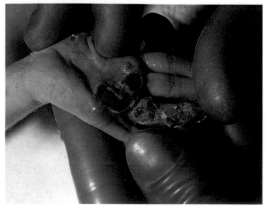
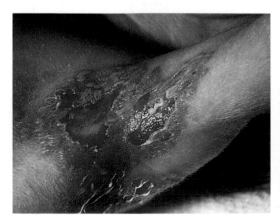

Figs 16.58–16.60 Neonatal HSV infection. Vesicles (**16.58**) and ruptured bullae (**16.59, 16.60**) with erosion in infant with neonatal HSV infection.

The rare infants infected in utero often have skin lesions at birth, including vesicles, bullae, pustules, erosions or scarrring (*Figs 16.58–16.60*). Chorioretinitis, microphthalmia, microcephaly, hydrocephaly, or other CNS involvement is seen in over 66% of these infants. Epidermal erosions simulating epidermolysis bullosa may occur (*Figs 16.61–16.63*).

The diagnosis of HSV infection can be confirmed by isolating HSV from cultures of the nasopharynx, conjunctivae, mouth, eyes, urine, blood, stool, rectum, CSF, and skin lesions, particularly vesicles. DNA amplification methods, such as PCR, are sensitive methods for detecting HSV DNA and are valuable for evaluating CSF specimens from cases of suspected herpes encephalitis.[49] Brain biopsy may be considered in infants with suspected HSV encephalitis if there are no lesions available and CSF HSV PCR is negative. The virus usually causes a cytopathic effect in tissue culture within 72 hours. Neonates with HSV infection have a variety of nonspecific laboratory abnormalities, including anemia, abnormal liver function tests, and CSF pleocytosis if there is CNS involvement.

CT scans may show cerebral swelling or focal hypodensities in perinatally acquired infections, and calcifications or cystic encephalomalacia in congenital infections (*Fig. 16.64*).

TREATMENT

Parenteral acyclovir should be administered empirically to all neonates with suspected HSV infection, regardless of clinical findings, after obtaining specimens for HSV culture[19] (*Table 16.20*). The best outcomes are observed among infants with disease limited to the eye, skin and mouth. Most infants treated for HSV encephalitis survive; however, most suffer considerable neurologic sequelae. Factors that increase the risk of mortality include dissemination, CNS involvement, coma, disseminated intravascular coagulation, prematurity, and pneumonitis. Factors associated with an increased risk of neurologic sequelae include skin, eye, and mucous membrane disease with three or more recurrent skin lesions after completion of acute therapy.

HUMAN PAPILLOMAVIRUS (HPV)

EPIDEMIOLOGY

Infections of the genital tract with HPV are probably the most common STDs in US adults (*see Chapter 14*). Genital warts, the most commonly recognized manifestation, are common,[3,52] and the incidence may have increased. Genital warts in women tend to become much larger during pregnancy or cell-mediated immunosuppression. Vaginal delivery may be complicated by the presence of large lesions.

VERTICAL TRANSMISSION

Maternal-to-infant HPV transmission appears to be rare and little is known about what factors increase transmission or progression to symptomatic disease in the newborn[52,53] About 50% of infants born to

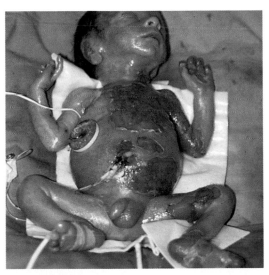
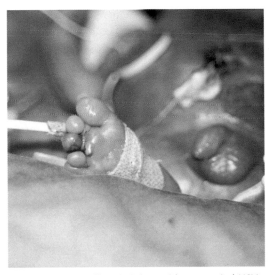
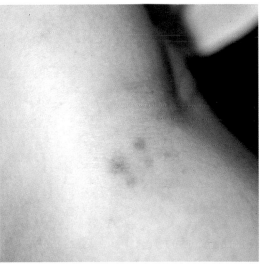

Figs 16.61 and 16.62 Severe epidermal erosions simulating epidermolysis bullosa in infant with congenital HSV infection. Courtesy of Sarkell B, Blaylock WK, Vernon H. *J Am Acad Dermatol* 1992; **27**: 817–821.

Fig. 16.63 Vesicle positive for HSV-2 on thigh of mother of infant seen in **16.61** and **16.62**. Courtesy of Sarkell B, Blaylock WK, Vernon H. *J Am Acad Dermatol* 1992; **27**: 817–821.

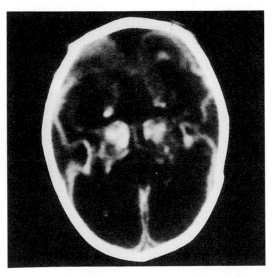

Fig. 16.64 Unenhanced CT scan of 4-day-old infant with congenital HSV-2 infection, showing intracranial calcifications, diffuse encephalomalacia, and poorly developed gyri. Courtesy of Bale JF, Murphy JR. *Ped Clin North Am* 1992; **39**: 669–690.

Acyclovir 60 mg/kg per day in 3 divided doses intravenously for 14 days if disease is limited to the skin, eye, and mouth and for 21 days if disease is disseminated or involves the CNS.

Topical antiviral ophthalmic drug (1–2% trifluridin, 1% iododeoxyuridine, or 3% vidarabine) for infants with ocular involvement, as well as intravenous acyclovir.

Source: American Academy of Pediatric (AAP). Herpes simplex. In: Pickering LK, ed. 2000 Red Book: Report of the Committee on Infectious Diseases. 25th ed. Elk Grove Village, IL 2000: 313.

Table 16.20 Treatment for suspected neonatal herpes simplex virus infection.

HPV-positive mothers are found to have HPV DNA. HPV transmission presumably occurs at birth due to contact with an infected birth canal. No effect of maternal HPV infection has been reported on pregnancy outcomes. Follow-up studies of patients whose mothers had anogenital warts have failed to show respiratory papillomatosis after 6 or more years of follow-up, suggesting that delivery through an infected canal alone may be insufficient to establish clinically apparent infection in the infant. Risk of infection detected by HPV DNA in the infants of mothers with HPV infection of the vaginal canal is less than 1%.

PREVENTION

Podophyllin and podofilox for the treatment of condylomata acuminata are contraindicated during pregnancy. Since lesions tend to proliferate and become friable during pregnancy, some experts advocate removal (*Table 16.21*). Cesarean delivery should not be performed solely to prevent transmission of HPV to the newborns, but only if the pelvic outlet is obstructed by genital warts, or if vaginal delivery would result in excessive bleeding.[19]

Cryotherapy with liquid nitrogen (not cryoprobes)

or

TCA 80–90% applied only to warts, powder with talc or sodium bicarbonate to remove unreacted acid if an excess amount is applied. Repeat weekly if needed.

Imiquimod, podophyllin and podofilox should not be used during pregnancy. Because genital warts can proliferate and become friable during pregnancy, many experts advocate their removal during pregnancy. HPV types 6 and 11 can cause laryngeal papillomatosis in infants and children. The route of transmission (i.e., transplacental, perinatal, or postnatal) is not completely understood. The preventive value of cesarean section is unknown; thus, cesarean delivery should not be performed solely to prevent transmission of HPV infection to the newborn. In rare instances, cesarean delivery may be indicated for women with genital warts if the pelvic outlet is obstructed or if vaginal delivery would result in excessive bleeding.

CDC 2002 STD Treatment Guidelines.

Table 16.21 Recommended treatment of genital warts during pregnancy.

CLINICAL MANIFESTATIONS

Oral and anogenital warts in early infancy are likely to be results of perinatal transmission (*Figs 16.65* and *16.66*). The most important manifestation of vertical transmission is laryngeal papillomatosis. This is the most common benign laryngeal tumor of infancy. The actual incidence of the disease in the USA is unknown, but is estimated at 1 in 100,000. Laryngeal papillomatosis has a bimodal age distribution. The first peak occurs from 2–5 years of age and the second, during adolescence.

Laryngeal papillomas appear as white, pink or red warty masses on the vocal cords (*Fig. 16.67*). Clinical symptoms generally develop prior to 4 years of age, consisting of hoarseness or abnormal cry, stridor, respiratory distress, and aphonia. Extension of disease from the larynx to the trachea occurs in up to 36% of cases; the risk increases to over 50% if the patient has undergone a tracheotomy to maintain an airway. Extension to the lung parenchyma is rare, difficult to manage, and often fatal. Malignant transformation is rare, and may be associated with radiation therapy.

Histologically, the papillomas are composed of vascular connective tissue cords covered by hyperplastic, stratified squamous epithelium. HPV 11 predominates in laryngeal papillomata, in contrast to genital condylomata, where HPV 6 predominates, suggesting that laryngeal tissues may be more susceptible to infection by HPV 11.[19,52,53]

TREATMENT

Laser surgical removal is the treatment of choice. The frequent regrowth of papillomas is not due to seeding of the virus during surgery, but to the fact that clinically uninvolved sites are often infected. Even biopsies from patients in remission often contain viral DNA. Tracheostomy and radiation therapy are contraindicated.

STDS IN CHILDHOOD

Non-sexual transmission of sexually transmitted pathogens is very unusual.[54] The diagnosis of an STD in a child is generally considered at least suspicious for, if not evidence of, abuse, if perinatal transmission can be excluded.[55] The evaluation for determining whether sexual abuse has occurred among children who have infections that can be sexually transmitted should be conducted in compliance with expert recom-

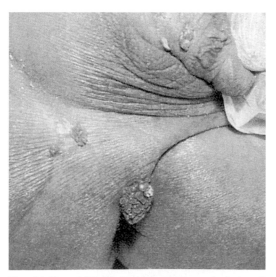
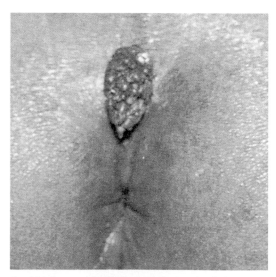

Figs 16.65 and 16.66 Condylomata acuminata in a 9-month-old infant, probably perinatally acquired. Courtesy of Boyd AS. *AJDC* 1990; **144**: 817–824.

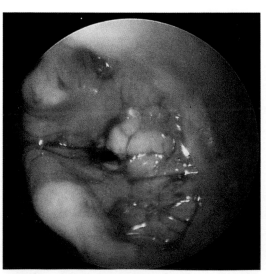

Fig. 16.67 Laryngeal papillomata presenting as warty growths almost occluding the larynx of a child with a history of chronic hoarseness. Courtesy of McBride TP, Davis HW, Reilly JS. Pediatric otolaryngology. In: Zitelli BJ, Davis HW (eds). *Atlas of Pediatric Physical Diagnosis*. 2nd edn. Gower Medical Publishing, 1992.

mendations by practitioners who have experience and training in the evaluation of abused children.[55] The diagnosis of non-vertically transmitted STDs in infants and children should be conducted using definitive techniques. Follow-up tests should be performed in cases of acute assault; the decision to evaluate the child for STDs must be made on an individual basis[19] (*Table 16.22*). The likelihood that an STD in a child confirms sexual abuse varies by type of STD (*Table 16.23*).[19,54,55]

EPIDEMIOLOGY

Sexual abuse appears to be common in all US racial and socioeconomic groups, and in most other countries where surveillance data exist.[52–59] It

may or may not coexist with other forms of maltreatment, and in only a minority of cases, are sexually transmitted diseases transmitted through abuse.[56–59] More than 1.0 million cases of suspected child abuse or neglect are reported each year in the USA, of which about 15% are sexual abuse cases. After a surge in the early 1990s, the total number of substantiated cases declined by 31% to 103,600 in 1999.[59] The number of perpetrators incarcerated in state facilities for sexual assault against children and adolescents rose by 39% between 1991–1997 to 60,700. In investigations undertaken by the United States Postal Inspection service from 1997–2000 in pursuit of child pornography, child molesters were identified in 36% of cases. At least 20% of US women and 10% of men report past abuse.[57] Signs of forcible coitus or overt physical trauma are

- Visual inspection of the genital, perianal, and oral areas for discharge, erythema, warts and ulcerative lesions.
- Cultures for *N. gonorrhoeae* specimens collected from the pharynx and anus in both boys and girls, the vagina in girls, and the urethra in boys. For boys, a meatal specimen of urethral discharge is an adequate substitute for an intraurethral swab specimen when discharge is present. Only standard culture systems for the isolation of *N. gonorrhoeae* should be used.
- Cultures for *C. trachomatis* from specimens collected from the anus in both boys and girls and from the vagina in girls. A urethral specimen should be obtained in boys if urethral discharge is present. Pharyngeal specimens for *C. trachomatis* are not recommended for either sex. Only standard culture systems for the isolation of *C. trachomatis* should be used.
- Cultures and wet mount of a vaginal swab specimen for *T. vaginalis* infection. The significance of bacterial vaginosis as an indicator of sexual exposure is unclear
- Collection of a serum sample to be evaluated immediately, preserved, and used as a baseline for comparison with follow-up serologic test. Agents for which suitable tests are available include *T. pallidum*, HIV, and HBV. The choice of agents for serologic tests should be made on a case-by-case basis
- Vaccination for HBV should be recommended if the medical history or serologic testing suggests that it has not been received (see Hepatitis B).

Source: American Academy of Pediatrics (AAP). In: Pickering LK, ed. 2000 Red Book: Report of the Committee on Infectious Diseases. 25th ed. Elk Grove Village, IL 2000, CDC 2001 STD Treatment Guidelines.

Table 16.22 Guidelines for screening for STDs in children suspected of having been sexually abused.

ST/SAI confirmed	Evidence for sexual abuse	Suggested action
Gonorrhea[1]	Diagnostic	Report[2]
Syphilis[1]	Diagnostic	Report[2]
Human Immunodeficiency Virus[3]	Diagnostic	Report[2]
Chlamydia trachomatis[1,]	Diagnostic	Report[2]
Trichomonas vaginalis	Highly suspicious	Report[2]
Condylomata acuminata (anogenital warts)[1]	Suspicious	Report[2]
Genital herpes	Suspicious	Report[2,4]
Bacterial vaginosis	Inconclusive	Medical follow-up

Adapted from American Academy of Pediatrics Committee on Child Abuse and Neglect. Guidelines for the evaluation of sexual abuse of children. Pediatrics 1999; 103: 186–191. Published correction Pediatrics 1999; 103: 149.
[1] *If not likely to be perinatally acquired.*
[2] *Reports should be made to the agency in the community mandated to receive reports of suspected child abuse or neglect.*
[3] *If not likely to be perinatally or transfusion acquired.*
[4] *Unless there is a clear history of autoinoculation.*

Table 16.23 Implications of commonly encountered sexually transmitted (ST) or sexually associated infections (SAI) for diagnosis and reporting of sexual abuse among infants and pre-pubertal children

Author/Journal		Total #	Female %	Abuse %	Gonorrhea +/tested (%)	Chlamydia +/tested (%)	Syphilis +/tested (%)	T. vaginalis +/tested (%)	BV +/tested (%)	HPV +/tested (%)	HIV +/tested (%)	HSV +/tested (%)
Robinson	Arch Dis Child 1998	319	76	100	3/159 (1.9)	2/131 (1.5)	0/6	4/159 (2.5)	3/159 (1.9)	1/242¶ (0.4)	0/6	—
Matthews	Ped Infect Dis J 1998	209	84	100	—	15/209 (7.2)	—	—	—	—	—	—
Larsen	Trans R Soc Trop 1998	191	96	61.5	20/91 (21.9)	1/91 (1.1)	6/91 (6.6)	9/87 (10.3)	14/87 (16.1)	17/91 (18.7)	1/91 (1.1)	1/91 (1.1)
Siegfried	Pediatrics 1998	40	73	100	0/38	5/38 (13)	0/14	—	—	2/34 (5.8)	—	—
Shapiro*	Pediatrics 1999	87	100	4.6	4/87 (4.6)	0/87	0/4	0/31	0/31	—	—	—
Stevens-Simon	Pediatrics 2000	31	100	100	—	—	—	—	—	5/31 (16.0)	—	—

*In this study, all patients known to have been abused, or where abuse was being considered were excluded; children were evaluated for STDs because of complaints of vaginal discharge, vaginal itching, and other vaginal complaints.
¶In this study, HPV was evaluated by examination for genital warts. In the others, PCR assays were used.

Table16.24 Studies of sexually transmitted disease (STD) prevalence, by pathogen, in children evaluated for possible sexually abuse and other children evaluated for STDs (published 1998–2000).

rare, but are more commonly seen among boys than girls; 20–25% of sexual abuse cases include penetration or oral-genital contact.[58] Girls predominate as victims, and their assailants are usually known to the child.

In children in whom sexual abuse is suspected or known, several investigations should be routinely performed, even in asymptomatic children.[19] Examination of the genitalia and the perianal area for warts, vaginitis, and evidence of trauma or other lesions should be undertaken. Speculum examination should not be performed on prepubertal girls. The most frequently diagnosed STD in sexually abused children is gonorrhea, but positive cultures for *C. trachomatis* and *T. vaginalis* are also common[56,59–64] (*Table 16.23*). Findings that increase the yield of STD testing include STDs in other children or adults in the household, genital discharge or other suggestive findings (*Table 16.22*).[19,63] In children with one sexually acquired infection, it is essential to test for others, and to investigate the possibility of abuse[19,56,64–69] (*Table 16.24*). Children may become HIV infected as a result of sexual abuse; 12 children reported with AIDS in 1999 in the US were infected by sexual abuse.[37] About 0.1–0.5% of abused children acquire HIV from their perpetrator; in studies of children with HIV, 6.3% and 15% had acquired the infection by abuse.[62,66] HIV transmission through sexual abuse is probably a far greater problem among children in very high prevalence communities.[62] Prevention of sexual abuse by child education is of limited value, though it tends to reduce the guilt of victims; interventions targeted at assailants are promising.

VULVOVAGINITIS

Vulvovaginitis is a common complaint in prepubertal girls, with an STD as the cause in only a minority of cases. Other frequent causes include *Candida*, *Streptococcus* or enteric organisms, and infestations (*Figs 16.68–16.69*). However, vaginitis is the most common presentation of gonococcal infection in children. The neutral-to-alkaline pH and the thin, atrophic nature of the prepubertal vagina predispose to diffuse vaginitis and dysuria.[63] The incubation period is brief. Some children are asymptomatic, but usually, a purulent, sometimes malodorous, discharge, accompanied by labial erythema develops (*Fig. 16.70*). Specimens for Gram stain and for culture on selective medium can be obtained from the first few millimeters of the vagina, without speculum examination, or from the discharge itself (*Figs 16.71–16.72*). Pelvic inflammatory disease occurs in about 6% of prepubertal children with gonococcal vaginitis. Suspicion of sexual abuse among children with gonococcal infections is virtually always confirmed; other STDs vary as to the likelihood that sexual abuse evidence will be uncovered (*Table 16.25*). Gram-stain evidence alone should not be considered evidence of gonococcal infection in pre-pubertal children.[19,23] Chlamydial infections are generally asymptomatic, but may present as vaginitis in prepubertal children. Cultures should be used to diagnose or confirm *C. trachomatis* infection in children who may have been sexually abused, because false-positive tests on non-amplified probes, direct fluorescent antibody and enzyme-linked immunoassays are common, and may have adverse medical, social and psychological consequences for the child and family.[19,28,61] Bacterial vaginosis and trichomoniasis can cause vaginal discharge, though some children with no history of sexual activity have evidence of bacterial vaginosis.

OTHER GONOCOCCAL INFECTIONS

Oropharyngeal gonococcal infection may present as an exudative tonsillitis, with soft-palate swelling and erythema and is seen in up to

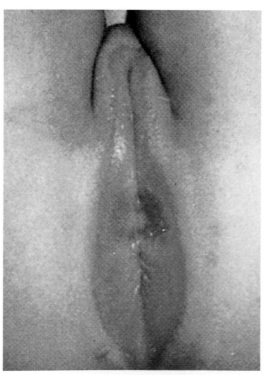

Fig. 16.68 Streptococcal vulvovaginitis presenting as sharply circumscribed erythema from the vulva to the perianal area. Courtesy of Murray P, Davis HW, Hamp M. Pediatric and adolescent gynecology. In: Zitelli BJ, Davis HW (eds). *Atlas of Pediatric Physical Diagnosis*. 2nd edn. Gower Medical Publishing, 1992.

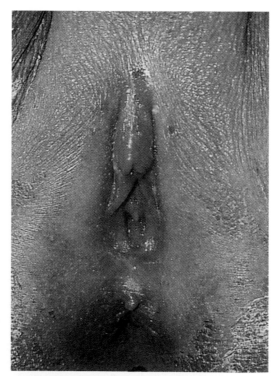

Fig. 16.69 Vulvar erythema and evident desquamation in a child with scarlet fever. Serosanguinous discharge is often seen in streptococcal vulvovaginitis. Streptococcal infections and other common nonsexually transmitted infection should be ruled out as part of the evaluation of vulvovaginitis. Courtesy of Murray P, Davis HW, Hamp M. Pediatric and adolescent gynecology. In: Zitelli BJ, Davis HW (eds). *Atlas of Pediatric Physical Diagnosis*. 2nd edn. Gower Medical Publishing, 1992.

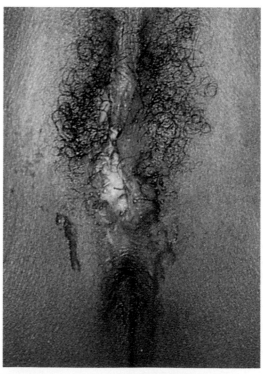

Fig. 16.70 Gonococcal vulvar erythema, edema, purulent vaginal discharge and Bartholin's cyst in a premenarchal sexually abused child. Rimaza B, Feingold M. Picture of the month. *AJDC* 1989; **143**: 381–382.

50% of sexually abused children in some series. Gonococcal arthritis is a common cause of bacterial arthritis in abused children; evaluation of children with arthritis should include cultures of synovial fluid, blood, oropharynx, rectum, vagina, and urethra for *N. gonorrhoeae* prior to initiation of antimicrobial therapy.[23]

ANOGENITAL LESIONS

Warts, chancres, ulcers and vesicular or pustular rashes should be evaluated for the diagnosis of condylomata acuminata, HSV infection, or syphilis.[19,52–54,56]

CONDYLOMATA ACUMINATA

HPV anogenital infection in prepubertal children typically presents as verrucous, flesh-colored or reddish papules; the most common location is perianal in either sex[53] (*Fig. 16.73*). The lesions may extend into the anal canal, the urethra, or hymen (*Figs 16.74–16.75*). The lesions are often asymptomatic, or may become infected, causing pain, bleeding, dysuria, pruritus, or vaginitis. Molluscum contagiosum, chronic benign pemphigus, histiocytosis X, neurofibromatosis, pseudoverrucous papules, nodules and skin tags must be considered in the differential diagnosis of anogenital condylomata (*Figs 16.76–16.77*). HPV DNA typing of anogenital warts may help in determining the mode of transmission of anogenital warts

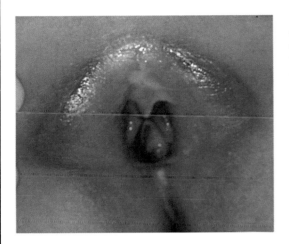

Fig. 16.71 Purulent discharge and vulvar erythema and edema due to gonococcal infection in a sexually abused child. Courtesy of Murray P, Davis HW, Hamp M. Pediatric and adolescent gynecology. In: Zitelli BJ, Davis HW (eds). *Atlas of Pediatric Physical Diagnosis.* 2nd edn. Gower Medical Publishing, 1992.

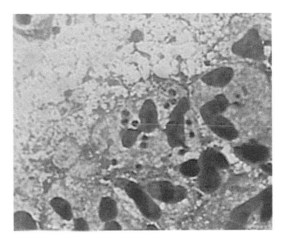

Fig. 16.72 Gram stain of vaginal discharge from patient in Fig 16.70, with sheets of polymorphonuclear leukocytes, several with intracellular Gram-negative diplococci. This finding, highly suggestive in a prepubertal child, should be confirmed by culture. Rimaza B, Feingold M. Picture of the month. *AJDC* 1989; **143**: 381–382.

Author/Journal		Total #	Female %	Abuse %	Gonorrhea +/tested (%)	Chlamydia +/tested (%)	Syphilis +/tested (%)	T. vaginalis +/tested (%)	BV +/tested (%)	HPV +/tested (%)	HIV +/tested (%)	HSV +/tested (%)
Handley	*Pediatr Dermatol* 1997	31	61	6.5	—	—	—	—	—	31/31 (100)	—	—
Lindegren	*Pediatrics* 1998	9,137	85	0.3	3/17 (17.6)	1/17 (5.9)	—	1/17 (5.9)	—	—	9,136/9,136 (100)	1/7 (35)
Connors	*Ped Emergency* 1998	3	33	66.0	0/2	0/2	3/3 (100)	—	—	—	0/2	—
Squires	*Arch Pediatr Adol* 1999	3	100	33.0	—	—	—	—	—	3/3 (100)	—	—
Christian	*Pediatrics* 1999	3	66	66.0	0/3	0/3	3/3 (100)	—	—	—	0/3	(0)

Table 16.25 Sexually transmitted disease (STD) prevalence, by pathogen, and prevalence of abuse as route of STD acquisition among children with symptoms or signs suggestive of STD, in studies published since January 1, 1997

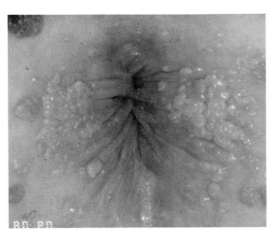

Fig. 16.73 Common presentation of perianal condylomata acuminata in a 6-year-old child. Courtesy of Frasier LD. *Ped Ann* 1994; **23**: 354–360.

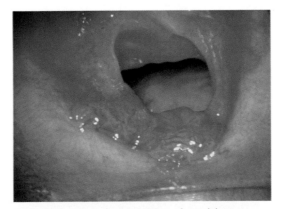

Fig. 16.74 Unusual presentation of condylomata acuminata in a 10-year-old sexually abused girl, with lesion appearing to extend from the vagina and erode the hymen. Courtesy of Frasier LD. *Ped Ann* 1994; **23**: 354–360.

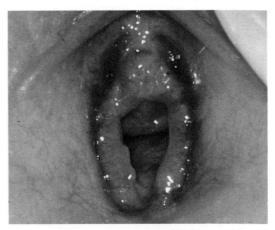

Fig. 16.75 Single condyloma in a 20-month-old girl, located on the posterior fourchette, with transection of the hymen consistent with sexual abuse. Courtesy of Frasier LD. *Ped Ann* 1994; **23**: 354–360.

in children.[65] Warts due to HPV types common in genital infection, including 6 and 11, are more likely to be associated with proven sexual or vertical transmission than those types commonly seen in skin warts, such as HPV-2. Nevertheless, evidence of sexual abuse is often found, even in children who have condylomata acuminata but deny abuse (*Fig. 16.77*). HPV type information should be interpreted together with other relevant information. HPV asymptomatic infection may be higher, among sexually abused children than non-abused children.[64] HPV infection diagnosed through nucleic acid amplification tests is not considered evidence of abuse.

SYPHILIS

Syphilis is rare among sexually abused children. When it occurs, it may present as condylomata lata, as isolated chancres, exanthems, or alopecia. Extragenital chancres are frequent in children with syphilis, including chancres of the lips, mouth, tongue, and thigh. Condylomata lata in children are generally perianal but may be perineal (*Figs 16.78–16.79*). They may be indistinguishable from condylomata acuminata on physical examination. Serologic tests for syphilis may be negative during primary syphilis or immediately after an isolated assault.[67] For these reasons, serologic tests for syphilis should be repeated one month after an assault if the assailant is unavailable for serologic testing and the prevalence of syphilis in the assailant's community justifies it.[19,54,55]

HSV INFECTIONS

Genital HSV infection presents in children generally as painful perineal ulcers, blisters, dysuria, vulvovaginitis and/or 'sores' (*Fig. 16.80*). Evidence of sexual contact is common among children with genital herpes.[49,54] Autoinoculation from oral lesions may result in genital herpes in

children who may not have been abused. This is more likely in children in whom the eruption of genital tract vesicles was immediately preceded by oral lesions. Generally, these are caused by HSV-1. Even in genital herpes due to HSV-1, evidence of sexual abuse is common, so such evidence should be sought in all cases of genital herpes in children, regardless of type. Occasionally, causes unrelated to abuse can simulate genital herpes, including allergic or contact dermatitis (*Figs 16.81–16.82*), and rarely, unilateral genital lesions caused by zoster.

TREATMENT

Because in prepubertal children, lower genital infections rarely ascend, prophylactic treatment is not usually offered. Sometimes, when parents and/or children feel strongly about needing treatment, or when it is very likely that the child has acquired a sexually transmitted infection, it may be considered on a case-by-case basis after samples for diagnostic tests have been collected. If a child has had a high-risk sexual exposure to an assailant(s) with, or at high risk of, HIV infection, within 72 hours of presenting, the provider should seek expert consultation and consider antiretroviral prophylaxis.[19,33,70] S/he should inform the child's guardians about the known adverse reactions, limited efficacy data, and need for adherence to the regimen, for the 28-day course of antiretroviral medication.[70]

STDS IN ADOLESCENTS

EPIDEMIOLOGY

In the United States, age-specific rates of STDs are highest among

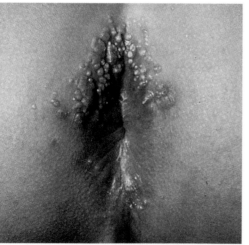

Fig. 16.76 Perianal molluscum contagiosum simulating condylomata acuminata in a 6-year-old male, necessitating biopsy confirmation. Courtesy of Frasier LD. *Ped Ann* 1994; **23**: 354–360.

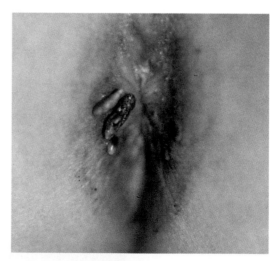

Fig. 16.77 Perianal condylomata acuminata in an 8-year-old boy. Hyperpigmented lesions were proven to be bowenoid papulosis by biopsy. Although the child had a rectal culture positive for *Chlamydia trachomatis*, confirming sexual abuse, he denied sexual activity. Courtesy of Frasier LD. *Ped Ann* 1994; **23**: 354–360.

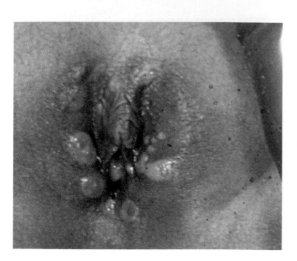

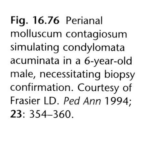

Figs 16.78 and 16.79 Childhood sexual abuse. Perineal flat condylomata lata in sexually abused girls. Fig. 16.79 courtesy of Dr. Angela Robinson, University College London Hospital.

adolescents, when controlled for sexual activity.[3,71] This is particularly striking with *N. gonorrhoeae* and *C. trachomatis* genital infections, which are highest among women between 15 and 19 years of age, exceeding those of adolescent males (*Figs 16.83–16.86*).[3] After years of decline, the gonorrhea rate increased by 13% in adolescents compared to approximately 9% for all ages between 1997 and 1999. STD rates among adolescents, like adolescent pregnancy rates, are much lower in other industrialized countries. Nevertheless, in the United Kingdom, the rates for gonorrhea, which are lower at 138.5 and 98.7 per 100,000 population for 16–19-year-old females and males, increased by 24% and 39%, respectively, from 1998 to 1999.[72] The trend in the United Kingdom over the last decade mirrors that in the United States with a decrease in the early 1990s and an increase in the late 1990s (*Figs 16.87–16.88*). In some African countries, gonorrhea prevalence ranges from 3.1–11.0% among adolescent and other young women screened during prenatal, family planning, and STD clinic care.[10,14] This is not much higher than rates of 4.1–9.9% among female adolescent and other youths screened in US prenatal and family planning clinics in high prevalence areas.[3,29]

C. trachomatis genital infection is the most common reportable infectious disease in USA with an estimated 3 million people contracting the infection each year.[71] Chlamydial infection is widespread regardless of race, ethnicity or gender; it is more concentrated among adolescents than any other sexually transmitted infection. Female adolescents have the highest rate of the order of 10–20% (*Fig. 16.86*).[3,29] The association between cervical ectopy (*see Chapter 4*), a normal finding during adolescence and the risk of chlamydial infection among exposed women in part explains the increased incidence among female adolescents.[3] Previously, oral hormonal contraceptives were believed to increase risk of *C. trachomatis* cervical infection, by increasing ectopy; however, this association may have reflected the increased likelihood of detection by methods of lower sensitivity (such as culture). Using NAATS, there is no association between oral contraception and *C. trachomatis* cervical infection.[73] In fact, because periodic screening is routinely done before prescribing oral contraceptives, these may actually be associated with decreased risk of *C. trachomatis* cervical infection.[29] There are less data on male adolescents, because the screening programs have been primarily directed at women; prevalences of more than 5% have been reported.[74] The prevalence of chlamydial infection is higher among male adolescents entering juvenile detention facilities and those that engage in commercial sex.[75] Rates of positive chlamydial

tests have risen between 1997 and 1999 in family planning clinics in eight of 10 regions of the United States; 40% of cases are reported among 15–19-year-olds, with a prevalence exceeding 10% (*Fig. 16.89*).[3] These changes may in part reflect the improved sensitivity of laboratory assays.[3] The highest rates are reported in southern states (*Fig. 16.90*). In the United Kingdom, chlamydial infection in 16–19-year-olds increased by 23% among males and 20% among females.[76,77] The age-specific rates per 100,000 population showed significant increases from those recorded in 1995 (*Figs 16.91–16.92*). Although this may reflect increased screening and case finding, increased incidence due to increased sexual transmission must be a contributing factor, as suggested by the accompanying rise in adolescent pregnancy rates.[76] Data from two pilot studies of widespread screening in women under 25 years of age showed a prevalence rate of up to 15% in adolescents.[77] In some African countries, the chlamydial infection rates among young women attending family planning or prenatal clinics (6.2–26%)[10,14] is similar to those among symptomatic women (18.5%), and among US adolescents.[3,29]

Pelvic inflammatory disease is the commonest complication of chlamydial and gonococcal infection. Chlamydial infection during adolescence is estimated to be approximately 10 times more likely to result in pelvic inflammatory disease than among older women.[78] In the United States, the trends towards decreasing numbers of first visits to physicians' offices and hospitalizations for pelvic inflammatory disease and ectopic pregnancies may be slowing.[3] In other developed countries, particularly Sweden, dramatic decreases in pelvic inflammatory disease among adolescents related to gonorrhea, and then to chlamydial infection, have been observed, with subsequent declines in ectopic pregnancy.[79,80] In the United Kingdom, rates continue to rise among adolescent women, whereas there has been a small decline for other age groups.[81] In young women in southern Africa, gonorrhea still appears to play a greater role in pelvic inflammatory disease than *C. trachomatis*, with prevalence rates of gonococcal PID ranging from 50–62%, and chlamydial PID rates from 11–30%.[14]

With the decline in syphilis incidence in the United States (*Fig. 16.93*), linked to declines in crack cocaine use, exchange of sex for drugs and money, and poverty, the disparity between rates among African Americans and Whites has decreased considerably[3] (*Fig. 16.93*). Investigation of a syphilis outbreak in an affluent Georgia suburb found, at its core, 18 White adolescent girls (12 of whom were <17 years of age) who engaged in non-commercial group sexual encounters and

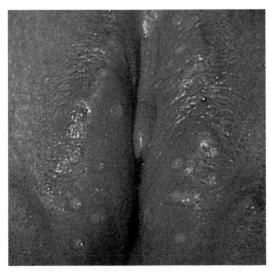

Fig. 16.80 Herpes simplex in a prepubertal child with dysuria and perineal pain. Courtesy of Murray P, Davis HW, Hamp M. Pediatric and adolescent gynecology. In: Zitelli BJ, Davis HW (eds). *Atlas of Pediatric Physical Diagnosis*. 2nd edn. Gower Medical Publishing, 1992.

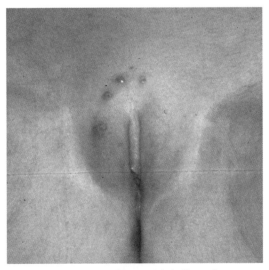

Fig. 16.81 Dermatitis due to nickel allergy from a bed-wetting alarm, simulating genital herpes. Courtesy of Hanks JW. *Pediatrics* 1992; **90**: 458–460.

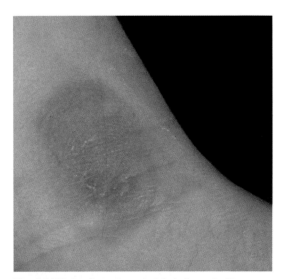

Fig. 16.82 Confirmation of nickel allergy in Fig. 16.81 given by patch-test on wrist. Courtesy of Hanks JW. *Pediatrics* 1992; **90**: 458–460.

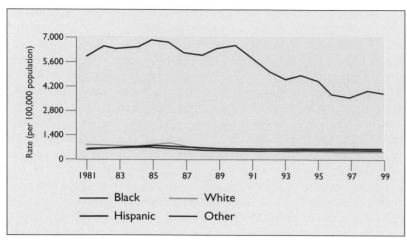

Fig. 16.83

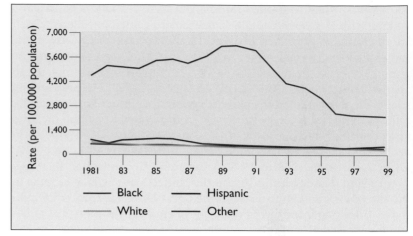

Fig. 16.84

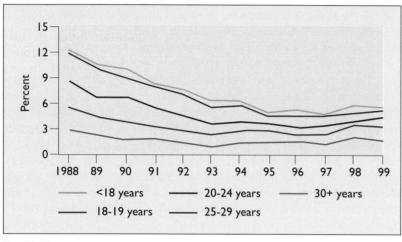

Fig. 16.85

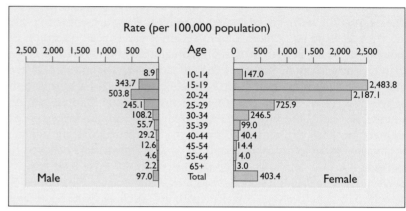

Fig. 16.86

Figs 16.83–16.86 Gonorrhea and Chlamydia incidence in selected adolescent and young adult populations, USA, 1980–1999: Reported gonorrhea among 15- to 19-year-old female adolescents (16.83) and male adolescents (16.84). Chlamydia positivity among women attending family planning clinics, by age groups (16.85), and Chlamydia, age and gender specific rates (16.86). Courtesy of DSTDP STD Surveillance 1999, CDC Atlanta, GA, 2000.

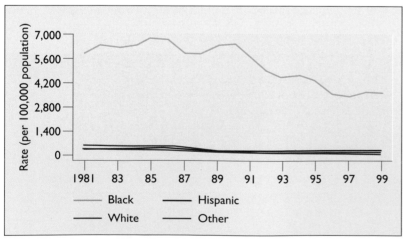

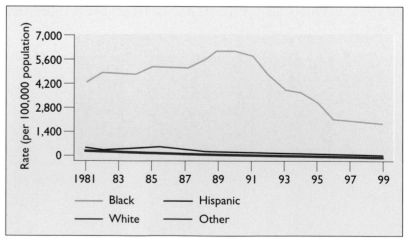

Figs 16.87 and 16.88 Gonorrhea rates, United Kingdom, 1990-1999. Courtesy of Dr. Angela Robinson University College London Hospital.

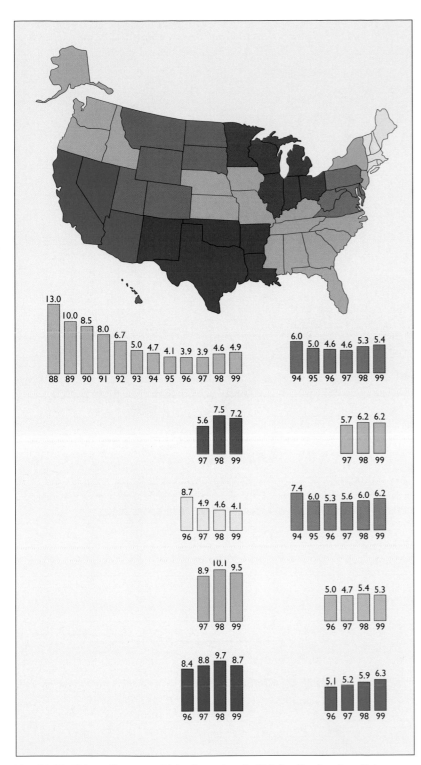

Fig. 16.89 Chlamydia test positivity, by region, in U.S. family planning clinics. Courtesy of DSTDP STD Surveillance 1999, CDC Atlanta, GA, 2000.

substance abuse with slightly older adolescents and men[82] (*Fig. 16.94*). Even in an era of very low syphilis prevalence, very intense, prolonged sexual mixing patterns can sustain syphilis transmission. Although syphilis prevalence in the United Kingdom is much lower than in the United States, there have been a number of outbreaks in both, indicating the possibility of resurgence.[82–86] In African countries, rates of syphilis seropositivity are extremely high and may exceed that of gonorrhea (*Fig. 16.3*).

The prevalence of HSV-2 infection in the US, as reflected by seroprevalence rates, has increased over the last decade.[87,88] From the previous National Health and Nutrition Survey (NHANES) II in 1976–1980, the prevalence of HSV-2 reported in NHANES III (1988–1994) showed an increase for all age groups, with a disproportionate increase among 12–19-year-olds, and 20–29-year-olds (*Fig. 16.95*). Although African Americans have a higher seroprevalence rate (45%) than Whites (17%), the increase among Whites noted in NHANES III was greater than that for African Americans. Data from genitourinary medicine clinics in the United Kingdom showed no overall increase in number of cases of genital herpes between 1998 and 1999; however, diagnoses increased among male and female adolescents by 9% and 3%, respectively.[72,81]

HPV infection is extremely common with an estimated 75% of the reproductive age population having evidence of infection, and a prevalence of 28–46% among women less than 25 years of age.[89] Approximately 14% of female college students in the United States are infected each year.[90] Fewer data are available for men, but prevalence rates appear to be similar to those of women. Genitourinary medicine clinics in the United Kingdom reported no change in the number of cases of genital warts among 16–19-year-old women, but an 11% increase among 16–19-year-old men.[72,81]

Most sexually transmitted infections have been shown to act as co-factors for HIV and HBV transmission and acquisition. Although there is an effective vaccine for hepatitis B, many adolescents at risk through sexual and drug-using behaviors have yet to be vaccinated. In one study, 70% had missed the opportunity for vaccination in the past.[91] The seroprevalence of hepatitis B is higher among African Americans (12%) than Mexican Americans (4.4%) and Whites (3%) (NHANES III).[88]

In the United States, as world-wide, HIV-related death has the greatest impact on young and middle-aged adults. At least half of all new HIV infections are among people under 25.[92] In 13–19-year-olds, 64% of reported HIV cases are among women, compared to 44% in the 20–24-year-old age group (*Fig. 16.96*). Most adolescents are infected sexually; among both female and male adolescents, the source of their infections is usually a male sexual partner(s). In female adolescents and young adults, most cases are acquired through heterosexual sex (*Fig. 16.97*). Surveillance data from 25 states of the United States with integrated HIV and AIDS reporting systems indicated that between January 1996 and June 1999 young people 13–24 years accounted for a greater proportion of HIV-positive (13%) than AIDS cases (3%). There has been no decline in the number of newly diagnosed HIV-positive cases in young people. The decline in AIDS cases related to use of highly active antiretroviral therapy has been greater among male than among female adolescents (*Fig. 16.98*), possibly because HIV infection is diagnosed in women later in the course of infection.

Of the estimated 1.5 billion young people aged between 10 and 24 years worldwide, 85% live in developing countries. Approximately one-third of all new STDs occurring in the world every year are in young people under the age of 25. In addition, the majority of new HIV infections occur among 15–24-year-old persons. Despite an overall decline in HIV incidence in Uganda, HIV prevalence in female adolescents is still higher than in males (*Fig. 16.99*).[12,93]

ADOLESCENT MEN WHO HAVE SEX WITH MEN (MSM) AND WOMEN WHO HAVE SEX WITH WOMEN (WSW)

Adolescence is the developmental stage where the formation of adult sexual identity takes place. Identity development, although an individualistic process, takes place in a social context in which culture, ethnicity, race and religion play major roles. For adolescent MSM and WSW, the recognized turmoil of this period is exacerbated by feelings of isolation and of being 'different' from peers. Many adolescents experience harassment and sometimes, open persecution, from peers and elders, and 'coming out' is such a difficult experience that MSM and WSW are vulnerable not only to high-risk sexual behavior, but also to depression, attempted suicide, under-achievement and substance abuse.[94–97] Of reported AIDS cases among 13–24-year-old men in the United States,

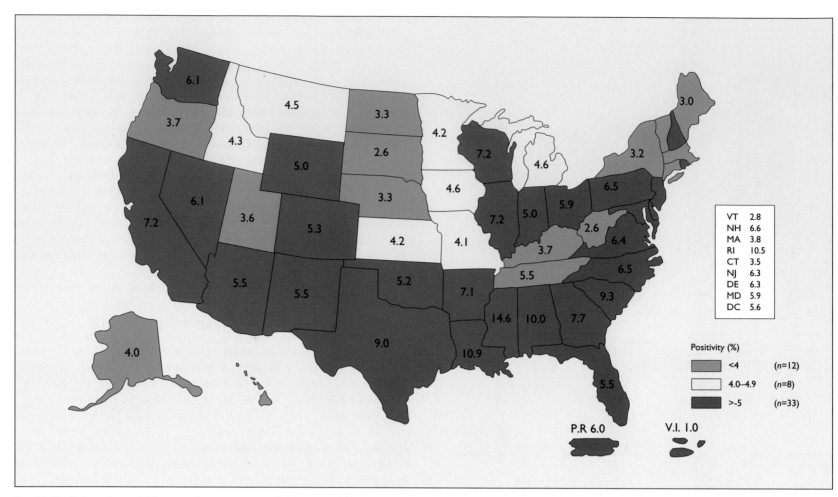

Fig. 16.90 Chlamydia positivity rates, by state, among 16–24 year old women, 1999. Courtesy of DSTDP STD Surveillance 1999, CDC Atlanta, GA, 2000.

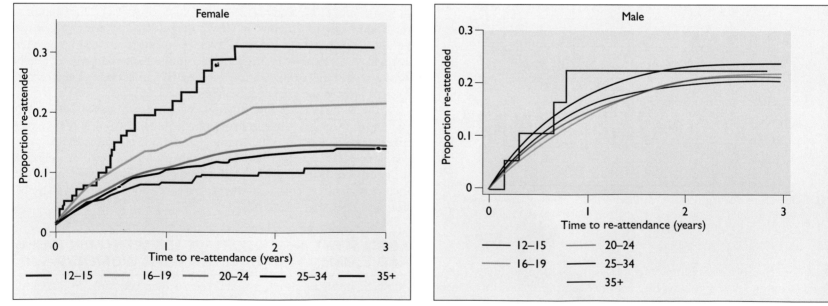

Figs 16.91 and 16.92 Chlamydia rates United Kingdom, 1990–1999. Courtesy of Dr. Angela Robinson University College London Hospital.

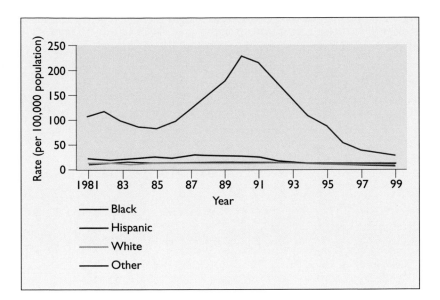

Fig. 16.93 Primary and secondary syphilis, US, by race, 1980–1999. Courtesy of DSTDP STD Surveillance 1999, CDC Atlanta, GA, 2000.

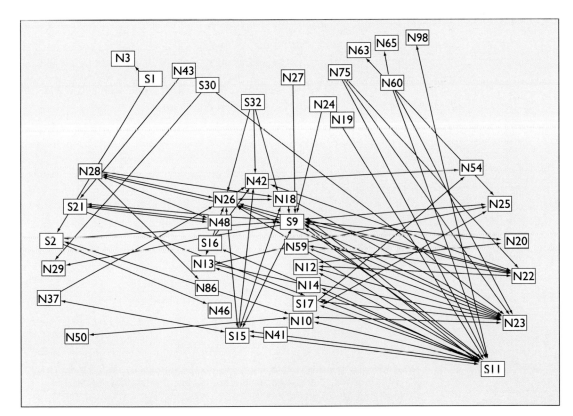

Fig. 16.94 Network diagram based on ethnographic assessment of relationships among major groups involved in syphilis transmission in a cluster in a Georgia suburb. The central group is composed of young white female adolescents. The group of six at the lower left are slight older white male adolescents. The group of six at the lower right are slightly older African-American male adolescents. Those above are persons associated with these primary groups. 'S' identifies people with syphilis, and 'N,' people without syphilis. Rothenberg RB, Sterk C, Toomey KE *et al. Sex Trans Dis* 1998; **25**: 154–160.

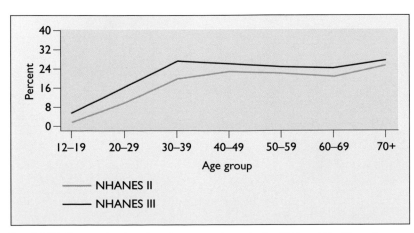

Fig. 16.95 Herpes simplex virus-2 seroprevalence in the National Health and Nutrition Surveys, II and III. Courtesy of DSTDP STD Surveillance 1999, CDC Atlanta, GA, 2000.

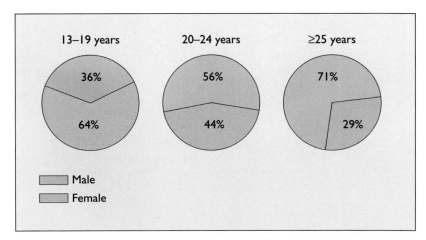

Fig. 16.96 New HIV infections among US males and females. CDC. *HIV AIDS Surveillance in Adolescents*, 1999. Atlanta, GA, USA.

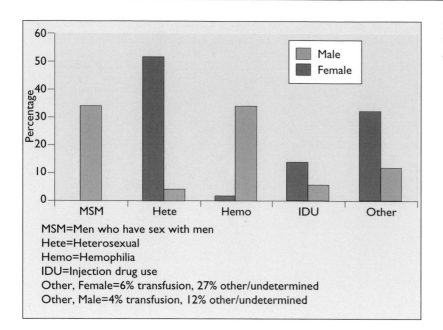

Fig. 16.97 AIDS cases among 13- to 19-year-olds by exposure category and sex, through 1999, United States. CDC. *HIV AIDS Surveillance in Adolescents*, 1999. Atlanta, GA, USA.

MSM=Men who have sex with men
Hete=Heterosexual
Hemo=Hemophilia
IDU=Injection drug use
Other, Female=6% transfusion, 27% other/undetermined
Other, Male=4% transfusion, 12% other/undetermined

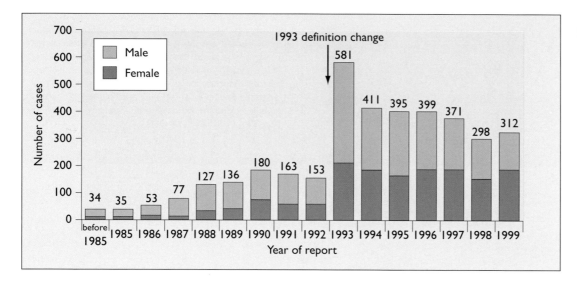

Fig. 16.98 AIDS in 13- to 19-year-olds, by sex and year of report, United States. CDC. *HIV AIDS Surveillance in Adolescents*, 1999. Atlanta, GA, USA.

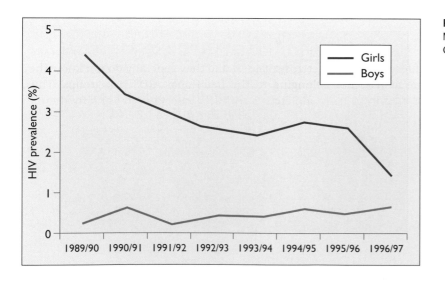

Fig. 16.99 HIV prevalence rate among 13- to 19-year-olds by sex, 1989 to 1997, Masaka, Unganda. Joint United Nations Programme on HIV/AIDS (UNAIDS). Geneva: Joint UN Programme on HIV/AIDS, 2000.

Fig. 16.100 Reattenders with STDs in 3 clinics in England. Courtesy of Dr. Angela Robinson, University College London Hospital.

Re-attendance with an acute STI
Crude rates and adjusted hazard ratios (HR) by sex and age group at initial presentation

Sex and age group	Rate per 100 person-years	HR§ (95% CI)	Sex and age group	Rate per 100 person-years	HR§ (95% CI)
Male*	14.1		Female†	8.9	
12-15	14.7	0.77 (0.19 to 3.12)	12-15	19.7	1.90 (1.13 to 3.18)
16-19	12.1	1.02 (0.77 to 1.35)	16-19	12.3	1.65 (1.32 to 2.05)
20–24‡	12.6	1	20–24‡	8.2	1
25–34	15.4	0.94 (0.80 to 1.10)	25–34	7.8	0.72 (0.57 to 0.91)
35+	13.7	0.70 (0.57 to 0.85)	35+	5.9	0.60 (0.40 to 0.88)

* $p = 0.001$, from likelihood ratio test of entire term in the model.
† $p < 0.001$, from likelihood ratio test of entire term in the model.
‡ Reference category.
§ Adjusted for all other variables.

Risk factors for adolescent STDs

- Age at first coitus
- Current sexual activity, multiple sexual partners
- Other behavioral risk factors (e.g. douching)
- Prevalence among partners
- Inconsistent use of barrier protection
- Biological factors (e.g.ectopy)
- Reduced access to reproductive health services and screening, treatment

Fig. 16.101 Risk factors for adolescent STDs. Courtesy of Beck-Sague CM, Santelli J, DRH, NCCDPHP, CDC.

75% have been in MSM.[92] However, younger age at identification as MSM was a strong predictor of pursuing HIV serologic testing.[98] Adolescent MSM typically acquire HIV infection soon after sexual debut; HIV seroprevalence in young MSM was found to be 2.0% among those aged 15–17 years and 6.8% among those 18–22 years.[99] In both groups, almost a third engaged in unprotected anal intercourse, associated with drug use. Most young men engaged in commercial sex work, which has been identified as a high HIV prevalence group, identify their sexual orientation as homosexual.[100,101] WSW exclusively are less likely to acquire many STDs; however, most WSW have, or in the past have had, sex with men. Sexually active adolescent WSW have higher rates of past pregnancy and STDs than other heterosexually active adolescent women.[94] Sexual HIV transmission from woman to woman has been reported,[102] and bacterial vaginosis may be sexually transmitted between WSW.[103]

SEXUAL ASSAULT

STDs in adolescents may be the first indication of sexual victimization. Establishing whether relationship(s) are consensual is an important part of medical evaluation of sexually active adolescents. Most survivors of sexual assault are under 25, with 60% being under 18 years of age.[104]

TREATMENT

Treatment of sexually transmitted infections should follow the guidelines for adults. However adolescents may not be as adherent with medication, and single-dose therapies are generally preferable.[19] Partner notification is an essential part of management, particularly among adolescents, to reduce their very high rates of re-infection. In some *C. trachomatis* screening programs, it has been estimated that 28% of infected persons were found via partner referral.[105] Among adolescent women treated for chlamydial infection, 6%, 11% and 17% were re-infected by 6, 12 and 24 months, respectively.[106] In Denmark, an intervention to increase adherence with partner treatment and risk reduction was associated with a risk of re-infection with *C. trachomatis* of 2.9% in one year, versus 6.6% in the control group.[107] In another study of re-infections undertaken in England, 20% of 12–15-year-old women presented with another STD within one year[108] (*Fig. 16.100*). Frequent re-screening of adolescents previously diagnosed with a sexually transmitted disease should be considered.

Many adolescents with HIV infection and AIDS are young women infected through heterosexual sex, and they generally do not know they are at risk, not belonging to the traditional AIDS risk groups. Thus, identifying female adolescents with HIV infection and linking them to specialized care, particularly timely anti-retroviral treatment to prevent progression to AIDS, has proven to be a challenge.[109] Identifying adolescents with HIV infection, regardless of gender or sexual orientation, requires willingness to take steps to make counseling and testing available in a much broader range of facilities, and to encourage discussion of sexual activity with a physician or counselor, since these factors have been strongly associated with pursuing HIV testing.[98,109] These facilities include family planning clinics, shelters for run-away and homeless adolescents, facilities for substance abuse counseling, and all other facilities providing services to sexually active adolescents, including those offering pregnancy testing and abortion counseling.

PREVENTION

Adolescents are a group at high risk of STD acquisition due to biological, psychological, behavioral and socio-economic factors, including

25-year study from an urban area of central Sweden. *Sex Transm Dis* 1996; **25**:384–391.

80. Kamwendo F, Forslin L, Bodin L, Danielsson D. Epidemiology of ectopic pregnancy during a 28 year period and the role of pelvic inflammatory disease. *Sex Transm Dis* 2000; **76**:28–32.

81. CDR Weekly. Young people bear the brunt of increasing sexually transmitted infections in England. *CDR Weekly 2000*; **10**:277–280.

82. Rothenberg RB, Sterk C, Toomey KE *et al.* Using social network and ethnographic tools to evaluate syphilis transmission. *Sex Trans Dis* 1998; **25**:154–160.

83. Centers for Disease Control. Resurgent bacterial sexually transmitted disease among men who have sex with men — King County, Washington, 1997–1999. *MMWR* 1999; **48**(No. 3):773–777.

84. CDSC. An outbreak of infectious syphilis in Bristol. *Commun Dis Rep CDR Wkly* 1997; **7**: 291.

85. CDSC. Increased transmission of syphilis in men who have sex with men reported from Brighton and Hove. *Commun Dis Rep CDR Wkly* 2000; **10**:177–180.

86. CDSC. Outbreak of heterosexually acquired syphilis in Cambridgeshire. *Commun Dis Rep CDR Weekly* 2000; **10**:401–404.

87. Fleming DT, McQuillan GM, Johnson RE. Herpes simplex virus type 2 in the United States, 1976 to 1994. *N Engl J Med* 1997; **337**; 1105–1111.

88. National Center for Health Statistics. *Plan and operation of the Third National Health and Nutrition Examination Survey, 1988–94. Vital and health statistics. Series 1.* No. 32. Washington, D.C.: Government Printing Office, 1994. (DHHS publication no. (PHS) 94–1308.).

89. Koutsky L. Epidemiology of Genital Human Papillomavirus Infection. *Am J Med* 1997; **102**(suppl 5A):3–8.

90. Ho GYF, Bierman R, Beardsley L *et al.* Natural history of cervicovaginal papillomavirus Infection in young women. *N Engl J Med* 1998; **338**(7):423–428.

91. Mast EE, Mahony FJ, Alter MJ, Margolis HS. Progress toward elimination of hepatitis B virus transmission in the United States. *Vaccine* 1998; (suppl): S48–S51.

92. Division of HIV/AIDS Prevention. *HIV Surveillance in Adolescents and Young Adults, 1999.* Centers for Disease Control and Prevention. Atlanta, GA.

93. Kamali A, Carpenter LM, Whitworth J, Grovera, James AG, Pool R, Ruberantwari A, Ojwiya. Seven-year trends in HIV-1 infection rates, and changes in sexual behaviour, among adults in rural Uganda. *AIDS* 2000; **14**:427–434.

94. Blake SM, Ledsky R, Lehman T, Goodenow C, Sawyer R, Hack T. Preventing sexual risk behaviors among gay, lesbian and bisexual adolescents: the benefits of gay-sensitive HIV instructions in schools. *Am J Public Health* 2001; **91**:940–946.

95. Bagley C, Tremblay P. Elevated rates of suicidal behavior in gay, lesbian and bisexual youth. *Crisis* 2000; **21**:111–117.

96. Perrin EC, Sack S. Health and development of gay and lesbian youths: implications for HIV/AIDS. *AIDS Patient Care & STDs* 1998; **12**: 303–313.

97. Stronski Huwiler SM. Remafedi G. Adolescent homosexuality. *Advances in Pediatrics* 1998; **45**:107–144.

98. Povinelli M. Remafedi G. Tao G. Trends and predictors of human immunodeficiency virus antibody testing by homosexual and bisexual adolescent males, 1989–1994. *Archives of Pediatrics & Adolescent Medicine* 1996; **150**(1):33–38.

99. Waldo Craig R, McFarland W, Katz MH, MacKellar D, Valleroy LA. Very young gay and bisexual men are at risk for HIV infection: The San Francisco Bay area young men's survey II. *J AIDS* 2000; **24**:168–174.

100. Boyer CB, Shafer MA, Teitle E, Wibbelsman CJ, Seeberg D, Schachter J. Sexually transmitted diseases in a health maintenance organization teen clinic: associations of race, partner's age and marijuana use. *Arch Pediatr Adolesc Med* 1999; **153**:838–44.

101. Boyer D, Male prostitution and homosexual identity. *J Homosex* 1989; **17**:151–184.

102. Chu SY, Buehler JW, Fleming PL *et al.* Epidemiology of reported cases of AIDS in lesbians, United States 1980–89. *Am J Public Health* 1990; **80**:1380–1381

103. Berger B, Kolton S, Zenilman JM *et al.* Bacterial vaginosis in lesbians: A sexually transmitted disease. *Clin Infect Dis* 1995; **21**:1402–1405

104. Kilpatrick DG, Edmunds CN, Seymour AK. *Rape in America: a report to the nation.* Charleston (SC): The National Victim Center and the National Crime Victims Research and Treatment Center at the Medical University of South Carolina, 1992.

105. Kretzschmar M, Welte R, van den Hoek A, Postma MJ. Comparative model-based analysis screening programs for *Chlamydia trachomatis* infections. *Am J Epidemiol* 2001; **153**:90–101.

106. Xu F, Schillinger JA, Markowitz LE, Sternberg MR, Aubin MR, St. Louis ME. Repeat *Chlamydia trachomatis* infection in women: analysis through a surveillance case registry in Washington State, 1993–1998. *Am J Epidemiol* 2000; **152**:1164–1167.

107. Ostergaard L, Andersen B, Moller JK, Olesen F. Home sampling versus conventional swab sampling for screening of *Chlamydia trachomatis* in women: a cluster-randomized 1 year follow-up study. *Clin Infect Dis* 2000; **31**: 951–957.

108. Hughes G, Bradey AR, Catchpole MA *et al.* Characteristics of those who repeatedly acquire Sexually Transmitted Infections: a retrospective cohort study of attenders at 3 urban sexually transmitted disease clinic in England. *STD* 2001; **28**:379–86..

109. Rudy BJ. Adolescents and HIV. *Handbook of Pediatric HIV Care* SL Zeichner, JS Read, Eds. Lippincott Williams & Wilkins, pp 178–188, Philadelphia, 1999.

110. Torkko KC, Gershman K, Crane LA, Hamman R, Baron A. Testing for *Chlamydia* and sexual history taking in adolescent females: results from a statewide survey of Colorado primary care providers. *Pediatrics* 2000; **106**:E32.

Infestations

S Morse and J Long

17

INTRODUCTION

Scabies and pubic lice are parasitic insects that live on or within the skin. The dermatidides that they produce are generally considered to be STDs, although they are also spread by nonsexual activity involving skin-to-skin contact. Sexual acquisition can often be assumed when the patient is a young adult with multiple sexual partners. Among young children, however, most cases do not imply sexual exposure.

SCABIES

Scabies is a pruritic dermatosis caused by the mite *Sarcoptes scabiei* var *hominis*. This condition, recognized for centuries as the 'seven-year itch' was associated with the mite as early as 1689. The casual relationship between the mite and the rash was much debated and not generally accepted until the nineteenth century.[1]

Sarcocptes scabiei is an arachnid that is highly adapted to a parasitic existence.[2] While free-living mites have a hard, rigid but jointed water-proof shell, scabies mites have a thin skin and are very susceptible to dehydration. Scabies mites lack the entire respiratory system possessed by typical free-living mites and obtain all oxygen through their thin skin. They also lack eyes and have short, stubby legs, which are sufficient to reach the walls of the tunnel in which they live. The female mite is primarily responsible for the rash and is the form most frequently recovered from infested patients (*Figs 17.1* and *17.2*). The adult female measures approximately 400 × 300 μm and is translucent and barely perceptible to the naked eye. Transverse grooves cover the body, and small denticles form a variable pattern on the dorsal surface. Although there is no distinct head, large, protruding jaws identify the anterior end (*Fig. 17.3*). Four pairs of legs are found in adult mites. In the female, the most posterior of these ends in long tendrils, while in the male the most posterior pair ends in suckers.

Sarcoptes scabiei from different hosts are morphologically indistinguishable, but biological evidence indicates that they are physiologically different and host-specific.[3] For example, scabies mites from dogs (var *canis*) can be experimentally transferred to rabbits, but scabies mites from humans (var *hominis*) cannot. Moreover, both experimental and clinical evidence indicate that *Sarcoptes scabiei* var *canis* cannot infest humans.[4] Based on host transfer experiments, most human and animal cross-infestations are probably self-limiting.[1]

On warm skin, the adult female can walk about 2.5 cm/min. Upon selecting a suitable site, the fertilized female uses her jaws and sharp blades on the first two pairs of limbs to dig into the horny layer of the skin, usually taking about an hour to submerge herself below the surface.[5] The mite digs down through the stratum corneum to the boundary with the stratum granulosum (*Fig. 17.4*), where she feeds on liquid oozing from cells which she has chewed and lays her eggs (*Fig. 17.5*). The stratum corneum is rich in lipids,[6] and scabies mites, especially adult females, are selectively attracted to several lipids that are found in human skin.[7] The lipids include odd-chain-length saturated (e.g., pentanoic and lauric) and unsaturated (e.g., oleic and linoleic) fatty acids as well as cholesterol and tripalmitin. Each day, the female mite extends the burrow by 0.5–5 mm and lays two to three eggs, each apparently stuck firmly to the lower surface of the burrow. Under optimal conditions, the mite will continue to burrow and lay eggs for a month or more, never returning to the skin surface. The burrow is confined to the stratum corneum. As this layer is being produced all the time, the burrow is pushed up nearer to the surface each day, and eventually the oldest sections may be lost as the surface of the epidermis is sloughed off.[5] After 3–4 days, the eggs hatch into larvae, which resemble the adults but have only three pairs of legs. The larvae leave the burrow after a day or so and move onto the surface of the skin. They soon burrow into the skin for shelter and to feed. After 3–4 days, the larvae molt to produce protonymphs. This stage is similar in appearance

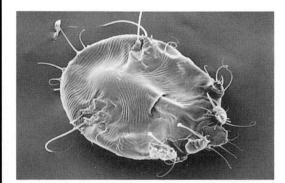

Fig. 17.1 Scanning electron micrograph of the ventral surface of a female *Sarcoptes scabiei* (× 300). A central bulge overlies the ovary, which contains a large egg. Courtesy of Patricianne Hurd, PhD, John Pietrahita, and Danny Blankenship, Fernbank Science Centre, DeKalb County Board of Education.

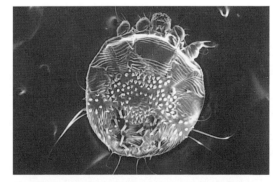

Fig. 17.2 Scanning electron micrograph of *Sarcoptes scabiei* showing the dorsal surface (× 200). Multiple small denticles are present except in a central bare area. Attempts to correlate the size of this bare area with biologic variants of the mite have had limited success. Courtesy of Patricianne Hurd, PhD, John Pietrahita, and Danny Blankenship, Fernbank Science Centre, DeKalb County Board of Education.

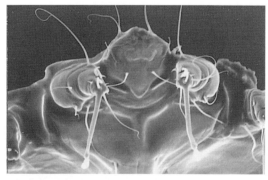

Fig. 17.3 Scanning electron micrograph of the jaw parts of *Sarcoptes scabiei* (× 1,000). These powerful jaws penetrate the skin and disrupt cells, producing a nutrient fluid on which the mite feeds. Courtesy of Patricianne Hurd, PhD, John Pietrahita, and Danny Blankenship, Fernbank Science Centre, DeKalb County Board of Education.

to the larva or adult, but has four pairs of legs. The protonymph lives on the skin or beneath the surface, and molts again in about 3 days to produce a second nymphal stage (tritonymph) (*Fig. 17.6*).

The adult appears 10–13 days after the egg is laid. The male is smaller than the female, and can be recognized because his fourth pair of legs end in suckers and not in bristles (*Fig. 17.6*). Young female mites burrow into the skin, apparently waiting to be found by a wandering male.[8] Copulation takes place in this temporary burrow; after copulation, the female emerges on the surface and wanders until she finds a suitable site for a permanent burrow. After fertilization, the developing ovaries swell the body to twice its previous volume.

If all eggs laid by a fertile female survived into adulthood, an infestation could produce about one million mites within 2 months. In fact, less than 10% of eggs survive to reach adulthood, even under the most favorable conditions. Scratching, bathing, and immunologic reaction all contribute to their poor survival. The average patient with scabies is infested with 11 mites, but about 50% of patients have no more than five (*Fig. 17.7*).

The clinical manifestations of scabies primarily reflect the host's immunologic response to the invading parasite. Under experimental conditions, 'virgin' volunteers infested with mites are asymptomatic with only minor erythema, even though burrows containing mites are

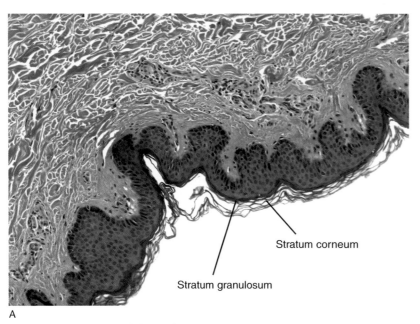
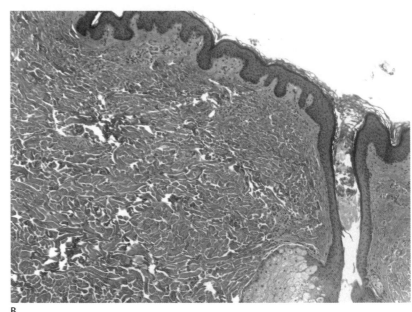

Stratum corneum

Stratum granulosum

A

B

Fig. 17.4 Thin sections of the epidermis stained with H & E showing the stratum corneum and stratum granulosum. Courtesy of Sherif Zaki, MD.

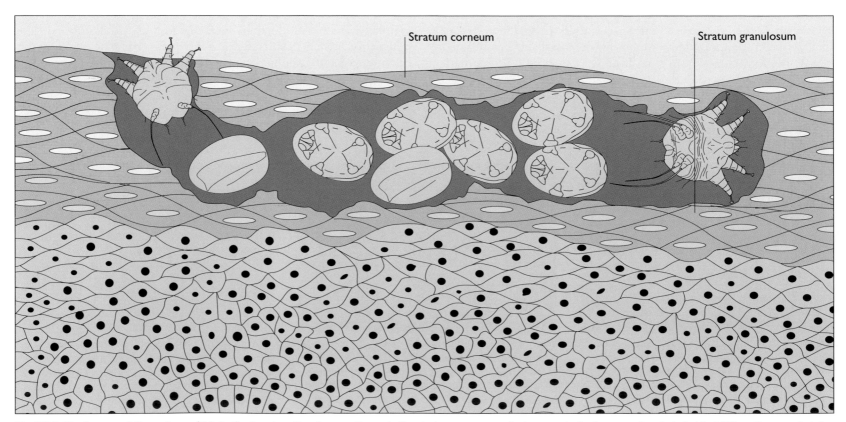

Stratum corneum

Stratum granulosum

Fig. 17.5 The burrow of *Sarcoptes scabiei*. As the female mite advances through the stratum corneum, she leaves a trail of eggs and scybala behind. When the eggs hatch, the larval forms emerge onto the skin surface.

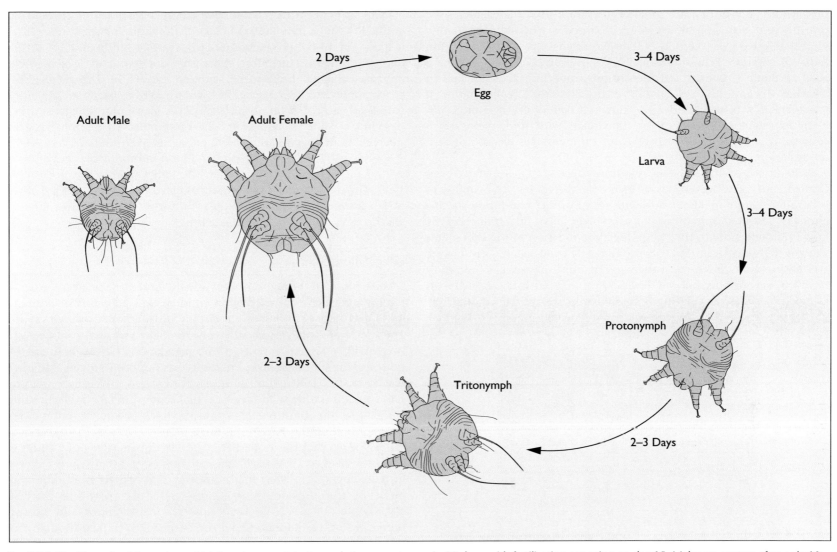

Fig. 17.6 The life cycle of *Sarcoptes scabiei*. Females complete the cycle from egg to egg in 19 days, with fertilization occurring on day 15. Males are mature after only 10 days.

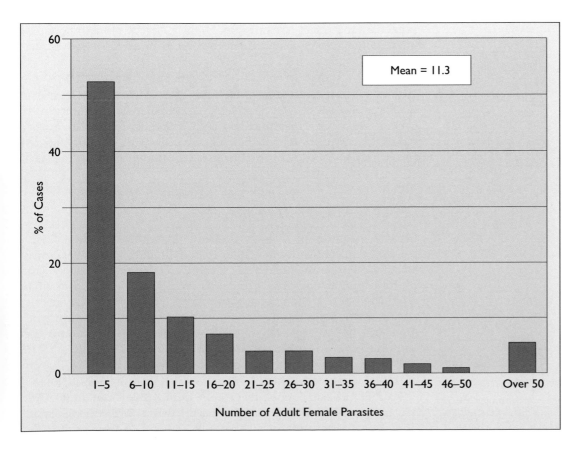

Fig. 17.7 The number of adult female mites recovered from a large series of carefully examined patients. Adapted from Orkin M, Maibach HI (eds): *Cutaneous Infestations and Insect Bites*. New York, Marcel Dekker, 1985.

present. It is not until a month after infestation that the characteristic pruritus and rash appear. However, volunteers who have been previously infested with the mite will develop signs and symptoms within a day of exposure. The number of mites infesting a patient reaches a peak at about 3 months and then begins to decline. It is not known whether the immune system can eventually clear the infestation if treatment is withheld. Under experimental conditions, it is more difficult to establish infestation in individuals with prior exposure to scabies. This suggests that there is an immunologic defense against reinfestation.

Several types of immunologic responses to the scabies mite have been studied, but investigations have been hampered by an inability to cultivate the mite in sufficient quantities to extract and purify specific antigens. The predominant response involves the cellular branch of the host's immune system. Histopathologic examination of the skin lesion shows a perivascular infiltrate, predominantly lymphocytes, histiocytes, and eosinophils (*Fig. 17.8*). Patients with impaired cellular immunity have fewer symptoms, but can develop a more severe infestation known as crusted scabies. Circulating immune complexes, vasculitis, and IgE-mediated reaction have also been associated with scabies.

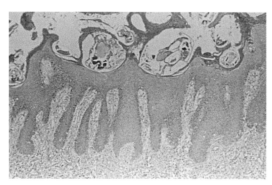

Fig. 17.8 Histology of a burrow and the inflammatory response of skin to scabies infestation. Typically, a superficial and deep perivascular infiltrate of lymphocytes, histiocytes, and eosinophils is present. When tissue sections do not reveal the mite, the pathologic pattern may be mistaken for a drug eruption, erythema multiforme, or malignant lymphoma. Courtesy of S.D. Glazer, MD.

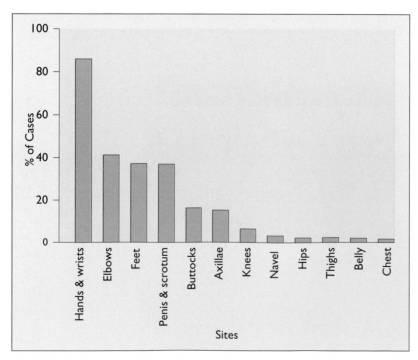

Fig. 17.9 The frequency with which various sites are infested with *Sarcoptes scabiei* from a large series of carefully examined patients. Adapted from Orkin M, Maibach HI (eds): *Cutaneous Infestations and Insect Bites.* New York, Marcel Dekker, 1985.

Many patients with scabies have elevated total serum IgE and IgE antibodies to the house dust mite, *Dermatophagoides pteronyssinus*.[9] This is likely due to the production of cross-reacting antibodies[10] to several different proteins, including those that are found in fecal particles (scybala). Rabbits immunized with an extract of *Dermatophagoides pteronyssinus* and *Dermatophagoides farinae* were resistant to infestation with *Sarcoptes scabiei* var *canis*.[10] One of the major mite allergens, which is found in mite excreta at a concentration of 10 mg/ml, has considerable homology to animal and plant cysteine proteases.[11]

Specific physical characteristics and local immunologic properties of skin at different sites may explain the mite's predilection for certain areas. The mite remains somewhat insulated from the full force of the host's immunologic response by burrowing only to the stratum granulosum, well away from the dermis.

EPIDEMIOLOGY

Scabies is known throughout the world. In underdeveloped countries, it is most prevalent among young children and adolescents, while in developed nations it is more uniformly distributed across age groups. The attack rate appears to be the same for males and females. Decreased susceptibility among various ethnic populations has been suggested; however, the idea of genetic immunity has not been proven. Although scabies is an STD, it is transmitted by prolonged, still, steady, skin-to-skin contacts[2] rather than specific sexual activity. In fact, holding hands is the most important of such contacts, which is why the mites are so commonly found in hands and fingers (*Fig. 17.9*). Scabies differs from other STDs in that it is not especially prevalent among young adults or homosexual men. The occurrence of scabies in infants and children further supports the view that nonsexual skin contact is an important mode of transmission. Most transmission occurs within families, although outbreaks have been observed in hospitals and nursing homes. Schools and fomites have not been shown to play an important role in the spread of scabies. Mites are subject to dessication, immobilized by cold, and killed by brief exposure to heat, so they seldom survive long away from the host. However, in a warm, moist environment they may survive for 2–3 days, suggesting at least the potential for indirect transmission. Fomites may be more important in institutional outbreaks, particularly when cases with large mite burdens occur.

It has been widely accepted that epidemics of scabies occur in 30-year cycles consisting of 15 years of high prevalence followed by 15 years of relatively few cases. Neither changes in population immunity nor a cyclical change in the mite has been found to explain this cycle. Recently, this phenomenon has been re-evaluated, and the apparent cycles may be more properly attributed to the great social upheavals caused by World Wars I and II.

CLINICAL MANIFESTATIONS

Clinical diagnosis of scabies requires a high index of suspicion. A patient's clinical history may offer important clues to the diagnosis of scabies. The typical patient seeks medical advice about 2–4 weeks after the onset of itching. The pruritus is usually most intense at night, especially upon first undressing and going to bed. Some patients itch only at night. Warmth intensifies the discomfort, and antipruritics may offer little relief. The rash typically begins on the hands and then spreads to the wrists, elbows, and other parts of the body (*Fig. 17.10*). The presence of a pruritic rash on the hands and trunk is very suggestive of scabies, as is a report that other family members are also itching.

A variety of skin lesions may result from scabies infestation (*Table 17.1*). Typical lesions of scabies are usually found on the flexor surfaces of wrists, elbows, anterior axillary folds, areolae in women, belt line,

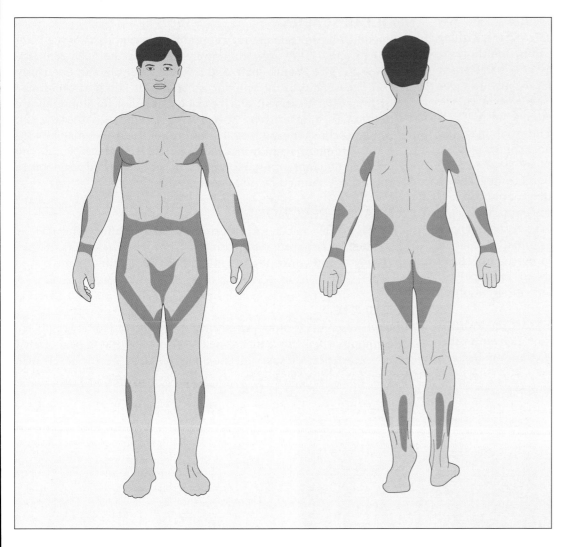

Fig. 17.10 Distribution of rash in *Sarcoptes scabiei* infestation. The rash does not correspond with the sites of election of the acari. Unshaded areas are rarely affected in healthy adults. Adapted from Johnson CG, Mellanby K: The parasitology of human scabies. *Parasitology* 1942; **34**:286, courtesy of Cambridge University Press.

Common	Unusual
Papules	Scaling crusts
Burrows	Urticaria
Excoriations	Vasculitis
Nodules	Attenuated or exaggerated lesions
Vesicles	
Pyoderma	
Eczema	

Table 17.1 Skin manifestations of scabies.

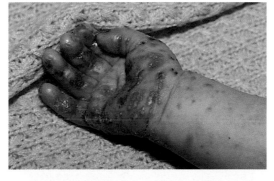

Fig. 17.11 Scabies of the palm with secondary pyoderma in an infant. Lesions on the palms, soles, head, neck and back are rare, except in infants and debilitated patients.

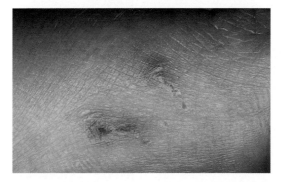

Fig. 17.12 Burrow of *Sarcoptes scabiei* on the side of a finger. Upper lesion shows the pathognomonic dirty-appearing wavy line extending out from an erythematous papule. In the lower lesion, the burrow has been nearly obliterated by excoriation.

lower portion of buttocks and upper thighs, and the male genitalia (*Fig. 17.10*). The back is conspicuously free of lesions except in infants and the debilitated.

In contrast to adults, infants often show heavy infestation of the palms, soles, head, neck, face, and back (*Fig. 17.11*). The individual papules and burrows maintain their characteristic appearances. Infants may refuse food and fail to grow because of scabies infestation. Secondary infection with bacterial flora associated with the anatomical sites of the lesions is common.[12]

Several specific types of skin lesions may be present in a single patient. The classically described burrow, although pathognomonic for the disease, is increasingly difficult to find. The burrow consists of a gray, dirty-appearing, 2–15 mm wavy line, usually seen on the wrist, interdigital web, or the side of a finger (*Fig. 17.12*). A tiny vesicle containing the mite may occasionally be seen at one end of the burrow (*Fig. 17.13*). The more typical lesion is a small, erythematous papule with surrounding erythema (*Fig. 17.14*). Lesions are usually sparse, but in some areas may become nearly confluent. These lesions are caused by larvae and nymphs that do not burrow.

In patients who bathe frequently, the manifestations of scabies may be subtle, with only a few lesions and rare burrows (*Fig. 17.15*). Bathing undoubtedly destroys many developing mites, thus limiting the number that reach maturity. Despite the paucity of characteristic lesions, the distribution and symmetry of the dermatitis provide a clue to diagnosis. In cases in which only a single body site is involved, the recognition of any infested contact may be the key to diagnosis.

Excoriation, denudation, eczema, and subsequent infection may alter the appearance of scabies lesions so that they resemble chronic eczema or pyoderma (*Fig. 17.16*). Infection, usually caused by *Staphylococcus aureus* or group A *Streptococcus pyogenes*, can produce local complications, including impetigo, ecthyma, furunculosis, and cellulitis, or more serious systemic disease such as bacteremia and internal abscesses. Secondary infection with group A streptococci can have serious consequences, with up to 2% of cases developing acute glomerulonephritis. Eczematous changes induced by scratching may be exacerbated by the irritant or drying effect of topical antipruritic and antiscabietic medications. Scratching may also cause trauma to superficial blood vessels, resulting in petechial or ecchymotic lesions (*Fig. 17.17*).

Manifestations of scabies may be altered by the presence of any other chronic or acute dermatosis. Scabies is frequently associated with other STDs. The diagnosis of scabies in sexually active individuals indicates a need to examine for other STDs.

NODULAR SCABIES

Firm, reddish-brown nodules may appear on covered parts of the body (*Figs 17.18* and *17.19*). Most commonly found on the male genitalia, including the glans penis, shaft, and scrotum, they are also frequently seen on elbows and in the anterior axillary folds. These nodules may persist long after treatment and probably represent an immunologic reaction to persisting antigens. Mite parts cannot be seen after the first month. Both clinically and histologically, nodular scabies may be confused with lymphoma and histiocytosis X. The inflammatory infiltrate is comprised of lymphocytes, histiocytes, plasma cells, and eosinophils. Giant cells and frank granulomas are uncommon.

URTICARIAL REACTIONS

A systemic allergic reaction to mite antigens may result in urticaria (*Fig. 17.20*). Such a response is not common, but when it occurs, it may completely overshadow the small number of scabies lesions. The urticaria resolves within a few days of antiscabietic therapy.

VASCULITIS

Although vasculitis is often present histologically, vasculitic lesions are not common. It is possible that some lesions that appear to be ulcerated due to excoriation or superinfection may actually be the result of a localized vasculitis (*Fig. 17.21*).

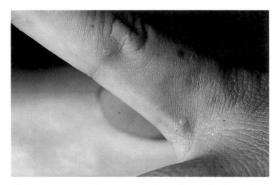

Fig. 17.13 Vesicular scabietic lesions on the lateral surface of a finger and interdigital web.

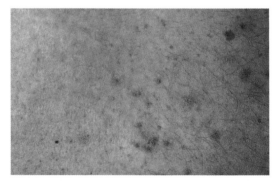

Fig. 17.14 Multiple larval papules on the abdomen. Such papules, which may be clustered or widely scattered, occur when immature mites penetrate the skin. These papules greatly outnumber burrows, which are formed only by the adult female mites.

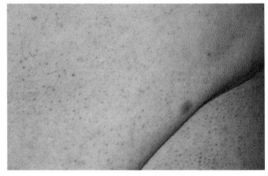

Fig. 17.15 Scabies in the clean patient. Frequent bathing kills immature mites and limits the severity of the infestation. This man had only a few pruritic papules such as this isolated lesion on the lower abdomen.

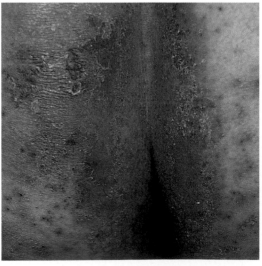

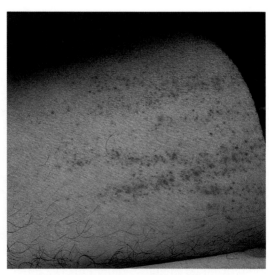

Figs 17.16 and 17.17 Excoriated lesions. (17.16) Eczema may result from repeated excoriation or from the irritating effect of topical medications. A scaling, pruritic rash on the buttocks is a common manifestation of scabies. (17.17) Petechiae and ecchymoses may also be caused by excoriation. These rows of petechiae resulted from capillary breakage during vigorous scratching.

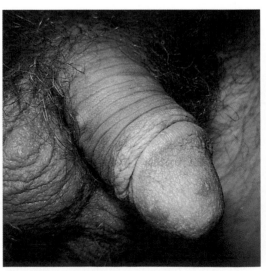

Fig. 17.18 Nodular lesions of scabies on the male genitalia. Nodules generally occur on covered parts of the body. In this patient, erythematous, indurated lesions are present on the glans, penile shaft, and scrotum.

CRUSTED SCABIES

Crusted scabies is characterized by lesions, resembling psoriasis, whose thick scales contain large numbers of mites (*Figs 17.22* and *17.23*). Pruritus is minimal. The disease is usually seen in immunologically incompetent or physically debilitated patients. It has also been associated with the use of topical fluorinated steroids (*Table 17.2*). Months are required for the generalized lesions of crusted scabies to develop. An impaired immune response or inability to scratch allows the mite to multiply unchecked. The shedding of tremendous numbers of mites causes this form of scabies to be extremely contagious.

SCABIES INCOGNITO

Topical application of steroids may markedly attenuate symptoms as well as reduce the number of lesions and alter their distribution. Such a presentation has been labeled scabies incognito (*Fig. 17.24*). Potent fluorinated steroids have also been associated with crusted scabies.

SCABIES AND AIDS

Patients with AIDS may have an atypical or exaggerated cutaneous response to many infections, including scabies infestation (*Fig. 17.25*). A disproportionately large number of AIDS patients develop crusted scabies.[15] The absence of burrows, an unusual distribution of lesions (i.e., face, scalp, and nails) and the scaling or crusted character of the dermatitis often delays diagnosis. Repeated treatments are required to eradicate the infestation, probably because of the large mite burden.

LABORATORY TESTS

An attempt should be made to confirm the diagnosis of scabies in all suspected cases. A number of techniques have been used to demonstrate the mite, its burrow, eggs or scybala (feces), any one of which is diagnostic. Although a positive diagnosis can probably be made in all cases if one searches with sufficient diligence, the success rates of various techniques are reported to range from 30–90%. Success with any technique increases with the skill and experience of the examiner.

SKIN SCRAPING

Preparation of a skin scraping is probably the most frequently used test for the scabies mite (*Figs 17.26–17.28*). First, the patient should be examined carefully in good light using a magnifying lens to select a burrow or papule that has not been excoriated. Lesions on the finger webs, wrists, or elbows are most likely to yield a positive diagnosis. Place a drop of mineral oil on the lesion and use a small disposable scalpel to scrape gently across the surface until the topmost layer of skin is removed. No bleeding should occur. Gently collect the mineral oil containing the flecks of skin onto the scalpel blade and transfer it to a glass microscope slide. Add a cover slip and examine under low magnification.

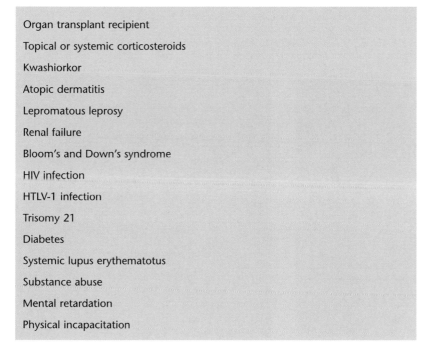

Organ transplant recipient

Topical or systemic corticosteroids

Kwashiorkor

Atopic dermatitis

Lepromatous leprosy

Renal failure

Bloom's and Down's syndrome

HIV infection

HTLV-1 infection

Trisomy 21

Diabetes

Systemic lupus erythematotus

Substance abuse

Mental retardation

Physical incapacitation

Table 17.2 Risk factors for developing crusted scabies.

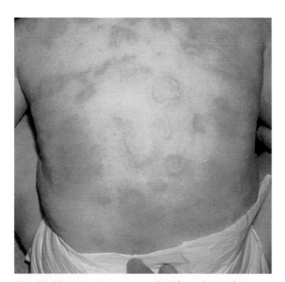

Fig. 17.19 Nodular scabies on the extensor surface of the elbow. Such lesions may persist long after antiscabietic therapy. Their clinical and histologic appearances have caused them to be mistaken for neoplasms. Courtesy of du Vivier A, McKee PH: *Atlas of Clinical Dermatology*. London, Gower Medical Publishing Ltd., 1986.

Fig. 17.20 Urticaria associated with scabies. This child had multiple wheals over the face, trunk, and extremities. Typical scabietic burrows on the palms and soles were initially overlooked. The urticaria disappeared 48 hours after treatment with lindane lotion. Courtesy of Chapel TA. Scabies presenting as urticaria. *JAMA* 1981; **246**:1441, with permission of the American Medical Association.

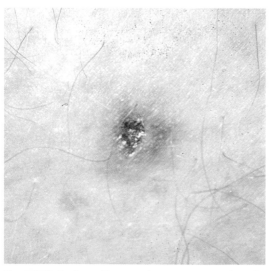

Fig. 17.21 Lesion with necrotic center suggestive of vasculitis. Histologic evidence of localized vascular inflammation is frequently present on biopsy, but a generalized vasculitic reaction is rare.

Visualization of any adult or larval mite forms, eggs, or scybala is diagnostic of scabies (*Figs 17.29–17.32*). Some clinicians prefer to omit the mineral oil and transfer the dry skin scrapings to a slide containing a drop of 10% KOH. Although this may help to disperse the cellular material for easier examination, it will destroy the fecal pellets that in some specimens are the only clues to the diagnosis. Fluorescence microscopy may also be helpful in identifying mites and ova.[16]

EPIDERMAL SHAVE BIOPSY

This technique offers improved sensitivity and may be less likely to cause injury in an uncooperative patient (*Figs 17.33–17.35*). Lift the selected lesion between the thumb and index finger. Gently shave off the outer layer of skin with a sterile scalpel. Use a fine sawing movement while holding the scalpel blade tangential to the skin surface. Transfer the shaving to a microscope slide, add a drop of mineral oil, apply a cover slip, and then examine under the microscope for mites, eggs, or scybala (*Figs 17.36* and *17.37*).

CURETTAGE

Use a small cutting curette to scrape the epidermal layer off a selected papule or burrow. This technique is particularly useful for infants or other uncooperative patients for whom the use of a scalpel might be hazardous. Place the scrapings on a slide with oil or KOH and examine.

BURROW INK TEST

Use a fountain pen to cover a papule with ink, then clean off the ink with alcohol (*Figs 17.38* and *17.39*). A positive result is seen when the ink penetrates the papule, revealing a dark, zigzag line running across and away from the papule (*Figs 17.40* and *17.41*). A positive ink test is specific for scabies; however, a shave biopsy on a positive lesion will demonstrate the actual mite. Topical tetracycline may be used instead of ink and washed off with alcohol after 5 minutes. A Wood's light will reveal burrows as areas of linear yellow-green fluorescence.

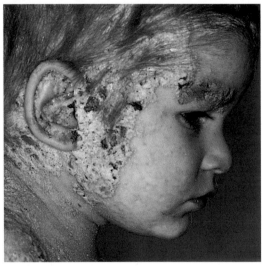

Fig. 17.22 Extensive crusted lesions of the face, neck, and scalp.

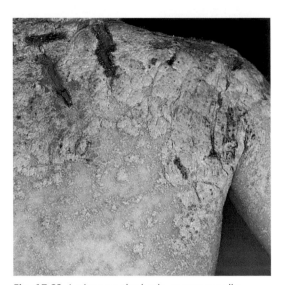

Fig. 17.23 Lesions on the back, an area usually spared in typical scabies.

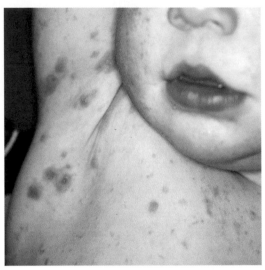

Fig. 17.24 Scabies incognito. Atypical lesions in a child treated with topical steroids. Steroids may either exacerbate or reduce the cutaneous response to infestation. Courtesy of Heidi Watts.

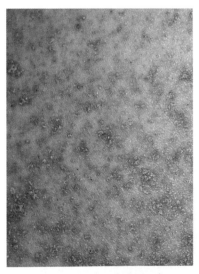

Fig. 17.25 Cutaneous lesions of scabies in a patient with AIDS. Lesions may be either diminished or exaggerated. In this patient, lesions on the back remained nearly confluent, even after multiple applications of scabicide.

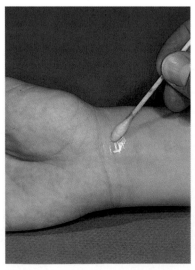

Fig. 17.26

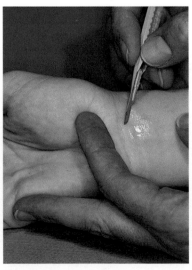

Fig. 17.27

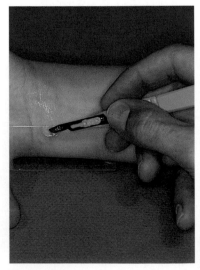

Fig. 17.28

Figs 17.26–17.28 Preparation of a skin scraping. (17.26) Select an unexcoriated burrow or papule, preferably on the hand or wrist. Cover the lesion with a thin layer of mineral oil. (17.27) Hold a sterile scalpel perpendicular to the skin. Gently scrape the lesion until the superficial skin is removed. Collect the mineral oil containing skin particles and mites onto the scalpel blade. (17.28) Transfer the mineral oil to a microscope slide and cover with a glass cover slip. Add another drop of oil if necessary to eliminate any air bubbles. Examine under a microscope with a low-power objective.

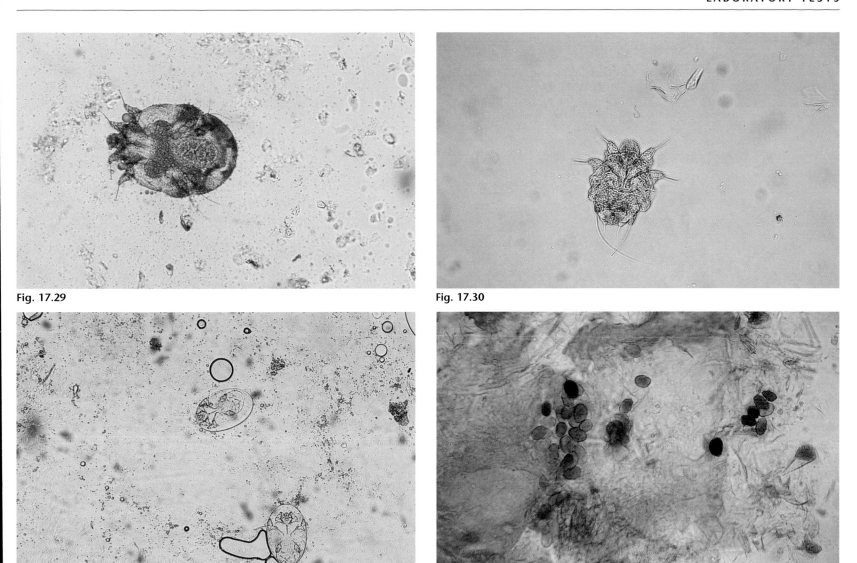

Fig. 17.29

Fig. 17.30

Fig. 17.31

Fig. 17.32

Figs 17.29–17.32 Positive skin scrapings. Any of the following are diagnostic of scabies infestation. (17.29) Adult female scabies mite. (17.30) Larval stage of scabies mite, which has only two hind legs. (17.31) *S. scabiei* eggs. (17.32) Feces of scabies are also called scybala. Figs 17.29 and 17.31 courtesy of Adele Moreland, MD.

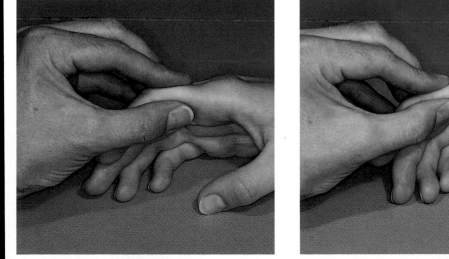
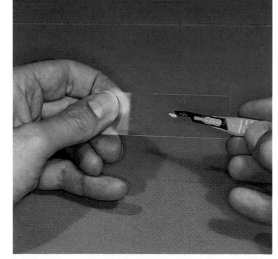

Fig. 17.33

Fig. 17.34

Fig. 17.35

Figs 17.33–17.35 Preparation of a shave biopsy. (17.33) Select a lesion and hold it firmly between the thumb and index finger, so that it is slightly elevated above the surrounding skin. (17.34) Hold a sterile scalpel with its blade parallel to the skin surface. Use a fine sawing motion to carefully shave off the outer layer of skin. (17.35) Use the scalpel blade to transfer the shaving to a microscope slide. Place a drop of oil over the specimen, then add a cover slip. Examine under a microscope using a scanning objective.

SEWING NEEDLE

An intact burrow must be present with the mite visible as either a dark point in Caucasian skin or a white point in Blacks. Using a needle or pin, perforate the burrow at this point and move the needle from side to side, holding it parallel to the skin. The mite will attach itself to the needle and can be transferred to a slide for examination.

GLUE STRIPPING

Place a drop of methacrylate glue on a glass slide and push down firmly over an intact lesion. Allow the glue to set, then strip the slide of the lesion briskly. Repeat the process two more times to obtain deeper organisms, then examine microscopically.

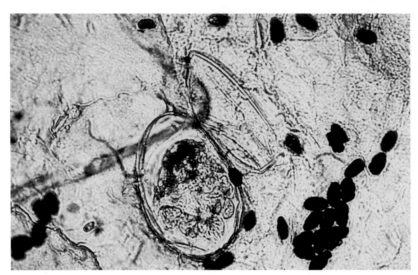

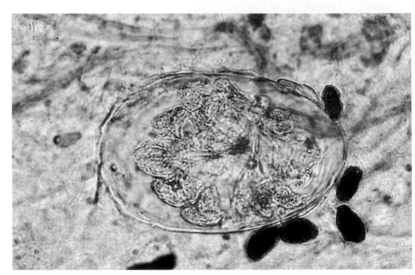

Figs 17.36 and 17.37 Positive shave biopsies. (17.36) Two eggs, one hatched and one containing a developing nymph, are visible within the skin shaving. Multiple small, dark fecal particles surround the eggs (× 50). (17.37) Egg and scybala under higher magnification. The egg contains a larva that is nearly ready to emerge (× 100). Fig. 17.37 courtesy of David Woodley, MD.

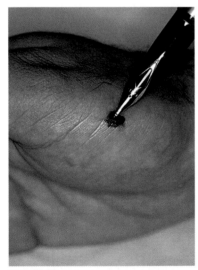

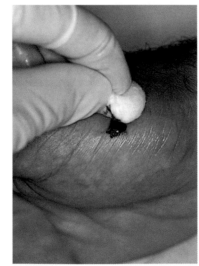

Figs 17.38 and 17.39 Burrow ink test technique. (17.38) Select an unexcoriated burrow or papule for the test. Cover the lesion with water-soluble ink from a fountain pen. (17.39) After 5 minutes, use an alcohol-soaked cotton ball to wash all the ink off the skin surface. Examine the lesion for evidence of ink remaining within the scabies burrow.

Fig. 17.38

Fig. 17.39

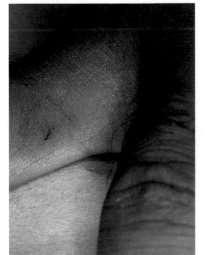

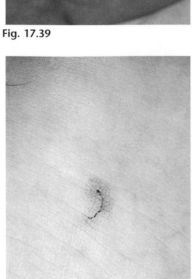

Figs 17.40 and 17.41 Positive burrow ink test. (17.40) An ink-filled burrow on the side of a finger is clearly visible after washing ink from the surface of the lesion. (17.41) A close-up view demonstrates the scabies burrow tracking across skin lines. The ink helps to define the morphology and limits of the burrow. Courtesy of Patricianne Hurd, PhD, John Pietrahita, and Danny Blankenship, Fernbank Science Centre, DeKalb County Board of Education.

Fig. 17.40

Fig. 17.41

Permethrin 5% cream
Apply from neck down and massage into skin. Wash off medication after 12 hours, usually overnight. One application is usually curative.

Lindane 1% lotion or cream
Apply a thin layer to entire body from the neck down and allow to dry. Wash off completely after 8–12 hours. One application is usually curative.

Crotamiton 10% cream
After bathing, massage cream into skin from neck down. Apply again after 24 hours. Wash off medication 48 hours after second application.

Precipitable sulfur 6% in petrolatum
Apply nightly from neck down for three nights. Wash off medication thoroughly 24 hours after final application. (May stain clothing.)

Benzyl benzoate 25% solution
Apply to entire body from neck down nightly for two nights. Wash off 24 hours after last application.

Malathion 0.5% aqueous lotion
Apply to whole body from neck down. Wash off medication after 12 hours, usually overnight.

Table 17.3 Treatment of scabies.

CELLOPHANE TAPE

Prepare the lesion by cleaning with ether, then apply a short length of clear cellophane tape. Briskly strip the tape from the skin and affix to a microscope slide. Repeat this several times for each lesion, using a new piece of tape each time.

PUNCH BIOPSY

If none of the above techniques is successful, a small 2-mm punch biopsy from an unexcoriated lesion may reveal the mite. Instruct the laboratory to make serial sections, all of which should be closely studied for evidence of the mite (see Fig. 17.8).

TREATMENT

Decisions in scabies therapy center on the choice of drug and on selection of contacts for prophylaxis. Because scabies may not become symptomatic until 1 month following infestation, it is essential to treat contacts prophylactically in order to prevent re-exposure. In general, all household and sexual contacts should be treated. Decisions on whether to treat other contacts should be based on the degree of skin-to-skin contact they have with the patient. Seven drugs are available to treat scabies: permethrin, lindane, crotamiton, sulfur, benzyl benzoate, malathion, and ivermectin (Table 17.3).[17]

PERMETHRIN

Permethrin, a synthetic pyrethroid, is available in a 5% cream and is effective with a single application. Permethrin should be applied from the neck to the feet, and then washed off after 12 hours, usually overnight. Adverse reactions are infrequent and generally consist only of local burning or stinging. Permethrin is a preferred treatment for children under 10 years of age, and pregnant or lactating women because it is not associated with CNS toxicity. Permethrin is the preferred treatment for scabies at the present time (compared to lindane and crotamiton).[17]

LINDANE

Lindane (hexachlorocyclohexane or gamma benzene hexachloride) in a 1% lotion or cream is cheaper than permethrin. After the patient bathes, lindane is applied to the entire body from the neck down. Eight to twelve hours later, it is washed off. A second treatment is not necessary unless there is evidence of treatment failure or reinfestation. Since lindane is toxic to the CNS and approximately 10% of the drug is absorbed through the skin, it should be used cautiously. To avoid overdose, only the amount actually needed (about 1 oz for an adult) should be prescribed. Applying lindane immediately after a bath may predispose to raising blood levels and should be avoided. Lindane should not be used by children under 10 years of age, pregnant women, lactating women, or patients with neurologic disorders because of the potential for toxicity. The low cost makes lindane a key alternative drug in many countries. Lindane resistance has been reported.[18]

CROTAMITON

Crotamiton, in a 10% cream, is an effective scabicide with minimal toxicity that is suitable for use in children under 10 years of age and pregnant or lactating women. It is applied nightly for 2 nights, then washed off 48 hours after the last application. Crotamiton is more likely than lindane to require a second course of therapy. Application of crotamiton cream may give symptomatic relief.[19]

SULFUR

Sulfur as 6% precipitated sulfur in petrolatum is an ancient therapy that remains effective, although it is seldom used because of its disagreeable odor and staining. It is applied nightly for 3 nights then washed off 24 hours after the last application. Upon completing the regimen of topical therapy, the patient should wash all clothes and bed linen used within the preceding 2–3 days.

BENZYL BENZOATE

Benzyl benzoate in a 25% solution has been used effectively for over 70 years to treat scabies. It is applied to the entire body from the neck down nightly for 2 nights then washed off 24 hours after the last application.

MALATHION

Malathion as a 0.5% aqueous solution has been recommended for the treatment of scabies.[19] No random clinical trials including malathion have been performed; however, non-controlled studies have suggested it is an effective treatment for scabies.[17]

IVERMECTIN

Ivermectin (200 µg/kg) is the only oral drug used in the treatment of scabies. It is also available as a 0.8% topical solution. A single dose was shown to be as effective as benzyl benzoate[20] and lindane,[21] but the number of individuals that were treated in these studies was small. Concerns have been raised about excess risk of death for elderly patients treated for scabies with ivermectin; however, this has not been confirmed.[22] Ivermectin has not received approval of the US Food and Drug Agency or the European Drug Agency for scabies.[22] Until approval is granted, ivermectin should be reserved for special forms of scabies (e.g., crusted scabies, HIV-related scabies) where it has been used successfully.[23,24]

Usually, pruritis begins to resolve within 2 days of therapy, but may not be completely resolved for several weeks. It is important that the patient knows what to expect because overuse of scabicides or other topical medications may lead to an irritant dermatitis that can be confused with treatment failure. Cases of apparent resistance to lindane and crotamiton are rare and may be due to improper use or reinfestation. Patients with crusted scabies may require multiple applications of scabicides over many weeks to eradicate infestation.

PHTHIRUS PUBIS

Phthirus pubis, the crab louse, is one of the three members of the order Anoplura that infests man. The other two are *Pediculus humanus* var *capitis*, the head louse, and *Pediculus humanus* var *corporis*, the body louse *(Fig. 17.42)*. Only *P. pubis* is primarily sexually transmitted. The blood-sucking lice are the most parasitic of all insects, because there is no free-living stage in the life-cycle at all.[2] Human lice feed only on blood drawn fresh from the host. Therefore, their diet is 100% liquid. *Phthirus pubis* is about 1 mm in length with a short, broad body and large, clawlike legs, which bear a remarkable resemblance to a crab, thus accounting for its common name *(Fig. 17.43)*. The head, conical and pointed anteriorly, contains stylets that can pierce human skin, enabling the louse to suck blood from its host. The louse has a thin semi-transparent cuticle through which the gut and its movements can

be clearly seen in living lice when under a microscope. During feeding, the body takes on a red-brown color. Three pairs of legs extend from the anterior abdomen. At the end of each leg, there is a hook-like claw and opposing thumb, which are specially suited for grasping hairs *(Fig. 17.44)*. Four sets of small, conical structures ending in bristles arise from the posterior abdomen.

The life cycle of *Phthirus pubis* includes five stages from egg to adult. The eggs, called nits, are encased in a cement substance and firmly affixed to the hair shaft. Each nit has a convex cap (operculum) containing air pores that comes off intact when the first nymphal stage emerges after 5–10 days *(Fig. 17.45)*. Nymphs resemble adults except for their smaller size and sexual immaturity. A tough, chitinous exoskeleton restricts the nymphs' growth, and a series of three molts is necessary to reach adulthood, a process requiring 2–3 weeks.[25] When lice reach adulthood, mating occurs after about 10 hours and continues

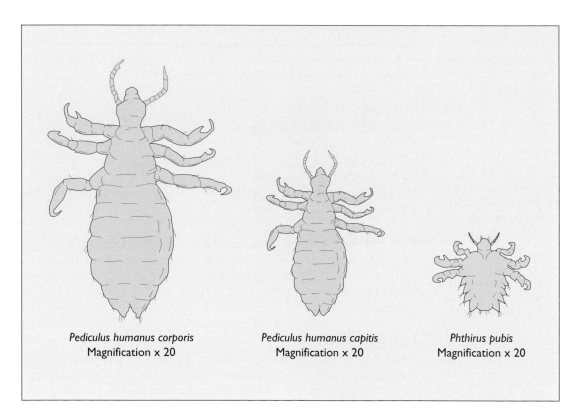

Pediculus humanus corporis
Magnification x 20

Pediculus humanus capitis
Magnification x 20

Phthirus pubis
Magnification x 20

Fig. 17.42 Lice that infest humans. The crablike appearance of *Phthirus pubis* makes it easy to distinguish from the head louse (*Pediculus humanus* var *capitis*) and the body louse (*Pediculus humanus* var *corporis*). *Phthirus pubis* may be found outside the pubic area, so diagnosis must be based upon the appearance of the louse rather than its site of infestation.

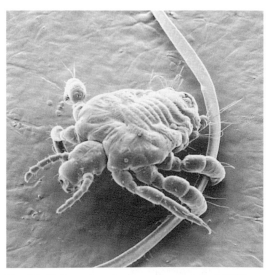

Fig. 17.43 Scanning electron micrograph of *Phthirus pubis* (× 50).

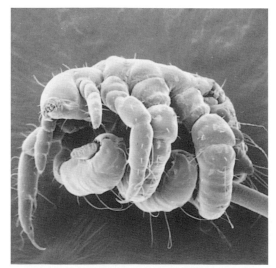

Fig. 17.44 Scanning electron micrograph of *Phthirus pubis* (× 100). Clawlike legs encircling a pubic hair produce a firm grip that can be difficult to dislodge.

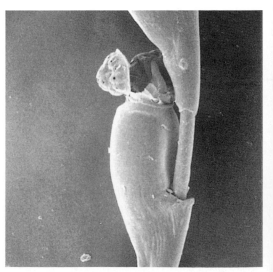

Fig. 17.45 Scanning electron micrograph of an egg, or nit, with nymphal stage of *Phthirus pubis* preparing to emerge. The cap (operculum) containing air pores is pushed off during this process (× 100).

until the lice dies. The female begins to lay eggs shortly after fertilization, producing approximately 4 eggs/day during her 3–4 week adult life.[25]

Crab lice are well adapted to its human host where infestation usually involves pubic, axillary and body hair, although beard, scalp, eyebrow and eyelash infestations have been reported.[26,27] Their preference for certain sites is probably related to hair spacing: the 2-mm spaces between pubic hairs match the span of the louse's hind legs, with which it grasps hairs. Pubic lice are usually sedentary, moving only a few millimeters per day. They seldom travel far from the initial area of infestation unless transferred to a new site by the host. To feed, the crab louse grasps hairs with its clawlike legs and pierces the skin to obtain blood from a capillary. It often remains attached and feeds intermittently for hours before moving to a new site. *Phthirus pubis* feeds exclusively on human blood and rarely survive more than 24 hours off a human host.

EPIDEMIOLOGY

Phthirus pubis spreads predominantly through intimate sexual contact. Transmission via nonsexual contact or fomites may occur occasionally, but it is unusual. Since *Phthirus pubis* infestation is not reportable in the USA, limited epidemiologic information is available. Many believe that the incidence of infestation has increased markedly during the past two decades, paralleling increases in other STDs during a period of changing sexual behavior. Most available epidemiologic information comes from STD clinics. However, such data certainly underestimate cases because the availability of effective nonprescription therapy makes it unnecessary to consult a physician for this disease.

The population with the highest incidence of crab lice is similar to that of gonorrhea and syphilis; single persons, ages 15 to 25 years;[28] the prevalence of infestation declines gradually to age 35 and is uncommon in persons older than age 35.

CLINICAL MANIFESTATIONS

Patients who present to a physician with *Phthirus pubis* infestation have usually seen lice or complain of severe pruritus in the pubic area. Excoriations and secondary infection are common findings in symptomatic patients. Ten or fewer adult lice are usually present at diagnosis.

In an STD clinic, half of infested patients are asymptomatic. The diagnosis is often made during examination for an unrelated problem. Occasionally the only complaint is the presence of multiple rust-colored spots on the patient's underclothes, resulting from bleeding at the sites of bites, or from excrement from the louse after a blood meal (*Fig. 17.46*). Most patients do not notice pruritis until 1 month after exposure to an infested partner. This incubation period is probably related to the development of the host's immunological response and growth of the lice population to a size sufficient to cause discomfort.

An uncommon manifestation of *Phthirus pubis* infestation is the macula caerulea, an asymptomatic bluish-gray macule that does not blanch under pressure. The lesion represents the bite of the louse and a resultant small hemorrhage into the skin. Most commonly seen are small punctate, red lesions near hair follicles that mark the sites of recent bites (*Fig. 17.47*). These lesions when inflamed and excoriated, resemble folliculitis. Excessive scratching may lead to super-infection.

LABORATORY TESTS

A diagnosis of *Phthirus pubis* infestation is usually straightforward and requires finding only one of the crab-like insects on the patient. The search is aided by good lighting and a magnifying lens. Their yellow-gray color makes the lice difficult to see on Caucasian skin, but after a blood meal they have a more visible rust color (*Fig. 17.48*). Occasionally, the lice are found only in extrapubic areas, such as the axillae, extremities, buttocks, scalp, and eyelashes (*Fig. 17.49*). Demonstration of adults, nymphs, or nits is sufficient for diagnosis. Nits are usually easiest to find, but may be confused with hair casts or scales of skin from seborrhea (*Fig. 17.50*). Nits may be distinguished from the latter by microscopy and by their firm adherence to the hair shaft. Unless removed with a special fine-tooth comb, nits will remain attached to the hair after therapy and move outward as the hair grows. If treatment failure or reinfestation is suspected, only those eggs close to the base of the hair shaft should be considered significant. Empty egg casings do not indicate active infestation, but can be distinguished from viable eggs only by microscopic examination (*Fig. 17.51*).

TREATMENT

Lindane and synergized pyrethrins are the drugs of choice for treatment of *Phthirus pubis* infestations and are equally effective (*Table 17.4*).

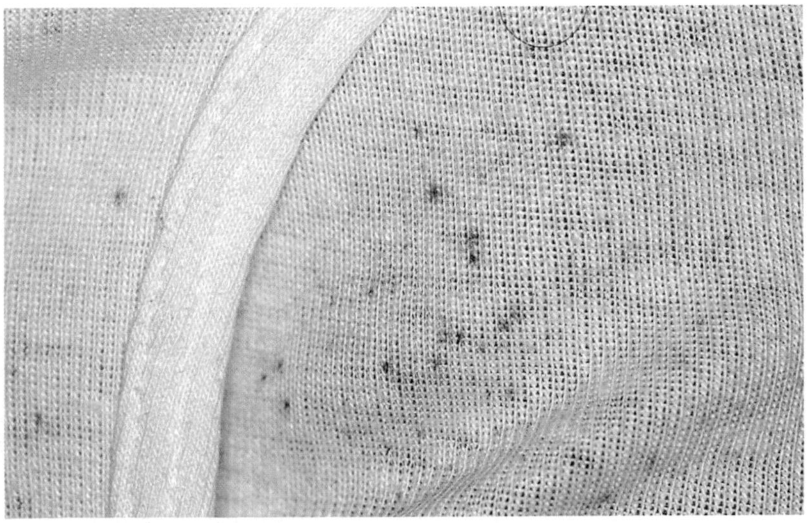

Fig. 17.46 Rust-colored spots on underclothing may result from bleeding at bite sites or from excrement from the louse after a blood meal. In patients without symptoms, these spots may be the first clue to the presence of infestation.

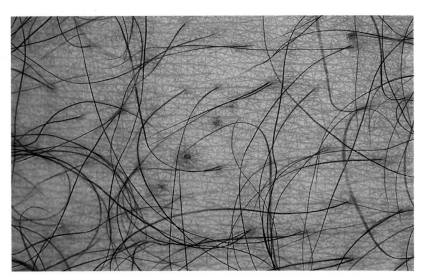

Fig. 17.47 Bite marks of *Phthirus pubis*. These punctate lesions with surrounding erythema are typical of the tiny papules that arise at sites of crab louse bites.

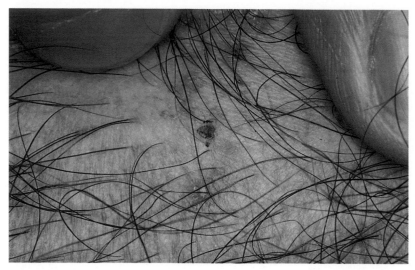

Fig. 17.48 *Phthirus pubis* feeding on its host. To obtain a meal of human blood, the crab louse uses its clawlike legs to grasp a hair on either side, then penetrates the host's skin with its mouth. Firmly anchored in this position, the louse may feed for hours. During feeding, the body takes on a red-brown color more easily seen against Caucasian skin.

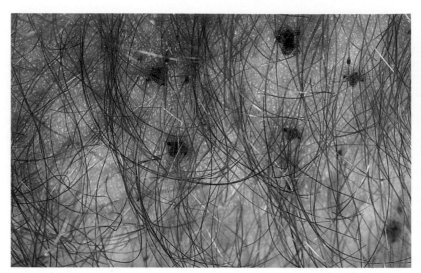

Fig. 17.49 Extrapubic infestation. *Phthirus pubis* may infest almost any area in hirsute individuals. This cluster of lice was present on the buttock of a patient whose pubic hair was not infested.

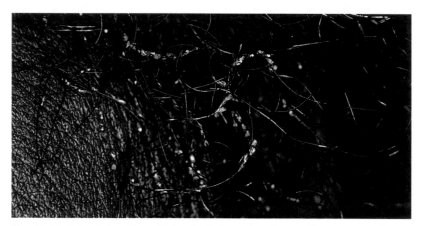

Fig. 17.50 Pubic hair with multiple nits. Hairs such as these with numerous nits are easily recognized as a sign of *Phthirus pubis* infestation. When only a few nits are present, a careful search with a magnifying lens may be necessary to establish the diagnosis.

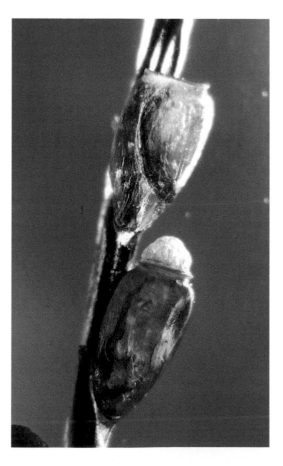

Fig. 17.51 Photomicrograph of two nits on a hair shaft. The upper egg is empty, but the lower one still contains a developing nymph. Empty nits may be a sign of past rather than current infestation. After therapy, unhatched nits at the base of hairs indicate treatment failure or reinfestation.

LINDANE 1% SHAMPOO

Apply shampoo to pubic hair and any other infested areas (except eyelashes). Add water to produce a thick lather; then wash off after four minutes. If the 1% cream or lotion is used, it should be washed off after 12 hours.

PERMETHRIN 1% CREAM RINSE

Cream rinse should be applied after washing hair, then rinsed out after 10 minutes.

PYRETHRIN WITH PIPERONYL BUTOXIDE

Lotion, gel, and shampoo preparations are available without prescription. Apply medication to thoroughly cover infested hair (except eyelashes). Wash off after 10 minutes.

PETROLATUM

Use only for infestation of the eyelashes. Apply twice daily for eight days. Any nits remaining after treatment can be physically removed.

Table 17.4 Treatment of *Phthirus pubis* infestation.

Lindane is available as a lotion, cream, or shampoo. The cream and lotion require a 12-hour application for complete killing of lice and ova, but the shampoo is effective in only 4 minutes. The use of lindane in children less than 2 years of age, pregnant or lactating women, and patients with extensive dermatologic or neurologic disorders should be avoided. However, if used correctly, the brief exposure to the shampoo presents a very limited opportunity for absorption of the drug. Pyrethrins synergized with piperonyl butoxide are available without prescription in lotion and shampoo forms. The infested hair must be covered with the lotion or lathered with the shampoo for 10 minutes, then washed with water. Toxicity is not a problem with this drug, which may be used safely during pregnancy.

Permethrin, a synthetic pyrethrin, is available without prescription as a 1% cream rinse. It should be applied to clean hair for 10 minutes, then rinsed out immediately. Effectiveness is comparable to lindane and synergized pyrethrins and less that 1% of patients require retreatment.

It is important to instruct the patient in the proper use of these medications. In most cases, treatment of the pubic and perianal hair is sufficient, although other sites should be inspected and treated if necessary. In individuals with much body hair, medication should be applied to the lower abdomen, thighs, and buttocks, regardless of whether or not lice are found in these areas.

After treatment, any clothing and bed linen used during the preceding 24 hours should be washed. Since the louse survives for less than a day away from the host, it is not necessary to treat furniture and other potential fomites with insecticide. In cases in which the eyelashes are involved, petrolatum applied to the lashes twice a day for 10 days is safe and effective. If nits remain after this treatment, they may be removed with forceps.

Sexual contacts should be examined and treated prophylactically; household contacts should be treated only if actually infested. Persons who are infested and are also infected with HIV should receive the same treatment regimen as those who are HIV-negative. Patients infested with *Phthirus pubis* should be examined for other STDs.

Resistance of *Phthirus pubis* to insecticides has not yet been reported. Most cases of treatment failure can be attributed to incorrect use of medication, failure to medicate all infested body sites, or re-exposure to an untreated partner. Persistant pruritis does not warrant additional therapy in the absence of active infestation. Repeated treatment with lindane may exacerbate the itching by causing a skin irritation. Delusions of parasitosis are not uncommon after successful therapy and frequently result in the overuse of medications.

References

1. Arlian LG. Biology, host relations, and epidemiology of *Sarcoptes scabiei*. *Ann Rev Entomol* 1989; **34**:139–161.
2. Maunder JW. Lice and scabies. Myths and reality. *Dermatol Clinics* 1998; **16**:843–845.
3. Arlian LG, Runyan RA, Estes SA. Cross infestivity of *Sarcoptes scabiei*. *J Amer Acad Derm* 1984; **10**:979–986.
4. Walton SF, Choy JL, Bonson A *et al*. Genetically distinct dog-derived and human-derived *Sarcoptes scabiei* in scabies endemic communities in Northern Australia. *Am J Trop Med Hyg* 1999; **61**:542–547.
5. Mellanby K. Biology of the parasite. In: Orkin M, Maibach HI, eds. *Cutaneous infestations and insect bites*. New York: Marcel Dekker, Inc; 1985:9–18.
6. Jenkinson DM. The basis of the skin surface ecosystem. In: Noble WC, ed. *The skin microflora and microbial disease*. Cambridge: Cambridge University Press; 1993:1–32.
7. Arlian LG, Vyszenski-Mohler DL. Response of *Sarcoptes scabiei* var *canis* (Acari: Sarcoptidae) to lipids of mammalian skin. *J Med Entomol* 1995; **32**:34–41.
8. Heilesen B. Studies on *Acarus scabiei* and scabies. *Acta Derm Venerol* 1964; **26**(suppl 14):1–370.
9. Falk ES, Bolle R. IgE antibodies to house dust mite in patients with scabies. *Br J Dermatol* 1980; **102**:283.
10. Arlian LG, Rapp CM, Morgan MS. Resistance and immune response in scabies-infested hosts immunized with *Dermatophagoides* mites. *Am J Trop Med Hyg* 1995; **52**:539–545.
11. Chua KY, Stewart GA, Thomas WR, Simpson, Dilworth RJ, Plozza TM, Turner KJ. Sequence analysis of cDNA coding for a major house dust mite allergen, *Der p* 1. Homology with cysteine proteases. *J Exp Med* 1988; **167**:175–182.
12. Brook I. Microbiology of secondary bacterial infection in scabies lesions. *J Clin Microbiol* 1995; **33**:2139–2140.
13. Dahl MV. The immune system in scabies. In: Orkin M, Maibach HI, eds. *Cutaneous infestations and insect bites*. New York: Marcel Dekker, Inc; 1985:75–83.
14. Walton SF, McBroom J, Mathews JD, Kemp DJ, Currie BJ. Crusted scabies: a molecular analysis of *Sarcoptes scabiei* variety *hominis* populations frompatients with repeated infestations. *J Infect Dis* 1999; **29**:1226–1230.
15. Orkin M. Scabies in AIDS. *Semin Dermatol* 1993; **12**:9–14.
16. Bhutto AM, Honda M, Kubo Y *et al*. Introduction of a fluorescent-microscopic technique for the detection of eggs, eggshells, and mites in scabies. *J Med Entomol* 1996; **33**:102–108.
17. Walker GJA, Johnstone PW. Interventions for treating scabies (Cochrane Review). In: *The Cochrane Library*, Issue 1, 2001. Oxford: Update Software.
18. Brown S, Becher J, Brady W. Treatment of ectoparasitic infections: review of the English-language literature, 1982–1992. *Clin Infect Dis* 1995; **20**(Suppl 1): S104–109.
19. Clinical effectiveness group. National guidelines for the management of scabies. *Sex Transm Inf* 1999; **75**(Suppl 1):S76–77.
20. Glaziou P, Cartel JL, Alzieu P, Moulia-Pelat JP, Martin PMV. Comparison of ivermectin and benzyl benzoate for treatment of scabies. *Trop Med Parasitol* 1993; **44**:331–332.
21. Chouela EN, Abeldano AM, Pellerano G et al. Equivalent therapeutic efficacy of ivermectib and lindane in the treatment of human scabies. *Arch Dermatol* 1999; **135**:651–655.
22. Chosidow O. Scabies and pediculosis. *Lancet* 2000; **255**:819–826.
23. Meinking TL, Taplin D, Hermida JL, Pardo R, Kerdel FA. The treatment of scabies with ivermectin. *N Engl J Med* 1995; **333**:26–30.
24. Corbett EL, Crossley I, Holten J, Levell N, Miller RF, De Cock KM. Crusted ('Norwegian') scabies in a specialist HIV unit: successful use of ivermectin and failure to prevent nosocomial transmission. *Genitourin Med* 1996; **72**:115–117.
25. Busvine JR. Pediculosis: Biology of the parasites. In: Orkin M, Maibach HI eds. *Cutaneous infestations and insect bites*. New York: Marcel Dekker, Inc. 1985:163–174.
26. Skinner CJ, Viswalingam ND, Goh BT. *Phthirus pubis* infestation of the eyelids: a marker for sexually transmitted diseases. *Int J STD & AIDS* 1995; **6**:451–452.
27. Clinical Effectiveness Group. National guidelines for the management of *Phthirus pubis* infestation. *Sex Transm Infect* 1999; **75**(Suppl 1):S78–79.
28. Billstein SA. Pubic lice. In: Holmes KK, Sparling PF, Mardh PA, Lemon SM, Stamm WE, Piot P, Wasserheit JN, eds. *Sexually transmitted diseases*, 3rd ed. New York: McGraw-Hill; 1999:641–644.

Syndromic Management

F Ndowa and R Ballard

INTRODUCTION

Sexually transmitted diseases (STDs) are caused by over 30 diverse pathogens, including bacteria, viruses, protozoan agents, fungal agents, and ecto-parasites. The different diseases are grouped together because sexual contact is epidemiologically important for their spread, though not necessarily the only mechanism through which the infections can be acquired. The World Health Organization (WHO) estimates that approximately 340 million incident cases of the four main curable STDs (gonorrhoea, chlamydia, syphilis, and trichomoniasis) occur every year, with 85 percent in resource-constrained countries.[1]

STDs impose an enormous burden of morbidity and mortality in many resource-constrained countries, both directly, through their impact on reproductive and child health, and indirectly, through their role in facilitating the sexual transmission of HIV. It has been estimated that in urban populations in sub-Saharan Africa 'classical' STDs, excluding HIV, are responsible for some 17% of the total burden of disease in women of reproductive age.

In recent years STDs have been accorded a priority disease by national ministries of health or by the international community on account of their strong cofactor effect on HIV transmission.

APPROACHES TO STD CASE MANAGEMENT

Prompt and effective treatment of STDs is an essential component of STD control as it renders an individual free of infection and aborts the likelihood of developing complications as well as the possibility of transmitting the infection further to any sex partners.

The traditional method for STD diagnosis has been through laboratory analysis to determine the etiological agent(s) either directly by microscopy, culture, antigen- or DNA-detection techniques, or indirectly by serology. While this is still the method of choice in many parts of the industrialized world, it is expensive both in terms of diagnostic equipment, reagents, infrastructure, and maintenance. Consequently, most health centers and dispensaries in resource-constrained countries do not have access to reliable laboratory facilities.

The other approach that has been commonly used is the presumptive clinical diagnosis through the identification of particular clinical features that an experienced physician interprets as clues to diagnosis. This method, however, has been shown to be inaccurate or incomplete for genital ulcers.[2-5] The reasons for this are similarities in clinical appearance of various etiologies, simultaneous infections with more than one organism causing the ulcer, atypical appearances due to longstanding disease, prior treatment or concomitant HIV infection. Furthermore, laboratory diagnostic tests to determine the etiology of genital ulcers are costly, technically sophisticated and time consuming.[6] The process would also require screening for a number of organisms at the same time in order not to miss mixed infections. Syndromic management is an option that has been shown to be highly sensitive and specific in both men and women presenting with genital ulcer disease.[7]

Thus, in order to deal with the limitations of both etiological and presumptive clinical diagnosis in the management of STDs, particularly for patients who attend the first level of primary health care, WHO developed and advocated the syndromic management approach.[8]

SYNDROMIC MANAGEMENT OF STD

The syndromic approach to STD case management is based on the identification of relatively constant combinations of symptoms and signs (syndromes) and on knowledge of the most common causative organisms of these syndromes and their antimicrobial susceptibility. Clinical algorithms (flow charts) are then developed to guide health-care workers to manage a patient who presents with a particular syndrome. The exact treatment is chosen typically to cover the major causative pathogens responsible for the syndrome in the specific geographic setting. Developed as a decision-making tool for the management of symptomatic STD patients the entry point for each algorithm is a clinical sign or symptom, such as urethral discharge, genital ulcer or vaginal discharge.

The syndromic approach does not only find application in the developing world, but also in some industrialized countries where it is used in the management of patients with pelvic inflammatory disease, as well as for the management of men with urethral discharge.[9] Syndromic management is also used in other conditions such as upper respiratory tract infections in the integrated management of childhood illness and in management of diarrheal diseases.

This approach has the advantages of providing immediate care and treatment at the patient's first visit and it is inexpensive in that no laboratory costs are incurred either by the patient or the service provider. Other advantages are that the algorithms help to standardize diagnosis, treatment and reporting and, on account of their simplicity, they can be used in a variety of outlets such as primary health-care facilities, family planning clinics and private practitioner consulting rooms as well as in STD clinics themselves.

One of the most commonly cited drawbacks of the syndromic approach is the inevitable over-treatment which occurs, to a greater or lesser extent, in patients who either do not harbor any of the presumed causative organisms or not all for which therapy is given. However, the cost of over-treatment, in terms of the cost of drugs and the hard to quantify risk of promoting antimicrobial resistance, should be weighed against the cost of complications, of continued STD transmission and of increased HIV transmission and the additional cost of either laboratory- or specialist-based diagnosis.[10,11] *Table A1.1* gives a summary of the advantages and disadvantages of the syndromic management of STD.

The syndromic approach performs well in the management of men with symptomatic urethral discharge (UD) and in the management of men and women with genital ulcer disease (GUD).[12-14] It has high to very acceptable cure rates, thus guaranteeing client satisfaction, prevention of sequelae and complications, as well as further transmission of STDs as well as HIV infection. In a multicenter study in Brazil the validity of presumptive clinical diagnosis and the national syndromic STD treatment recommendations were determined against a laboratory gold standard in symptomatic men with urethral discharge. The syndromic approach had the highest sensitivity of the three approaches.[15]

Advantages	Disadvantages
• Simple • Rapid • No laboratory required • Treatment given at first visit, preventing complications and further transmission • Simplifies reporting and supervision	• Leads to over-treatment, especially in women • May lead to problems with partner notification, especially in women who are told they have an STD when they do not • Only applies to patients with symptoms

Table A1.1 Advantages and disadvantages of syndromic management of STDs.

Requirements	Components

• Accurate diagnosis
• Treatment at first encounter
• Rapid cure with effective drugs
• Simplicity
• Integration
• Modifying risk behavior
	• History taking and symptoms
	• Examination
	• Treatment
	• Health education
	  – nature of infection
	  – compliance
	  – risk reduction
	• Counseling
	• Condoms
	• Partner notification
	• Follow-up, if necessary

Table A1.2 Requirements and elements for comprehensive STD case management.

The syndromic approach probably performs well in the management of women with vaginitis, although further validation of the current vaginal discharge algorithm is required.[16] The algorithms currently available for the management of cervical infection are, however, far from ideal. Initially it was thought that the finding of abnormal vaginal discharge (VD) would be indicative of both vaginal and cervical infection, but it has become clear that while VD is indicative of the presence of vaginitis, it is poorly predictive of STD-induced cervicitis due to the latter's frequently asymptomatic nature. Thus, the first-generation VD algorithms had a low sensitivity and specificity for the management of cervicitis. Cervicitis seems to be more frequently associated with the presence of cervical mucopus, cervical erosions, cervical friability and bleeding between menses or during sexual intercourse and with a number of risk factors.[17–19] A number of studies in different settings have shown a significant association between cervical infection and some demographic and behavioral factors, referred to as *risk factors*, such as being single, younger age of below 20 or 25 depending on setting, more than one sex partner in the previous 3 months and male sex partner having a urethritis. These risk factors vary with each setting. Thus, while an abnormal discharge in terms of quantity, color or odor is most commonly due to a vaginal infection, combining it with both clinical and demographic risk factors can improve the validity of the algorithm in predicting cervical infection. Another approach to improve the performance of this algorithm is a non-hierarchical score-driven approach, where multiple risk factors and signs which provide multiple entry points are considered, as opposed to a single entry point.[17] In Malawi a local modification that increased the sensitivity of the algorithm in detecting cervical infection was the expansion of the entry point into the algorithm from vaginal discharge alone to genito-urinary complaints, which included vaginal discharge, dysuria and vulvar odor, itching, soreness and swelling.[20] Although adding these signs and a risk assessment to the VD algorithm does increase the specificity and thus the positive predictive value, the latter remains low, especially when the algorithm is applied to populations with relatively low rates of infection. It should be noted that such risk factors are usually specific for the population group for which they have been identified and validated, and cannot be reliably extrapolated to other populations or to other countries. In many cases, however, the use of these algorithms does improve case management by standardizing and rationalizing treatment decisions, or by offering treatment where currently none is provided.

Although the positive predictive values (PPVs) of such an algorithm in women are invariably low, it should be borne in mind that such PPVs are comparing syndromic algorithms with a laboratory gold standard. Such laboratories are either not available or, if they are, could not cope with the workload in settings of high STI prevalence. Syndromic management of vaginal discharge, therefore, though not ideal, is the minimum that should be used in any setting without a functional laboratory service.

Syndromic management algorithms were developed for use in symptomatic individuals. Not surprisingly, when attempts were made to use them as screening and case-finding tools, as well as for case management in asymptomatic infections, especially in women, the results were unsatisfactory, producing low rates of sensitivity and specificity.

COMPREHENSIVE STD CASE MANAGEMENT

Definition: STD case management is the care of a person with an STD-related symptom, clinical sign, or syndrome, or with a positive test for one or more STDs.

Syndromic management of STDs is only a component of comprehensive patient care. The requirements and elements of comprehensive case management are shown in *Table A1.2*, and the elements are briefly described in the next few paragraphs.

HISTORY TAKING

History taking is important for a number of reasons. If properly done and privacy is assured, the process of taking a history establishes a rapport between health-care provider and patient. History can give early clues to the possibility of the presence of an STD, traumatic lesions, previous treatments and allergies. History will also assess the patient's risk behavior and duration of infection, and will help identify the sex partners who may have exposed the patient or have been exposed by him/her.

EXAMINATION

Whatever the mode of diagnosis used, but more so with the syndromic approach, examination of the patient is a must. It is important to examine the patient in good light and on an examination couch. The examination of either male or female patient while standing is not recommended as the patient will not be relaxed and a thorough examination of the genital area cannot be easily accomplished. Furthermore, a proper examination may reveal another condition that the patient may not have been aware of.

IDENTIFICATION OF THE STD

This can be done through clinical diagnosis, syndromic diagnosis, or laboratory testing, as discussed earlier. In this instance a combination of the presenting symptoms and the findings on examination will mark the entry point for the established syndrome, whether genital ulcer, urethral discharge or lower abdominal pain.

ANTIBIOTIC TREATMENT FOR THE STD SYNDROME

Availability and use of effective antibiotics is essential for STD control. Single-dose or short-duration regimens are preferable as they improve compliance.[21] The most effective drugs must be available at the first point of contact with the patient. The use of ineffective or partially effective drugs may result in escalation of costs as patients repeatedly seek treatment for the same condition or its complications. Partially effective treatments may also be responsible for the rapid appearance of resistant strains of pathogens and persistent sub-clinical infections in individuals. As the syndromic management will be used at the lowest level of health-care drug choices should be clearly defined in terms of first-line drugs, alternatives in case of allergies or other contra-indications, and treatment failures.

EDUCATING THE PATIENT

Health education is preferably provided by a trained health educator, nurse, or counselor, in a separate room during one-on-one discussions, rather than a physician who may have very little time in a busy clinic. There are compelling reasons for spending sufficient time on health education with a patient with STD. Firstly, a person who has presented for STD care at a health center is at his/her most receptive for education about the nature of the infection, its consequences, and risk reduction to prevent future infections. Secondly, the person is at higher risk, if not educated, of becoming re-infected and spreading the infection. Finally, educating the patient about the nature of his/her infection will enhance patient co-operation with the health-care worker's advice.

Reinforcement of key education messages is necessary and can be achieved by giving the patient an information leaflet, which should be designed in a way and translated in a language that is easy to understand and relevant for the population.

The following topics should be addressed during one or several sessions:

- infectious nature of STDs
- transmission through sexual intercourse
- increased risks of infertility and other complications
- importance of completing treatment, even after improvement
- reasons for reporting back to the clinic
- risk of re-infection by the partner and reason for sexual abstinence or using condoms while under treatment
- advantages and importance of treating sex partner(s)
- messages and information on future risk reduction

COUNSELING THE PATIENT

Counseling relates more to issues of anxiety and coping with the infection and its social consequences. Thus, counseling is important in discussing, identifying, and dealing with issues such as:

- informing the partner or spouse about the STD diagnosis
- learning about and coming to terms with worrisome complications, e.g., infertility
- coping with chronic/incurable infections, e.g., HIV, genital herpes, and genital warts

CONDOM PROMOTION AND SUPPLY

Although the STD consultation provides an opportunity for the promotion and supply of condoms, as the patient should be more receptive to understanding their usefulness in decreasing future exposure to STD/HIV, there should be mechanisms for people to access condoms in different outlets outside of the health center. Three issues must be covered in condom education and supply, namely, condom demonstration, condom supply and information and advice on further sources of condoms in the community and/or at the health center. This forms part of a prevention strategy. Condom use should then be clearly demonstrated using a penis model, allowing the patient to try the process out as well, even if they are familiar with condoms. This will tend to dispel any embarrassment during the discussions. Condom use will require some negotiating skills with sex partners. Ideally, such skills should be taught by a trained counselor, but this may not be possible at the first visit and may require further visits or referral to other community services.

PARTNER NOTIFICATION AND MANAGEMENT

Contacting or notifying sex partners of STD patients, persuading them to present for STD screening and examination, with subsequent immediate treatment for any STD diagnosed as well as treatment for the same condition as in the index patient, is an integral part of comprehensive STD case management. The objectives of partner notification are to notify partners at risk, to protect the uninfected and decrease transmission among the infected, interrupt the chain of transmission in the community and to reduce the pool of asymptomatic STD in the population.

Particular attention should be paid to the social and cultural acceptability of partner notification in order to avoid ethical and societal problems, especially for women who may be rejected or subjected to physical abuse. Moreover, the lack of specificity of genital symptoms in women makes it difficult to distinguish between common vaginal or endogenous infections, which often are not sexually acquired and thus would not warrant treatment of partner(s), and sexually acquired infections for which treatment of sex partner(s) is required. Thus, in the absence of a specific laboratory diagnosis caution should be exerted before initiating partner notification for female index patients. Health-care workers need to be properly trained in undertaking partner notification in a sensitive and confidential manner. Partner notification should not be compulsory. Treatment of index patient should not be conditional upon sex partners being divulged or brought forward.

CLINICAL FOLLOW-UP

In some settings it may be logistically difficult for patients to return for follow-up. Where feasible, follow-up should be encouraged, particularly in situations where symptoms and/or signs have persisted. During the follow-up visit messages of prevention can be reinforced and, should there be persistence of disease, treatment could be restarted if compliance seems to have been a problem, or alternative treatment given if failure of first-line treatment is suspected. Or, indeed, the patient may be referred to another level of care if second-line drugs are not available, or if the condition warrants it. Explicit referral guidelines should be defined for each level of care.

STD SYNDROMES

It is important to define the main STD syndromes in any setting before embarking on the development of management protocols. There are six major STD syndromes:

- Urethral discharge in men (suspected urethritis). This is commonly due to *Neisseria gonorrhoeae* and/or *Chlamydia trachomatis* and/or non-gonococcal/non-chlamydial pathogens e.g., *Mycoplasma genitalium*
- Testicular pain and swelling (suspected epididymo-orchitis). This is commonly due to *N. gonorrhoeae* and/or *C. trachomatis*.
- Abnormal vaginal discharge (vaginitis and/or cervicitis). This

syndrome is caused predominantly by organisms causing vaginal infection, such as *Trichomonas vaginalis, Candida albicans* or bacterial vaginosis, but *N. gonorrhoeae* and *C. trachomatis* (which are of greater public health importance for their complications) can cause a cervical discharge and consequently manifest as vaginal discharge. 'Abnormal' discharge refers to a change in abundance, color, odor, or consistency of genital secretions as perceived by the patient and confirmed by a trained health provider.

- Lower abdominal pain in women (suspicion of pelvic inflammatory disease [PID]). This condition is due to *N. gonorrhoeae* and/or *C. trachomatis* and/or anaerobic pathogens.
- Genital ulcers. The genital ulcer syndrome can be caused by a number of pathogens including, *Haemophilus ducreyi* (chancroid), *Treponema pallidum* (syphilis), Herpes simplex virus (HSV) type-2 (sometimes also HSV type-1). Donovanosis (caused by the agent *Calymmatobacterium granulomatis*) may be important in some settings (e.g., South India, South Africa, and Papua New Guinea), as can be lymphogranuloma venereum (LGV) caused by specific strains L1–L3 of *C. trachomatis*, which, however, produce only transient and mild ulcerations.
- Inguinal bubo. This syndrome is associated with chancroid (*H. ducreyi*) or LGV (*C. trachomatis* L-serovars).

SYNDROME OF URETHRAL DISCHARGE

One or all of the following symptoms may be an indication of inflammation of the urethra (urethritis) in men: urethral discharge, dysuria and itching at the tip of the urethra. Characteristically, urethral discharge is the physical sign observed. The major pathogens causing urethral discharge are *N. gonorrhoeae* and *C. trachomatis*. In less-industrialized tropical countries the commonest causative organism of urethral discharge in men is *N. gonorrhoeae*. For example, in India 75% of 525 men with symptoms of urethritis had *N. gonorrhoeae*.[22] In a study of 206 men with urethritis in Malawi gonorrhea was found to be the commonest cause, accounting for 64% of the isolated pathogens.[23] In rural Zimbabwe gonorrhea was isolated in 64% of men presenting with genital discharge, and 8% had *T. vaginalis* isolated.[24] In a study in Thailand, among men presenting with urethritis 32.6% had gonorrhea as the commonest causative organism followed by *C. trachomatis* (23.3%) and *T. vaginalis* (1.8%).[25] In Bandung, Indonesia, a study among men with urethral discharge found gonorrhea as the commonest cause in 67% of the patients, followed by *C. trachomatis* in 33% of the patients. In this study 42% of the urethritis patients had only gonorrhea, 8% had only chlamydia infection and 25% had concomitant gonococcal and chlamydia infections.[13] In a multicenter study in Brazil gonorrhea was the most frequently detected pathogen in men with urethral discharge. In this study 472 men presented with urethral discharge, and gonorrhea was diagnosed in 44% (210) of the patients, chlamydia alone in 7%, *T. vaginalis* alone in 2% while concomitant gonococcal and chlamydia infections were found in 8%.[15]

Although *N. gonorrhoeae* is the commonest pathogen causing urethritis it is noted that there is a high frequency of co-infection with *C. trachomatis*. Syndromic management, therefore, recommends that treatment of this syndrome should cover both organisms. In settings where *T. vaginalis* is found to be significantly frequent, a site-specific modification of the algorithm may include the treatment of this organism in the syndromic management.

MANAGEMENT

Throughout the tropics an increasing number of isolates of *N. gonorrhoeae* show both plasmid and chromosomally mediated resistance to penicillin and other cheap antibiotics such as tetracycline and co-

Treatment options for gonorrhoea	PLUS	Treatment options for chlamydia*
Ciprofloxacin 500 mg po, as a single dose OR Ceftriaxone 125 mg im, as a single dose OR Cefixime 400 mg po, as a single dose OR Spectinomycin 2 g im, as a single dose		Doxycycline 100 mg po bid for 7 days OR Azithromycin 1 g po as a single dose *Not given when azithromycin used for treatment of gonorrhea

Based on the WHO recommended treatment options for uncomplicated anogenital gonococcal infection.[27]

Table A1.3 Syndromic treatment options for urethral discharge.

trimoxazole.[26] Therefore, it is important to monitor local in vitro gonococcal susceptibilities, as well as the clinical efficacy of recommended regimens. Based on such global reports and monitoring of gonococcal susceptibility to antibiotics WHO updated the recommended treatment options for gonorrhea.[27] Ideally gonorrhea should be treated with a single-dose oral antibiotic. The dose administered should give a serum level of at least three times the minimum inhibitory concentration for 8 or more hours. To any one of the options of antibiotics chosen for gonorrhea must be added treatment to cover chlamydia infection. For chlamydia the treatment recommendations for uncomplicated urethral, endocervical, or rectal infections are tetracylines, such as doxycycline, and macrolides such as erythromycin and azithromycin (*Table A1.3*).[28,29]

SYNDROME OF ABNORMAL VAGINAL DISCHARGE

The three most prevalent causes of vaginal discharge are *T. vaginalis*, bacterial vaginosis and *C. albicans*. *N. gonorrhoeae* and *C. trachomatis*, which infect the endocervix rather than the vagina in adult women, are less commonly associated with a symptomatic discharge. However, it is not possible to distinguish consistently between these infections on clinical grounds. A microscopic examination of a wet preparation made from a swab collected from the vaginal posterior fornix can usually distinguish between candidiasis, trichomoniasis and bacterial vaginosis, but a microscopic identification of *N. gonorrhoeae* from a cervical swab is more difficult while *C. trachomatis* identification requires more sophisticated laboratory tests. Thus, while vaginal discharge is indicative of vaginitis, it is poorly predictive of cervical infection due to either *N. gonorrhoeae* or *C. trachomatis*.

SYNDROMIC MANAGEMENT OF VAGINAL DISCHARGE

As vaginal discharge is more indicative of vaginitis rather than cervicitis women presenting with this complaint should receive treatment for vaginitis. Subsequently, further assessment should be done to exclude or implicate gonococcal or chlamydial cervical infection. If such cervical infection is suspected, treatment for cervicitis should be added to the vaginitis treatment.

Based on this principle WHO recently updated the vaginal discharge algorithm to emphasize the role of infections causing vaginitis (*Fig. A1.1*).[27] With this algorithm, all women presenting with vaginal discharge would receive treatment for trichomoniasis and bacterial vaginosis. Then, the next step is to identify those women with an increased likelihood of being infected with *N. gonorrhoeae* and/or *C. trachomatis* by incorporating locally determined risk factors. This also requires a good knowledge of the prevalence of gonococcal and/or chlamydia in women presenting with vaginal discharge within the setting. The higher the prevalence, the stronger the justification for adding treatment for cervical infection. Risk-assessment-positive women have a higher likelihood of cervical infection than those who are risk-negative. With this process women with vaginal discharge and a positive risk assessment are, therefore, offered additional treatment for gonococcal and chlamydia cervicitis on top of the treatment for vaginitis.

The recommended treatment regimen for vaginitis discharge is shown in *Table A1.4*. The recommended additional treatment for cervical infection will be as shown for urethritis in *Table A1.3*.

Whereas trichomoniasis is a sexually transmitted infection, bacterial vaginosis is an endogenous reproductive tract infection. Treatment of sex partners has not been demonstrated to be of benefit in the latter.

SYNDROME OF LOWER ABDOMINAL PAIN IN WOMEN

Salpingitis is the most common, and of most important public health concern, of all complications of gonorrhea and chlamydia infections in women. Acute salpingitis, or pelvic inflammatory disease (PID) is an

Drug options for BV*	Drug options for TV*	Drug options for CA
Metronidazole 400 or 500 mg po bid for 7 days	Metronidazole 2 g po as a single dose	Miconazole or Clotrimazole 200 mg intravaginally for 3 consecutive days
	OR	OR
Alternatives Clindamycin vaginal 2% cream, 5 g at bedtime intravaginally for 7 days	Tinidazole 2 g po as a single dose OR Metronidazole 400 or 500 mg po bid for 7 days	Fluconazole 150 mg po as a single dose
OR Metronidazole 0.75% gel twice daily intravaginally for 5 days	OR Tinidazole 500 mg po bid for 5 days	
OR Clindamycin 300 mg po bid for 7 days		

Based on the WHO recommended treatment options for vaginal infection.[27]

Table A1.4 Treatment options for vaginal discharge. BV, bacterial vaginosis; TV, trichomoniasis; CA, Candidiasis.

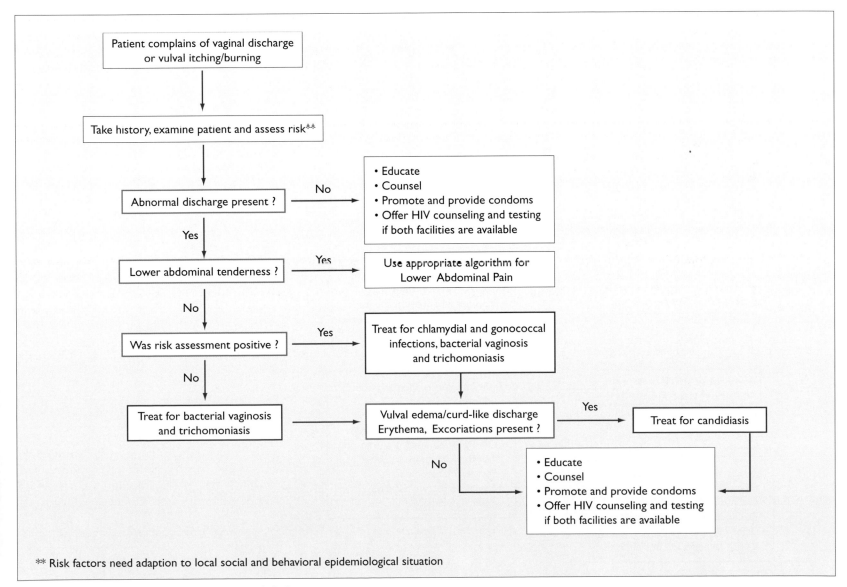

Fig. A1.1 Algorithm for the management of vaginal discharge.

inflammatory disorder of the female upper genital tract, including any combination of endometritis, salpingitis, tubo-ovarian abscess and pelvic peritonitis. Women with this complication present with lower abdominal pain and tenderness. A perihepatitis (Fitz–Hugh–Curtis syndrome) may also occur. PID is described as occurring in about 10–20% of women with acute gonococcal infection, however, the actual incidence in developing countries is not known.[30]

Untreated or asymptomatic infection may lead to long-term problems of chronic PID, and increased risk of ectopic pregnancy (increased tenfold after a single episode of salpingitis). Sterility may complicate both overt and asymptomatic infection in either sex. In a study from Central Africa, fallopian tube occlusion was present in 83% of infertile women.[31] Acute salpingitis has been estimated to produce sterility in 17% of patients, the risk rising with multiple episodes or more severe inflammation. PID is the commonest cause of admission to gynecology wards in Africa.[32] Ectopic pregnancy as a sequel of PID is up to three times as common in Africa as in Europe, and tubal infertility, another common sequela, is widespread, with up to 20% of women affected in some regions of Africa.[33]

Clinically, patients present with a non-specific spectrum of symptoms, such as fever, nausea and vomiting, lower abdominal pain, vaginal discharge, dysmenorrhoea, irregular menstrual bleeding and dyspareunia. A few patients may be asymptomatic.

PID results predominantly from the spread of micro-organisms such as *C. trachomatis* and *N. gonorrhoeae*, genital mycoplasmas, endogenous vaginal flora (anaerobic and aerobic bacteria), and aerobic streptococci[34] from the lower to the upper genital tract. An association between PID and bacterial vaginosis has also been demonstrated in the absence of *C. trachomatis* and *N. gonorrhoeae*.[35]

Unmistakably, therefore, the syndromic diagnosis of PID is imprecise.

At the same time it can be seen that a precise diagnosis would require laboratory diagnostic capability, including invasive procedures in some cases. Though not ideal, syndromic diagnosis seems to be the option for most settings in the world. Given the seriousness of the consequences of untreated PID, overdiagnosis and overtreatment from syndromic management can be justified in order to ensure appropriate antibiotic treatment early in the course of the disease. Care should be taken to exclude competing surgical diagnoses such as appendicitis and ectopic pregnancy.

The management of PID for ambulatory patients should, therefore, cover *N. gonorrhoeae*, *C. trachomatis* and anaerobic bacteria. Analgesics are given for pain. The duration of treatment is prolonged as this is a complication; thus, for example, a single dose of ceftriaxone 125 mg by intramuscular injection, a 14-day course of doxycline 100 mg twice daily and a 14-day course of metronidazole 400–500 mg twice daily should lead to a resolution of disease. In severe cases, patients with PID should be admitted into hospital and given more intensive treatment.

SYNDROME OF GENITAL ULCER

The relative prevalence of causative organisms for genital ulcer disease varies considerably in different parts of the world and may change dramatically over time.

After examination to confirm the presence of genital ulceration, treatment appropriate to local etiologies and antibiotic sensitivity patterns should be given. For example, in areas where both syphilis and chancroid are prevalent, patients with genital ulcers should be treated for both conditions at the time of their initial presentation to ensure adequate therapy in case of loss to follow-up. In areas where donovanosis or LGV is prevalent, treatment for these conditions should be included.

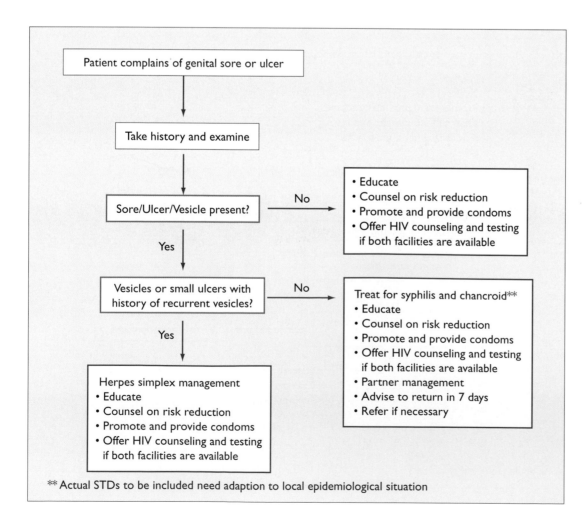

Fig. A1.2 In this flow chart the entry point is a genital ulcer or sero. After history and examination a decision is made according to the findings. The exit from each decision box is either a "yes" or "no".

** Actual STDs to be included need adaption to local epidemiological situation

HSV2 infection is the primary cause of genital herpes. It is highly prevalent in human populations in many parts of the world, and is the most common cause of worldwide. It is the major cause of GUD in the developed world, where it is a major public health concern in its potential role as an important co-factor for HIV transmission.[36] Where HIV infection is prevalent, an increasing proportion of cases of GUD is likely to harbor herpes simplex virus. In such settings there is increasing frequency of treatment failure when using the current syndromic algorithm for GUD, even if the antibiotics given will have successfully treated and cured other co-existing pathogens such as *H. ducreyi* and *T. pallidum*. This shift in the frequency of HSV2 may mean the addition of antiviral therapy to the GUD algorithm. One such antiviral product is acyclovir which has been the standard treatment for genital herpes in industrialized countries for the past decade. For the developing world the current main constraint to the widespread use of acyclovir is the cost of the drug. It will be of public health importance that this drug be made more readily available in the future.

The algorithm (*Fig. A1.2*) demonstrates the steps to be followed in the syndromic management of GUD. *Table A1.5* gives a summary of the key management elements and *Table A1.6* gives syndromic treatment options for GUD.

THE SYNDROME OF TESTICULAR PAIN AND SWELLING

Inflammation of the epididymis (epididymitis) usually manifests itself by an acute onset of unilateral testicular pain and swelling, often with tenderness of the epididymis and vas deferens and occasionally with erythema and edema of the overlying testicular skin. The adjacent testis is often also inflamed (orchitis), giving rise to epididymo-orchitis. In men under the age of 35 years the sexually transmitted pathogens of *N. gonorrhoeae* and *C. trachomatis* are the most common etiologies of acute epididymitis.[37,38] When the epididymitis is accompanied by urethral discharge, it should be presumed to be of a sexually transmitted origin.

The syndromic treatment, therefore, is similar to that of urethritis, covering both *N. gonorrhoeae* and *C. trachomatis*. Adjuncts to this treatment are bed rest and scrotal support until local inflammation and fever subside. If not effectively treated, STI-related epididymitis may lead to infertility.

Genital ulcer disease management	Herpes simplex management
• Treat for syphilis, and, depending upon local epidemiology, either chancroid, donovanosis or lymphogranuloma venereum • Aspirate any fluctuant glands (surgical incision should be avoided) • Educate and counsel on risk reduction • Offer syphilis serologic testing and HIV serologic testing where appropriate facilities and counseling are available • Review if lesion not fully healed	• Advise on basic care of the lesion (keep clean and dry) • Provide or prescribe specific antiviral herpes treatment according to local policy • Educate and counsel on compliance and risk reduction • Offer syphilis and HIV serologic testing where appropriate facilities and counseling are available • Promote and provide condoms • Advise to return in 7 days if lesion is not fully healed, and sooner if there is clinical deterioration; if so, treat for other causes of GUD as per guidelines

Table A1.5 Genital ulcer disease. Key elements for management of GUD.

Drug options for syphilis	Drug options for chancroid	Drug options for donovanosis	Drug options for LGV	Drug options for genital herpes
Benzathine penicillin 2.4 million Units IM, single dose	Ciprofloxacin 500 mg orally b.i.d. for 3 days OR Erythromycin 500 mg orally 4 times a day for 7 days OR Azithromycin 1 g orally as a single dose	Azithromycin 1 g orally on day 1 then 500 mg once daily OR Doxycycline 100 mg orally b.i.d. UNTIL LESIONS ARE HEALED	Doxycycline 100 mg orally b.i.d. for 14 days OR Erythromycin 500 mg 4 times daily for 14 days	Acyclovir Valaciclovir Famciclovir
Alternatives	**Alternatives**	**Alternatives**	**Alternatives**	
Procaine benzylpenicillin 1.2 million Units IM daily for 10 days	Ceftriaxone 250 mg IM as a single dose	Erythromycin 500 mg orally 4 times daily OR Tetracycline 500 mg 4 times daily OR Trimethoprim (80 mg)/ Sulfamethoxazole (400 mg) 2 tablets daily orally UNTIL LESIONS ARE HEALED	Tetracycline 500 mg orally 4 times daily for 14 days	
Penicillin allergy and not pregnant				
Doxycycline 100 mg orally b.i.d. for 15 days OR Tetracycline 500 mg orally 4 timesa day for 15 days				

Note 1. The decision to treat for chancroid, granuloma inguinale or LGV depends on the local epidemiology of the infections.
Note 2. Specific treatment for herpes genitalis is recommended as it offers clinical benefits to most symptomatic patients. Health education and counselling regarding the recurrent nature of genital herpes lesions, the natural history, sexual transmission, probable perinatal transmission and available methods to reduce transmission are an integral part of genital herpes management.

Table A1.6 Genital ulcer. Treatment options for syndromic management.

It is important to consider other non-infectious causes of scrotal swelling, such as trauma, testicular torsion and tumor. Testicular torsion, which should be suspected when onset of scrotal pain is sudden, is a surgical emergency that needs urgent referral.

THE SYNDROME OF INGUINAL BUBO

Inguinal and femoral buboes are localized enlargements of the lymph nodes in the groin area, which are painful and may be fluctuant. They are frequently associated with LGV and chancroid. In many cases of chancroid an associated genital ulcer is visible, but occasionally may not be. Non-sexually transmitted local and systemic infections can also cause swelling of inguinal lymph nodes. Therefore, it is important to exclude infections of the lower limb, an inguinal staphylococcal abscess and other systemic infections such as tuberculosis. The recommended syndromic treatment is ciprofloxacin, 500 mg orally, twice daily for 3 days and doxycycline, 100 mg orally twice daily for 14 days (or erythromycin, 500 mg orally four times daily for 14 days). Some cases may require a longer duration of treatment. Fluctuant lymph nodes should be aspirated through healthy skin. Incision and drainage or excision of nodes may delay healing and should not be attempted.

OUTSTANDING ISSUES AND LABORATORY

The syndromic approach does not address subclinical and asymptomatic infections. As with laboratory diagnosis the syndromic approach requires that the patient presents at a health center. Therefore, strategies for improving people's health-care-seeking behavior need to be put in place. Such strategies will include public education to promote awareness of STI symptoms and increased access to acceptable and affordable services. Asymptomatic infections will require other strategies such as screening programs (which would require laboratory facilities), presumptive treatment of partners of index cases and conceivably presumptive treatment of specific groups shown to be high-frequency transmitters of infection. Above all, prevention strategies need to be intensified, especially for young people, in order to prevent acquisition of infection in the first place.

The adoption of syndromic management does not exclude use of laboratories. Laboratory services will be important at the public health level where they contribute to the development and validation of national STI case management guidelines, and assist in the necessary epidemiological and microbiological monitoring and in training of health-care providers. At the individual level simple laboratory tests are used for case finding, for example, in pregnant women attending antenatal care. In this case syphilis detection is both feasible and cost-effective.

References

1. World Health Organization. Global prevalence and incidence of selected curable sexually transmitted infections: Overview and Estimates. *WHO/HIV-AIDS/2001.02, Geneva 2001.*
2. Chapel TA, Brown WJ, Jeffries C *et al.* How reliable is the morphological diagnosis of penile ulceration? *Sex Transm Dis* 1977; **4**:150–152.
3. Ndinya-Achola JO, Kihara AN, Fisher LD *et al.* Presumptive specific clinical diagnosis of genital ulcer disease (GUD) in a primary health care setting in Nairobi. *Int J STD AIDS* 1996; **7**:201–205.
4. O'Farrell N, Hoosen AA, Coetzee KD *et al.* Genital ulcer disease: accuracy of clinical diagnosis and strategies to improve control in Durban, South Africa. *Genitourin Med* 1994; **70**:7–11.
5. Dangor Y, Ballard RC, Exposto F da L *et al.* Accuracy of clinical diagnosis of genital ulcer disease. *Sex Transm Dis* 1990; **17**:184–189.
6. Bruisten SM, Cairo I, Fennema H, Pijl A *et al.* Diagnosing genital ulcer disease in a clinic for sexually transmitted diseases in Amsterdam, The Netherlands. *J Clin Microbiol* 2001; **39**:601–605

7. Htun Y, Morse SA, Dangor Y *et al.* Comparison of clinically directed, disease specific, and syndromic protocols for the management of genital ulcer disease in Lesotho. *Sex Transm Inf* 1998; **74**:(Suppl 1):S23–28.
8. World Health Organization. Global programme on AIDS. Management of sexually transmitted diseases. *WHO/GPA/TEM/94.1* Geneva: WHO, 1994.
9. Ryan CA, Holmes KK. Editorial: how should clinical algorithms be used for syndromic management of cervical and vaginal infections? *Clin Infect Dis* 1995; **21**:1456–1458.
10. Over M, Piot P. HIV infection and sexually transmitted diseases. In: *Disease Control Priorities in Developing Countries*, Jamison DW, Mosley H *et al* (eds), New York, Oxford University Press, 1993, Chapter 20.
11. Islam MQ, Latif A *et al.* Analysis of the cost effectiveness of different approaches to STD case management. *Sex Transm Dis* 1994; **21**(suppl 2):S138.
12. La Ruche G, Lorougnon F, Digbeu N *et al.* Therapeutic algorithms for the management of sexually transmitted diseases at the peripheral level in Côte d'Ivoire: assessment of efficacy and cost. *Bull World Health Organ* 1995; **73**:305–313.
13. Djajakusumah T, Sudigdoadi S *et al.* Evaluation of syndromic patient management algorithm for urethral discharge. *Sex Trans Inf 1998*; **74**(Suppl 1):S29–S33.
14. Hanson S, Sunkutu RM, Kamanga J *et al.* STD care in Zambia: an evaluation of the guidelines for case management through a syndromic approach. *Int J STD AIDS* 1996; **7**:324–332.
15. Moherdaui F, Vuylsteke B, Siqueira LFG *et al.* Validation of national algorithms for the diagnosis of sexually transmitted diseases in Brazil: results from a multicentre study. *Sex Transm Inf* 1998; **74**(Suppl 1):S38–43.
16. Behets FM-T, Williams Y, Braithwaite A *et al.* Management of vaginal discharge in women treated at a Jamaican sexually transmitted diseases clinic: use of diagnostic algorithms versus laboratory testing. *Clin Infect Dis* 1995; **21**:1450–1455.
17. Vuylsteke B, Laga M, Alary M *et al.* Clinical algorithms for the screening of women for gonococcal and chlamydial infection: evaluation of pregnant women and prostitutes in Zaire. *Clin Infect Dis* 1993; **17**:82–88.
18. Mayaud P, Grosskurth H, Changalucha J *et al.* Risk assessment and other screening options for gonorrhoea and chlamydial infections in women attending rural Tanzanian antenatal clinics. *Bull World Health Organ* 1995; **73**:621–630.
19. Daly CC, Maggwa N, Mati JK *et al.* Risk factors for gonorrhoea, syphilis and trichomonas infections among women attending family planning clinics in Nairobi, Kenya. *Genitourin Med* 1994; **70**:155–161.
20. Costello Daly C, Wangel AM, Hoffman IF *et al.* Validation of the WHO diagnostic algorithm and development of an alternative scoring system for the management of women presenting with vaginal discharge in Malawi. *Sex Transm Inf* 1998; **4**(Suppl 1):S50–58.
21. Wright MW, Htun Y, Leong MG *et al.* Evaluation of the use of calendar blister packaging on patient compliance with STD syndromic treatment regimens. *Sex Transm Dis* 1999; **26**:556–563.
22. Ray K, Bala M, Kumar J *et al.* Trend of antimicrobial resistance in *Neisseria gonorrhoeae* at New Delhi, India. *Int J STD AIDS* 2000; **11**:115–118.
23. Cohen MS, Hoffman IF, Royce RA *et al.* Reduction of concentration of HIV-1 in semen after treatment of urethritis: implications for prevention of sexual transmission of HIV-1. *Lancet* 1997; **349**:1868–1873.
24. Le Bacq F, Mason PR, Gwanzura L *et al.* HIV and other sexually transmitted diseases at a rural hospital in Zimbabwe. *Genitourin Med* 1993; **69**:352–356.
25. Chandeying V, Skov S, Tabrizi SN *et al.* Can a two-glass urine test or leucocyte esterase test of first-void urine improve syndromic management of male urethritis in southern Thailand? *Int J STD AIDS* 2000; **11**:235–240.
26. Van Dyck *et al.* Antimicrobial susceptibility patterns of *N. gonorrhoeae* in Bénin. *Int J STD AIDS* 2001; **12**:89–93.
27. World Health Organization. Guidelines for the management of sexually transmitted infections. *WHO/HIV_AIDS/2001.01*, Geneva 2001.
28. Wehbeh HA, Ruggeirio RM, Shahem S *et al.* Single-dose azithromycin for Chlamydia in pregnant women. *J Reprod Med* 1998; **43**:509–514.
29. Steingrimsson O, Olafsson JH, Thorarinsson H *et al.* Single-dose azithromycin treatment of gonorrhea and infections caused by *C. trachomatis* and *U. urealyticum* in men. *Sex Transm Dis* 1994; **21**:43–46.
30. Holmes KK, Eschenbuch DA, Knapp JS. Salpingitis: Overview of etiology and epidemiology. *Am J Obstet Gynecol* 1980; **138**:893.
31. Collet M, Reniers S, Frost E *et al.* Infertility in Central Africa: infection is the cause. *Int J Gynaecol Obstet* 1988; **26**:423–428.
32. Muir DG, Belsey MA. Pelvic inflammatory disease and its consequences in the developing world. *Am J Obstet Gynecol* 1980; **138**:913–928.
33. Cates W, Farley TMM, Rowe PJ. Worldwide patterns of infertility: is Africa different? *Lancet* 1985; **2**:596–598.
34. Simms I, Stephenson JM. Pelvic inflammatory disease epidemiology: what do we know and what do we need to know? *Sex Transm Inf* 2000; **76**:80–87.

35. Sweet R. Role of bacterial vaginosis in pelvic inflammatory disease. *Clin Infect Dis* 1995; **20**:S271–275.

36. O'Farrell N. Increasing prevalence of genital herpes in developing countries: implications for heterosexual HIV transmission and STI control programmes. *Sex Transm Infect* 1999; **75**(6):377–384.

37. Kristensen JK, Scheibel JH. Etiology of acute epididymitis presenting in a venereal disease clinic. *Sex Transm Dis* 1984; **11**:32–33.

38. Berger RE, Kessler D, Holmes KK. Etiology and manifestation of epididymitis in young men: correlations with sexual orientation. *J Infect Dis* 1987; **155**:1341–1343.

Selection and Evaluation of Diagnostic Tests

J Lewis

PURPOSE AND SELECTION OF DIAGNOSTIC TESTS

DIAGNOSIS OF DISEASE

The process of diagnosis requires two essential steps. The first is the establishment of a differential diagnosis (i.e., diagnostic hypotheses) followed by attempts to arrive at a single diagnosis by progressively ruling out specific diseases. This process requires very sensitive tests. Such tests, when normal (i.e., negative), permit the physician to confidently exclude the disease. The next step is the pursuit of a strong clinical suspicion for a specific disease. This process requires a very specific test. Such a test, when abnormal (i.e., positive), should essentially confirm the presence of the disease.

SCREENING

The primary use of screening tests in asymptomatic patients is to detect diseases whose morbidity can be reduced by early detection and treatment and to reassure patients found to be free of disease. There are several important principles in applying screening tests. First, the disease in question should be common enough to justify the effort to detect it. Next, if not treated, it should be accompanied by significant morbidity and effective therapy should exist to alter its natural history. Finally, detection and treatment of the presymptomatic state should result in benefits beyond those obtained through treatment of early symptomatic disease. Once these criteria are met, the issue can be examined from the standpoint of laboratory tests. An acceptable test is one that will be abnormal (i.e., positive) in almost all individuals with the disease and provide the physician with confidence that the patient is free of disease when the test is normal (i.e., negative).

PATIENT MANAGEMENT

Tests are commonly repeated for one or more of the following purposes:

1. To monitor the status of a disease process

2. To identify and reverse complications of treatment
3. To ensure therapeutic levels of one or more drugs
4. To aid in prognosis
5. To check an unexpected test result

For these purposes, the reproducibility of the test is the most important characteristic.

DETERMINATION OF DISEASE DISTRIBUTION

The purpose of a diagnostic test is to discriminate between patients with a particular disease and those who do not have the disease. However, most diagnostic tests measure some disease marker or surrogate (e.g., an antibody that is variably associated with the disease) rather than the presence or absence of the disease itself. The performance level of a diagnostic test depends on the distribution of the marker being measured in diseased and nondiseased patients and on the technical performance characteristics of the test itself (i.e., precision and reliability).

Each disease marker has a distribution in populations of diseased and nondiseased patients. Unfortunately, these distributions frequently overlap so that measurement of the marker in question does not usually permit a complete separation of the two populations (*Fig. A2.1*).

EVALUATION OF DIAGNOSTIC TESTS

The first step in evaluating a diagnostic test is to determine its technical performance. Does the test measure what it claims to measure? Is the test replicable? (Replicability, or precision, reflects the variance in a test result that occurs when the test is repeated on the same specimen). A highly precise test exhibits little variance among repeated measurements; an imprecise test exhibits great variance. The greater this variation, the less faith one has in results based on a single test. However, a precise test is not necessarily a good test. A test may exhibit a high level of replicability yet be in error. If the test is reliable (i.e., unbiased), it must exhibit agree-

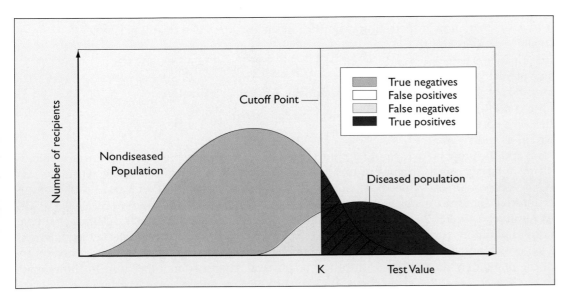

Fig. A2.1 Relationship of test value to diseased and nondiseased populations for a hypothetical diagnostic test.

ment between the mean test result and the true value of the biologic variable being measured in the sample. Evaluations of clinical tests should consider both the replicability and the reliability of the test.

The three most commonly used measures of diagnostic test performance are sensitivity, specificity, and predictive value (*Table A2.1*). These test characteristics deal with the ability of the diagnostic test to identify correctly subjects with and without the condition of interest.

SENSITIVITY

Sensitivity, which measures the ability of a test to detect infection when it is present, is of maximum concern in patient populations having a high prevalence of disease, such as STD clinics. Sensitivity measures the proportion of all infected patients exhibiting a positive test.

SPECIFICITY

Specificity, which measures the ability of a test to correctly exclude infection in uninfected patients, is of maximum concern when testing in patient populations having a low prevalence of disease, such as family planning clinics and most private practice settings. Specificity measures the proportion of uninfected patients with a negative test.

Sensitivity and specificity have been adopted widely because they are considered to be stable properties of diagnostic tests when properly derived from a broad spectrum of infected and uninfected patients. That is, their values are thought not to change significantly when applied in populations with different prevalences, presentations, or severity of disease. If diagnostic tests do not have a broad population base, their sensitivities and specificities change as the prevalence and severity of disease vary in the populations tested.

PREDICTIVE VALUES

When a test is to be used in a large, unselected population, it is important to know what its predictive value will be — that is, what is the likelihood that a person with a positive test result actually has the disease and, conversely, what is the likelihood that a person with a negative test result does not have the disease. This likelihood cannot be directly estimated from the test sensitivity and specificity value obtained in the preliminary evaluation since the predictive value is related to the actual prevalence of the disease in the total population.

Taken alone, test sensitivity and specificity do not reveal how likely it is that a given patient really has the condition in question if the test result is positive, or how likely it is that a given patient is not infected if the test result is negative. The fraction of those patients with a positive test result who actually are infected is called the predictive value positive (PVP) of a test. The fraction of patients with a negative test result who are actually free of the disease is called the predictive value negative (PVN).

The PVP and PVN of a diagnostic test measure, respectively, how likely it is that a positive or negative test result actually represents the presence or absence of disease in a given population of patients with a given prevalence of disease. The positive and negative predictive values of a diagnostic test, however, are not stable characteristics of that test. Rather, they depend strongly on the prevalence of the condition being examined in the population being tested. Where the disease prevalence (pretest likelihood of disease) decreases, the proportion of individuals with a positive test result who actually are infected falls and the proportion of uninfected patients falsely identified as being infected rises. Conversely, as the prevalence of disease increases, the proportion of patients with a positive test result who are in fact infected increases, while the proportion of patients with a negative test result who are not suffering from the disease falls. This fact has enormous implications for all diagnostic tests, particularly when they are used in populations with a low prevalence of disease, such as in screening for the presence of an uncommon disease.

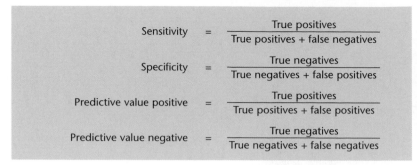

Table A2.1 Characteristics of diagnostic tests.

Actual disease prevalence (%)	Predictive values	
	Positive (%)	Negative (%)
1	16.1	99.9
2	27.9	99.9
5	50.0	99.7
10	67.9	99.4
20	82.6	98.7
50	95.0	95.0
75	98.3	83.7
100	100.0	–

Table A2.2 Predictive values of positive and negative test results at varying disease prevalences when sensitivity and specificity each equal 95%.

The following example will illustrate this principle: A test for gonorrhea is evaluated in 100 individuals who are known to have gonorrhea and in 100 normal control subjects with no evidence of the disease or of any factor known to result in increased risk for the disease. It is found that 95% of the infected individuals had positive test results (sensitivity, 95%), whereas only 5% of the control group had positive test results (specificity, 95%). In comparison with other tests, this test is considered highly accurate. What is the accuracy of a positive test in predicting gonorrhea in an unselected sample of 10,000 subjects in whom the actual prevalence of gonorrhea is 2%?

By simple arithmetic, there are 200 infected individuals in a population of 10,000 subjects with a 2% prevalence of gonorrhea, 190 of whom will have a positive test and 10 a negative test. There are 9,800 uninfected persons in this population, 9,310 of whom will have a negative test and 490 a positive test. Therefore, the predictive value of a positive test in detecting gonorrhea in the total population will be:

$$\frac{190}{(190 + 490)} = 27.9\%$$

The predictive value of a negative test will be:

$$\frac{9,310}{(9,310 + 10)} = 99.9\%$$

Table A2.2 shows the effect of disease prevalence on the predictive values of positive and negative test results when the sensitivity and specificity of the test are both 95%. The PVP of a test result increases with increasing disease prevalence; when the disease prevalence is 50%, PVP equals sensitivity and PVN equals specificity. Although higher disease prevalences are unlikely to occur in unselected populations, they may be obtained by preselection of the group to be tested on the basis of historical or physical data or some other test. In the example given above, the actual PVP in the positive reactor group was shown to

Specificity (%)	Sensitivity							
	50%	60%	70%	80%	90%	95%	98%	99%
50	2.0	2.4	2.8	3.2	3.5	3.7	3.8	3.9
60	2.5	3.0	3.4	3.9	4.4	4.6	4.8	4.8
70	3.3	3.9	4.5	5.2	5.8	6.1	6.2	6.3
80	4.8	5.8	6.7	7.6	8.4	8.8	9.1	9.2
90	9.2	10.9	12.5	14.0	15.5	16.2	16.7	16.8
95	17.0	19.7	22.2	24.6	26.9	27.9	28.6	28.8
98	33.8	38.0	41.7	44.9	47.9	49.2	50.0	50.2
99	50.5	55.0	58.8	62.0	64.7	66.0	66.7	66.9

A

Specificity (%)	Sensitivity							
	50%	60%	70%	80%	90%	95%	98%	99%
50	98.0	98.4	98.8	99.2	99.6	99.8	99.9	99.9
60	98.3	98.6	99.0	99.3	99.7	99.8	99.9	100.0
70	98.6	98.8	99.1	99.4	99.7	99.8	99.9	100.0
80	98.7	99.0	99.2	99.5	99.7	99.9	99.9	100.0
90	98.9	99.1	99.3	99.5	99.8	99.9	99.9	100.0
95	98.9	99.1	99.4	99.6	99.8	99.9	100.0	100.0
98	99.0	99.2	99.4	99.6	99.8	99.9	100.0	100.0
99	99.0	99.2	99.4	99.6	99.8	99.9	100.0	100.0

B

Table A2.3 Predictive value of a positive test (PVP) (A) and a negative test (PVN) (B) over a range of sensitivities and specificities when actual disease prevalence is 2%.

be 27.9% under the conditions described (*Table A2.2*). However, PVN of a test is not affected except at very high disease prevalences.

The value of PVP when actual disease prevalence is 2% is given for a range of sensitivities and specificities in *Table A2.3A*. It is seen that the predictive value of a positive test is primarily dependent on the specificity of the test, but at this disease prevalence PVP has a maximal value of 66.9% even at very high sensitivity (99%) and specificity (99%). The values of PVN in a population with a 2% disease prevalence are shown in *Table A2.3B*. Sensitivity and specificity have relatively little effect on this parameter.

One must be careful when applying results obtained during the preliminary evaluation of diagnostic tests using groups of known infected and uninfected individuals to unselected groups because of the magnification of false-positive errors by the generally low prevalences of disease in the general population. The concepts of sensitivity and specificity are not in themselves adequate to predict test reliability under these circumstances. This may be done, however, if the parameters of PVP and PVN are employed in unselected populations. These parameters take into account the known or assumed actual prevalence of disease in the general population.

Errors can be minimized by increasing the specificity of the test and by preselecting subjects at high risk of disease. This will produce a higher disease prevalence in the population to be tested. The preselection of the population by the first test will increase greatly the predictive value of the second test.

A good example is the screening use of the Rapid Plasma Reagin (RPR) or Venereal Disease Research Laboratory (VDRL) test to 'enrich' the group of positives, which are then subsequently tested with the Fluorescent Treponemal Antibody Absorption (FTA-ABS) test for confirmation. A similar situation exists for the human immunodeficiency virus (HIV) enzyme-linked immunosorbent assay (ELISA) and Western blot tests. Use of the FTA-ABS or Western blot as a screening test is not indicated. These tests are no better than the screening tests for evaluation and are much more expensive and difficult to interpret.

A major problem in determining performance characteristics of many diagnostic tests is the lack of an appropriate reference standard, known as 'gold standard,' against which to judge the test. In practice, one is often forced to accept the best available, albeit imperfect, diagnostic test as a pseudo-reference standard. Diagnostic tests should always be evaluated in terms of their use with, and contribution to, other diagnostic tests and not merely in terms of their absolute accuracy in isolating already-known clinical information.

The effectiveness of a program to control STDs depends upon its effectiveness to detect STDs. Although most laboratories will employ a number of different tests, the range that is available is rapidly increasing.

Laboratory services are an integral part of all disease control programs, and the availability of laboratory tests considerably improves the quality of patient care. The most important characteristic and justification for the use of a laboratory test is its ability to provide information to assist patient management. The types of tests a laboratory can offer will depend on the level of its competence and its responsibilities (*Table A2.4*).

QUALITY CONTROL

Quality control of diagnostic tests depends on adherence to recommendations regarding refrigeration and/or shelf life of antibiotics, culture medium, and test reagents. More important are measures of outcome. Among these are the percentage of patients who have follow-up examinations and are found cured for each treatment regimen and, whenever possible, the level of agreement between different diagnostic tests for the same disease. For example, all intermediate and central laboratories should develop methods for comparing results of Gram-stained smears and cultures for *Neisseria gonorrhoeae*. This is the only practical way to continuously monitor the quality of gonorrhea diagnostic techniques that begins with medium production and ends with transmittal of results to patients.

Bibliography

Griner PF, Mayewski RJ, Mushlin AI, Greenland P. Selection and interpretation of diagnostic tests and procedures. *Ann Intern Med* 1981; **94**:553.

Hart G. *Epidemiologic Aspects of Venereal Disease Control. US Dept of Health and Human Services publication No. 00–3633.* Atlanta, Centers for Disease Control, 1980.

Hart G. The role of treponemal tests in therapeutic decision making. *Am J Public Health* 1983; **73**:739.

Holmes KK, Mårdh P-A, Sparling PF, Wiesner PJ. *Sexually Transmitted Diseases*, ed I. New York, McGraw-Hill Book Co, 1984, pp 992–998.

Rothenberg RB, Simon R, Chipperfield E, Catterall RD. Efficacy of selected diagnostic tests for sexually transmitted diseases. *JAMA* 1976; **235**:49.

Swartz JS. *Assessing Medical Technologies*. Washington, DC, National Academy Press, 1985, pp 70–175.

Vecchio TJ. Predictive value of a single diagnostic test in unselected populations. *N Engl J Med* 1966; **274**:1171.

Whittington WL, Cates W Jr. Checking out the new STD tests. *Contemp Obstet Gynecol* 1984; **23**:135.

World Health Organization — VDT 85.437. *Simplified approaches for sexually transmitted disease (STD) control at the primary health care (PHC) level.* Report of a WHO working group. Geneva, Sept. 24–28, 1984.

Disease	Agent	Laboratory test	Sensitivity	Specificity	Recommended Level of availability* P	I	C
Syphilis	*Treponema pallidum*	Dark-field microscopy	80–90	<100	+/–	+	+
		VDRL (nontreponemal) test	71–100†	79–98‡	+	+	+
		RPR card (nontreponemal) test	73–100†	79–98‡	+	+	+
		FTA-ABS (treponemal) test	85–100†	95–100‡	–	+	+
		TP-PA (treponemal) test	70–100†	96–100	–	+	+
		Direct FA	90–95	>98	–	+/–	+
		#PCR	>95	>99	–	–	+
Gonorrhea	*Neisseria gonorrhoeae*	Gram stain					
		Urethral, symptomatic	90–85	95–99	+	+	+
		Urethral, asymptomatic	50–70	85–87	+	+	+
		Endocervix	45–65	90–99	+	+	+
		Conjunctiva	95		+	+	+
		Vagina	Not recommended		–	–	–
		Anal canal	Not recommended		–	–	–
		Pharynx	Not recommended		–	–	–
		Culture					
		Urethral discharge	94–98	>99	+/–	+	+
		Urethral, asymptomatic	80–85		+/–	+	+
		Endocervix	85–95	>99	+/–	+	+
		Conjunctiva	95		–	+	+
		Vagina	50–85		–	+	+
		Anal canal	70–85		–	+	+
		Pharynx	50–70		–	+/–	+
		Disseminated infection					
		Gram stain					
		Blood	Not recommended		–	–	–
		Joints	5–10		+	+	+
		Lesions	5–10		+	+	+
		Culture					
		Blood	25–75		–	+/–	+
		Joint	25–75		–	+	+
		Lesions	2–5		–	+	+
		Direct antigen detection					
		Urethra	90–95	81–99	–	+/–	+
		Endocervix	60–85	76–99	–	+/–	+
		Rectum	Not recommended		–	–	–
		Pharynx	Not recommended		–	–	–
		β-lactamase tests	>99		–	+/–	+
		Direct FA	90–95	95–99	–	+/–	+
		DNA probes	85–90	99	–	+/–	+
		Confirmatory tests	95–99	>95	–	+	+
		Antimicrobic susceptibility					
		Disk diffusion			+/–	+	+
		Minimum inhibitory concentration (MIC)			–	–	+
		PCR					
		SDA					
		Urethra	>95	>99	–	–	+
		Endocervix	90–95	>99	–	–	+
		Urine	>95	>99	–	–	+
		Hybrid capture					
		Urethra	>95	>99	–	–	+
		Endocervix	90–95	>99	–	–	+
		Urine	>95	>99	–	–	+
		TMA					
		Urethra	>95	>99	–	–	+
		Endocervix	90–95	>99	–	–	+
		Urine	>95	>99	–	–	+
		LCR					
		Endocervix	>95	>99	–	–	+
		Urine	90–95	>99	–	–	+

continued

Disease	Agent	Laboratory test	Sensitivity	Specificity	Recommended Level of availability*		
					P	I	C
Genital herpes	Herpes simplex virus types 1 and 2	Tzanck test	40–50	>95	–	+/–	+
		Papanicolaou smear	30–40	>95	–	+/–	+
		Direct FA	70–80	>95	–	+/–	+
		Culture	25–90†	>99	–	+/–	+
		Neutralizing antibody	65–70	x	–	–	+
		Direct EIA	85–90	>99	–	–	+
		Direct FA	>90	>98	–	+/–	+
		PCR	>95	>95	–	–	+
Trichomoniasis	Trichomonas vaginalis	Wet mount/saline	50–75	>99	+	+	+
		Culture	80–90	>99	–	+	+
		FA	85–90	>99	–	+/–	+
		EIA	90–95	>99	–	+/–	+
		DNA probe	>95	>99	–	–	+
		PCR					
		Vaginal swab	>95	>99	–	–	+
		Urine	87–90	>99	–	–	+
Candidiasis	Candida albicans	Wet mount/10% KOH	40–60	>99	+	+	+
		Culture	70–80	>99	–	+	+
		Latex agglutination	71–81	96–98	–	+	+
		DNA probe	85–90	>99	–	+	+
Chancroid	Haemophilus ducreyi	Gram stain	<50	50–70	+	+	+
		Culture	30–80	100	–	+/–	+
		Serology	70–80	80–90	–	–	+
		PCR	>90	>99	–	–	+
Bacterial vaginosis	Gardnerella vaginalis and others	Wet mount/saline	70–90	95–100	+	+	+
		Gram stain	60–80	95–100	+	+	+
		pH	75–80	60–70	+	+	+
		Culture	80–90	>99	–	+/–	+
		DNA probe	>90	>99	–	–	+
		Rapid pH (FemCard)	80–85	85–90	+	+	+
		Rapid Amine (Femcard)	85–90	85–90	+	+	+
		Rapid PIP (G. vaginalis)	80–85	90–92	+	+	+
Donovanosis	Calymmatobacterium granulomatis	Direct stain/Wright–Giemsa	40–50	<50	+	+	+
		Culture	5–10	>99	–	–	10
		PCR	Not available	Not available	–	–	+
Chlamydia (also lympho-granuloma venereum)	Chlamydia trachomatis	Culture	60–80	>99	–	–	+
		EIA					
		Urethral	60–70	>99	–	–	+
		Endocervix	60–70	>99	–	–	+
		Direct antigen-FA	75	>99	–	+	+
		Giemsa stain	45	95	–	+	+
		Papanicolaou stain	62	96	–	+/–	+
		Conjunctiva Giemsa stain	95	90–95	–	–	+
		Conjunctiva culture	95	>99	–	–	+
		Micro-IF antibody	60–80	95	–	–	+
		Complement fixation for LGV	40–50	85	–	+/–	+
		DNA probes	75	>99	–	+/–	+
		PCR					
		Endocervix	88–95	>99	–	–	+
		Urine	92–96	>99	–	–	+
		Urethral	90–95	>99	–	–	+
		LCR					
		Endocervix	87–94	>99	–	–	+
		Urine	94–96	>99	–	–	+
		Urethral	>95	>99	–	–	+
		SDA					
		Endocervix	90–95	>99	–	–	+
		Urine	>95	>99	–	–	+
		Urethral	90–95	>99	–	–	+

continued

Disease	Agent	Laboratory test	Sensitivity	Specificity	Recommended Level of availability*		
					P	I	C
Chlamydia (also lympho-granuloma venereum)	*Chlamydia trachomatis*	Hybrid capture					
		Endocervix	90–95	>99	–	–	+
		Urine	90–95	>99	–	–	+
		Urethral	90–95	>99	–	–	+
		TMA					
		Endocervix	90–95	>99	–	–	+
		Urine	>95	>99	–	–	+
		Urethral	90–95	>99	–	–	+
Genital mycoplasma infections	*Mycoplasma hominis*	Culture	75–80	95–97	–	+/–	+
		Serology	Not recommended		–	–	–
	Ureaplasma urealyticum	Culture	90–95	90–92	–	+/–	+
		Serology	Not recommended		–	–	–
AIDS	Human immunodeficiency virus (HIV-1)	EIA	>99	>99	–	+/–	+
		Western Blot	>99	>99	–	+/–	+
Genital warts	Human papillomaviruses (HPV)	DNA probes	88–92	96–98	–	+/–	+

*Peripheral (P) = outpatient clinics or primary practitioner's laboratory (facilities limited); intermediate (I) = regional, state, hospital laboratory; central (C) national research of reference laboratory.
†Varies with stage of disease
‡Varies with population being tested
#For investigational use only

Table A2.4 Laboratory tests commonly performed in the diagnosis of sexually transmitted infections.

L M Mahilum-Tapay and H Lee

The successful cultivation, isolation, characterization and identification of infectious agents depend largely on the quality of the specimen that one collects. Furthermore, many infectious agents are slow-growing and often occur in mixed populations of organisms. Thus, it is oftentimes necessary to use enriched or selective media to favor their growth and suppress the undesirable contaminating organisms. Once they are in pure culture or even *in situ*, any specialized structures or unique features may be enhanced using special stains and test procedures. From this perspective, this appendix attempts to give a comprehensive list and detailed information on transport and culture media, reagents, test procedures and stains which are either standard or reference tests or which the authors of the various chapters deemed important. It should be noted that inclusion or exclusion of manufacturers of reagents does not constitute endorsement or disapproval of any manufacturer or product.

This appendix is divided into three sections: 1) Transport and Culture Media, 2) Reagents and Test Procedures and 3) Stains. Under each section, the entries are arranged alphabetically.

TRANSPORT AND CULTURE MEDIA

A8 AGAR
Growth medium for *Mycoplasma hominis* and *Ureaplasma urealyticum*.

Trypticase soy broth (BD Diagnostic Systems, Sparks, MD, USA)	2.4 g
$CaCl_2 \cdot 2H_2O$	0.014 g
Putrescine dihydrochloride	0.166 g
Distilled water	80 mL
Agar, bacteriological grade (Difco Laboratories, Detroit, MI, USA)	1.05 g

Dissolve ingredients (except agar) and adjust pH to 5.5 with 2N HCl. Add agar, autoclave at 121°C for 15 min and equilibrate at 56°C. Add the following filter-sterilized, combined supplements to the basal agar medium:

Unheated, pooled normal horse serum	20 mL
CVA enrichment	0.5 mL
Yeast extract (25% aqueous extract of pure dry yeast), pH 6.0	1.0 mL
Urea solution, 10%	1.0 mL
L-cysteine-HCl (2% solution)	0.5 mL
GHL tripeptide (20 μg/mL solution)	0.1 mL
Penicillin G, potassium (100,000U/mL solution)	1.0 mL

Inoculate plate and then incubate at 37°C in a CO_2 incubator until growth is observed. Typical colonies of *Mycoplasma hominis* and *Ureaplasma urealyticum* appear as pinpoint colonies.

BIPHASIC BLOOD AGAR
Isolation medium for *Gardnerella vaginalis*.
Basal layer

CNA agar base (Columbia Agar, BD Diagnostic Systems, Sparks, MD, USA)	7 mL

Colistin	10 μg
Nalidixic acid	15 μg
Amphotericin B	2 μg/mL

Overlay medium

Basal layer medium	14 mL
Human blood	5% (v/v)

Make serial dilutions of the sample and plate aliquots of each dilution on the plate. Incubate at 37°C for 24–48 hr or until colonies appear.

Gardnerella vaginalis colonies are pinpoint after 24 hr becoming 0.4–0.5 mm in diameter after 48 hr, opaque and smooth. They become larger after 48 hr but lose their viability rapidly.

BLOOD AGAR
Growth medium for *Mycoplasma* spp.

Blood agar base No. 2 (Oxoid, Hampshire UK)	40 g
Dextrose	5.0 g
Thallous acetate (or thallous sulfate)	0.125 g
Distilled water	1000 mL
Penicillin	100,000 U
Horse serum	200 mL

Boil first three ingredients in distilled water to dissolve and autoclave at 121°C for 15 min. Cool to 50°C and add penicillin and horse serum. Mix well and pour thick plates. Inoculate and incubate separate plates at 37°C, for up to 5 or 6 days, under aerobic and anaerobic conditions simultaneously.

Mycoplasma appear as pinpoint colonies.

CHLAMYDIA TRANSPORT MEDIUM
This medium is used for the transport of specimens for isolation of *Chlamydia*.
Per liter of distilled water:

Sucrose	74.60 g
L-glutamic acid	0.72 g
Potassium diphosphate	0.51 g
Potassium monophosphate	1.24 g
HEPES	4.76 g
Fetal bovine serum	100 mL
Phenol red	3.00 mg
Gentamycin	50.00 mg
Nystatin	30.00 mg
Amphotericin B	2.50 mg

Sterile filter and aseptically dispense the medium in small volumes. Keep at 2–8°C.

CO-CULTIVATION TECHNIQUE FOR GROWING *CALYMMATOBACTERIUM GRANULOMATIS*
Materials:

Histopaque 1077 (Sigma Chemicals, St. Louis, MO, USA)
Blood sample from a healthy donor

Hank's Balanced Salt Solution (Gibco Invitrogen Co, Carlsbad, CA, USA)

Growth medium (RPMI-1640 supplemented with L-glutamine, Gibco Invitrogen Co Carlsbad, CA USA, and 10% autologous serum)

Shell vials, 5-ml

Cover slips (to fit the shell vial)

Amikacin (10 mg/L)

PBS, pH 7.2

Procedure:

Cell culture

1. Isolate peripheral blood mononuclear cells (PBMCs) from a healthy blood sample by layering blood onto equal volume of Histopaque 1077.
2. Centrifuge at 1200 rpm for 20 min.
3. Carefully remove plasma and then collect the PBMCs which would form a white ring between the plasma and Histopaque layer.
4. Rinse PBMCs in about 25 ml HBSS and centrifuge at 1200 rpm for 5 min.
5. Gently resuspend pellet in growth medium.
6. Inoculate to shell vials containing coverslips and incubate at 37°C for 1 hr in 5% CO_2.

Inoculation

1. Pre-treat specimens with amikacin (10 mg/L) for 2 hr.
2. Rinse with PBS, homogenize and suspend in growth medium.
3. Inoculate 0.5 ml of the suspension onto PBMC monolayers and incubate at 37°C in 5% CO_2.
4. After 48 hr, prepare subcultures onto fresh monolayers.
5. After incubation, fix coverslips in methanol and stain with appropriate stain. Organisms appear as elongate bacilli with a characteristic bipolar appearance. On subculture in PBMC, large, elongated coccobacillary forms with a characteristic safety-pin appearance are seen.
6. Inoculate specimens onto a variety of cell-free media, such as Horse Blood Agar (HBA; Oxoid, Hampshire UK) and MacConkey Agar plus crystal violet (Oxoid, Hampshire UK), and incubate at 37°C for 48 hr.

CHOCOLATE AGAR

A complex non-selective medium used for cultivating fastidious micro-organisms such as *Neisseria gonorrhoeae*.

Solution A

GC Agar base (BD Diagnostic Systems, Sparks, MD, USA)	7.2 g
Distilled water	100 mL

Mix and boil for 2 min. Autoclave at 121°C for 15 min. Cool to 50°C.

Solution B

Hemoglobin	2.0 g
Distilled water	100 mL

Mix the hemoglobin with 2–3 mL of distilled water to form a smooth paste. Continue mixing and gradually add all the water. Autoclave at 121°C for 15 min and cool to 50°C.

Aseptically combine solutions A and B. Add 2 mL IsoVitalex (BD Diagnostic Systems, Sparks, MD, USA). Mix and pour 20–25 mL per Petri dish.

DULANEY SLANTS

A medium used for cultivating *Calymmatobacterium granulomatis*.

Aseptically separate yolks from 5–8-day hen egg embryos and place in an equal volume of sterile Locke solution containing glass beads. Mix vigorously and dispense homogenate into slanted tubes. Steam at 80°C for 15 min to coagulate the mixture.

GC II AGAR BASE

(BD Diagnostic Systems, Sparks, MD, USA) Basal medium used for the preparation of selective media for *N. gonorrhoeae* and *Haemophilus ducreyi*.

Pancreatic digest of casein	7.5 g
Selected meat peptone	7.5 g
Corn starch	1.0 g
K_2HPO_4	4.0 g
KH_2PO_4	1.0 g
Sodium chloride	5.0 g
Agar	10.0 g
Distilled water	1000 mL

The final pH should be 7.3 ± 0.2.

GC-LECT

(BD Diagnostic Systems, Sparks, MD, USA) A selective medium for *N. gonorrhoeae*.

ISOVITALEX

(BD Diagnostic Systems, Sparks, MD, USA) A supplement for media used for the isolation of *N. gonorrhoeae* and *H. ducreyi*.

Per liter of distilled water:

Vitamin B12	0.01 g
L-glutamine	10.0 g
Adenine	1.0 g
Guanine HCl	0.03 g
ρ-aminobenzoic acid	0.013 g
Diphosphopyridine nucleotide, oxidized (coenzyme 1)	0.25 g
Cocarboxylase	0.1 g
Ferric nitrate	0.02 g
Thiamine HCl	0.003 g
L-cysteine HCl	25.9 g
L-cystine	1.1 g
Dextrose	100.0 g

Each vial of IsoVitaleX enrichment is supplied with a vial of sterile rehydrating fluid diluent containing approximately 10% dextrose. The composition of this enrichment is similar to that of Vitox (Oxoid, Hampshire UK).

JEMBEC

This medium is used for the transport and selective growth of *N. gonorrhoeae*. The Jembec plate allows the investigator to add the CO_2 required for the growth of *N. gonorrhoeae*, after the specimen has been inoculated by placing a CO_2-generating tablet in a well provided in the plate. Plates containing either modified Thayer-Martin or Martin-Lewis medium are available ready-to-use according to the manufacturer's specifications.

MARTIN-LEWIS MEDIUM

A selective medium for *N. gonorrhoeae* identical to modified Thayer-Martin medium except for substituting anisomycin (10 µg/ml) for nystatin.

MODIFIED DIAMOND'S MEDIUM

This is a culture medium for *Trichomonas vaginalis*.

Trypticase (BD Diagnostic Systems, Sparks, MD, USA)	20.0 g

Yeast extract	1.0 g
Maltose	0.5 g
L-cystine HCl	0.5 g
L-ascorbic acid	0.02 g
Distilled water, make up volume to	90.0 mL

Adjust pH to 6.5 and autoclave at 121°C for 15 min, cool to 48°C, and add the following:

Sodium penicillin G	1000 U/mL
Streptomycin sulfate	1.5 mg/mL
Amphotericin B	2 µg/mL
Horse serum (inactivated at 56°C for 30 min)	10 mL

Aliquot 5-mL amounts into sterile tubes and store at 4°C for up to 14 days. Warm to 35°C before inoculation. This medium, without the horse serum, may be stored at –20°C.

MODIFIED CHLAMYDIAL CULTURE TECHNIQUE FOR *CALYMMATOBACTERIUM GRANULOMATIS*

Materials:

Human epithelial cell line, Hep-2
Growth medium
RPMI 1640

Fetal calf serum	10 %
NaHCO$_3$	0.2 %
Vancomycin.HCl	20 mg/L
Benzylpenicillin	100 U/L

Cycloheximide stock solution
Shell vials, 5-ml
Coverslips (which fit the vials)

Procedure:

1. Put swab in 1 ml of transport medium. Keep at –70° for 2–14 da until ready for use. Immediately prior to testing, thaw in a 37°C water bath.
2. Grow Hep-2 cells on 4 coverslips contained in a 5-ml shell vial containing 1-ml of growth medium. Incubate at 37°C in a 5% CO$_2$ incubator for 24-hr or until a monolayer is formed.
3. Inoculate monolayer with 25 to 50 µl of the specimen (in transport medium).
4. Centrifuge vial at 1000 × g at 33°C for 45 min. Just prior to inoculation, add 0.7 mg/L cycloheximide to inhibit further growth of Hep-2 cells.
5. Incubate at 35°C in 5% CO$_2$ for 24 to 72 hr.
6. After incubation, fix one cover slip with methanol and stain overnight with 1% Giemsa stain. Organisms resembling Donovan bodies appear as pleomorphic bacilli with a halo. The characteristic bipolar staining and safety-pin appearance may be apparent in elongated forms of the organism, some of which may be dividing.
7. The other coverslips may be used for other tests while another one may be stored at –70°C for subsequent passaging.
8. For verification, inoculate specimens onto a variety of cell-free media, such as Horse Blood Agar (HBA; Oxoid, Hampshire UK) and MacConkey Agar plus crystal violet (Oxoid, Hampshire UK), and incubate at 37°C for 48 hr. *C. granulomatis* does not grow in cell-free medium.

MODIFIED NYC MEDIUM

A selective medium for *N. gonorrhoeae*.

GC agar base	36 g
Bio-enrichment	10 mL
30% lysed horse red blood cells	200 mL
Horse plasma	120 mL

Dextrose	5.0 g
Colistin	5.0 mg
Vancomycin	2.0 mg
Amphotericin B	1.2 mg
Trimethoprim lactate	3.0 mg
Distilled water	1000 mL

N. gonorrhoeae colonies appear as gray/brown and measure 0.25–2 mm after 24 hr of incubation. With further incubation to 48 hr, the colonies may grow bigger and measure 1–3 mm in diameter.

MYCOPLASMA BROTH

This is a transport medium for *Mycoplasma* spp.

Mycoplasma broth base	70 mL
Yeast extract (1 part)	30 mL
Horse serum (2 parts)	60 mL

Mix and add the following:

0.4% Phenol red	0.5 g
Penicillin (100,000U/mL)	0.5 mL
Polymyxin (5000 µg/mL)	1.0 mL
Amphotericin (5000 µg/mL)	0.1 mL

Adjust pH to 6.0 with 1 N HCl, sterile filter and dispense into 1-ml aliquots.

MYCOPLASMA BROTH BASE

A component of media used for transport and culture of *Mycoplasma* spp.

Beef heart infusion	50.0 g
Peptone	10.0 g
NaCl	5.0 g
Distilled water	1000 mL

Autoclave at 121°C for 15 min and store at 4°C.

NICKERSON MEDIUM

(Bacto BiGGY Agar, Difco Laboratories, Detroit, MI USA) A selective medium recommended for the detection, isolation and differentiation of *Candida* spp.

Bacto yeast extract	1.0 g
Glycine	10.0 g
Bacto dextrose	10.0 g
Bismuth sulfite indicator	8.0 g
Bacto agar	20.0 g
Distilled water	1000 mL

Final pH should be 6.8. Dissolve ingredients in distilled water with heating. Do not boil for longer than a few minutes as overheating will destroy the selective properties of the medium. *Do not autoclave*. The medium contains a flocculent precipitate that should be evenly dispersed by swirling the medium in flask prior to dispensing in tubes or plates. Prepared medium should be stored at 4°C if not to be used right away.

Inoculated plates are incubated at 30°C for 48–72 hr. *Candida* spp. appear as dark colonies.

SABORAUD DEXTROSE AGAR

This culture medium is recommended for growing *Candida albicans* and other fungi.

Glucose	40.0 g
Neopeptone or polypeptone (BD Diagnostic Systems, Sparks, MD, USA)	10.0 g
Agar	15.0 g
Demineralized water	1000 mL

Final pH should be 5.6. Heat the mixture to dissolve completely. Dispense into tubes (18–25 mm diameter) and autoclave at 121°C for 15 min. *Candida* and other yeasts appear as cream (or colored, in some other yeasts) opaque colonies while multicellular fungal colonies may form cottony growth.

SHEPARD'S 10 B BROTH

Growth medium for *Mycoplasma hominis* and *Ureaplasma urealyticum*.

PPLO broth (without crystal violet) (Difco Laboratories, Detroit, MI USA)	1.47 g
Distilled water	73 mL

Dissolve powder and adjust pH to 5.5 with 2N HCl. Autoclave at 121°C for 15 min. The following supplements may be combined, filter sterilized, and added to the basal broth after cooling to room temperature.

Unheated normal serum	20 mL
Yeast extract, 25%	10 mL
L-cysteine HCL stock solution, 2%	0.5 mL
Urea stock solution, 10%	0.4 mL
CVA supplement	0.5 mL
Sodium phenol red solution, 1%	0.1 mL
Penicillin G potassium, 100 000 U/mL	1.0 mL

The final pH of the complete 10B broth should be approximately 6.0. The medium is aseptically dispensed in convenient small volumes and stored at –20°C.

SP-4 MEDIUM

Growth medium for *Mycoplasma hominis* and *Mycoplasma genitalium*.
Liquid medium:

Mycoplasma broth base	1.0 g
Bacto-peptone (Difco Laboratories, Detroit MI, USA))	1.6 g
Bacto-tryptone (Difco Laboratories, Detroit MI, USA)	3.0 g
Distilled water	197 mL

Dissolve ingredients and adjust pH to 7.8 (0.6 mL 2N NaOH). Autoclave at 121°C for 30 min and cool to room temperature. Add the following sterile components:

Phenol red (0.5% solution)	1.2 mL
Penicillin G potassium (100 000U/mL)	3.0 mL
Yeastolate (Difco) 2%	30.0 mL
CMRL-1066 (10X) (with glutamine, without NaHCO$_3$) (Gibco Invitrogen Co, Carlsbad CA, USA)	15.0 mL
Fresh yeast extract (25%)	10.5 mL
Fetal bovine serum (heat-treated, 56°C for 1 hr)	50.0 mL
Glucose (50% solution)	3.0 mL

Final pH should be 7.4.
Solid medium:
Add 2.4 to 6.8 g Difco Noble agar (depending on spiroplasma) to autoclavable fraction, before autoclaving and after adjusting pH. After autoclaving, cool to 56°C and allow non-autoclavable portion to warm to 56°C. Combine both fractions aseptically before pouring plates.

2SP MEDIUM

This is a transport medium recommended for *Chlamydia trachomatis* or *Mycoplasma* spp.

Sucrose	0.2 M
Phosphate buffer, pH 7.2	0.02 M
Gentamycin	2 µg/mL
Amphotericin	0.5 µg/mL
Vancomycin	10 µg/mL

THAYER-MARTIN AGAR

A selective medium for the isolation of *N. gonorrhoeae*.

To the complete chocolate agar (see p. 382), add 1 mL of VCN inhibitor containing (per mL):

Vancomycin	300 µg
Colistin	750 µg
Nystatin	1250 µg

A modified Thayer-Martin agar may be prepared by adding trimethoprim lactate at a final concentration of 5 µg/mL. Typical *N. gonorrhoeae* growth would appear as translucent, non-pigmented to brownish colonies measuring 0.5 to 1.0 mm in diameter.

TRANSGROW MEDIUM

This is a transport and selective growth medium for *N. gonorrhoeae*.

GC agar base (BD Diagnostic Systems, Sparks, MD, USA)	7.2 g
Glucose	0.3 g
Agar	2 g
Distilled water	100 mL

Autoclave at 121°C for 15 min. Cool to 50°C and keep in the water bath.

Hemoglobin	2.0 g
Distilled water	100 mL

Mix the hemoglobin with 2–3 mL of the distilled water to form a smooth paste. Continue mixing and gradually add all the water. Autoclave at 121°C for 15 min and then cool to 50°C. Aseptically combine both solutions and then add 1 mL of VCN inhibitor. Aseptically dispense into sterile bottles, gas with 20% CO$_2$ in air, and tighten caps securely.

TRANSPORT MEDIUM FOR HERPES SIMPLEX VIRUS

Hank's balanced salt solution with 2% fetal calf serum (and antibiotics to prevent bacterial growth) (Gibco Invitrogen Co, Carlsbad, CA, USA).

TRANSPORT MEDIUM FOR DONOVANOSIS SPECIMENS

Glucose phosphate buffer, 0.2 M, pH 7.2, sterile	1 L
Fetal calf serum	10 %
Vancomycin hydrochloride	20 mg
Amphotericin B	2.5 mg

TRYPTICASE SOY BROTH + 0.5% BOVINE SERUM ALBUMIN

This is a transport medium for *Mycoplasma* spp.

Trypticase soy broth (BD Diagnostic Systems, Sparks, MD, USA)	3 g
Bovine serum albumin	0.5 g
Distilled water	100 mL

Dissolve by mixing thoroughly and warming gently until solution is complete. Dispense and autoclave at 121°C for 15 min.

TRYPTICASE SOY BROTH + 15% GLYCEROL

This is a freezing medium for storage of Neiserriae at –70°C.

Trypticase soy broth (BD Diagnostic Systems, Sparks, MD, USA)	30 g
Distilled water	500 mL
Glycerol	150 mL
Distilled water, make up volume to	1000 mL

Dissolve trypticase soy broth in 500 mL of water by mixing thoroughly and warming gently. Add glycerol and make up solution to 1000 mL. Dispense into individual tubes and autoclave at 121°C for 15 min.

Procedure:

1. Grow *Neisseria* culture to logarithmic phase (24–48 hr).
2. Harvest cells by centrifugation (if grown in liquid culture) or by gently scraping growth from agar surface (be careful not to include agar bits). Resuspend the cells in freezing medium previously cooled in an ice bath.
3. Aliquot 1 ml (containing 10^7 to 10^8 cells) into a cryovial. Keep in a –70°C freezer. For long storage, it is recommended that vials are kept in a liquid nitrogen tank.

YEAST EXTRACT, 25%

(Difco, Laboratories, Detroit, MI, USA; Oxoid, Hampshire UK) This is a component of a medium used for the growth of *Mycoplasma* spp.

Sprinkle 250g active baker's yeast onto the surface of 1 L distilled water in a 2-L beaker. Heat the mixture to boiling, then clarify it by centrifuging at 1000 g for 1 hr. Adjust the pH to 8.0 with 1N NaOH and filter sterilize.

REAGENTS AND TEST PROCEDURES

ACETIC ACID (3%)
(Acetowhitening)

Glacial acetic acid	3.0 mL
Distilled water, make up volume to	100 mL

ANTIMICROBIAL SUSCEPTIBILITY TESTING (AST)

Antimicrobial sensitivity testing is simple and yet as accurate as other tests if carried out with proper controls. A number of basal media recommended for AST such as the Mueller-Hinton Agar, Diagnostic Sensitivity Agar, and the Iso-Sensitest Agar.

There is no single world standard method for AST although the NCCLS (National Committee for Clinical Laboratory Standards, NCCLS Publications, Villanova, PA, USA) method is widely accepted and adopted by many countries. The reader is therefore advised to adopt the method accepted in his/her country.

The following are some of the more common media used in AST:

DIAGNOSTIC SENSITIVITY AGAR
(Oxoid, Hampshire UK)

Proteose peptone	10.0 g
Veal infusion solids	10.0 g
Glucose	2.0 g
Sodium chloride	3.0 g
Disodium phosphate	2.0 g
Sodium acetate	1.0 g
Adenine sulphate	0.01 g
Guanine hydrochloride	0.01 g
Uracil	0.01 g
Xanthine	0.01 g
Aneurine	0.00002 g
Agar	12.0 g
Distilled water	1 L
pH 7.4 ± 0.2	

Add 40 g to 1 L of distilled water. Bring to a boil and dissolve completely. Autoclave at 121°C for 15 min.

For blood agar, cool the base to 50°C and add 7% of defibrinated horse blood. Mix with gentle rotation and pour into petri dishes or other containers. Reconstitution and mixing should be performed in a flask at least 2.5× the volume of medium to ensure adequate aeration of the blood.

ISO-SENSITEST MEDIUM

(Oxoid, Hampshire UK) Required medium for AST in Australia.

Hydrolysed casein	11.0 g
Peptones	3.0 g
Glucose	2.0 g
Sodium chloride	3.0 g
Soluble starch	1.0 g
Disodium hydrogen phosphate	2.0 g
Sodium acetate	1.0 g
Magnesium glycerophosphate	0.2 g
Calcium gluconate	0.1 g
Cobaltous sulfate	0.001 g
Cupric sulfate	0.001 g
Zinc sulfate	0.001 g
Ferrous sulfate	0.001 g
Manganous chloride	0.002 g
Menadione	0.001 g
Cyanocobalamin	0.001 g
L-Cysteine hydrochloride	0.02 g
L-Tryptophan	0.02 g
Pyridoxine	0.003 g
Pantothenate	0.003 g
Nicotinamide	0.003 g
Biotin	0.0003 g
Thiamine	0.00004 g
Adenine	0.01 g
Guanine	0.01 g
Xanthine	0.01 g
Uracil	0.01 g
Agar	8.0 g
pH 7.4 ± 0.2	

Suspend 31.4 g in 1 litre of distilled water and bring to a boil to dissolve the agar. Sterilise by autoclaving at 121°C for 15 minutes.

MUELLER-HINTON MEDIUM

(Oxoid, Hampshire UK). For antimicrobial sensitivity testing for *N. gonorrhoeae*, the formula of which has been modified to meet internationally recognized standards.

Beef, dehydrated infusion from	300.0 g
Casein hydrolysate	17.5 g
Starch	1.5 g
Agar	17.0 g
Distilled water	1 L
pH 7.4 ± 0.2	

Add 38 g to 1 L of distilled water. Bring to a boil and dissolve the medium completely. Sterilize by autoclaving at 121°C for 15 min.

ALKALINE PHOSPHATASE TEST

ρ-Nitrophenyl phosphate disodium tetrahydrate	100.0 mg
Distilled water, make up volume to	100 mL

Dissolve the substrate and add 25 mL of a solution containing 0.1 M glycine and 0.001 M $MgCl_2$, pH 10.5. Filter sterilize, dispense into 0.3 mL aliquots and store at –20°C. To detect alkaline phosphatase production, inoculate the substrate-containing solution with test organism and incubate at 35°C for 6 hr. Development of a yellow color is indicative of a positive test.

β-LACTAMASE TEST

Cefinase is available from BD Diagnostic Systems, Sparks, MD, USA. Use according to manufacturer's instructions.

CATALASE TEST

Add a drop of 3% H_2O_2 to a loopful of growth placed on a glass slide. A positive test is recorded when brisk bubbling occurs upon addition of H_2O_2.

IMMUNO-BASED ASSAYS

A number of immunological assays in various formats (enzyme immunoassay, lateral flow strip or Western blot) are FDA- or CDC-approved for use in diagnostic testing of STD agents. The following table lists some of these products and their manufacturers.

Target	Trademark	Manufacturer
Chlamydia trachomatis	Micro Trak Chlamydia	Trinity Biotech Plc, Wicklow Ireland
	Clearview Chlamydia MF	Unipath Ltd, Bedford UK
	Quik Vue Chlamydia Test	Quidel, San Diego CA USA
	Chlamydia OIA	Biostar, Boulder CO USA
Neisseria gonorrhoeae	Micro Trak Neisseria gonorrhoeae Culture Confirmation Test	Trinity Biotech Plc, Wicklow Ireland
Treponema pallidum	ASI RPR Card Test VDRL Test	Arlington Scientific Inc, Springville UT USA
HIV	Genetic Systems HIV-1/HIV-2 (rDNA or peptide) EIA	Bio-Rad Laboratories Blood Virus Division, Redmond WA USA
	Genetic Systems rLAV EIA	Bio-Rad Laboratories Blood Virus Division, Redmond WA USA
	HIV-1 Western Blot kit	Chiron Corporation, Emeryville CA USA
	Genetic Systems HIV-1 Western Blot	Bio-Rad Laboratories Blood Virus Division, Redmond WA USA
Hepatitis C virus	VITROS Anti-HCV assay	Ortho-Diagnostics, Raritan NJ USA
	Abbott HCV EIA 2.0	Abbott Laboratories, Abbott Park IL USA
	Chiron RIBA HCV 3.0 Strip Immunoblot assay	Chiron Corporation, Emeryville CA USA
Hepatitis B virus	Genetic Systems HBsAg EIA 2.0	Bio-Rad Laboratories Blood Virus Division, Redmond WA USA
	HBsAg ELISA System	Ortho-Diagnostics, Raritan NJ USA
	HBsAg Confirmatory Test	Ortho-Diagnostics, Raritan NJ USA
	VITROS Anti-HCV assay	
Herpes virus	POCkit HSV-2 Rapid Test	Diagnology, Belfast Northern Ireland
	HerpeSelect	Focus Technologies, Cypress CA USA

KOH (10%)

KOH	10.0 g
Distilled water, make up volume to	100 mL

KOVAC'S REAGENT

ρ-Dimethylaminobenzaldehyde	5.0 g
Amyl alcohol	75.0 mL

Dissolve completely by warming the solution in a 56°C water bath. Slowly add 25.0 mL concentrated HCl. Dispense into a brown bottle and store at 4°C. The reagent should be a light color.

LOCKE SALT SOLUTION

Sodium chloride	0.900 g
Calcium chloride	0.024 g
Potassium chloride	0.042 g
Sodium carbonate	0.020 g
Glucose	0.250 g
Distilled water	100 mL

NITRATE REDUCTASE TEST

Nitrate broth:

Heart infusion broth	25 g
Potassium nitrate C.P.	2.0 g
Distilled water	1000 mL

Adjust pH to 7.0. Dispense into 4.0 mL aliquots in 15×125-mm tubes containing inverted Durham fermentation tubes, autoclave at 121°C for 15 min, and store at 4°C.

Reagent 1:

Sulfanilic acid	2.8 g
Glacial acetic acid	100 mL
Distilled water	250 mL

Reagent 2:

Dimethyl-α-naphthylamine	2.1 mL
Glacial acetic acid	100 mL
Distilled water	250 mL

Inoculate the broth with the test organism and incubate at 35°C for 48 hr. Add 5 drops of each of the reagents 1 and 2 consecutively and examine for the presence of a pink to red color. If negative (i.e. medium remains colorless), add a small amount of zinc dust and incubate at room temperature for 5 min to detect any nitrate that has not been reduced. A red color at this point indicates that the nitrate has not been reduced (a negative test for nitrate reduction); however, if the broth remains colorless, the nitrate has been completely reduced (a positive test for nitrate reduction).

NUCLEIC ACID-BASED TESTS

There is increasing use of nucleic acid-based assays for the diagnosis of micro-organisms due to their increased sensitivity compared to traditional tests such as culture or enzyme immunoassays. They are particularly effective in detecting asymptomatic infection or individuals at early phase of seroconversion. The following table lists some of the assays currently available in the market.

Target	Trademark	Manufacturer
Chlamydia trachomatis	BD Probetec ET BD Be Aware TM	BD Diagnostic Systems, Sparks, MD USA
	LCx Chlamydia	Abbott Laboratories, IL USA
	Amplicor	Roche Diagnostics Corporation, Indianapolis INUSA
Neisseria gonorrhoeae	Gen Probe PACE 2	Gen-Probe, San Diego CA USA
	BD ProbeTec ET BD Be Aware TM	BD Diagnostic Systems, Sparks, MD USA
	LCx Neisseria gonorrhoeae	Abbott Laboratories, IL USA
	Amplicor Neisseria gonorrhoeae	Roche Diagnostics Corporation, Indianapolis IN USA
Mycoplasma	Mycoplasma Plus PCR primer set	Stratagene, La Jolla CA USA

Target	Trademark	Manufacturer
Gardenerella vaginalis, *Trichomonas vaginalis* and *Candida*	BD MicroProbe and Affirm VP III Microbial identification Test	BD Diagnostics, Sparks MD USA
HIV	Amplicor HIV-1 Monitor	Roche Diagnostics Corporation, Indianapolis IN USA
	LCx HIV-1 RNA Quantitation Assay	Abbott Laboratories, IL USA
	NucliSens® HIV-1 QT	bioMerieux, Raritan NJ USA
	UltraQual HIV-1 RT-PCR Assay	National Genetics Institute, Los Angeles, CA USA
	VERSANT HIV-1 Quantitative Assay	Bayer Diagnostics, Tarrytown NY USA
Human Papillomavirus	Hybrid Capture-II HPV DNA Assay	Digene Diagnostics, Gaithersburg MD USA
Hepatitis C virus	Amplicor HCV-Monitor	Roche Diagnostics Corporation, Indianapolis IN USA
	Chiron RIBA HCV 3.0	Chiron Corporation, Emeryville CA USA
	UltraQual HCV-RT-PCR-Assay	National Genetics Institute, Los Angeles, CA USA
	VERSANT HCV RNA Quantitative Assay	Bayer Diagnostics, Tarrytown NY USA
Hepatitis B virus	Amplicor HBV-Monitor	Roche Diagnostics Corporation, Indianapolis IN USA
	VERSANT HBV DNA Quantitative Assay	Bayer Diagnostics, Tarrytown NY USA

OXIDASE TEST

Tetra-methyl-ρ-phenylenediamine dihydrochloride	1.0 g
Distilled water	100 mL

Saturate a filter paper contained in a petri dish with the reagent. Pick a portion of the colony to be tested using a platinum wire and rub it on the filter paper. A positive reduction is indicated by a deep purple color appearing in 10 seconds.

PHOSPHATE BUFFER, M/15, pH 6.4

KH_2PO_4	6.63 g
Na_2HPO_4	2.56 g
Distilled water, make up volume to	1000 mL

PORPHYRIN TEST

Delta-aminolevulinic acid hydrochloride	0.034 g
$MgSO_4 \cdot 7H_2O$	0.02 g
Phosphate buffer, 0.1 M, pH 6.9	100 mL

Filter-sterilize, dispense into 0.5 mL aliquots and store at –20°C.
Test Procedure:

1. Add a very heavy loopful of the test organism to the substrate solution.
2. Incubate at 35°C for 4 hr.
3. Examine under a Woods lamp for a red fluorescence. A red fluorescence indicates a positive reaction. If no fluorescence is observed, incubate reaction mixture overnight and re-examine.
4. If no fluorescence is observed after an overnight incubation, add an equal volume of Kovac's reagent.
5. Shake vigorously and allow the aqueous and alcohol phases to separate. The development of a red color in the lower aqueous phase indicates a positive reaction.

PRODUCTION OF EXOPOLYSACCHARIDE FROM SUCROSE

Strains of some *Neisseria* spp. (*N. sicca*, *N. subflava* biovar *perflava*, *N. mucosa*, *N. flavescens*, *N. polysaccharea*) produce a polysaccharide from sucrose that can be detected by the addition of iodine to the colonies. Traditionally the polysaccharide test is performed by the incorporation of 5% (w/v) sucrose into a medium, such as tryptic soy agar, which does not contain starch (which will give a positive test). Strains of *Neisseria* spp. are inoculated by the streak-plate method or spotted onto the medium and incubated at 35°C for 5 days. However, some strains may be inhibited by 5% sucrose. Alternatively, the test may be performed on tryptic soy agar containing 1% (w/v) sucrose after incubation for 24 hr. A drop of Lugol's iodine (Gram's iodine diluted 1:4) is added to the growth. If polysaccharide has been produced, the colonies, and often the surrounding medium will turn a dark blue, brown, or black.

Note: It is important that the recommended time of incubation is not exceeded. Many strains that produce polysaccharide metabolize it, and if the incubation is carried out for longer than recommended, the polysaccharide may be completely consumed and thus no longer detectable. It is also possible to detect the polysaccharide in traditional sucrose-containing media in which acid production is detected. The polysaccharide may be detected as a brown-to-black precipitate when one or two drops of Lugol's iodine are added to the sucrose-containing medium. The precipitate will range from fine brown to a coarse black flocculent precipitate. The reaction will fade if the test is allowed to sit at room temperature, but may be rejuvenated with fresh Gram's iodine that has been made according to the original formula; aged Gram's iodine and commercially prepared iodine will give negative results. The polysaccharide production test may not be performed using the rapid tests for the detection of acid production from sucrose.

SUPEROXOL TEST

Add a drop of 30% H_2O_2 to a colony of the organism on a chocolate agar plate. A positive superoxol test is recorded when brisk bubbling occurs immediately when the 30% H_2O_2 is added to the colonies. A delay of 3 sec before a bubbling is observed is interpreted as a negative superoxol test. Although all human *Neisseria* spp. and *Branhamella catarrhalis* are catalase-positive, strains vary in their reactions in the superoxol test. Strains of *N. gonorrhoeae* are superoxol-positive whereas strains of other species vary in their reactions in this test. Strains of *N. meningitidis* serogroup A, *N. lactamica*, and *B. catarrhalis* may give positive superoxol tests. Thus the superoxol test must be used in combination with other tests to accurately identify strains of *N. gonorrhoeae*. It also must be noted that, similar to the catalase test, the superoxol test should not be performed on medium containing unheated blood, which will react with the H_2O_2.

STAINS

ACRIDINE ORANGE STAIN

This stain is useful for the detection of bacteria in clinical specimens. At pH 4.0, bacteria stain red-orange while eukaryotic cells stain green-yellow.

Materials:

Glass slide
Specimen
0.5% acridine orange in 0.15 M acetate buffer, pH 4.0

Procedure:

1. Make a smear of the specimen onto a clean glass slide.
2. Air dry and fix by immersion in absolute methanol for 2 min.
3. Flood the slide with acridine orange stain for 2 min.
4. Rinse the slide with water, air dry and examine in an ultraviolet-equipped microscope at 400–1000× magnification.

FLUORESCENT/IMMUNOPEROXIDASE ANTIBODY STAINS

Commercial reagents for either direct or indirect fluorescent or enzyme-conjugated monoclonal antibody are available for detection of STD agents. The following table lists some of them.

Target	Trademark	Manufacturer
Chlamydia trachomatis	Bartels Chlamydiae Fluorescent Monoclonal Antibody Test	Trinity Biotech Plc, Wicklow Ireland
	Bartels Chlamydiae Immunoperoxidase Test	Trinity Biotech Plc, Wicklow Ireland
	DAKO IDEIA Chlamydia	DAKO, Denmark
Neisseria gonorrhoeae	Micro Trak Neisseria gonorrhoeae Culture Confirmation Test	Trinity Biotech Plc, Wicklow Ireland
	Bacto FA N. gonorrhoeae	Difco Laboratories, Detroit, MI USA
Herpes virus	Micro Trak HSV Culture Identification/Typing Test and bartels HSV Monoclonal Antibody Test	Trinity Biotech Plc, Wicklow Ireland
Treponema pallidum	MarDx FTA-ABS Test System	Trinity Biotech Plc, Wicklow Ireland

GIEMSA STAIN

Materials:

Glass slide
Methanol, absolute
Specimen
Stain

1. Stock solution:

Giemsa powder	0.5 g
Glycerol	33.0 mL
Methyl alcohol, absolute, acetone-free	33.0 mL

Dissolve the powder in glycerol in a water bath (55–60°C) for 90 minutes. Once the crystals have dissolved completely, add the methanol. Store at room temperature.

2. Working solution (Must be prepared fresh just prior to use):

Stock solution	1 mL
Phosphate buffer	23 mL

3. Phosphate buffer:

Solution 1

Na_2HPO_4	9.47 g
Distilled water, make up to	1000 mL

Solution 2

KH_2PO_4	9.08 g
Distilled water, make up to	1000 mL

Mix 72 mL of solution 1 with 28 mL of solution 2. Add 900 mL of distilled water.

95% ethyl alcohol

Procedure:

1. Make a smear on a clean glass slide. Air dry and fix with methanol for at least 5 min. Air dry.
2. Flood the smear with the stain working solution for 1 hr.
3. Rinse the slide rapidly in ethyl alcohol.

4. Dry and examine under the microscope for the presence of the typical intracytoplasmic inclusion bodies. The elementary bodies stain purple, whereas reticulocyte bodies are slightly more basophilic and tend to stain toward blue. There is some variability in commercially available prepared stock Giemsa solutions; these commercial products should be screened before being used. Modifications of the Giemsa stain are used to stain protozoa (parasites) and *Dermatophilus* spp. and to detect intracellular Donovan bodies in tissues.

GRAM STAIN

Materials:

Glass slide
Reagents

a. Crystal violet

Solution 1:

Crystal violet	10 g
5% Ethyl alcohol	100 mL

Solution 2:

Ammonium oxalate	0.8 g
Distilled water	80 mL

Mix solutions 1 and 2 and store overnight at room temperature. Filter through Whatman filter paper

b. Gram's iodine

Iodine	1 g
Potassium iodide	2 g
Distilled water	300 mL

c. Decolorizer

95% Ethyl alcohol

d. Counterstain

Stock solution

Safranin-O	2.5 g
95% Ethyl alcohol	100 ml

Working solution

Stock solution	10 mL
Distilled water	90 mL

Procedure:

1. Prepare a smear on a clean glass slide.
2. Heat-fix briefly by passing over a small flame 3–5x.
3. Cover the smear with the crystal violet stain for 1 min.
4. Rinse in running tap water and blot dry.
5. Flood the smear with Gram's iodine.
6. Decolorize until no blue-violet color comes off the slide.
7. Apply counterstain on the smear for 30 sec.
8. Rinse in running water and blot dry.
9. Examine under the microscope. Gram-positive bacteria stain blue-violet while gram-negative bacteria stain pink or light red.

Ready-to-use Gram stain kits are also available from manufacturers of microbiological laboratory media and reagents.

HEMATOXYLIN AND EOSIN STAIN

Materials:

Specimen sections, cut at 5 mm, mounted on clean glass slide
Xylol

Ethanol, absolute, 95%, 90%, 80%, 60%
Distilled water
Harris hematoxylin stain

Hematoxylin	100 mL
Glacial acetic acid	5 mL

Picro-eosin solution
Neutral xylol-damar

Procedure:

1. Dip slide in two changes of xylol for 2 min.
2. Dip slide in two changes of absolute alcohol, 1 min each.
3. Change to 95% ethanol and dip for 1 min.
4. Dip in 90% alcohol for 0.5 min.
5. Change to 80% alcohol and dip for 0.5 min.
6. Change to 50% alcohol and dip for 0.5 min.
7. Rinse in distilled water, twice or more until the slides have cleared.
8. Cover with the hematoxylin stain for 1–2 min.
9. Rinse in distilled water.
10. Place the slide in tap water containing 20–40 drops of ammonium hydroxide for 3 sec (*Note: the section will turn blue immediately*).
11. Rinse in two changes of tap water to remove the ammonia.
12. Counterstain in picro-eosin solution for 30 sec.
13. Dip in two changes of 95% alcohol, 1 min each followed by
14. Two changes in absolute alcohol for 1 and 2 min, respectively.
15. Dip in two changes of xylol for 1 min each.
16. Mount in neutral xylol-damar. Let it dry.
17. Examine under the microscope.

JONES' IODINE STAIN
Materials:

Glass slide
Specimen
Stain

Potassium iodide	5 g
Iodine crystals	5 g
Absolute methanol	50 mL
Distilled water	50 mL

Combine reagents and mix well until in solution. Store at room temperature in a brown bottle. Before use, filter through a Whatman No. 41 ashless filter paper.

METHYLENE BLUE STAIN
Materials:

Glass slide
Specimen
Stain

Methylene blue	0.3 g
Ethanol	30 mL
Distilled water	100 mL

Dissolve the dye in ethanol. Add the distilled water.
Procedure:

1. Prepare and fix a smear on a clean glass slide.
2. Flood slide with the stain for 1 min.
3. Wash the stain off the slide in running tap water.
4. Air dry and examine under the microscope.

MODIFIED ACID-FAST STAIN FOR *CRYPTOSPORIDIUM* OOCYSTS IN STOOL SPECIMENS
Materials:

Glass slide
Stool specimen
Stain

Primary stain

Basic fuchsin crystals	4 g
Ethanol	25 mL
Phenol, liquefied	12 mL
Glycerol	25 mL
DMSO (dimethylsulfoxide)	25 mL
Distilled water	75 mL

Dissolve the crystals in ethanol and then add the liquefied phenol. Mix well with a glass stirring rod. Then add glycerol, DMSO and distilled water. Mix well and allow to stand for 30 min. The stain may be used immediately or kept indefinitely at room temperature in an amber glass bottle.

Counter-stain

Malachite green	4.4 g
Distilled water	220 mL
Acetic acid, glacial	30 mL
Glycerol	50 mL

Dissolve malachite green in distilled water and then add acetic acid and glycerol. Mix well and may be kept indefinitely at room temperature in a closed container.
Procedure:

1. Smear the fecal material over a 2.5 × 3.0-cm area of a clean, flamed glass slide.
2. Air dry on a warming plate.
3. Fix the smear by dipping in a Coplin jar of absolute methanol for 5–10 sec.
4. Stain with primary stain in a Coplin jar for 5 min.
5. Rinse in running tap water until excess stain no longer runs off.
6. Dip in a Coplin jar containing the counterstain for 1 min or until a green background appears.
7. Rinse in running tap water for 10 sec.
8. Drain, blot and place on a warming plate until thoroughly dry.
9. Examine under the microscope under 4× magnification: oocysts appear as brilliant pink to fuschia against a pale green background.
10. Examine the oocysts closely at 100× for the internal vacuole and material clumped to one side of the 4- to 5-μm oocyst.

MODIFIED DIENES' STAIN
Materials:

Glass slide
Specimen
Scalpel
Petrolatum-paraffin mixture (1:1)
Stain

Methylene blue	2.50 g
Azure II	1.25 g
Maltose	10.0 g
Na$_2$CO$_3$	0.25 g
Distilled water	100 mL

Mix the ingredients well and then prepare a 3% dilution of the stain in water and filter through a 0.22 μm filter.
Procedure:

1. Cut out a one-cm square of agar containing suspected colonies.
2. Mount the agar block on a glass slide with the colonies facing up.

3. Make a petrolatum-paraffin seal around the agar section, slightly higher than the agar block.
4. Completely cover the agar block with 1 to 4 drops of the stain.
5. Place a cover slip over the stained agar block, allowing it to contact the petrolatum seal. The cover slip should be as close as possible to the agar surface without touching it.
6. Examine under the microscope at 100x magnification: *Mycoplasma* colonies stain **blue**, whereas most bacterial and fungal colonies appear colorless.

RAPID GIEMSA STAIN FOR DONOVAN BODIES

Ideal for the diagnosis of donovanosis in busy STD clinics in the developing world.
Materials:

Cotton-tipped swab
Glass slides
RapiDiff Giemsa staining kit (Clinical Science Diagnostics Ltd, Booysens 2016, South Africa)
PBS, pH 6.8

Procedure:

1. Prepare a smear by rolling the specimen (on a swab) on a glass slide.
2. Dip the smear (6 times) in RapiDIff fixative for 15 sec.
3. Dip the smear in RapiDiff 1 solution (Eosin Y) 6 times for 15 sec.
4. Dip in RapiDiff 2 solution (Thiazine Dye Mixture) 6 times for 15 sec.
5. Rinse in PBS, air dry and examine by light microscopy under oil immersion (1000 × magnification).
6. Stained Donovan bodies appear as pink-purple bacilli with unstained capsule.

SLOW GIEMSA STAINING TECHNIQUE FOR DONOVAN BODIES

Materials:

10% formaldehyde
Paraffin
Xylene
Absolute alcohol
1% Giemsa stain (Prepared by mixing 13.2 g Giemsa powder with 66 ml methyl alcohol and equal volume of glycerine. The working Giemsa stain solution is made fresh by using 0.5 ml stock Giemsa, 1.5 ml methyl alcohol, and 50 ml distilled water.)
1% acetic acid

Procedure:

1. Fix tissue in 10% formaldehyde.
2. Embed in paraffin at 62°C.
3. Cool the block rapidly in tap water.
4. Cut sections in a microtome at 4–5µm thickness.
5. Pass through xylene and absolute alcohol for deparaffinization.
6. Pass through absolute alcohol and 95% alcohol to prevent dehydration. Then pass through running and distilled water.
7. Place sections in 1% working Giemsa solution overnight (about 16 hrs).
8. Treat section with 1% acetic acid until it appears purplish-pink to sky-blue when examined under the microscope.
9. Rinse twice in absolute alcohol and xylene.
10. Mount in either 'Clarite' or 'Permount' mountants.
11. Examine under oil immersion objective: Donovan bodies appear as purplish-blue to reddish-pink; nuclei are blue against the faint blue cytoplasm of the inflammatory cells; and collagen appears pink in color.

TZANCK SMEARS

This is useful in the demonstration of multinucleated giant cells.
Materials:

Specimen
95% ethyl alcohol
Wright's or Giemsa stain

Procedure:

1. Prepare a smear from the underside of an air-dried snip biopsy taken from the periphery of a lesion.
2. Fix with 95% alcohol for 5 min.
3. Stain with Wright's or Giemsa's stain.
4. Examine under the microscope: A positive preparation shows the Donovan bodies in a deep blue cytoplasm.

WARTHIN-STARRY SILVER STAIN

Materials:

Acidulated water	
Triple distilled water	
Citric acid, 1% or less to bring solution to pH 3.8 to 4.4	
2% silver nitrate	
silver nitrate	2 g
acidulated water	100 ml
1% silver nitrate	
silver nitrate	1 g
acidulated water	100 ml
0.15% hydroquinone	
hydroquinone	0.15 g
acidulated water	100 ml
5% gelatin	
gelatin	5 g
acidulated water	100 ml
Developer solution (Note: Mix when ready to use)	
2% silver nitrate	9 ml
5% gelatin	22.5 ml
0.15% hydroquinone	12.0 ml
Acid-cleaned glassware	

Procedure

1. Prepare and heat solutions to 56°C. Deparaffinize specimen and hydrate to distilled water.
2. Place in 1% silver nitrate (in a Coplin jar) at 56°C for 1 hr.
3. Drain off 1% silver nitrate stain and keep slides in the Coplin jar in the water bath.
4. Mix developer and pour into the Coplin jar through the side.
5. Remove slides from developer when tissues turn yellow to light brown (about 1–3 minutes).
6. Rinse quickly in hot tap water.
7. Dehydrate, clear and mount in synthetic mounting medium. Donovan bacilli and spirochetes appear black against a pale yellow to light brown background.

WRIGHT'S STAIN
Materials:

Glass slide
Mortar and pestle
Phosphate buffer, pH 6.4
Stain

Wright's stain (powder form)	3 g
Glycerol (C.P.)	30 mL
Absolute methanol (acetone-free)	970 mL

Place the Wright's stain in a large mortar. Add approximately 5 mL glycerol and 30 mL methanol and grind to dissolve. Add the rest of the glycerol and methanol gradually until the dye is completely dissolved. Store in a dark, tightly stoppered bottle, and age for approximately 2 weeks. Filter before use.

Procedure:

1. Prepare smear on a glass slide. Air dry.
2. Flood the smear with the stain for 2 min.
3. Add 2–3 mL of phosphate buffer to the stain, blowing to mix stain and buffer.
4. Rinse with buffer until all the purple stain is removed.
5. Air dry and examine under the microscope.

ZIEHL-NEELSEN CARBOL-FUCHSIN STAIN

Materials:

Glass slide
Specimen
Absorbent paper, strips
Stain

Basic fuchsin	0.3 g
Ethanol, 95%	10 mL
Phenol, 5% aqueous solution	90 mL

Dissolve stain in ethanol and add solution to phenol. Store reagent in stoppered bottles to prevent evaporation. If crystals form during storage, filter the reagent prior to use.

Acid alcohol

| HCl, concentrated | 3 mL |
| Ethanol, 95% | 97 mL |

Aqueous methylene blue

| Methylene blue chloride | 0.3 g |
| Distilled water | 100 mL |

Procedure:

1. Prepare smear and heat-fix it.
2. Cover the smear with a strip of absorbent paper.
3. Add enough stain (4–5 drops) to saturate the paper.
4. Gently heat the bottom of the slide until the stain begins to steam.
5. Continue heating for 5 min but do not allow the stain to boil or dry. Add more stain if necessary.
6. Carefully lift absorbent paper from the slide with forceps.
7. Rinse smear with running tap water.
8. Flood the smear with acid alcohol for 2 min.
9. Rinse smear with tap water and flood slide with aqueous methylene blue for 1–2 min.
10. Rinse in tap water, drain and dry.
11. Acid-fast bacilli appear red against a blue background.

Application of Nucleic Acid-based Technologies in STD Diagnostics

H Lee and E Nadala

A variety of strategies are available for the detection of bacterial and viral nucleic acids in sexually transmitted diseases, which differ in sensitivity, specificity and reproducibility. In terms of sensitivity, nucleic acid-based tests are generally more sensitive than enzyme immunoassays (EIA). The amplified nucleic acid technologies have a theoretical limit of one copy of target, while the non-amplified technologies require about 10,000 copies (*Fig. A4.1*).

Nucleic acid tests can be divided into three stages: sample preparation, hybridization/amplification and detection (*Fig. A4.2*). The overall performance of the test depends largely on what kinds of technologies are used in each of these stages.

In sample preparation, although the tests use standard methods for isolating nucleic acids from organisms and clinical material, test performance would depend on the efficiency of the extraction, and on the presence of nucleases and inhibitors in the sample. For instance, although nucleic acid amplification assays are theoretically capable of detecting as little as one target in a sample, this sensitivity is rarely achieved because of sample inhibition. Certain samples may contain factors that inhibit the enzyme activity needed for the amplification reaction. During the hybridization/amplification stage, test sensitivity would depend on whether the target and/or signal are amplified or not. A continuum of sensitivity can result, based on the technology utilized. In the detection stage, variations in sensitivity and specificity can result based on the type of label used, the efficiency of labeling, and the method of detection. Most amplified nucleic acid tests use enzyme-labeled nucleic acid probes to detect the resulting amplified material. A chemiluminescent substrate is commonly used to reveal the presence of the enzyme because of its high sensitivity.

Nucleic acid tests have been in use for over a decade, mostly in research laboratories but increasingly in clinical microbiology laboratories as well. Some examples of FDA-approved nucleic acid tests for sexually transmitted diseases (STD) are shown in *Table A4.1*. Nucleic acid tests for hepatitis C virus and hepatitis B virus are also available for research use.

AMPLIFIED NUCLEIC ACID TECHNOLOGIES

Amplified nucleic acid technologies offer superior performance in terms of sensitivity over the direct (non-amplified) probe-based tests. Nucleic acid amplification provides the ability to selectively amplify specific targets present in low concentrations to detectable levels (*Fig. A4.3*).

Commercial amplification-based molecular diagnostic systems for sexually transmitted diseases have focused largely on systems for detecting *Neisseria gonorrhoeae, Chlamydia trachomatis,* human immuno-deficiency virus (HIV), hepatitis B virus (HBV), hepatitis C virus (HCV) and human papilloma virus (HPV). In addition to qualitative detection of viruses, quantification of viral load in clinical specimens is now recognized to be of great importance for diagnosis, prognosis and

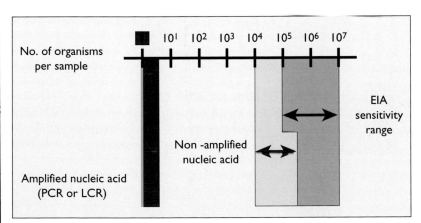

Fig. A4.1 Sensitivity comparison of various diagnostic technologies.

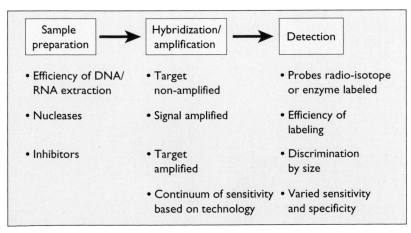

Fig. A4.2 Probe diagnostics combine multiple technologies.

Target organisms	Technology	Company
Chlamydia trachomatis (CT) detection	PCR	Roche
	LCR	Abbott
	TMA	Gen-Probe
	HC	Digene
Neisseria gonorrhoeae (NG) detection	PCR	Roche
	LCR	Abbott
	HC	Digene
CT/NG screening/detection	HPA	Gen-Probe
	SDA	Becton-Dickinson
HPV screening	HC	Digene
HIV detection/quantification	PCR	Roche
Gardnerella, Trichomonas, and *Candida*	Hybridization	Becton-Dickson

Table A4.1 Examples of FDA-approved Nucleic Acid Tests for STD.

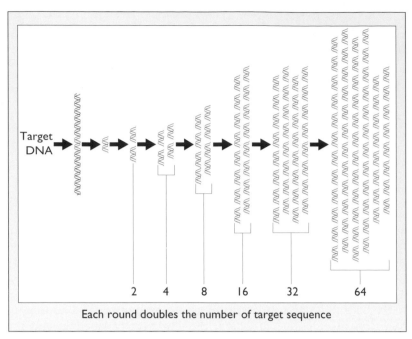

Fig. A4.3 DNA amplification.

Technology	Company	Isothermal	Target	Enzymes
PCR	Roche	No	DNA	DNA polymerase
LCR	Abbott	No	DNA	DNA ligase
TMA	Gen Probe	Yes	RNA	Reverse transcriptase and RNA polymerase
NASBA	Organon Teknika	Yes	RNA	Reverse transcriptase, RNase H, RNA polymerase
SDA	Becton Dickinson	Yes	DNA	DNA polymerase and restriction endonuclease

Table A4.2 Nucleic acid amplification technologies.

therapeutic monitoring for HIV, HBV and HCV. The nucleic acid amplification technologies are listed in *Table A4.2* along with the companies that market the technology, whether it is isothermal or not, the type of target, and the enzymes they use.

POLYMERASE CHAIN REACTION (PCR)

PCR was the first target DNA amplification technique to be developed. It was also the first technique to be used successfully in research laboratories for detection of STDs. Subsequent improvements and modifications to the technique later allowed it to be used for quantification of viral load. Because of its flexibility and ease of performance, it remains the most widely used molecular diagnostic technique in both research and clinical laboratories.

The PCR reaction uses two oligonucleotide primers that hybridize to opposite strands and flank the target DNA sequence that is to be amplified. The elongation of the primers is catalyzed by a heat-stable DNA polymerase (such as Taq DNA Polymerase). A repetitive series of cycles involving template denaturation, primer annealing, and extension of the annealed primers by the polymerase, results in exponential accumulation of a specific DNA fragment (*Fig. A4.4*). Because the primer extension products synthesized in a given cycle can serve as a template in the next cycle, the number of target DNA copies approximately doubles every cycle; thus, 20 cycles of the PCR will yield about a million copies of the target DNA.

DNA amplicons generated in a PCR reaction can be detected by ethidium bromide-stained gel electrophoresis. Newer amplicon detection techniques include the use of capture and enzyme-labeled detection probes in a microwell format (*Fig. A4.5*). In this detection technique, the PCR product is initially immobilized on the surface of the microwell plate by specific hybridization with a capture probe linked to BSA that is bound to the microwell surface. Immobilized PCR products are then detected by means of a biotinylated detection probe, that hybridizes to a specific sequence of the PCR product, and subsequently binds to an enzyme-labeled streptavidin conjugate via its biotin label. The presence of the enzyme conjugate is revealed following the addition of a chemiluminescent substrate.

LIGASE CHAIN REACTION (LCR)

LCR is a probe amplification technique with sensitivity similar to that of PCR. It differs from polymerase-based nucleic acid amplification

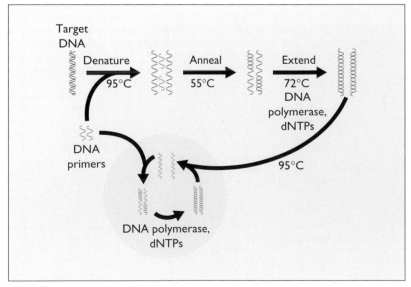

Fig. A4.4 PCR.

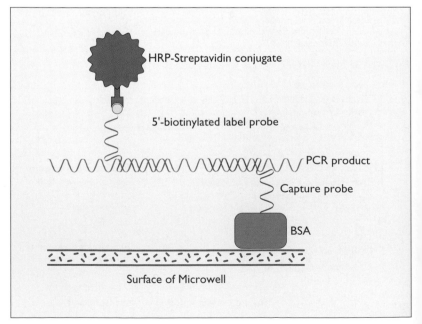

Fig. A4.5 PCR-product detection.

methods (PCR, NASBA, SDA) in that there is no requirement for the synthesis of new DNA or RNA. In the former, in vitro synthesis of new nucleic acid molecules provides templates for additional extension reactions. In LCR, the target sequence is not duplicated; it simply provides a template for the binding of preexisting probe sequences. Once bound and ligated, these probe sequences become the substrates for additional DNA ligase-mediated joining reactions (*Fig. A4.6*).

LCR relies on repeated cycles of oligonucleotide hybridization and ligation to generate multiple copies of nucleic acid sequences of interest. Two complementary pairs of oligonucleotide probes (probes A and A' and probes B and B') are required to initiate the reaction. Probes A and B, and Probes A' and B' hybridize at adjacent positions on each strand of the target DNA. The target-bound probes provide a substrate for joining by the nick-sealing activity of DNA ligase. After ligation, the target-ligation product duplex is separated by thermal denaturation. Both the single-stranded target DNA and the ligated probe products are then available to act as templates for the hybridization and ligation of additional probes. Each cycle of oligonucleotide hybridization and ligation results in a doubling of the number of templates with sensitivity similar to that of PCR.

The LCR products can be detected by autoradiography using radioactively labeled probes or by enzyme immunoassay using hapten-labeled probes with corresponding monoclonal antibodies. Because LCR is basically a series of ligation reactions, LCR primers are labeled with two different labels such that ligation products can be detected using a sandwich-type immunoassay. One such assay is a magnetic particle-based sandwich enzyme immunoassay illustrated in *Fig. A4.7*. Double-labeled LCR products are captured by antibody-coated magnetic particles via one label and detected (after washing steps) using an antibody-enzyme conjugate via the other label. The presence of the enzyme antibody conjugate is revealed by a chemiluminescent substrate.

TRANSCRIPTION-MEDIATED AMPLIFICATION (TMA)

TMA is an isothermal target RNA amplification technology that enables the production of billions of RNA amplicons from a single target molecule in less than one hour. The technique uses two enzymes

(reverse transcriptase and RNA polymerase) and two primers, one containing a promoter sequence for the RNA polymerase. There are two main series of steps in TMA. The first series involves the generation of RNA amplicons using the original target RNA as template. The second series involves the reentry of newly synthesized RNA amplicons into the TMA process to serve as templates for a new round of replication leading to an exponential expansion of the RNA amplicons (*Fig. A4.8*).

The RNA amplicons produced in the TMA reaction are detected using the hybridization protection assay (HPA) technique to be described in the next section on non-amplified DNA technologies.

NUCLEIC ACID SEQUENCE-BASED AMPLIFICATION (NASBA)

NASBA amplification technology is very similar to TMA except that it relies on the simultaneous activity of three (instead of two) enzymes: AMV-RT (Avian Myoblastosis Virus–Reverse Transcriptase), RNAse H and T7 RNA polymerase. Their concerted action, along with those of specific primers, enables the amplification of the nucleic acid sequence of interest (*Fig. A4.9*).

Amplified RNA is detected by probe hybridization using the electro-chemiluminescence (ECL) technique. NASBA technology can be used for both quantitative and qualitative assays of HIV-1 RNA.

STRAND-DISPLACEMENT AMPLIFICATION (SDA)

SDA is an isothermal amplification process that utilizes DNA polymerase, a restriction enzyme and a series of primers to exponentially amplify the unique target nucleic acid sequence. It consists of two stages: target generation followed by exponential amplification. During

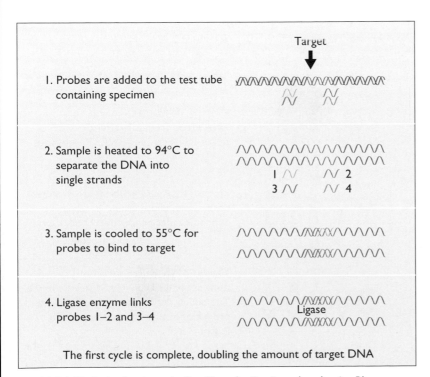

Fig. A4.6 LCR. Probe 1 = A; probe 3 = A'; probe 2 = B; and probe 4 = B'.

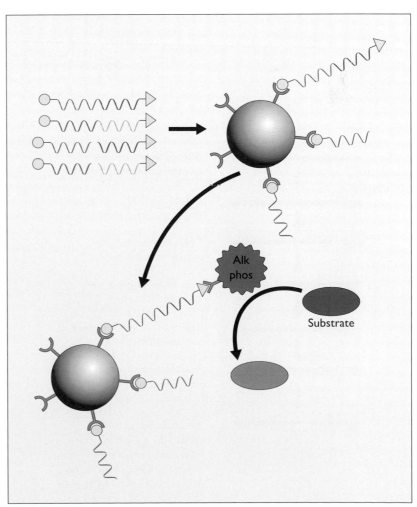

Fig. A4.7 LCR product detection.

target generation, the double-stranded target DNA is heat denatured, creating two single-stranded copies. A series of specially manufactured primers (amplification primers for copying the base sequence and bumper primers for displacing the newly created strands) combine with DNA polymerase to form altered targets capable of exponential amplification. These altered targets go into the amplification phase (*Fig. A4.10*), where several billion copies of the partial DNA target segment is produced in just minutes.

SDA is highly specific because the amplification reaction involves recognition of six distinct regions on the template DNA. The extremely high amplification efficiency enables detection of minute amounts of nucleic acid in about half an hour. SDA amplification products are detected by a solid-phase hybridization sandwich system utilizing capture probes and enzyme-labeled detector probes revealed through chemiluminescence, similar to the one described for detection of PCR products (*Fig. A4.5*).

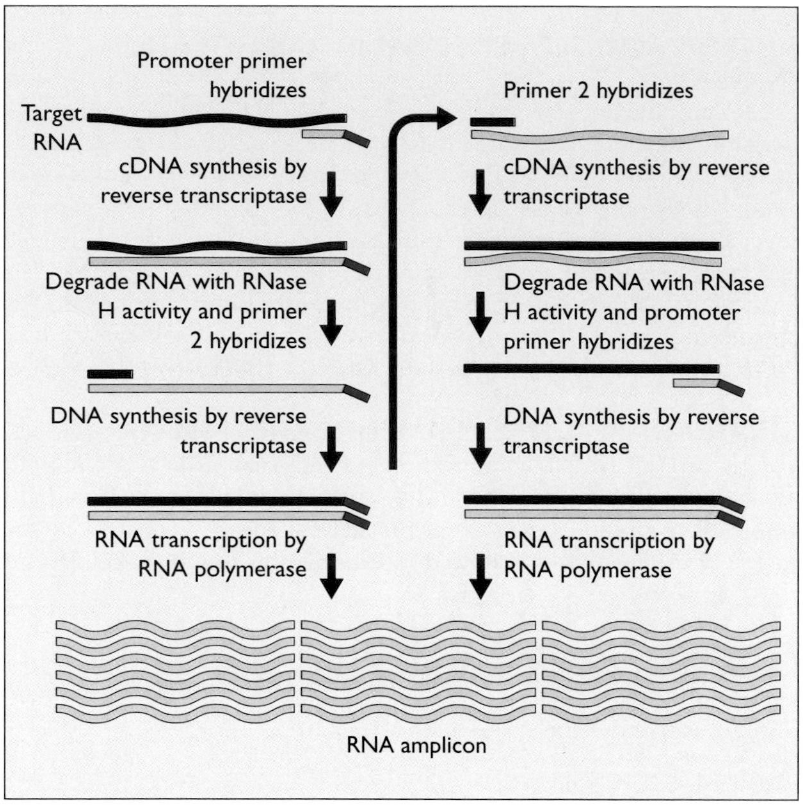

Fig. A4.8 TMA.

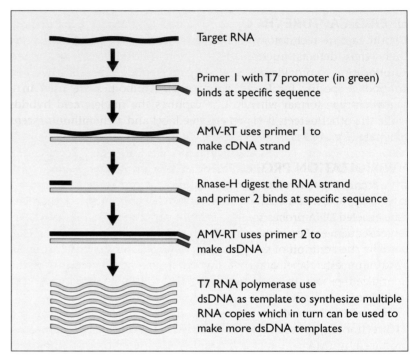

Fig. A4.9 NASBA.

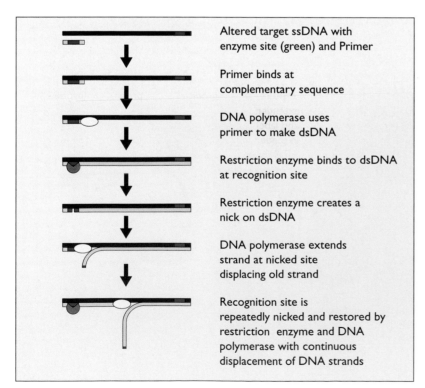

Fig. A4.10 SDA.

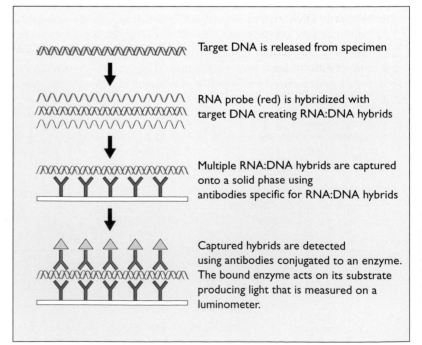

Fig. A4.11 Hybrid capture.

NON-AMPLIFIED NUCLEIC ACID TECHNOLOGIES

Non-amplified nucleic acid technologies are usually rapid and simple to perform, although they are considerably less sensitive than the amplified technologies. Most direct probe detection assays require at least 10^4 copies of nucleic acid per microliter for reliable detection.

Amplification of the detection signal after probe hybridization improves sensitivity to as low as 500 target copies per microliter and provides quantitative capabilities. This approach has been used extensively for quantitative assays of viral load (HIV and HBV). Its sensitivity exceeds that of culture or immunologic methods but does not match the analytical sensitivity of target amplification-based methods.

HYBRID CAPTURE (HC)

Hybrid capture technology (HC) is a quantitative hybridization-based assay that detects nucleic acid targets directly and uses signal amplification to provide increased sensitivity. The technology relies on antibodies specific for DNA-RNA hybrids. Antibodies are used in a sandwich-type format wherein one captures the nucleic acid hybrids while the other detects it via an enzyme label and a chemiluminescent substrate (*Fig. A4.11*).

HYBRIDIZATION PROTECTION ASSAY (HPA)

HPA technology involves detection of RNA or single-stranded DNA targets by means of a chemiluminescent DNA probe. These acridinium ester-labeled DNA probes are added and allowed to hybridize to specific target sequences. Separation of hybridized from unhybridized probes is done by the addition of selection reagent (alkali) which hydrolyzes the acridinium ester label on the unhybridized probes. The label on the hybridized probes is protected within the double helix and is not hydrolyzed. No light is emitted from the unhybridized probes, whereas light is emitted and detected from the hybridized probes (*Fig. A4.12*). HPA technology is used to detect *Chlamydia trachomatis* RNA amplicons produced by TMA.

BRANCHED-CHAIN DNA HYBRIDIZATION (bDNA)

Branched-chain DNA hybridization technology relies on a series of probes to achieve signal amplification. Target nucleic acid is first captured on a solid substrate (microwell plate) using capture probes and then hybridized in sequence to a series of probes that build up a branched-chain DNA structure (*Fig. A4.13*). This structure enables a large number of labeled probes to hybridize to a single target molecule thereby enhancing sensitivity. Enzyme-labeled probes are detected using the chemiluminescence technique. The bDNA hybridization technology has been used for detection and quantification of HIV, HBV and HCV.

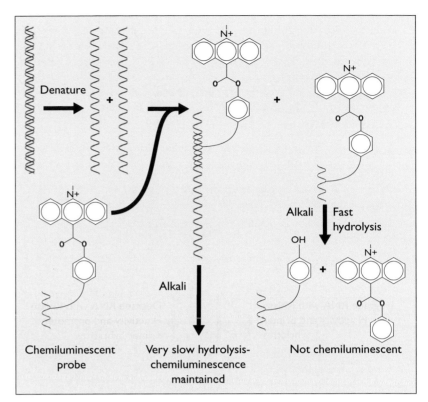

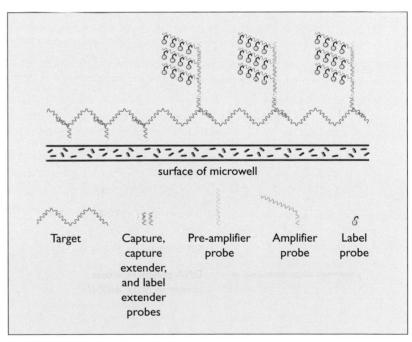

Fig. A4.12 Hybridization protection assay.

Fig. A4.13 bDNA signal amplification.

Web Sites For Reference

GUIDELINES/REPORTS

1. http://www.who.int/HIV_AIDS/ *WHO guidelines for the management of sexually transmitted infections.*
2. http://www.hivatis.org *Guidelines for the use of antiretroviral agents in HIV-infected adults and adolescents.*
3. http://www.cdc.gov/nchstp/dstd/dstdp.html *2002 STD treatment guidelines.*
4. http://www.unaids.org/publications/documents/impact/std/una97e6.pdf *Policies and Principles for Prevention and Care.*
5. http://www.unaids.org *Report on the global HIV/AIDS epidemic, June 2000, Geneva.*
6. http://www.cdc.gov/std/stats *USA STD surveillance data.*

ORGANIZATIONS

1. www.iusti.org *International Union Against Sexually Transmitted Infections.*
2. www.isstdr.org *International Society for STD Research.*
3. www.ashastd.org *American Social Health Association.*
4. http://www.phls.co.uk *Public Health Laboratory Service, UK.*

DISEASE-SPECIFIC INFORMATION

1. http://www.who.int/HIV_AIDS/ *HIV/AIDS.*
2. http://www.cdc.gov/health/std.htm *Scabies and trichomoniasis.*

REFERENCE/RESEARCH

1. http://www.stdgen.lanl.gov/ *Database of genome sequences of STD pathogens.*
2. http://www.cochrane.org/cochrane/revabstr/g460index.htm *Cochrane reviews on STD-related subjects.*
3. http://www.who.int/health-topics/std.htm *WHP publications on STD-related subjects.*
4. http://www.nlm.nih.gov/medlineplus/sexuallytransmitteddiseases.html *STD-related research information.*
5. http://www.niaid.nih.gov/factsheets/stdinfo.htm *Fact sheets on STDs.*
6. http://www.virology.net *The Big Picture Book of Viruses.*
7. http://www.dermis.net/doia *Dermatological conditions.*

Index